THE SHOULDER AND NECK

by

JAMES E. BATEMAN, M.D., F.R.C.S. (C)

Diplomate American Board of Orthopedic Surgery;
Surgeon-in-Chief, Orthopedic and Arthritic Hospital, Toronto

Formerly Fellow and Instructor in Surgery, University of Toronto;
Chief of Orthopedic Surgery, Scarborough General Hospital
Consultant Workmens' Compensation Board of Ontario, Department
of Veterans' Affairs, Sunnybrook Hospital, Peel Memorial Hospital,
Belleville General Hospital, Northwestern General Hospital,
Toronto, Ontario

Drawings by Louise Gordon and Dorothy Irwin

W. B. Saunders Company • *Philadelphia* • *London* • *Toronto*

W. B. Saunders Company: West Washington Square
                            Philadelphia, Pa.   19105

                            12 Dyott Street
                            London, WC1A   1DB

                            833 Oxford Street
                            Toronto 18, Ontario

The Shoulder and Neck   ISBN 0-7216-1570-8

Print No.:   9   8   7   6   5   4   3   2

To my Mother,
Mental, moral, and spiritual lifetime example

PREFACE

Interest in injuries and diseases of the shoulder region has increased considerably over the past decade. Associated with this has been a realization of the important influence that disorders of the cervical spine exert on this area. No investigation of complaints in either region is complete without assessment of both zones. Specific shoulder derangements have been brought more clearly into focus. The incidence and significance of cervical disorders, particularly the nerve root syndromes, have been elucidated, and appropriate surgical measures now have a fixed place in our armamentarium.

In this volume emphasis has been placed on methods of diagnosis and clinical investigation based on identification of pain patterns. In considering disorders affecting the whole forequarter, a reliable system of identification is most helpful in sorting the various entities; an analysis of the pain pattern is a useful and rapid guide to differential diagnosis. The section on clinical entities clearly demarcates four groups according to the pain pattern: those having dominant neck pain, those having shoulder-neck pain, those having predominant shoulder pain, and those conditions presenting as shoulder plus radiating pain. Pathology, treatment and rehabilitation have been outlined in each case. New surgical procedures, particularly a utility approach applicable to most glenohumeral reconstruction, have been presented.

A new approach to the study of injuries of the shoulder and neck has been made based on the influence of environment. It matters considerably whether a given fracture has occurred in an athlete or in a workman or whether it has resulted from a household accident or been caused by a violent motor mishap. For this reason, there are separate discussions of athletic, industrial and automobile injuries.

Basic sciences, embryology, anatomy, and physiology of the shoulder and neck have been considered extensively. Interaction of the shoulder and neck elements has been emphasized in demonstration of anthropological development, anatomical units and overall physiological influence.

A section has been devoted to general systemic diseases such as rheumatoid arthritis which implicate the shoulder and neck, with consideration being given to proper planning of the sequence of rehabilitation and reconstruction in these lesions.

Particular attention has been paid to the assessment of disability and the estimation of permanent impairment, since employers, insurance companies and courts increasingly demand that the doctor be able to predict the course of healing and intelligently estimate residual defects.

JAMES E. BATEMAN, M.D.

Appreciation

Development and growth of a special institution, the Orthopaedic and Arthritic Hospital in Toronto, has made possible application of the author's continuing interest in problems of the shoulder region. The assembling of clinical material and the availability of assistance from all departments has been of inestimable help in this project. Dr. C. S. Wright, Administrator; Miss Patricia O'Connor, Head Nurse; Miss Stephanie Debreczeny, Record Librarian; Mr. John Pearce, Photographer; and Model, Mrs. Janis Van Iperen merit very special thanks for enabling the complilation of this work.

Assistance from the Clinical Staff has also been significant. Dr. J. Munn, Radiologist, added importantly to the material initially so painstakingly assembled by Dr. H. M. Worth. Contributions on rheumatology from Drs. Norrie Swanson and Dan Mehta, on metabolic medicine from Dr. Jack Olin, on electromyography from Dr. E. W. M. Howes, and clinical examples from Drs. J. C. Colwill and W. J. Virgin have all contributed greatly.

Untiring residents have helped at all stages: Drs. M. Kohanim, J. Bernal, V. G. Raghavan, H. M. Cheema, and E. Vasquez-Vela have been particularly involved.

The fine foundation of art work and illustrations, so well introduced by Mrs. Louise Gordon in the original volume, has been most ably continued by Mrs. Dorothy Irwin.

Colleagues of many years' standing helped appreciably. Dr. Julius Neviaser most graciously contributed importantly to the section on fractures and dislocations. Experience and principles gleaned from association with "shoulder greats" like Fred Mosley, Charlie Neer, Carter Rowe, Tony DePalma, Arthur Eyere-Brooke, as well as the stimulus from younger ones like Charles Rockwood, John Hazlett, and Virgil May, has helped to provide a wealth of background material.

All who aspire to produce manuscripts of this order must have efficient and understanding secretaries such as Miss Mary Manna or the task could never be completed.

The patience, advice, and constant assistance of a superlative publisher, W. B. Saunders Company, so ably executed by Mrs. Charlotte Brick and Mr. John Dusseau, at all stages of the project are most gratefully acknowledged.

JAMES E. BATEMAN, M.D.

CONTENTS

Section IV Trauma to the Neck and Shoulder

Section V Systemic Disorders of the Shoulder and the Neck

Section VI Tumors of the Shoulder and the Neck

Section VII   Disability Evaluation of the Shoulder and the Neck

Introduction

CORRELATION OF SHOULDER
AND NECK LESIONS

Disorders of modern times have dictated a new interpretation of clinical states based more on regional concepts of body structure. In the realm of musculoskeletal disorders, disease specifically related to the shoulder has been pre-eminent, but an appreciation of the contribution of pathologic changes in the neck to these disorders is now emerging. In the past the role of the neck seemed somewhat secondary in its precise contributions to the shoulder system. Although the neck has long been accepted as playing a part in forequarter disorders, its significance has now become much clearer. This does not mean that many clinical entities have heretofore been wrongly interpreted, but it does mean that we have a more valid explanation for some less well understood changes. The significance of cervical spondylosis, intervertebral disc changes, foraminal disorders and nerve root syndromes has become much more apparent. The tendency to be avoided, and the one which has been frequent in many areas of medicine in the past, is not to overuse this new knowledge and distort its true place; enthusiasm over a new concept almost always leads to overemphasis on its actual importance.

Time distills clinical impressions and inexorably assesses the success of therapeutic measures, both medical and surgical. Most surgical procedures related to the shoulder are standing this test of time in principle, but new approaches, new tools and new guide lines of application have enhanced their effectiveness significantly. In this presentation nearly all major procedures have undergone some degree of technical modification, with consequent improvement in results.

Environmental influences have assumed new significance for our way of life. Specific aspects are contributed to trauma, for example, depending on whether the injury took place at work, on the playing field or in an automobile. It is true that a broken clavicle is much the same, no matter how it occurred, but

1

the treatment which is best will depend on whether it occurred in a workman or an athlete. The possibility of complications in "stop-light" sprain require the same careful diagnosis and therapy as the headlong tumble of the workman.

In an effort to more accurately pinpoint specific treatment rather than simply state already proved axioms, injuries have been considered in this presentation according to environmental causes; we have separated industrial injuries, athletic injuries and automobile injuries so that emphasis may be placed on the peculiarities contributed to the clinical states by the mechanism of the injury.

Progress is reflected also in abandonment of certain long accepted terms because of their inaccuracy. Peritonitis, a once favorite diagnosis of abdominal ills, is now used rarely; when it is, it precisely delineates the primary source. The term bursitis, a shotgun denotation of many shoulder lesions, has undergone a similar change. The dominant zone of pathological change is the tendon of the shoulder rotators, with the other zones of frailty embracing the acromioclavicular joint and the bicipital mechanism; all these implicate the shoulder peritoneum, but each requires a different management. A complication of any of these states may be freezing of the glenohumeral joint, which then requires treatment also, but cannot be fully cured without eradication of the primary flaw.

Overshadowing these pure shoulder lesions are the long suspected influences of cervical spine changes. Cervical root syndromes from many sources and cervical myelopathy due to spondylosis have both been clearly demarcated and their role in the forequarter's ailments more specifically defined.

Nowhere in medicine is there offered a more fruitful field for the combined effort of specialties than in the treatment of arthritis. The advances made by rheumatologists have opened vast fields for contributions by orthopedists; this is as true in the shoulder-neck region as elsewhere in the body. Related biochemical and biophysiological processes offer still further and better avenues of therapeutic control.

Regardless of chemistry, physics and local influences, accurate interpretation of pathology, surgical anatomy and technical advances continue to be paramount. The approach now entails a broader regional concept when zones like the shoulder and the neck exist in an environment of such constant interplay.

Section

I

BASIC SCIENCES AS RELATED TO THE SHOULDER AND THE NECK

Chapter I

EVOLUTION, EMBRYOLOGY AND CONGENITAL ANOMALIES

Many evolutionary changes have been evoked by the need for a prehensile extremity in man. Two primary problems have been met as the shoulder-neck region has evolved: one group of changes has been concerned with the development of new parts, while the other process has been the integration of these parts with the already existing structures.

The development of the neck as a ribless mobile zone is an example of the compromises in structure that have taken place. Large nerves from the segments opposite the appendage require unobstructed passage outward to reach the hand so that ribs disappear in the cervical region (Fig. 1–2). A similar process operates in relation to the lumbar plexus and the lower limbs. Since we are upright and our eyes look forward, work is done in front of the body; for this to be possible, rotation of the upper limb has occurred (Fig. 1–1).

As these adaptive changes have taken place, some parts of the body have had to change more radically than others. Due to the new position the arm takes up, the supraspinatus

no longer pulls from behind forward, but instead acts at an admittedly poorer mechanical advantage by pulling from below and upward (Fig. 1–1). Because of this it is exposed to much greater mechanical stress (Fig. 1–3).

Elements of the shoulder and neck may first be identified in cartilaginous fishes, which have a dorsal or scapular segment and a ventral or coracoid element; the space in between eventually represents the shoulder joint. Steps in evolution demarcate the neck and the shoulder and eventually separate the appendage more definitely from the body. Some transitional forms representative of this stage may be recognized. The neck and fin are connected by a solid element as an intermediate step prior to complete separation. In human beings, examples of this stage are the various anomalies of incomplete descent of the scapula. In some there is a definite bone, the omovertebral bone, connecting the scapula to the neck; in further stages of this process, there may simply be a high riding scapula with some underlying fibrous bands (Fig. 1–4).

Mobility of the neck is a property of the

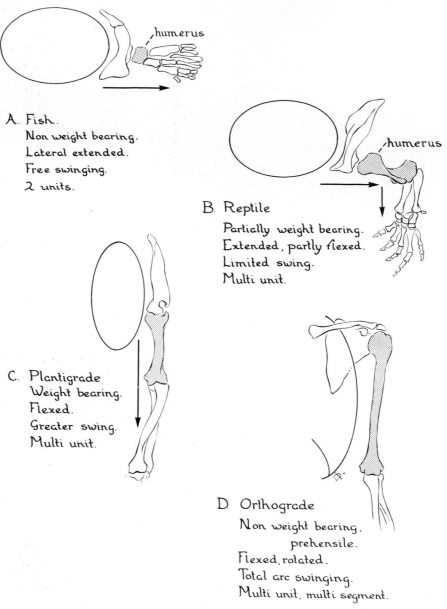

Figure 1–1   Upper extremity development through geological time.

higher mammals. The heavy bony elements which buttress the forelimb in lower forms gradually disappear so that both the upper limb and the neck segments assume greater separation and much greater mobility (Fig. 1–5). In addition to the bony changes, extensive shifting occurs in the attachment of the primary muscles that move the appendage in its new position.

Evolutionary changes rotate the upper limb so that it can function in front of the body rather than at the side. The scapula shows the greatest degree of change from primitive forms to more specialized groups; it becomes the base of the arm and shifts from the cervical position over the chest, carrying the limb with it. As it does so, it rotates so that its axillary border changes to the present position from one which originally related to the position of the posterior spinous processes.

The supraspinous portion of the scapula is a property of higher mammals; there is no corresponding part in the lower limb. As

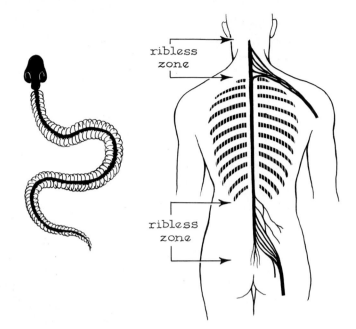

Figure 1–2 Ribless zones developed to allow unobstructed innervation of extremities.

the mobility of the neck develops, the upper portion of the scapula becomes attenuated while the lower portion enlarges. The muscle masses attached to these zones change accordingly, so that there is developed a much smaller supraspinous and a much larger infraspinous muscle area (Fig. 1–6).

As the fully upright position is assumed,

greater stress falls on the smaller supraspinatous. Rotation of the girdle as a whole takes place between the scapula and the chest, but further rotation due to the torsion of the humerus also occurs. In lower mammals like sheep or dogs the biceps splits the lateral surface of the head of the humerus evenly; but as the upper limb is rotated in man, the

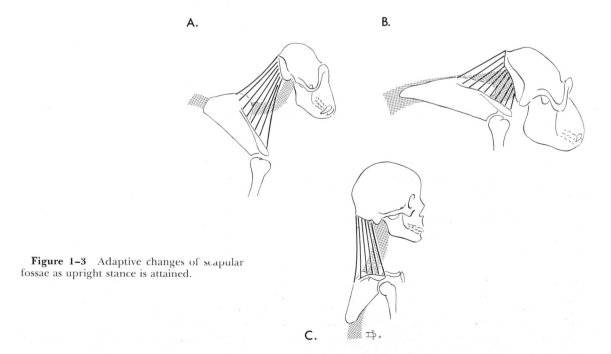

Figure 1–3 Adaptive changes of scapular fossae as upright stance is attained.

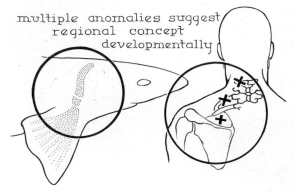

multiple anomalies suggest
regional concept
developmentally

Figure 1–4 Incomplete descent of scapula with multiple anomalies suggests regional concept of development.

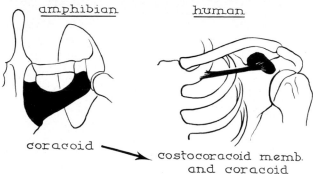

amphibian   human

coracoid → costocoracoid memb. and coracoid

Figure 1–5 All that remains in man of heavy precordial element of lower forms is the thin costocoracoid membrane.

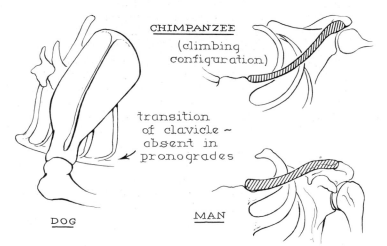

CHIMPANZEE
(climbing configuration)

transition
of clavicle –
absent in
pronogrades

DOG   MAN

Figure 1–6 Clavicle development is an important property of man, providing free hanging of upper extremity.

biceps swings to the front so that greater stress then falls on the much smaller and lesser tuberosity (Fig. 1–7).

ANOMALIES OF THE BONES OF THE SHOULDER AND NECK

In man the upper limb bud appears a little earlier than the lower, at about the fifth week of embryonic life. There develops a mesenchymal core which condenses into a rod about the sixth week. The centers of chondrification for all the main bones appear in this rod during the ensuing two weeks. Lying around the skeleton is a periskeletal mesenchyme which develops into the muscular elements (Fig. 1–8).

The limb continues to migrate, following a course from a parallel position into a right angle, then to adduction and, finally, to flexion plus lateral rotation. From a cervical position the scapula then moves down over the ribs, taking up its resting position about the third month. In its descent, muscles are

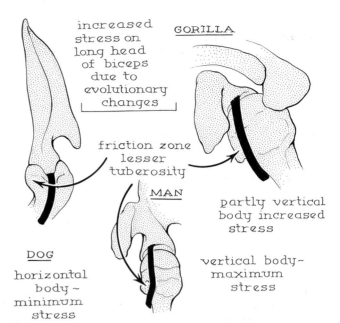

Figure 1-7 Bicipital mechanism profoundly influenced by upper limb evolution.

pulled down, extending their attachment from the cervical spine to the humerus. A prime example of this pattern of migration is the latissimus dorsi, which extends from the cervical spine to the humerus and carries its nerve supply with it. Once the initial developments are over and fundamental relationships have been established, a further stabilization and molding occurs in the bone joints, muscles, nerves and vessels. This process not only continues throughout embryonic life, but is not really completed until puberty (Fig. 1–9).

CONGENITAL ABNORMALITIES OF THE SHOULDER AND NECK

Etiology of Malformations

Knowledge of the source of congenital malformations has increased extensively since the discovery by Greg in 1941 that German measles affecting a mother during early pregnancy could cause abnormalities in the embryo. Approximately 10 per cent of all known human malformations are due to environmental factors and another 10 per cent to genetic and chromosomal factors; the remaining 80 per cent may be the result of an interplay of both of these influences.

Among environmental factors of known influence may be listed German measles, which can lead to abnormalities of the eye, internal ear, heart and teeth. Mental retarda-

tion and certain cerebral abnormalities have also been identified in children born to mothers who have had rubella during pregnancy. Other viral infections such as measles, mumps, hepatitis, poliomyelitis and chickenpox have also been implicated as contributing to fetal abnormalities.

The probable dangers of radiation have been underlined by studies that followed the atomic bomb explosions over Hiroshima and Nagasaki. Upwards of 25 per cent of the children born to Japanese women pregnant at the time of the atomic bomb explosions had abnormalities of the central nervous system such as microcephaly and mental retardation. An accumulated dose of radiation also has been suspected of causing abnormalities in children born in later years to parents who had been exposed to the radiation.

The increased incidence of amelia and phocomelia led to studies which implicated drugs such as thalidomide. Defects produced by thalidomide include absence or gross deformities of the long bones, intestinal atresia and cardiac anomalies. Other drugs with teratogenetic properties include aminopterin, used in treatment of leukemia, and tolbutamide, used in diabetes.

Hormones that are possible causes of congenital abnormalities include progesterones and cortisone. Defects may also be caused by certain antibodies, vitamin deficiencies, chromosomal and genic factors.

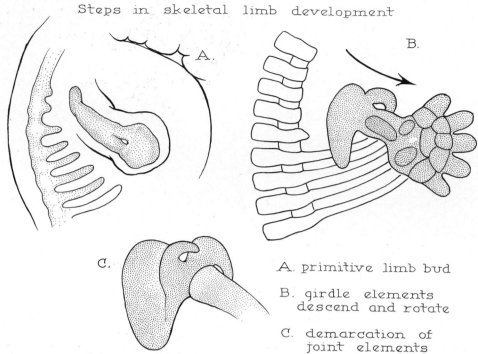

Figure 1–8 Development of upper limb. (After Keibel and Mall.)

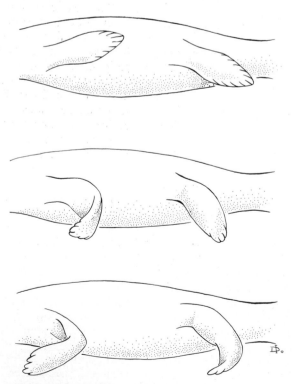

Figure 1–9 Migration and rotation of limbs for prehensile action.

DEVELOPMENT OF THE NECK

During the third week of embryonic life, the spinal cord, as the notocord, extends as a continuous rod; by the fifth week, differentiation of individual segments is apparent. At the same time sclerotomes invest the notocord and the neural tube as a sheath, becoming the vertebral elements. At the end of the fifth week chondrification starts, with separate centers for centrum, neural arches and costal processes in each segment. About the eighth week centers of endochondral ossification appear. The notocord shrinks and eventually disappears except at the interbody levels, where it persists to form the nucleus pulposus area of the intervertebral disc. Initially the head is acutely flexed on the pericardial region; during the second month this zone elongates to form the neck. Four arches develop in the foregut and constitute the branchial arches; as they grow, the head is straightened and the intervening neck zone is formed (Fig. 1–10). The internal grooves constitute the pharyngeal pouches and ultimately produce the middle ear and the eustachian tube from arch I, the tonsillar fossa from arch II, the thymus gland and inferior parathyroid gland from arch III, and the superior parathyroid from arch IV. Anomalies and vestiges of these elements lead to the branchial cysts and sinuses encountered clinically.

CONGENITAL ANOMALIES OF THE BONES OF THE NECK

Abnormalities of the bony elements show wide variation in the neck. Severe aberration

Table 1–1 ANOMALIES OF THE NECK

1. Anomalies of Suboccipital Region
   a. Interparietal bone
   b. Platybasia
   c. Synostosis with Atlas

2. Anomalies of Atlas
   a. Absence of Posterior Arch
   b. Segmental Replacement with Occipital Bone

3. Anomalies of Axis
   a. Ossiculum terminale
   b. Os odontoideum
   c. Rudimentary odontoid
   d. Absence of odontoid

4. Cervical Spondylolisthesis

5. Congenital Scoliosis

6. Klippel-Feil Syndrome

7. Spina Bifida

8. Congenital Fusions

9. Anomalies of Joints

is seen in anencephaly, in which the nape of the neck and the adjacent occipital zone are distorted to a degree incompatible with postnatal survival. In this state the vertebrae are decreased in number, vertebral bodies fail to fuse or they are markedly distorted. Similar extensive neural changes are often apparent with occipital anencephaly and a short or absent cervical spinal cord. Only a few forms of this severely altered pattern are compatible with survival. One less severe form, the Klippel-Feil syndrome, or congenital brevicollis, is sometimes encountered; this is a

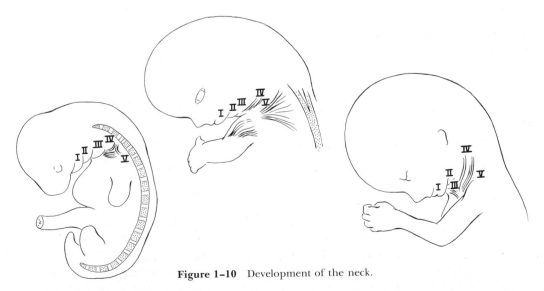

Figure 1–10 Development of the neck.

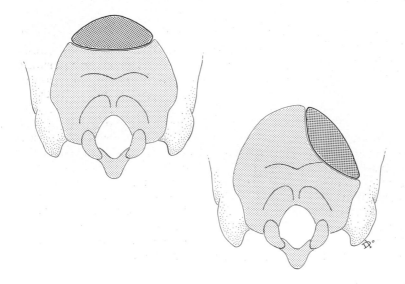

Figure 1-11 Anomalies of the occipital region.

fusion of vertebral bodies with or without fusion of corresponding arches and obliteration of apophyseal joints. This anomaly most commonly involves C.2 and C.3. As a rule, congenital fusion of vertebral bodies produces few symptoms but may come to light following injury or routine investigation. A somewhat less flexible neck is present but, as a rule, only two segments are implicated and the cervical spine is able to compensate adequately for this aberration.

ANOMALIES OF THE SUBOCCIPITAL REGION

Aberrations in the growth and development of the suboccipital region contribute to clinical abnormalities. The occipital bone is in four parts at birth. The upper or squamous portion develops from two centers which have united (interparietal) and a lower portion (supraoccipital); these unite to form the complete squamous portion. The condylar portions ossify from a single center on each side; the basilar part, from a further single center. About the fourth year the squamous portions unite with the condylar portion, and at about the sixth year the basilar portion unites with the rest of the bone to form a single unit (Fig. 1–12). The commonest congenital deviation is the persistence of a portion of the upper section of the squamous area as a separate bone, the interparietal bone.

Distortion of the foramen magnum may result from abnormalities of the condylar and basilar portions, leading to pressure from the odontoid process, which then lies at an abnormally high level. This condition

is similar to the platybasia encountered in osteomalacia, Paget's disease and rickets. Further abnormalities of this area consist of a very rare synostosis of occiput and atlas which is usually bilateral. Variations in the development of the arch of the atlas occur; one side may be absent, with the occipital bone taking the form of an extended segment to replace the loss of the arch.

ANOMALIES OF THE ATLAS

The atlas develops in two separate segments, an anterior and a posterior, which subsequently fuse. Absence of the posterior part of this ring has been identified clinically; a portion or all of this segment may be missing. The anomaly frequently comes to light only after injury of some type has focused attention on the area. Clinical in-

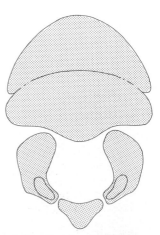

Figure 1–12 Development of the occiput.

stability cannot be detected beforehand and even stress x-rays taken in flexion and extension may fail to show any abnormal excursion of the atlas. In cases that have been reported, no extensive neurological signs or symptoms have been noted.

ANOMALIES OF THE AXIS

Failure of normal development of the odontoid process is the source of numerous anomalies of the axis. The process develops from two centers. A further epiphysis for the apex appears and usually unites with the first two centers by age two. The whole unit then unites with the axis by age 18. Alterations in this development lead to several separate abnormalities including (1) ossiculum terminale, (2) os odontoideum, (3) rudimentary odontoid, and (4) absence of odontoid (Fig. 1–13).

Ossiculum Terminale

Anomalies of the cranial tip of the odontoid are the rarest of this group and perhaps represent a pro-atlas found in some lower forms such as birds and reptiles. In these lower vertebrates the separate piece lies forward between the foramen magnum and the odontoid, but in man, when the tip of the odontoid remains as a separate ossicle, this position is changed to a more vertical one.

Cases have been reported of severe atlanto-axial instability when this anomaly is present. A small, almost flake-like tip of the odontoid lies above and somewhat anterior to a rudimentary odontoid. The curative treatment is occipitovertebral arthrodesis.

Os Odontoideum

Failure of fusion of the odontoid and the arch centers produces an os odontoideum,

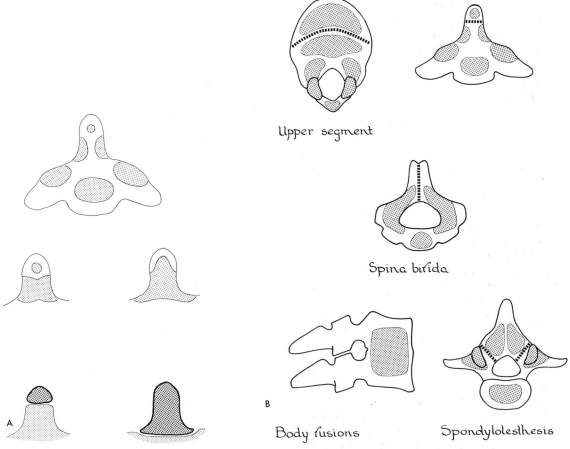

Upper segment

Spina bifida

Body fusions

Spondylolesthesis

A

B

Figure 1–13   *A,* Anomalies and development of the odontoid. *B,* Anomalies of the neck.

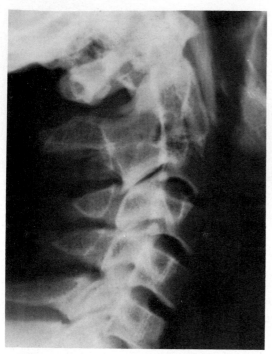

Figure 1-14 Congenital anomaly of the axis.

which is a frequent and important anomaly (Fig. 1–13B). The odontoid develops to normal proportions, but union with the axis is deficient. The anomaly may be present throughout life without producing symptoms, but may come to light following cervico-occipital trauma. The clinical picture consists of local neck discomfort, with extension of pain to the shoulder region, pain in the suspensory muscles and recurrent stiffness on rotation. Transient paralysis may also occur. Lateral roentgenograms demonstrate the subluxation of the atlas on the axis, particularly on flexion and extension films, which should be made with considerable care. Treatment consists of stabilization if there is any suggestion of neurological changes. Stabilization should also be provided for those patients engaged in heavy labor in which recurring trauma is possible.

Rudimentary Odontoid

An abnormally small odontoid may occur, favoring atlanto-axial instability. Trauma to the posterior aspect of the head and neck results in local pain and headache and sometimes a transient quadriplegia. Lateral roentgenograms made in flexion and extension identify the instability by showing increased space between the anterior arch of the atlas

and the odontoid. The degree of normal anteroposterior motion between the atlas and the axis has been carefully studied; the usual distance is 2 to 3 mm. If this is increased, cord impingement is possible. The distance is greater in children, in whom 4 to 5 mm. may be the upper limit. Treatment is by stabilization of the atlanto-axial joint.

Absence of Odontoid

This anomaly is not particularly rare and may be present without producing serious symptoms. Injury, however, can precipitate significant changes. Displacement of the atlas on the axis can be identified in lateral roentgenograms. Symptoms of local pain, headache, restriction of rotation and transient cord signs may develop. Treatment is by skeletal traction, followed by fusion of the upper three cervical vertebrae.

CERVICAL SPONDYLOLISTHESIS

Spondylolisthesis occurs in the cervical spine, usually in association with a spina bifida. The commonest level is the sixth cervical vertebra but the lesion has been identified as involving the fourth and fifth levels also. As a rule, there is a characteristic bilateral defect in the intra-articular portion of the vertebral arch, but without significant slipping of the vertebral body (Fig. 1–13B).

The anomaly may be an incidental finding or may be discovered in patients who have suffered neck trauma. Occasionally it is the source of separate neck symptoms, including local neck pain with radiation to the suboccipital region or to the shoulders. Some restriction in motion also may be present.

In many instances the spine is sufficiently stable that, when symptoms come to light as the result of slight trauma, conservative measures will control the abnormality. These include a period of traction if there are radiating symptoms, followed by the application of a cervical collar. When there is a suggestion of instability, spinal fusion should be carried out.

CONGENITAL SCOLIOSIS

Hemivertebra is the common developmental error producing this deformity (Fig. 1–15). It may occur as a single anomaly and be interpreted as a simple torticollis, causing little difficulty apart from slight tilting of the

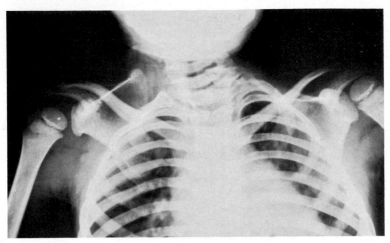

Figure 1–15 Congenital hemivertebra with cervical scoliosis.

head. Symptoms may not be noted until the patient is well along in life. In addition to local neck discomfort, these patients may develop a neurovascular type of radiating pain. When symptoms develop from this abnormality, particularly in the early stage, a program of muscle education is initiated. If the deformity increases, plaster splint correction and stabilization may be necessary, but careful study should be made of any compensatory thoracic curve. In later stages a program of rest, intermittent use of a cervical splint and physiotherapy are required.

KLIPPEL-FEIL SYNDROME OR CONGENITAL BREVICOLLIS

In this anomaly the neck is short as the result of the fusion of several vertebrae. Correspondingly, the posterior hairline appears very low and, hence, the name brevicollis. There may be fewer cervical vertebrae than normal, the shape may be distorted, or a posterior spina bifida caused by failure of ossification centers may frequently be present (Fig. 1–16).

The skull rests at a lower level than normal. The hairline is lower and excess folds of skin extend from the mastoid to the acromion process, adding to the broadened, squat appearance. The bony abnormalities may cause very little disturbance, apart from some limitation of movement. If the skin folds are obvious, they give a bat-like appearance; sometimes thickened subjacent bands are identified in the folds. Plastic reconstruction can materially improve the appearance of the patient.

CERVICAL SPINA BIFIDA

Localized defect of one of the lower vertebral arches may occur in the cervical spine, but much less frequently than in the

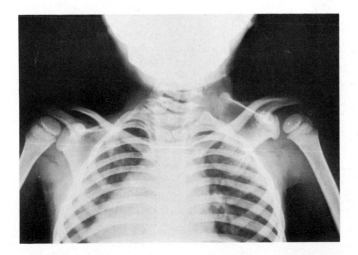

Figure 1–16 Congenital brevicollis.

lumbosacral region (Fig. 1–17). The primary flaw rests in the development of the neural tube rather than its overlying bony skeleton. When this lesion is situated superiorly, it is a form of anencephaly, essentially a Klippel-Feil syndrome. In the lower cervical area, C.6 and C.7 may be similarly involved, but extensive neural abnormalities are rare. The lesion comes to light during routine investigation or following injury and, as a rule, does not require other than conservative treatment (Fig. 1–18).

CONGENITAL ANOMALIES OF THE SCAPULA

The scapula participates prominently in the severest congenital aberration of the shoulder-neck region.

CONGENITAL ELEVATION OF THE SCAPULA

In 1891 Sprengle first described this deformity and explained it as a failure of normal descent of the limb bud in relation to the trunk. The scapula comes to ride at an abnormally high level, often with a bony or ligamentous connection to the spine and a

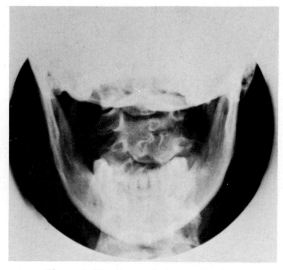

Figure 1–18 Congenital anomaly of C3.

corresponding aplasia of some of the related muscles (Fig. 1–19).

Clinical Picture

The principal feature of this disorder is asymmetry of the neck-shoulder region. This disturbance is at the root of the neck, between the neck and the shoulder, rather than at the point of the shoulder. The involved side appears to start out from the neck at a higher level than normal, particularly when the patient is viewed from the front (Fig. 1–20). At the back there appears a ridge or hump, leading from the region of the angle of the scapula up to the back of the neck. Closer inspection shows the scapula lying near the midline, higher than normal and with the inferior angle tilted backward, making it more prominent than usual. When the deformity is present on both sides it gives the appearance of a short neck with web-like folds. The presence of an abnormal bony connection with the spine is a severer phase of the deformity that, when it is present significantly, interferes with shoulder motion (Fig. 1–21). The scapula is fixed much more securely than normal, so that abduction and circumduction are hampered. Forward rotation is not implicated so much. Weakness is present because of the faulty development of the lower portion of the trapezius, rhomboid and serratus muscles. The failure of descent probably results in a decrease of adequate attachment of the primitive muscle mass. In addition, the restricted

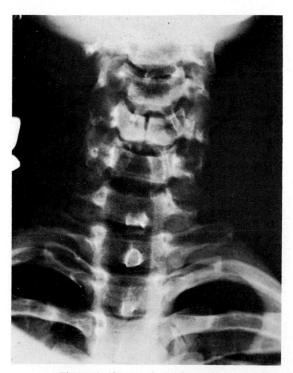

Figure 1–17 Cervical spina bifida.

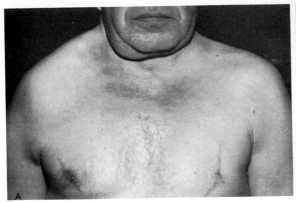
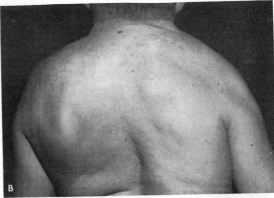

Figure 1–19 Sprengel's deformity. Appearance in an adult of uncorrected congenital elevation of the scapula.

Table 1–2 ANOMALIES OF SHOULDER BONES

1. Anomalies of Scapula

   a. Sprengel's deformity
   b. Bipartite acromion
   c. Aplasia of glenoid

2. Anomalies of Clavicle

   a. Congenital coracoclavicular bar
   b. Congenital clavicular fossae
   c. Segmental defects of clavicle
   d. Cleidocranial dysostosis
   e. Congenital pseudo-arthrosis of clavicle
   f. Congenital neural foramina

3. Anomalies of Humerus

   a. Aplasia of head of humerus
   b. Congenital retroversion
   c. Bicipital groove aberrations

4. Anomalies of Glenohumeral Joint

   a. Congenital dislocation
   b. Epiphyseal separation

Figure 1–20 Congenital elevation of the scapula. Note the filling of the neck-shoulder angle by the omo-vertebral bone on the right.

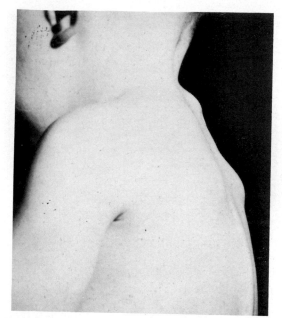

Figure 1–21 Lateral view highlights deformity of body of the scapula in Sprengel's deformity.

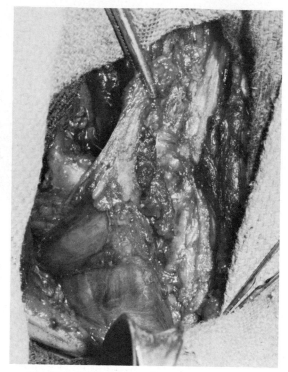

Figure 1–22 Omovertebral bone at operation.

motion leads to lessened development and power in all the muscles of the shoulder girdle.

The size and fixation of the bony bar vary considerably and, consequently, so does the muscle aplasia. Not all patients have extensive limitation of motion. Associated deformities such as cervical scoliosis may mask the lesion or be the dominant embryological error. The only condition with which it may be confused is pterygium colli, a disorder of superficial structures without associated bony abnormalities. In the x-ray the scapula appears smaller than normal; when there is a bony bar present, it appears as a short, thick density, extending from the cervical spine, outward and downward, toward the angle of the scapula. In the lateral view it may appear as an elongated portion of the spine of the scapula.

Pathological Findings

The important findings are centered about the omovertebral bone, which is encountered in roughly half the patients (Figs. 1–22 and 1–23). The most extensive series of these abnormalities has been described by Giannestras, who carefully summarized the operative findings in 21 patients. In ten of these the bone was resected.

There are variations in size, in consistency and in both the medial and lateral attach-

ments. In some cases it is continuous with the spinous processes, laminae or transverse processes of the cervical spine. Occasionally a marrow cavity may be identified in the omovertebral bone. The bar is broader medially

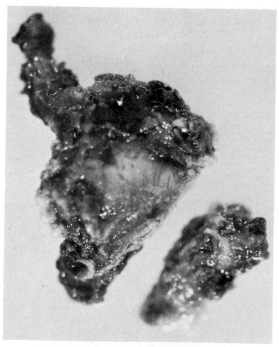

Figure 1–23 Omovertebral bone resected.

and tapers toward a point close to the scapula. At the lateral end it may be continuous with the scapula or form a separate joint or end in a cartilaginous knob. When the bar is incomplete it is usually connected to the scapula by a fibrous cord. In addition to the omovertebral bone, abnormalities of the scapula and related muscles are present. The scapula is smaller than normal and may be distorted in shape. The upper border projects forward. The infraspinous fossa is shorter and smaller and the inferior angle is blunter. The muscles arising from the medial aspect and the inferior angle are weak or absent. The lower segment of the trapezius muscle is most frequently lacking, along with the rhomboids and a portion of the serratus anterior.

Treatment

An effort is made to improve both the appearance and the function of the shoulder. In girls particularly, the distortion may constitute a serious cosmetic defect. In the less severe forms, conservative measures are employed. The earlier the lesion is recognized, the better is the prognosis.

Conservative Program. The principal impairment is lack of abduction. When the appearance is not significantly distorted, efforts to improve abduction and mobilize the scapula at the spine by a proper program of physiotherapy are started. Accessory movements about the shoulder also are emphasized to compensate for the rigidity and the decreased motion of the girdle as a whole. The exercise program includes shrugging of the shoulder to develop the trapezius; pulling the shoulder upward to improve the rhomboid muscles; abduction and external rotation exercises at the glenohumeral joint; and general exercises to improve girdle mobility. These patients need to be followed for some time. The exercise program is continued for at least a year and, in some instances, may be beneficial if followed over a considerably longer period.

Operative Treatment. In those patients with significant deformity or in whom there is an omovertebral bone, surgical therapy is preferable. The aims of the operation are to excise the bony obstruction, to mobilize the scapula so that it can come to rest at a lower level, and to stabilize it to improve its anchoring function in the new position. A program of muscle education and exercises must be conscientiously followed after operation.

TECHNIQUE. The patient is placed on the operating table face down. With the patient under general anesthesia, a curvilinear incision is made, extending from the base of the neck distally to beyond the medial angle of the scapula. Care must be taken not to cut the accessory nerve in the upper portion of the wound. The omovertebral bone lies beneath the fibers of the trapezius muscle, which may be separated along their length; the bone is exposed by periosteal dissection. After careful exposure of the strut, it is excised as completely as possible. Usually, tight bands are adjacent to the strut and these are also cut. The upper border of the scapula is dissected free and frequently is resected, allowing the scapula to fall through a lower level. A note of caution must be sounded against too radical an effort to restore the normal contour by pulling downward violently on the scapula. Brachial plexus paralyses have been reported from a too rugged manipulation of this type. Extensive periosteal dissection around the medial border of the scapula is also discouraged.

No fixation is applied following operation, and exercises are started as soon as the wound is healed (Figs. 1–24 and 1–25).

Woodward Procedure. An alternative operative procedure has been suggested by Woodward. A midscapular longitudinal incision is made from above the angle to below the tip of the scapula. The trapezius and rhomboid muscles are dissected free from their attachments to the scapula. The omovertebral bone, if it is present, is also dissected free and removed along with a corner of the scapula. The scapula is then depressed to a more normal level and held in this position. The trapezius and the rhomboid muscles are then attached to the scapula in its new position.

CONGENITAL DEFORMITIES OF CLAVICLE

There are several congenital abnormalities of the clavicle which frequently do not come to light until middle life. Serious symptoms are not often associated with these abnormalities, and sometimes it is a routine radiological investigation that brings them to light.

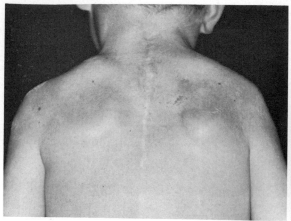

Fig. 1–24 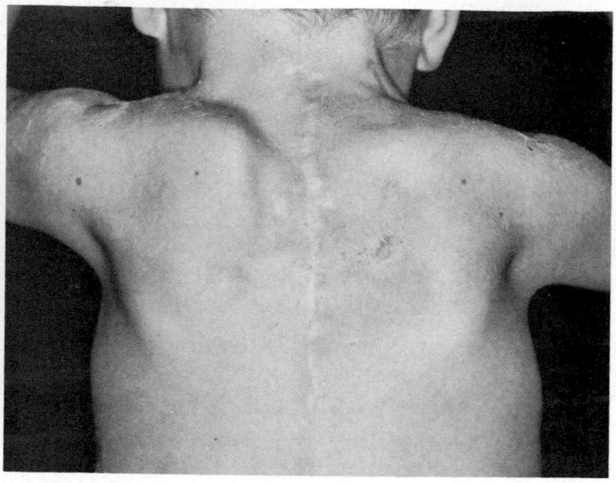   Fig. 1–25

Figure 1–24   Appearance following correction of congenital elevation of the scapula.
Figure 1–25   Motion possible following resection of omovertebral block.

Congenital Coracoclavicular Bar or Joint

A bar of bone may persist between the clavicle and the coracoid process. This may be discovered as an incidental finding in routine x-rays of the chest. It has been reported as having an incidence of 1 to 1.2 per cent (Figs. 1–26 and 1–27). In the lowest vertebral forms the coracoid process is an extensive bar of bone; this gradually disappears until it is represented, in most mammals, by a small stub and the costocoracoid ligament. This ligament varies in size and may contain islands of cartilage. The presence of this ligament has been linked to neurovascular syndromes caused by a compression of the neurovascular bundle, particularly when a congenital coracoclavicular joint is present. Clinically some restriction of shoulder motion is present because of interference with scapular rotation. In patients carrying on strenuous circumduction activities, irritation of the neurovascular bundle may develop. If the bar is sufficiently thick to fix the clavicle, arthritic changes in the acromioclavicular joint are prone to appear because of the restricted rotatory motion.

Treatment. In patients with an established bony bar who have persistent symptoms, surgical excision of the bar should be carried out.

The area is exposed through a short transverse incision just below the clavicle, the coracoid process is again identified, and the bony bar is followed from the top of the coracoid up to the clavicle. It is usually identified by digital dissection, pressing backward along the upper border of the coracoid. There may or may not be a joint between this bony projection and the clavicle. The bar and the intervening joint are excised as completely as possible. In some instances the bar is present on both sides, but usually it is only the master arm which is affected clinically. Removal of the bar is followed by relief of discomfort in a high percentage of patients.

Cleidocranial Dysostosis

This is a relatively rare hereditary condition in which there has been ineffective ossification of the skull and the clavicles. There is only a small portion of the frontal or occipital bone present at birth, and this leads to delayed closure of the fontanelles. A varying degree of clavicular aplasia is present; this controls the signs and symptoms that develop related to the shoulder. The lesion is always bilateral, and when the clavicles are com-

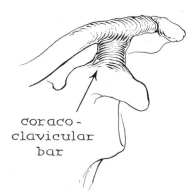

coraco-
clavicular
bar

Figure 1–26   Congenital coracoclavicular bar.

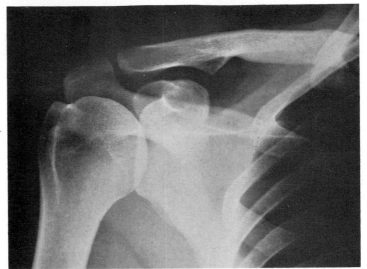

Figure 1-27 Congenital coracoclavicular bar.

pletely absent, it is possible to swing the two shoulders to the front with the arms touching, presenting a grossly deformed appearance (Figs. 1-28, 1-29, 1-30, 1-31, and 1-32). Even when this extreme deformity can be produced, the amount of altered function is not so extensive as might be anticipated.

In some instances only the central part of the clavicle may be absent, resulting in what amounts to a pseudoarthrosis in the center of the clavicle and leading to some instability and increased mobility of the shoulder. The defect is one which principally involves bone and there are very few, if any, corresponding soft tissue disturbances, which tends to mini-

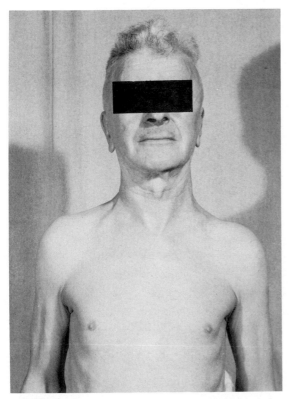

Figure 1-28 Cleidocranial dysostosis. Note shortened shoulder breadth.

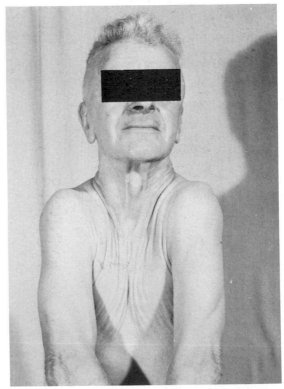

Figure 1-29 Rudimentary clavicles allow shoulders to be swung almost together in front.

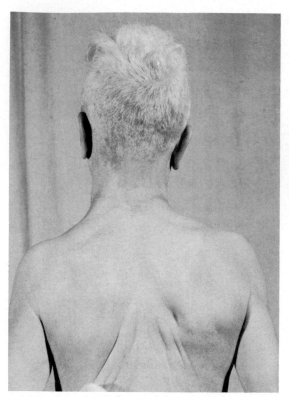

Figure 1–30 Posterior appearance in cleidocranial dysostosis.

mize the deleterious effects considerably. No treatment apart from postural and strengthening exercises is necessary.

Congenital Clavicular Fossae

A small oblong fossa directed obliquely may develop at the sternal end of the clavicle (Fig. 1–33). It is nearly always present on both sides and may be erroneously interpreted as an infectious or neoplastic process. No symptoms have been reported arising from this abnormality and no treatment is required.

Local Congenital Defects of the Clavicle

Abnormalities in the appearance of the centers of ossification of the clavicle lead to the development of local defects. The clavicles may be absent on both sides without significant abnormality related to the skull. The outer third of the clavicle may be missing, the inner two thirds may be missing or the center portion may be absent. As a rule, not so ex-

tensive clinical disturbance is present as might be anticipated, and frequently the only abnormality is some increase in the normal mobility of the shoulder. Injury may bring the weaknesses into focus. The explanation of these clinical forms lies in the process of ossification of the clavicle. The ossification spreads inward and outward from two centers which appear at the junction at the middle and outer thirds. When neither center appears, the clavicle is absent. If the outer center fails to develop, the lateral third of the clavicle is lacking. Failure of the inner center is less common but leads to absence of the inner two thirds. In some instances a branch of the supraclavicular nerve perforates the clavicle at the junction of the ossifications, spreading from the epiphyseal centers (Fig. 1–34).

Congenital Pseudoarthrosis of the Clavicle

A frank pseudoarthrosis of the midportion of the clavicle, without any other congenital

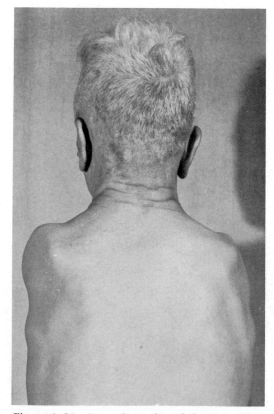

Figure 1–31 Gross shortening of shoulder breadth apparent posteriorly in cleidocranial dysostosis.

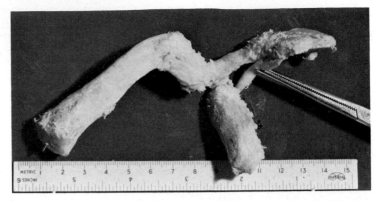

Figure 1–32 Specimen in cleido-cranial dysostosis.

stigmata such as accompany cleidocranial dysostosis, is commonly encountered.

Etiology. Centers of cartilaginous development appear in the embryo during the seventh and eighth weeks in the isolated mass of mesenchyme which forms the clavicle. These start at the junction of the outer third and the inner two thirds, with growth proceeding toward each end. A gap may persist between these two centers, and this development has been interpreted as the source of a congenital pseudoarthrosis.

Clinical Picture. An abnormal swelling develops along the clavicle, usually on one side, and is quite painless but presents a feeling of looseness on palpation because of movement of the two segments. It contrasts with the exuberant callus and pain of a birth fracture, and there are no associated changes in other structures as in cleidocranial dysostosis. The x-rays show a pseudoarthrosis, with enlarged ends and sclerotic edges.

Treatment. Autogenous bone grafting is the treatment of choice and is followed by a much higher rate of success than when such procedures are followed for similar conditions in the tibia (Fig. 1-35).

Subluxation of the Acromioclavicular Joint

A state of congenital luxation of the acromioclavicular joint has been recognized. Grieve first called attention to this condition when he reported seven cases discovered during routine acromioclavicular examinations. It is a bilateral abnormality in which the outer end of the clavicle is prominent and the joint is lax. It must be differentiated from simple enlargement of the outer end of the stable clavicle, which is encountered in later life. As a rule, there is no history of injury preceding the development or the discovery of this lesion. Congenital subluxation usually comes to light on routine clinical or x-ray examination or when consultation is sought because of the unusual appearance of the bone.

Examination shows the outer end of the clavicle riding above the acromion, and it appears to bounce in a vertical direction on pressure. A subluxation amounts to a variation of 0.5 to 1.0 cm. Little disability results; pain and limitation of movement are not prominent, and the suspensory ligaments are not involved. The origin of this abnormality is related to faulty development of the outer end of the clavicle or the adjacent zone of the acromion. This has been corroborated by Smith, who reported a case of subluxation of the clavicle in which there was a congenital distortion of the acromion.

Treatment is not necessary unless the subluxation is sufficient to distort the appearance. When the disturbance is of cosmetic

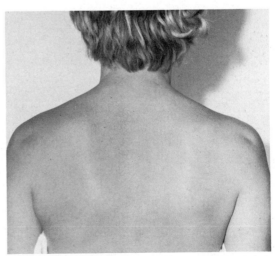

Figure 1–33 Congenital supraspinous fossae. Slight tendency toward prominence of acromioclavicular joints also.

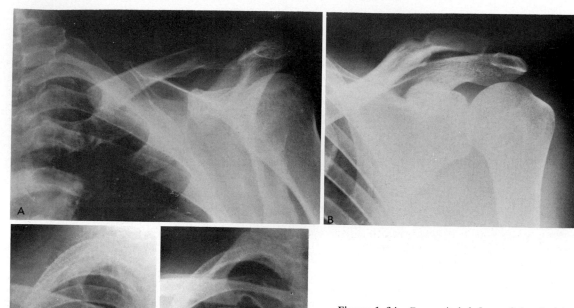

Figure 1-34 Congenital defects of the clavicle. *A*, Absence of inner third. *B*, Neural hiatus. *C*, incomplete hiatus. *D*, Congenital fossa.

concern, the outer end is stabilized as for traumatic acromioclavicular dislocation. Excision of the outer end of the clavicle is not recommended unless the joint is damaged, because this may increase the deformity unless measures are taken to stabilize the clavicle. Recognition of the lesion is important in medicolegal and compensation problems. Demonstration of the abnormality on both sides indicates the true nature of the condition (Figs. 1–36 and 1–37).

CONGENITAL ABNORMALITIES OF THE HUMERUS

In a study of the progress of developing mammalian forms, significant changes can be recognized relative to the upper end of the humerus. The principal alteration involves the head. The position is changed, and the upper end of the humerus twists so that in man, instead of facing dorsally, it comes to face medially. The presence of this torsion explains the altered size of the tuberosities of the humerus and the subsequent shift of the bicipital groove medially, which leaves

a greater lateral and a much smaller lesser or medial tuberosity.

The new position of the tuberosities also alters the position of certain muscles such as the biceps so that they come to lie on the front instead of the side, and the tendon follows a much more tortuous or right angle course than formerly. This more medial position places extra strain on the lesser tuberosity and the transverse humeral ligament.

Ossification of the Humerus. The humerus develops as a typically long bone from a core of cartilage for the shaft, which later is encased in a sheath of bone from the periosteum (Fig. 1–38). The upper end is an epiphysis of solid cartilage in which ossification begins in the head during the first year, then in the greater tuberosity at three years, and in the lesser tuberosity at five years. These fuse by the age of six and unite with the shaft at age 20. The upper end of the humerus unites after the lower end so that growth continues longer at the shoulder than at the elbow. The time of union of the epiphyses has been thought to affect the frequency of development of primary malignancies. This means that with growth going

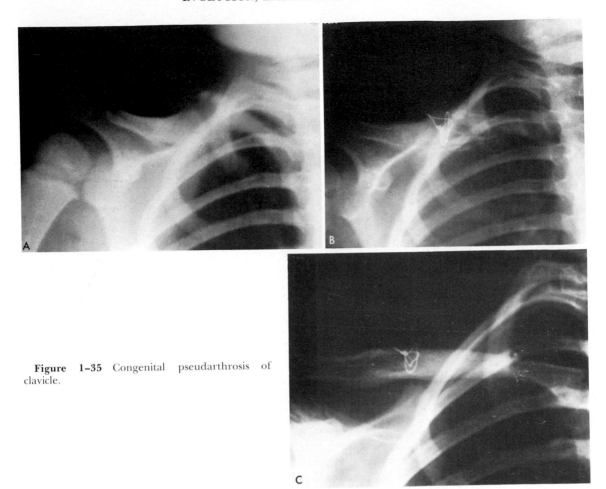

Figure 1–35 Congenital pseudarthrosis of clavicle.

on longer in the shoulder, the incidence of neoplasms is greater in this region than at the elbow. At birth the upper end of the humerus is completely cartilaginous; in x-rays taken at this time no upper end is visible.

Severe abnormalities of the upper end of the humerus are not common. The head of the humerus may be completely absent, and this aplasia may be associated with similar maldevelopment of the glenoid. Abnormalities in the degree of rotation of the humeral head occur more frequently. In some instances excessive internal rotation of the head of the humerus or humerus varus develops; this explains the development of congenital recurrent posterior dislocation of the shoulder. When the head of the humerus is rotated inward to a greater degree than normal, as the arm is flexed, the head has a tendency to rotate internally to an abnormal degree so that, instead of facing the glenoid fossa in the usual application, it tends to rotate farther posteriorly and slips out of the glenoid as the arm is flexed. The author has corrected congenital recurrent posterior dis-

location by carrying out an external rotation osteotomy of the upper end of the humerus, bringing the distal segment inward to prevent the recurrent posterior luxation.

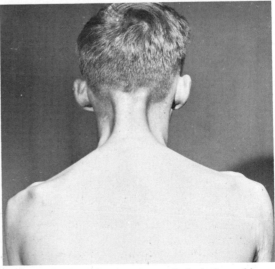

Figure 1–36 Congenital acromioclavicular subluxation.

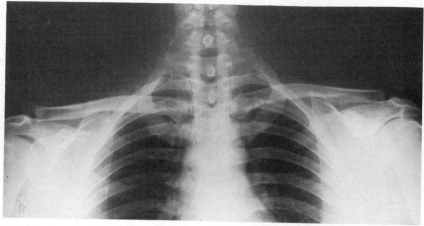

Figure 1–37   Distinct prominence of outer end of clavicle clinically and radiologically in congenital acromioclavicular subluxation.

Variations in the size and shape of the bicipital groove may be recognized and have considerable clinical significance. A shallow groove may be present, and a correspondingly large tendon may easily slip from the groove. The converse may be true, and the groove may be deeper than normal and end as a deep cleft, holding a small tendon so that constriction and undue restriction easily result. Fortunately the long head of the biceps is an extremely pliable structure and accommodates well to a great many variations of the position of its groove and the tuberosities; otherwise, clinical disturbance would be much more frequent.

ANOMALIES OF THE SHOULDER JOINT

The joint cavities, synovium and associated ligaments of the shoulder arise from the embryonic ray of tissue between the elements of the humerus and the scapula (Fig. 1–39). In the developing joint a central translucent area appears at the ends of this zone and remains continuous with the bone ends. This layer of tissue then forms the capsule and thus becomes continuous with the periosteum. In this fashion strong hinges develop, forming protection for the articular surfaces yet remaining rigidly adherent to the bone ends. The origin of the capsule with its extremely strong attachment to bone has been recognized as the mechanism protecting the shoulder joint from dislocation, reducing, in particular, the frequency of congenital dislocation as compared with that of the hip joint.

The tendon of the long head of the biceps invaginates the capsule and then is enveloped in a synovial layer. This layer later disappears,

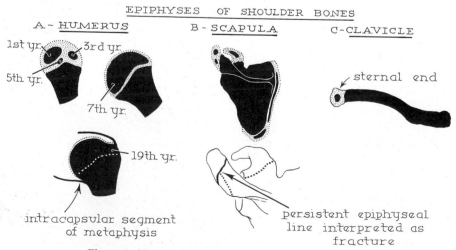

Figure 1–38   Development of bones about the shoulder.

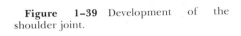
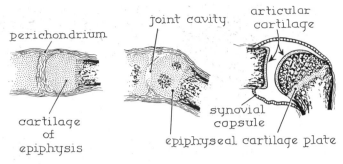

Figure 1–39 Development of the shoulder joint.

leaving the tendon free within the joint cavity, lying on bare cartilage. The line of attachment of capsule demarcates intra-articular from extra-articular structures. That portion of the bone which develops adjacent to the cavity zone persists, covered with cartilage and protected with capsule. That portion outside of the capsular attachment is free of capsule and has no articular cartilage. When rotation and descent of the upper extremity occur, the line of capsule attachment alters so that more of the inner aspect of the humerus adjacent to the head comes within the capsule and the attachment extends farther down the neck. There is no such change in the case of the scapula, so that the attachment of the capsule remains close to the articular margin around the perimeter of the glenoid, blending with the labrum. The process of capsule development with continuity to perichondrium explains the secure attachment of labrum to the glenoid also.

Capsule attachment is at the edge of the cartilage, except at the inferomedial aspect, where the change in position of the head of the humerus due to rotation allows it to shift down the shaft. This brings a short piece of the metaphysis or the upper end of the shaft of the humerus to lie within the joint. The clinical significance lies in the fact that infection of the upper end of the humerus in children, which commonly implicates the metaphysis, may then spread into the joint proper because of the inclusion of this small portion of metaphysis.

The firm attachment of the capsule to the glenoid is maintained throughout life, and use is made of it in certain surgical maneuvers. By means of this firm attachment it is possible to exert a pull on the glenoid and so reduce fractures in this region which otherwise would be difficult to manipulate and tedious to expose. (See the chapter on fractures.)

Congenital Dislocation of the Humerus

Congenital dislocation of the shoulder is extremely uncommon, and many authors have questioned its ever occurring. Many of the cases which have been reported as congenital are really paralytic or are caused by trauma at birth. There is a condition of maldevelopment of the scapulohumeral mechanism which results in abnormal relation of the head of the humerus to the glenoid. The name congenital dislocation should be reserved for conditions of this type. A type of congenital dislocation in cases of arthrogryposis has been identified, but this condition is bilateral and is accompanied by many other deformities elsewhere. The primary defect is an abnormal development of the

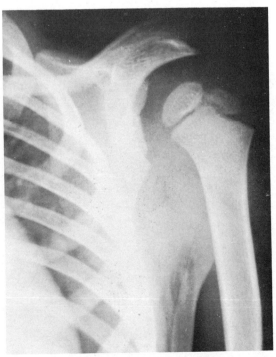

Figure 1–40 Epiphyseal abnormalities.

glenoid cavity, which may fail to attain normal proportions but may retain normal position. In some instances the position is abnormal, and the relationship with the head of the humerus is distorted. In the first instance, incongruity between the humerus and the glenoid resembles the aplasia of the acetabulum in congenital dislocation of the hip (Figs. 1–40 and 1–41, *A*). The infantile glenoid assumes an anterior position, and the head of the humerus, which develops normally, has a tendency to ride posteriorly. The more frequent mechanism has to do with an abnormal position of the glenoid and subsequent aberration of the development of the coracoid. The coracoid process extends farther forward and points laterally, forcing the glenoid face backward. The head of the humerus is carried backward with the glenoid cavity so that an atopic articulation results. Greater distortion of the upper portion of the glenoid also occurs in this deformity.

The reason that the inferior aspect of the glenoid is not involved so much is that is does not share in the rotation because it develops from the scapula without a separate epiphysis. In both conditions the joint is not really dislocated but is carried backward to an abnormal site. The pathological findings consist of an abnormally shaped scapula with an elongated spine and a somewhat irregular acromion. The glenoid fossa is distorted and loses its normal oval shape (Fig. 1–42). The upper portion is convex and closely related to the coracoid; the lower portion is concave and more nearly normal in shape. Only the lower part of the humerus is in contact with the rudimentary cavity, and the remaining articular surface is misshapen. The coracoid is directed horizontally and laterally without any normal vertical or horizontal limb. The spine of the scapula is also distorted and becomes twisted at its base so that the upper surface faces forward and the

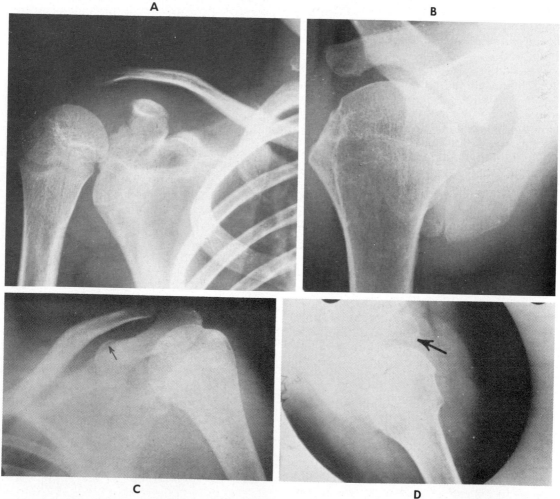

Figure 1–41 Developmental defects of upper end of the humerus and related area of the scapula as reported in congenital dislocation of the shoulder. *A*, Glenoid. *B*, Metacromion showing persistent ununited distal end. *C* and *D*, Coracoid anomaly with persistent ununited distal end.

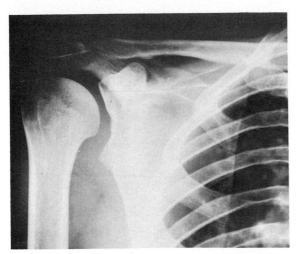

Figure 1–42 Aplasia of glenoid and retroversion of humeral head.

lower surface backward. The acromion is deformed, tending to be more horizontal than oblique. The upper portion of the body of the scapula is straight and not angled and the whole body of the scapula may be altered.

Congenital Posterior Dislocation of the Humerus

An entity which should be differentiated from severe congenital dislocation is congenital posterior dislocation, which is sometimes described as congenital posterior subluxation (Fig. 1–43). Frequently the condition does not become apparent until five to seven years of age, and it then takes a form of recurrent posterior laxity of the shoulder joint.

Frequently the patient complains initially only of the catching sensation in the shoulder, but then gradually becomes conscious of a posterior projection. Eventually flexion action of any degree initiates the prominence of the head of the humerus posteriorly. If the arm is held in external rotation and abducted, there is less tendency to luxation. It is the act of internal rotation which alters the normal relationship of the head of the humerus to the glenoid.

Pathological Considerations. In this condition very few bony abnormalities can be demonstrated, in contrast to severe congenital dislocation. In some instances slight hypoplasia or aplasia of the glenoid is apparent. In many instances there is retroversion of the head of the humerus so that, as the arm is flexed, there is a tendency for posterior rota-

tion and the humerus faces the posterior capsule, leading to a posterior prominence.

The condition is almost always bilateral, with the master arm exhibiting the greater tendency to subluxation.

Treatment. Many operations have been devised in treatment, including fascial and capsuloplasty of the posterior aspect, posterior bone block and combinations of these procedures. In the author's hands the most effective procedure has been a rotation osteotomy to correct the malalignment of the upper end of the humerus.

SURGICAL TREATMENT. Through a longitudinal incision along the lateral aspect in the lateral bicipital groove, the upper end of the humerus is exposed over a distance of about 5 inches. A transverse rotation osteotomy is performed, and the distal segment is rotated internally about 20 degrees. Fixation in this position is then carried out with a compression plate and screws. The arm is immobilized in a shoulder spica for eight to ten weeks until union is satisfactory (Figs. 1–45 and 1–46).

Paralytic Dislocations

Paralytic dislocation is not a true congenital dislocation, but it is a commoner occurrence

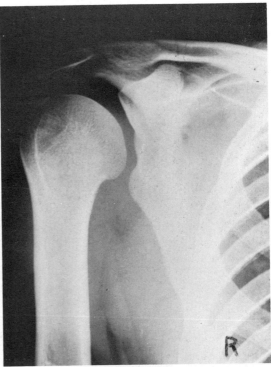

Figure 1–43 Congenital posterior dislocation of the humerus.

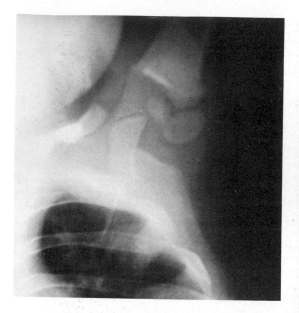

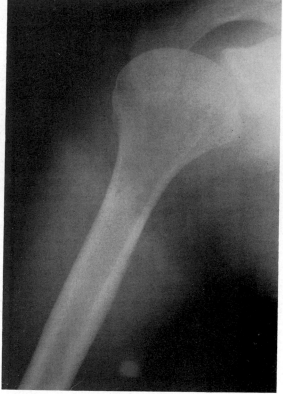

Figure 1–44 Developmental posterior dislocation of the humerus.

than the latter. In injuries to the brachial plexus, particularly the upper roots, C.5 and C.6, extensive loss of muscle power and soft tissue stability occurs and gradual subluxation with anterior dislocation of the head of the humerus may develop. Any dislocation should be reduced and maintained in correct position, either by a body swathe or a single Kirschner wire. Once the paralytic dislocation has improved, soft tissues become more stable and the subluxation comes under control. Further discussion of the management

of the nerve injury is found in the chapter on nerve injuries.

Epiphyseal Separation

The embryological development of the shoulder joint explains the likelihood of epiphyseal separation being greater than true glenohumeral congenital dislocation. The primitive capsule forms a stout layer over the joint and becomes continuous with the periosteum. This, then, constitutes a strong hinge, protecting the articular por-

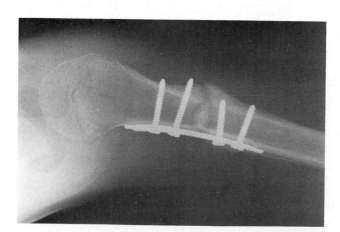

Figure 1–45 Retroversion corrected by osteotomy.

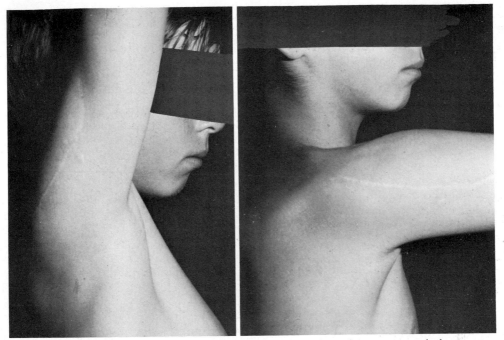

Figure 1–46 Correction in patient in Figure 1–45, shown here postoperatively.

tion of the contiguous bones and becoming rigidly adherent just beyond the cartilaginous line. This process of capsular development and continuity with the perichondrium explains the secure attachment of the labrum to the glenoid. The epiphyseal belt closely follows the lower edge of the articular cartilage and constitutes a much weaker zone during the period of early growth than does the intra-articular capsular covered area. For this reason, when strong force is applied to the shoulder joint the humerus is more likely to give way through the soft epiphyseal zone than it is through the strongly anchored capsule. In experimental efforts to produce congenital dislocation, the deformity which has resulted has been a fracture through the shaft or a displacement through the epiphysis rather than separation of the joint surfaces. The injury is treated by reduction and fixation. It is not difficult to restore the alignment, but it should be remembered that this needs to be carried out largely by palpation since no shadow of the epiphysis of the head is apparent in the x-ray at birth. In the very young, fixation by a soft sling and bandage dressing, with the arm at the side for two weeks, is all that is necessary; a shoulder spica should be applied to more mature bones.

ANOMALIES OF THE MUSCLES

The muscles of the shoulder are extremely important since they not only provide power but permit precision control of the joint. Many muscles acting on the upper limb retain their primitive attachment to the vertebral column, the skull and the iliac crest, which adds to mobility and at the same time exerts extensive control. Such a mechanism provides powerful leverage, and yet a complete circle of motion is feasible. The muscles of the lower limb, in contrast, do not reach above the iliac crest, minimizing their influence.

An orderly pattern of development synchronizes the various groups of girdle muscles. In the beginning the base is made secure,

Table 1–3 CONGENITAL ANOMALIES OF MUSCLES

1. Development of Muscles
2. Clinical Significance of Muscle Embryology
3. Development of Trapezius and Sternomastoid
4. Development of Latissimus Dorsi and Pectoralis
5. Development of Deltoid, Spinatae and Teres Muscles
6. Development of Biceps and Coracobrachialis

and then motion for the base is provided; this is followed by the development of muscles to move the upper arm on the base, and, finally, structures to control the more distal portion of the lever are fabricated. This sequence progresses from the neck outward. Muscles connected with the neck appear first in the premuscle mass of mesenchyme. Structures such as the trapezius and sternomastoid muscles may be identified at the beginning and are followed by the development of the serratus anterior, levator scapulae and rhomboids. A group that connects the girdle to the trunk, such as the latissimus dorsi and the pectoralis, may then be identified. There then develops the collection of muscles in the shoulder girdle group such as the deltoid, the supraspinati and the teres. The last group to appear are those, like the biceps and coracobrachialis, which connect the shoulder girdle to the arm.

CLINICAL SIGNIFICANCE OF THE MUSCLE EMBRYOLOGY

Development of the primitive muscle mass producing these muscles can be followed through the evolution of amphibia, reptiles and mammals. The assumption of the upright position produced profound changes in the configuration of these structures. In the pronogrades, in which the anterior limb is used for locomotion and weight bearing, the axis of pull on these muscles is almost parallel to the limb. In orthograde forms, when the arm drops to the side, the line of pull alters. The pull in the upright mammalian position is almost at right angles to the primitive angle and, therefore, is much less mechanically efficient. In this process the supraspinatus shows the greatest degree of change.

As the scapula elongates, the infraspinatus increases in size and bulk, but the supraspinatus does not follow suit. Upward elongation of the scapula would interfere with movement of the neck and shoulder so that the supraspinatus zone remains relatively small. In addition to this lack of development, the rotation of the extremity produces a further strain on the supraspinatus tendon because it comes to pull in much less of a straight line than in the lower animal forms. Added to these two detrimental embryological developments is the increased stress placed upon the supraspinatus by the assumption of the upright posture and the necessity for man to do much work at shoulder level or above. The combination of these factors produces a congenitally relatively weak muscle which has to assume a constantly increasing burden. In analysis of the many clinical syndromes affecting the shoulder it is to be expected that degenerative changes will appear first in this region.

An anomaly of similar importance is related to the muscles, such as the biceps, which extend from the arm to the shoulder girdle. When the head of the humerus rotates, following the glenoid cavity, the trough containing the long head of the biceps shifts medially also. This changes the direction of pull so that instead of being squarely over the lateral surface of the head of the humerus, it is shifted medially. In this site it is in a less secure position, and increased tension is placed on the fibers which hold this tendon in position. The intertubercular fibers resist a constant tendency toward dislocation of the long head of the biceps, particularly in acts of flexion and external rotation. The application of sudden force in this arc may then rupture this retaining ligament, allowing the tendon to slip out of the groove. A much more frequent but less dramatic change is the constantly increased wear to which the bicipital tendon is exposed by these embryonal changes. In this instance also it can be anticipated that wear and tear changes will frequently be encountered in this region in the adult.

Development of the Trapezius and Sternomastoid

The first muscles connected to the shoulder girdle develop from a sheet of primitive tissue growing tailward from the occiput to the arm bud. This sheet splits, forming the trapezius posteriorly and the sternomastoid anteriorly. The split remaining between these muscle masses then becomes the posterior triangle of the neck in the adult (Fig. 1–47). In the migration from the occiput to the base of the arm bud, the nerve supply of these muscles trails along, which explains the extensive course of the accessory nerve. The sternomastoid muscle arises from the anterior portion of this primitive muscle sheet. It develops as a strap-like layer extending from the mastoid process to the sternum and the inner end of the clavicle.

Abnormalities at birth in the sternomastoid have long been recognized as the cause of

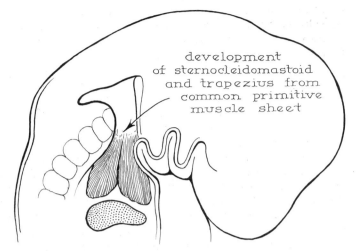

Figure 1–47 Development of the trapezius and sternomastoid, leaving the posterior triangle between.

torticollis. In some instances interference with the blood supply has been described, whereas in others traction or pressure on the muscle has been blamed. The treatment of this lesion has been presented in Chapter 13.

Development of the Latissimus Dorsi and Pectoralis

In our remote ancestors climbing muscles were extremely vital. The latissimus dorsi and pectoralis major are examples of powerful muscles attached to the body but extending to the upper limb and, therefore, of great use in climbing (Fig. 1–48). They developed during the arboreal era, enabling the body to be pulled upward by the arm. This phase of existence and the resultant necessities of anatomical development are reflected also in the shape of the chest (Fig. 1–49). Continued use of these muscle groups at the front and the back led to compression of the chest in an anteroposterior direction, so that it was altered from the round shape of forefooted specimens such as the dog to the more oval or kidney-shaped cross section essential for the upright stance.

The latissimus dorsi is the muscle mass which arises on the posterior aspect of the shoulder and migrates to the present attachment to the humerus during the phase of rotation of the shoulder girdle and the humerus. The lengthy course which its nerve follows has been thought to be the result of migration.

The anterior counterpart to the latissimus dorsi is the pectorals. These develop in close relationship to the arm bud, but in the front of the chest. In this position the mass becomes

attached to the humerus, coracoid, clavicle and upper ribs in sequence. A horizontal split appears in the primitive muscle mass, eventually demarcating the pectoralis major and the pectoralis minor. The pectoralis major develops from the superficial layer, retaining its attachment to the humerus, crossing from the chest. As the humerus rotates, the muscle insertion is drawn with it and eventually is folded over on itself, explaining the appearance of this tendon in the adult. The pectoralis minor develops from a split in this mass and does not rotate so extensively on its long axis, so there is no folding over of this tendon. The pectoralis minor has gradually assumed a much less important role as evolutionary progress has

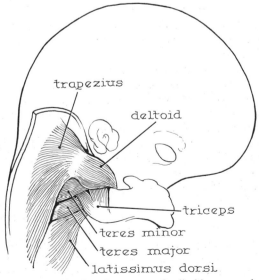

Figure 1–48 Development of climbing muscles.

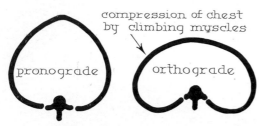

Figure 1–49 Chest shape developed in the upright stance.

been made from flying forms to plantigrade and orthograde levels. Originally this muscle mass extended to the movable portion of the extremity through the coracoid and was associated with a heavy precoracoid element. In orthogrades this element is represented by the costocoracoid membrane only, replacing the heavy buttress form found in amphibians and flying forms. Abnormalities of this group of muscles are encountered in man. In some instances the pectorals are poorly developed, and not infrequently they are completely absent on one side (Fig. 1–50).

Development of Deltoid, Spinati and Teres Muscles

Lying a little more toward the tip of the limb bud there is a further primitive mass of muscle lying in the same layer as the previous group which ultimately produces the deltoid, the spinati and the teres muscles. This group develops largely in the region of the limb bud and extends proximally to gain attachment to the shoulder girdle (Fig. 1–51). The anterior portion fans out as it grows, becoming attached to the clavicle and acromion in sequence; it eventually constitutes

the deltoid muscle. The teres muscles develop a little farther distally, migrating in a similar fashion from the limb bud to the girdle elements.

Development of Biceps and Coracobrachialis

The biceps and coracobrachialis arise from a common V-shaped muscle mass which extends proximally from around the central bony core to attachment to the bones of the shoulder girdle. As growth of the limb proceeds, a gap develops at the proximal end of this muscle, creating long and short heads. The larger portion remains on the lateral aspect and the small part extends to the coracoid. Occasionally encountered embryonal errors in the division of the proximal end of this mass result in three or four heads of the biceps instead of the usually encountered two.

Development of the Triceps

The muscle mass at the back of the limb develops in a similar fashion so that corresponding muscles appear. The muscle mass extends proximally and splits to make its attachment on the humerus and then spreads to the shoulder girdle. As the limb grows these proximal attachments separate, forming the three heads of the triceps.

DEVELOPMENTAL ANOMALIES OF NERVES OF THE SHOULDER-NECK REGION

The nerves of the limb spring from the nerve column opposite the limb bud and ex-

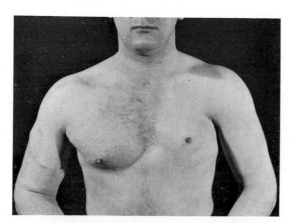

Figure 1–50 Congenital absence of pectorals.

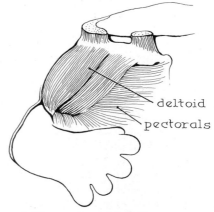

Figure 1–51 Development of deltoid and pectorals.

tend outward as a sheet (Fig. 1–52). The tips of this nerve sheet advance into the limb core and the fibers come to lie among the layers of primitive muscle substance. As the tips of the nerves become attached to the primitive muscle, they follow the muscles in between the layers of the muscle substance. As the limb grows, nerves from the plexus branch into individual muscles, and the site of this point of innervation exerts some control over further muscular development. In this way main nerve trunks develop along intervertebral paths, while nerve branching occurs in the intermuscular septa of the individual muscles. The muscle masses receive their nerves at an early date; as they develop, they draw the nerves along with them to keep pace with the skeletal maturation. This explains the intricate and lengthy course of the supply to such muscles as the trapezius and the latissimus dorsi.

The base of the limb bud of the arm lies opposite the lower four cervical and first thoracic segments. This relationship of vertebral bodies to arm axis may vary and, consequently, different nerves will then extend into the limb bud. There may be a variation of as much as three segments in the origin of the segmental nerves entering the limb, in which case this is referred to as a pre- or postfixed plexus (Fig. 1–53). The brachial plexus consists of a continuous sheet of fibers extending distally into the limb bud; it splits into dorsal and ventral divisions as it meets the humerus. The ventral division produces the anterior and medial cords, and these cords, in turn, break up into large branches, passing among the intramuscular spaces. From the ventral or anterior split arise the musculocutaneous, median and ulnar nerves. The posterior segment produces the axillary and radial nerves.

The pattern of embryonal development is

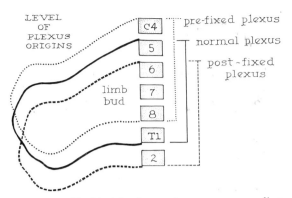

Figure 1–53 Limb level may vary as to corresponding body and nerve segments, producing plexus anomalies.

reflected in individual muscle innervation, since the course within the muscle is determined by the direction of the development of the muscle fibers. In a muscle composed largely of parallel fibers, the innervation has a longitudinal pattern, with the main nerve entering the proximal portion and extending distally. When fibers are disposed somewhat differently, the innervation is at right angles, and the nerve crosses midway between the points of attachment of the muscles to attain the most efficient pattern of distribution. For example, the nerve for the coracobrachialis, which has long parallel fibers, comes in at the upper end and gives off branches from a parallel-running, intermuscular septum. The nerve for the deltoid, on the other hand, enters at right angles to maintain an efficient branching pattern. The importance of these relations becomes apparent when one must make incisions in the muscles. If the biceps and coracobrachialis are cut transversely near the top they will become completely paralyzed. The deltoid, however, may be split its entire length on the inner side, and the only loss would be to a portion of the fibers on the medial aspect of this incision.

ANOMALIES OF THE BRACHIAL PLEXUS

The neck in man is developed as a ribless zone so that innervation from the neural segments opposite the limb bud may extend down into the limb. Large nerves from the segments opposite the appendage require unobstructed passage outward to reach the hand (Fig. 1–54). Since the limb bud may develop at different levels in relation to the spinal column, it follows that the nerve segments which may enter the limb will vary also. When the bud lies higher, a larger con-

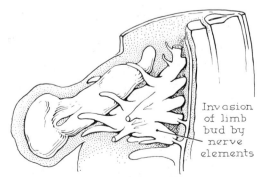

Figure 1–52 Invasion of muscle mass by nerve elements.

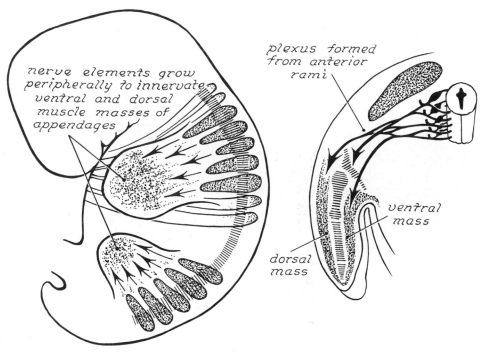

Figure 1–54 Formation of the brachial plexus.

tribution may be expected from the upper segments, C.4 and C.5, and consequently less from T.1. When this occurs, there is less obstruction to the developing rib elements at the lower level of C.7, and frequently a primitive costal segment will then be free to develop. A rib which then appears in relation to the seventh cervical vertebral body will be closely related and can easily exert an upward pressure on the lower root of the plexus, which must then arch upward and over this obstruction to reach the limb. Conversely, when the limb bud develops farther tailward in relation to the vertebral column, a greater contribution can be expected from the second thoracic nerve; this has been termed a postfixed plexus. No cervical rib should be expected to develop under these circumstances, since there is increased obstruction by the outgrowing nerves.

DEVELOPMENT AND ANOMALIES OF THE VESSELS IN SHOULDER-NECK REGION

Knowledge of development of the vascular pattern is not so complete as in the case of bone, muscle and nerve. However, the vessels do not play quite so important a part from the standpoint of congenital anomalies as do these other structures. The primary artery of the limb is an axial stem which develops from an arterial network, taking shape near the base of the limb bud. Capillaries arise from the lateral side of the primitive aorta and this network gradually extends outward into the limb bud (Fig. 1–55). The network continues to develop and, as it progresses peripherally, unnecessary communications disappear so that gradually one main vessel is left, corresponding to the limb. In the case of the arm this means that three or four segmental stems or subclavian vessels, one for each of the body segments, are initially present in the embryo and undergo consolidation. The vessel of the seventh, or central, segment of the group survives as the main vessel or subclavian artery of the fetus, and the rest disappear. In some instances evidence of the primitive network persists and there is a plexiform arrangement of smaller vessels rather than one main subclavian vessel. In normal development the artery perforates the primitive nerve segments that eventually constitute the brachial plexus. When there are more channels because of the persistence of some parts of the primitive vascular network, there may be two or more subclavian arteries. The presence of vascular anomalies is more frequent if other anomalies are present, particularly

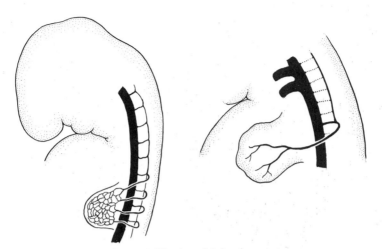

Figure 1–55   Arterial development.

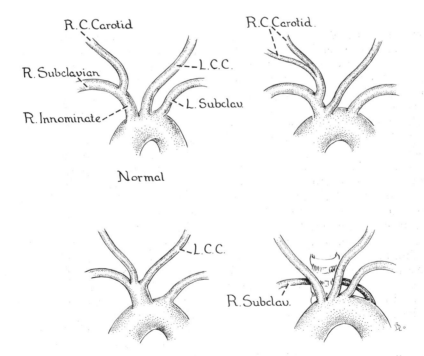

Figure 1–56   Vascular anomalies.

any involving the development of the brachial plexus. In some instances, when there is a cervical rib perforating the plexus, there may be two subclavian arteries. Alternatively, some of the adjacent large vessels may take over a greater portion of the subclavian supply than normal and become much larger in size and superficial in position, in which case the subclavian artery is very small. In surgical procedures such as scalenotomy, exploration of the brachial plexus or excision of the cervical rib, these possible vascular anomalies should be kept in mind (Fig. 1–56).

REFERENCES

Babitt, D. P., et al.: Obstetrical paralysis and dislocation of the shoulder in infancy. J. Bone Joint Surg. (Amer) 50:1447–1452, 1968.

Bardeen, C. A., and Lewis, W. H.: Development of limbs, body wall and back. Amer. J. Anat. 1:1, 1901.

Browne, D.: Congenital deformities of mechanical origin. Proc. Roy. Soc. Med. 29:1409, 1936.

Cattell, H. S., et al.: Pseudosubluxation and other normal variations in the cervical spine in children. A study of 160 children. J. Bone Joint Surg. (Amer) 47:1295–1309, 1965.

Chandler, F. A., and Altenburg, A.: Congenital muscular torticollis. J.A.M.A. 125:476, 1944.

Chevrel, J. P.: Occipitalization of the atlas. Arch. Anat. Path. (Paris) 13:104–108, 1965.

Desgrez, H., et al.: Congenital abnormalities of the arch of the atlas. J. Radiol. Electr. 46:819–826, 1965.

Fleming, C., and Hodson, C. J.: Os odontoideum. J. Bone Joint Surg. 37B:622, 1955.

Francis, C. C.: Variations in the articular facets of the cervical vertebrae. Anat. Rec. 122:589, 1955.

Gardner, E.: The prenatal development of the human shoulder joint. Surg. Clin. N. Amer. 43:1465–1470, 1963.

Giannestras, N. J., et al.: Congenital absence of the odontoid process. Case report. J. Bone Joint Surg. (Amer) 46:839–843, 1964.

Gjorup, P. A., et al.: Congenital synostosis in the cervical spine. Acta Orthop. Scand. 34:33–36, 1964.

Grieve, J.: Bilateral subluxation of acromioclavicular joint. Lancet 2:424, 1942.

Haas, W. H., et al.: The coracoclavicular joint and related pathological conditions. Ann. Rheum. Dis. 24 :257–266, 1965.

Honkomp, J., et al.: Total fusion of the atlas and epistropheus. Z. Orthop. 100:183–186, 1965.

Jain, K. K., et al.: Congenital anomaly of the cervical spine, simulating fracture-dislocation—a case report. J. Canad. Ass. Radiol. 18:328–329, 1967.

Jinkins, W. J.: Congenital pseudoarthrosis of the clavicle. Orthopedics 62:183–186, 1969.

Jones, M. D., et al.: Occipitalization of atlas with hypoplastic odontoid process: A cineradiographic study. Calif. Med. 104:309–312, 1966.

Kruff, E.: Occipital dysplasia in infancy. The early recognition of craniovertebral abnormalities. Radiology 85:501–507, 1965.

Lahl, R., et al.: A rare combined malformation of the upper cervical spine. Zbl. Neurochir. 26:50–56, 1965.

Michaels, L., Prevost, M. J., and Crang, D. F.: Pathological changes in a case of os osdontoideum (separate odontoid process). J. Bone Joint Surg. (Amer) 51: 965–972, 1969.

Moore, M. T., et al.: Congenital cervical ependymal cyst. Report of a case with symptoms precipitated by injury. J. Neurosurg. 24:558–561, 1966.

Obrador, S.: Clinical and surgical aspects of occipitocervical malformations. Rev. Clin. Esp. 101:321–328, 1966.

Oxnard, C. E.: The functional morphology of the primate shoulder as revealed by comparative anatomical, osteometric and discriminant function techniques. Amer. J. Phys. Anthrop. 26:219–240, 1967.

Piccoli, N.: Partial absence of the posterior arch of the atlas. Arch. Sci. Med. (Torino) 120:85–94, 1965.

Ribstein, M., et al.: Cervical spinal synostosis and fusions. Critical study of 7 cases. J. Med. Bordeaux 142:948–953, 1965.

Ribstein, M., et al.: Congenital blocks of the cervical spine and neurological manifestations. Neurochirurgie 11:604–607, 1965.

Sanerkin, N. G., et al.: Birth injury to the sternomastoid muscle. J. Bone Joint Surg. (Brit) 48:441–447, 1966.

Sassu, G., et al.: Morphological variations of the atlas in adult Sardinians. Stud. Sassar 43:228–237, 1965.

Seze, S. de, et al.: Ageing of the cervical spine. Rev. Rhum. 32:654–662, 1965.

Shehata, R.: Occipitalization of the atlas (case report). Kyushu J. Med. Sci. 15:109–113, 1964.

Shinomura, H., et al.: Case of congenital defect of the dens epistrophei. Orthop. Surg. (Tokyo) 16:1239–1242, 1965.

Singh, S.: Variations of the superior articular facets of atlas vertebrae. J. Anat. 99:565–571, 1965.

Smith, R. W.: Dublin Quart. J. Med. Sci. 50:474, 1870.

Symposium on the Clavicle. Clin. Orthop. May–June, 1968.

Chapter II

SURGICAL ANATOMY OF THE SHOULDER AND NECK REGION

Anatomy of the shoulder and neck region is presented here from the standpoint of clinical examination and surgical approach. Accurate visualization of the vital soft structures can be accomplished only by following identification of the bony landmarks. In a thin patient this is easy, but in the plump or heavily muscled individual only the most prominent parts are accessible for assessment, so that one must be aware of the critical surgical relations.

Some system should be followed in examination of this region, and the simplest is to assess it systematically from the front and then the back. The two fields are roughly triangular in shape and contain all the vital parts. Such a plan allows plotting of surgical approaches and measurement and recording of ranges of motion.

ANTERIOR LANDMARKS

Usually the region of the shoulder and neck is inspected by initial examination of one segment or the other. In this presentation examination of the shoulder is made first (Figs 2–1, 2–2, and 2–3).

Because of wide variation in the thickness of the soft structures covering this region,

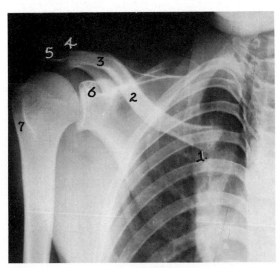

Figure 2–1 X-ray of shoulder landmarks from the front.

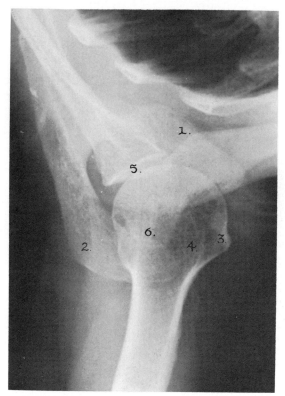

Figure 2–2 X-ray of shoulder landmarks from the top.

it is essential to have a central landmark such as the acromioclavicular joint (Fig. 2–1, *4*; Fig. 2–2, *6*) to which the·other structures may be accurately related. The acromioclavicular joint can always be identified precisely by running the fingers laterally along the clavicle (Figs. 2–1 and 2–3, *2*) and lifting the head of the humerus (Fig. 2–1, *7*) upward with the arm at the side. The cleft between acromion (Fig. 2–1, *5*) and clavicle (Fig. 2–1, *3*) can be both seen and felt. When this is used as the central landmark, just in front of the joint lies the coraco-acromion ligament and beneath it the critical "zone of impingement." This crescentic area is encroached upon by frayed or torn cuffs, redundant bursae, bursal fringes, lax bicipital tendons or irregularities of the tuberosities.

A finger's breadth forward is the greater tuberosity (Fig. 2–2, *3*); a finger's breadth medially is the long head of the biceps in its groove (Fig. 2–2, *4*). The point of the shoulder is the lateral aspect of the head of the humerus. The angle of the acromion lies posteriorly (Fig. 2–2, *2*) and is the landmark for injecting the subacromial recess from the back in such procedures as contrast studies.

The point of the coracoid process (Figs.

2–2 and 2–3, *1*) is so often overlapped by the deltoid that it can only be made out by digging deeply into the soft tissues with the fingers. The neurovascular bundle can be compressed beneath the tip, but the fingers must press medially against the rib cage to detect the subclavian pulsation.

Above the clavicle three zones should be identified, the sternomastoid muscle, the anterior edge of the trapezius and, in between these two structures, the posterior triangle containing the brachial plexus. The trapezius and the sternomastoid develop from the same muscle mass in the embryo and spread apart like the door of an Indian tepee as growth proceeds. In this hiatus the brachial plexus may be felt if the head and neck are gently pushed to the opposite side (Fig. 2–4). The plexus appears from between the scalenes and crosses the triangle to disappear under the clavicle. Important lymph glands are palpable just about the center of the triangle and, with deep pressure, the transverse processes of the middle cervical vertebrae can be made out in this region. These glands are important because the accessory, the lesser occipital and the greater auricular nerves lie below and often intermingle with the glands. The scalene point lies under the lateral border of the sternomastoid about 1 inch above and lateral to the medial end of the clavicle. Farther medially the sternoclavicular joint is palpated, and above this the thyroid, trachea, coracoid, thyroid cartilage and hyoid can be felt. Pressure beneath the medial border of the sterno-

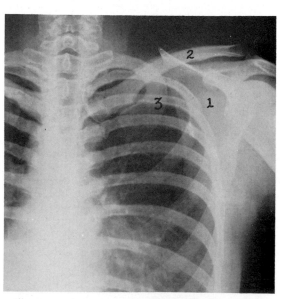

Figure 2–3 X-ray of shoulder landmarks from the back.

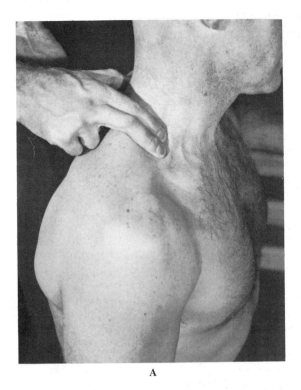

A

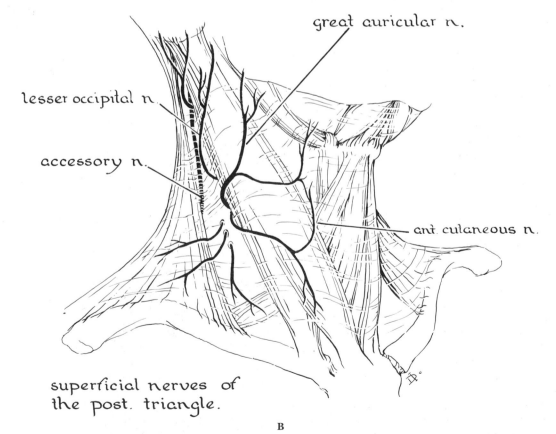

great auricular n.

lesser occipital n.

accessory n.

ant. cutaneous n.

superficial nerves of
the post. triangle.

B

Figure 2–4 *A*, Trunks of the brachial plexus may be palpated on the superior aspect. *B*, Superficial structures of importance above the clavicle.

mastoid identifies the carotid sheath and its contents.

Pressure medially shifts the trachea and esophagus so that the anterior corners of the vertebral bodies can be felt.

GLENOHUMERAL JOINT

The glenohumeral joint is the "universal" of the shoulder mechanism. The shoulder as a whole is really a system of joints embracing five principal moving mechanisms. In addition to the glenohumeral there are the acromioclavicular and sternoclavicular joints. The other two moving mechanims of extreme importance are the bicipital and the scapulothoracic. Although these are not synovial joints in the proper sense, they are true moving mechanisms participating in the shoulder complex. The intimate relationship dictates a common effect on shoulder function, and each mechanism influences a specific sphere. The three cardinal components are pervaded so often by a common pathological process that the whole region is linked as a unit. The glenohumeral, acromioclavicular and bicipital apparatuses are so closely associated that frequently it is necessary to bring all three into view at once at operation to correct a derangement.

The glenohumeral joint is a ball-and-socket mechanism that relies entirely on soft tissues for its stability. Unless soft tissue mechanisms can be protected and repaired, preservation of articular elements means very little. This dictum governs surgical approaches to the shoulder.

SUPERO-ANTERIOR APPROACH TO THE SHOULDER

A shoulder strap incision extending from just behind the acromioclavicular joint, over it, and continuing in this line for 2 to 3 inches reveals all the important structures of the three principal mechanisms of the shoulder (Fig. 2–5). The deltoid fibers are separated along their grain just lateral to the cephalic vein, which is retracted medially as it extends to the deltopectoral groove. The capsule of the acromioclavicular joint is apparent superiorly just distal to this, and beneath the deltoid is the subacromial bursa (Figs. 2–6 and 2–15).

Just below and medial to the acromioclavicular joint is visible the coraco-acromial ligament, which extends to the coracoid. The anterior portion of the rotator cuff comprising the conjoint area of subcapularis and supraspinatus is identified beneath the bursa, and on the medial aspect lies the bicipital groove.

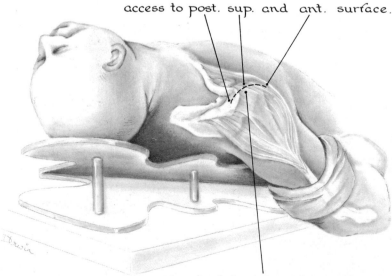

Table position for shoulder surgery.

access to post. sup. and ant. surface.

standard incision for most shoulder reconstruction.

Figure 2–5 Table position for shoulder surgery.

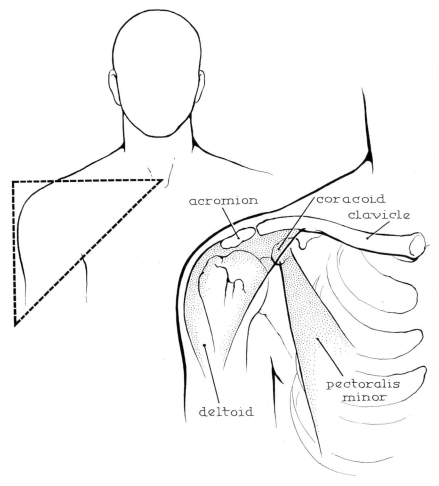

Figure 2–6   Anatomy of the anterior approach to the shoulder.

SUBACROMIAL BURSA

Lying over the top and front of the joint is the largest bursa in the extremities. It is hung from the undersurface of the acromion, coraco-acromial ligament and deltoid. It flows under the coracoid and the muscles attached to it and over the subscapularis. It spreads over the greater tuberosity and medially over the rotator cuff.

The bursa continues under the deltoid muscle; the subacromial bursa is usually understood as including the subdeltoid bursa. Deep to the bursa are elements of the rotator cuff and the greater tuberosity of the humerus. Normally it is thin walled, less than a quarter inch in depth, and does not communicate with the shoulder joint (Figs. 2–7 and 2–8).

In this position the bursa cushions the greater tuberosity, preventing impingement on the overhanging coraco-acromion arch. Roughening or irregularity of the tuberosi-

ties and underlying cuff serves as an irritant. If the irritation persists, the bursa becomes redundant and its walls thickened, constituting a further obstacle to abduction and rotation of the head of the humerus. Abduction and flexion then may be blocked or checked at the point of tuberosity contact as it rotates under the arch. The bursa has been compared to the abdominal peritoneum as an indicator of disease. It is exposed in the

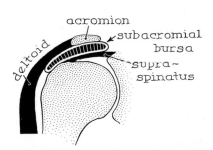

Figure 2–7   Subacromial bursa.

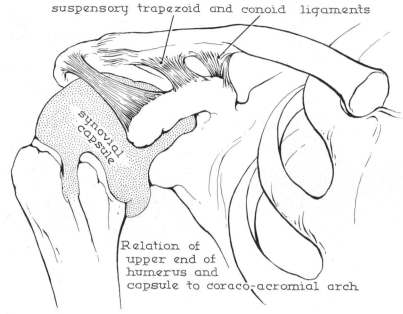

Figure 2–8 Relationship of bursa and capsule to coracoacromial arch and suspensory ligaments.

routine supero-anterior incision described previously. When it is thickened and redundant it may be excised; if possible when carrying out repairs of the rotator cuff, it is preserved and resutured on top of the cuff repair to provide and enhance a smooth surface for movement beneath the coraco-acromial arch (Fig. 2–8). It is not necessary to remove the acromion to excise the bursa but, as a rule, the coraco-acromial ligament is resected; in such an exposure a great deal of the bursa will come into view as the arm is abducted.

CAPSULE OF THE GLENOHUMERAL JOINT

The most important structure of the shoulder mechanism lies beneath the sub-acromial bursa. It consists of the rotator cuff and the capsule of the shoulder joint (Figs. 2–9, 2–10, and 2–11).

The capsule and the cuff participate in some measure in an overwhelming number of shoulder disabilities. There are weaknesses in other major joints in our bodies, such as the menisci and patellae in the knee and the blood supply of the head of the femur in the hip; in the shoulder the capsule is the vulnerable structure. The fibrous capsule is so intimately blended with the rotator tendons that it is best to consider the combination as a single structure. It extends as a sleeve from around the glenoid cavity to embrace the head of the humerus. Superiorly it is attached to the anatomical neck, but inferiorly it extends for a half inch beyond the articular cartilage. At the glenoid it is attached just beyond the rim, and in the front the line of attachment is some distance back of the edge so that a portion is reflected along the bone blending with the labrum. As indicated in the description of the embryo-

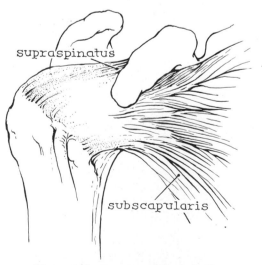

Figure 2–9 Rotator cuff from the front.

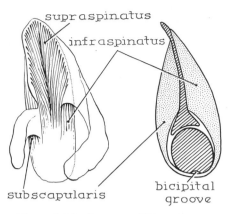

Figure 2-10   Rotator cuff from the top.

logical development, it is securely anchored to the bone at all parts.

Superior Capsule

Clinically this is the most important portion of the mechanism. Three muscles extend from the back over the top of the head of the humerus, blending into a cartilaginous sheet anchored in the region of the greater tuberosity just beyond the articular surface (Fig. 2-12). Such a musculotendinous sleeve provides protection and also serves as a lever for the rotator and short abductor muscles. From a quite broad fleshy area the tendons narrow and blend into a homogeneous strip. The insertions of the muscles are inti-

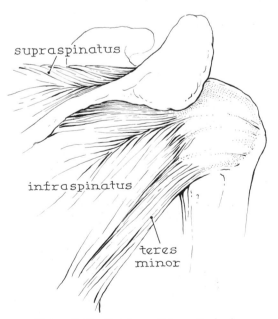

Figure 2-11   Rotator cuff from the back.

mately incorporated with the capsule and with each other so that individual tendons are not well demarcated except in young people.

The cuff normally is a quarter of an inch thick, and the surface is extremely smooth. The mechanism of attachment is such that it is made around a circle without a wrinkle and, as the muscles pull from their origins, tension may be focused at the front, the top or the back. Normally no defect is present, and the joint is sealed completely from the subacromial bursa. Extensive pathological changes are encountered in this aspect of the capsule in injury, in metabolic disturbances and as a result of degenerative processes.

Anterior Portion of the Capsule

The anterior wall of the capsule lies under the subscapularis tendon at the front (Fig. 2-13). There is a prolongation that forms a synovial sheath for the tendon of the long head of the biceps. The subscapularis tendon is broad and short, about an inch in width, and the tendons are 3/4 to 1 inch long, blending closely with the capsule. In a complete anterior exposure of the front of the joint, this tendon is reflected medially.

The subscapularis bolsters the anterior aspect as it passes from the undersurface of the scapula to the distal portion of the inferior tuberosity. As it traverses the glenoid, there is a slight notch which gives the kidney shape to the glenoid. A large bursa separates it from the capsule anteriorly and connects with the joint medially. The capsule under the subscapularis is a somewhat loose outpouching; superiorly, this recess extends to just below the coracoid process.

Variations occur in the attachment of the medial aspect of the capsule, and this is of particular significance in conditions such as recurrent dislocation of the shoulder. When the attachment of the capsule is beyond the labrum and along the neck of the scapula, greater freedom for movement of the head of the humerus is present and resultant ballooning of the capsule allows more room for the head to slip from the glenoid.

Inferior Portion of the Capsule

The weakest part of the capsule is the inferior aspect and, as such, it has important

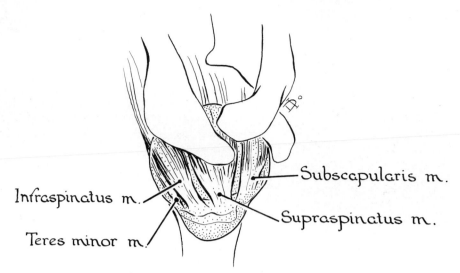

Figure 2–12 Diagram of cuff attachment.

clinical associations. The capsule and synovial reflection are loose and redundant, and the synovium lies in accordian-like pleats extending from the anatomical neck well below the articular margin to just beyond the glenoid rim. Normally, with the arm at the side, the thumb may be inserted easily between the capsule and the lower joint margin. This slack is taken up as the arm is abducted and rotated. The inferior redundance is obliterated in conditions such as adhesive capsulitis, in which the capsule becomes plastered to the articular surface, from which it may be peeled like adhesive tape.

No supporting ligament or tendon lies below this inferior aspect, and it is through this zone that the head of the humerus slips in antero-inferior dislocation of the shoulder. When the arm is abducted the long head of the triceps is the sole support at the bottom; the circumflex nerves are closely related to the inferior aspect and pass through a space bounded by the long head of the triceps and the teres major muscles. The axillary nerve and branches to the triceps are also related to the capsule at this point. In abduction the triceps and teres become taut, like the opening of the crotch of a pair of scissors, thereby providing support for the head of the humerus.

ACROMIOCLAVICULAR JOINT

The most important accessory articulation is exposed at the top of the supero-anterior incision (Fig. 2–15). It is identified by feeling the outer end of the clavicle and the cleft just beyond, between the clavicle and the acromion. A somewhat slack capsule, the acromioclavicular ligament, covers it. A stronger band reinforces this capsule posteriorly and a much weaker one anteriorly.

Many variations in the obliquity of the acromioclavicular joint line are encountered. These extend from a quite vertical to an almost horizontal joint cleft (Fig. 2–16). The

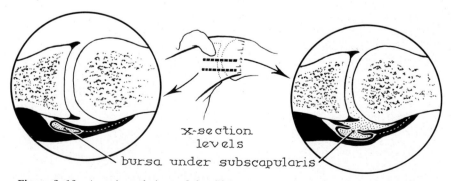

Figure 2–13 Anterior relations of shoulder capsule, subscapularis muscle and bursa.

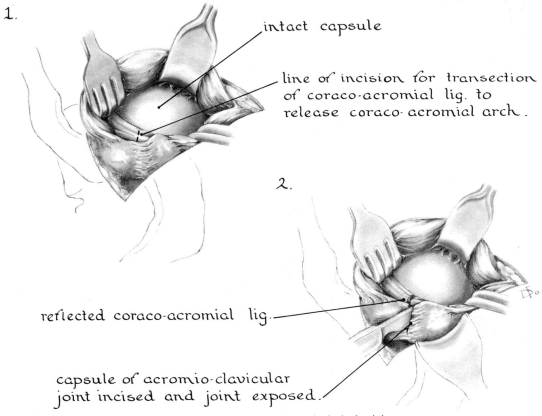

1.

intact capsule

line of incision for transection of coraco-acromial lig. to release coraco-acromial arch.

2.

reflected coraco-acromial lig.

capsule of acromio-clavicular joint incised and joint exposed.

Figure 2–14 Approach to acromioclavicular joint.

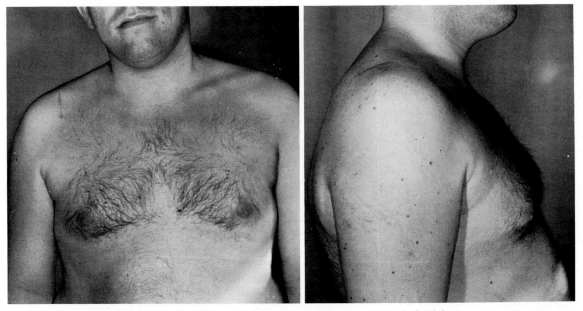

Figure 2–15 Utility incision used to expose acromioclavicular joint.

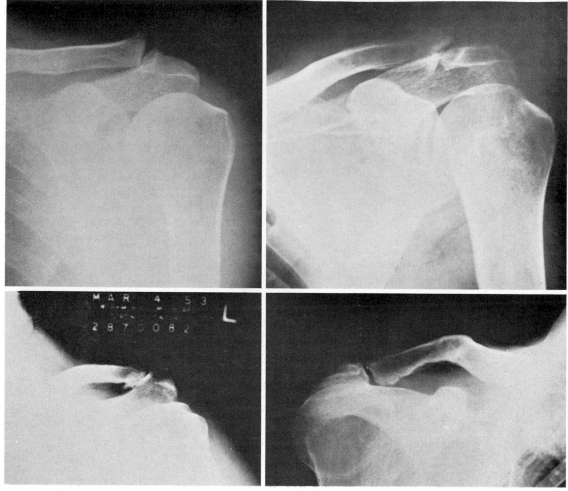

Figure 2–16 X-rays of acromioclavicular joints.

lateral end of the clavicle frequently is bulbous, enlarged and overriding. A small cartilaginous disc is present before the age of 20 and partially divides the joint into two segments. It is closely attached to the lateral articular surface.

The contiguous surfaces of acromion and clavicle are not symmetrical. As viewed from above, the clavicle articulates with the acromion in a small segment of an arc (Fig. 2–17).

The acromion rotates about the lateral end of the clavicle, gliding forward and backward and also upward and downward. The joint is quite stable unless injured. Because of this, the lateral half inch of the clavicle may be resected, leaving the posterior capsular reinforcement in place, without causing significant instability in the zone. The rotator cuff and subacromial bursa are closely applied to the undersurface, so close that spurs on the joint may dig directly into the bursa and the capsule.

THE CORACO-ACROMIAL LIGAMENT

An important ligament lies directly in front of the acromioclavicular joint. It is a flat band extending from the acromion to the lateral aspect of the coracoid, triangular in shape and with its base at the medial end. Normally enough space is present to permit insertion of the little finger in between this ligament and the cuff. Damage to structures like the bursa lying underneath or to the farther subjacent cuff decreases this space so that the ligament is rubbed as the head of the humerus is abducted and rotated.

The coraco-acromial ligament is a vestigial structure representing the former continua-

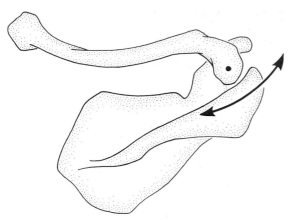

Figure 2-17 Acromioclavicular relations and appearance from above.

tion of a pectoralis minor across the coracoid to the acromion. It is a weak defence against upward dislocation of the head of the humerus and it can be resected with impunity. Removal increases the space for rotation of the head of the humerus and decreases obstruction, so that it is often deliberately excised in repairing cuffs or in general debridement of the area (Fig. 2–18).

BICIPITAL MECHANISM

Below and medial to the coraco-acromial ligament, the long head of the biceps may be palpated beneath the capsule. It is held in the groove by the transverse humeral ligament, a thickened prolongation of the cap-

sule extending between the lesser and greater tuberosities. The critical zones in this structure are the point at which the tendon arches over the humeral head and at which the floor on which it glides changes from bony cortex to articular cartilage (Fig. 2–19).

Dimensions of the groove vary widely. Deep narrow apertures favor constriction of the tendon, and shallow flat grooves tend to allow slipping and luxation of the tendon. If the cuff zone at the top of the groove is torn, the tendon may slip out of the groove, particularly if the arm is abducted and rotated externally. Similarly, if strong force is applied in this position, the tendon may be wrenched out of the groove.

SUBSCAPULARIS TENDON AND ITS RELATIONS

The subscapularis forms the lower anterior part of the shoulder casing. It is best felt by externally rotating the humerus a little; it is identified as a firm band roofing the bicipital groove. A prolongation of the capsule extends between the tuberosities along the bicipital tendon for a variable length (Fig. 2–13).

The tendon is heavy and indents the glenoid as it arches across anteriorly to the glenoid labrum. The muscle does not have a long tendon, so that incisions allowing reflection must be placed carefully toward the lateral aspect; otherwise, it will be difficult to

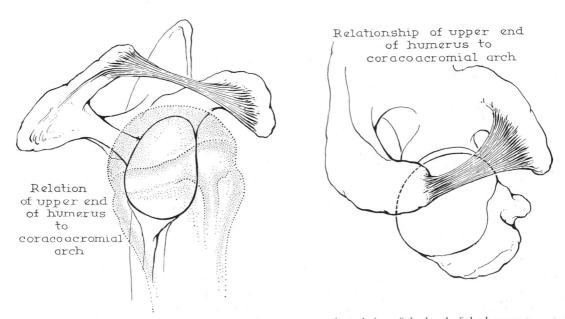

Figure 2-18 Coracoacromial ligament; an important superior relation of the head of the humerus.

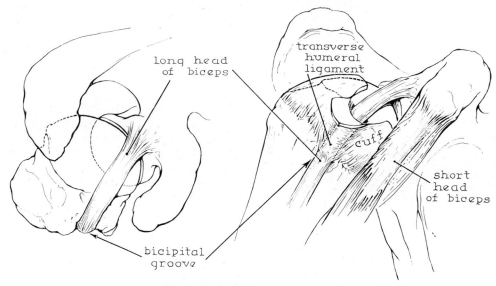

Figure 2-19 Bicipital mechanism.

resuture the fleshy fibers to the tendinous portion.

GLENOID LABRUM

A fibrocartilaginous lip sits along the margin of the glenoid cavity, deepening it considerably. Superiorly it blends with and is intimately attached to the long head of the biceps. The labrum is triangular in cross section, tough and firmly anchored to the bone. It is subject to pathological changes from injury and the wear and tear of degeneration. In many joints, zones of separation, fraying, roughness and sometimes fragmentation may be found, particularly on the anterior aspect. In recurrent dislocation of the shoulder, separation of the labrum or fracture is found in a high percentage of patients. Sometimes pieces are broken off and lie free in the joint as loose bodies similar to those seen from a torn meniscus in the knee. The joint capsule is attached to the scapula beyond the labrum, extending farther anteriorly and superiorly than posteriorly and inferiorly.

INFERIOR OF GLENOHUMERAL JOINT

In exploring the glenohumeral joint the incision is made through the anterior capsule medial to the long head of the biceps. About one half of the humeral head is then visible, and more becomes apparent with external rotation. The head of the humerus looks disproportionately large when com-

pared with the glenoid, and the articular surface of the glenoid can hardly be seen through this exposure. Strong retraction and external rotation are necessary to visualize the articular cartilage of the glenoid.

The labrum may be felt deep in the incision as a fibrocartilaginous lip sitting on the anterior rim of the glenoid. It blends with the long head of the biceps above and is less prominent as it is traced toward the lower aspect of the glenoid. Extensive variation in position and size of the labrum occurs; it may be partly detached or torn, or there may be loose pieces found directly within the joint. Sometimes very little labrum can be felt.

ANATOMY OF THE POSTERIOR ASPECT OF THE SHOULDER AND THE CERVICAL SPINE

The posterior aspect of this region functionally includes structures related to both the neck and the shoulder (Fig. 2-20).

Pathological processes producing pain interpreted as implicating the shoulder in general are common in this region.

SURFACE ANATOMY

The important structures in this region lie largely in a compact area that is triangular in outline. The tips of the spines of the cervical vertebrae and the upper thoracic vertebrae form the medial boundary. The

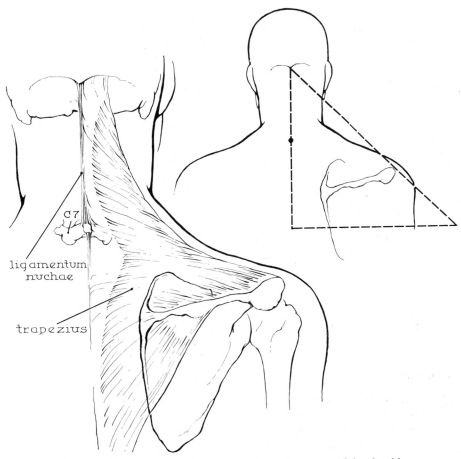

Figure 2–20   Anatomy of the neck and posterior aspect of the shoulder.

base is horizontal and level with the lower border of the scapula. The apex is the suboccipital region.

In the center of this triangular area is the spine of the scapula, which curves upward and forward like a hockey stick, ending in the acromion and forming the bony contour of the shoulder. The prominent spine of C.7 can be palpated level with the top of the shoulder. The scapula lies opposite the first eight ribs, with the base of the spine usually opposite T.3.

LIGAMENTUM NUCHAE

Forming the upper medial border of this triangular area is a thick, tough ligamentous band which extends from the occiput to the tip of the posterior spinous process of C.7. At the top it fashions a bony elevation, the external occipital protuberance, and below it is firmly anchored to the posterior spinous process of C.7. Between these two anchoring points, the heavy portion of the ligament skips the cervical tips but is connected to

them by slender slips. It looks a little like the string of a bow arching the cervical spine forward. In man this ligament is the representative of a powerful elastic structure that holds the head up in plantigrade form. It is triangular in cross section, and superficial layers blend with the aponeurosis of the trapezius. Cutaneous nerves pierce the aponeurotic zone close to the midline, coming from the posterior rami of spinal nerves (Fig. 2–21).

The attachments of the ligamentum nuchae explain certain symptoms and their localization in certain injuries. In the extremely common whiplash or extension-flexion rear impact syndrome, the slender slips may be avulsed from the tips of the spinous processes.

Powerful flexion when the neck muscles are tense may lead to avulsion of the C.7 spinous process because the ligament is so strongly anchored that bone gives way instead of the ligament.

More extensive changes are often found at the superior portion of this attachment

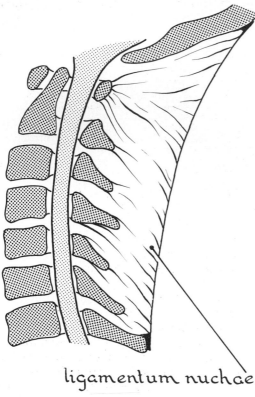

ligamentum nuchae

Figure 2–21 Ligamentum nuchae and relations.

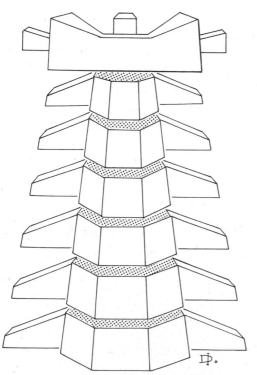

Figure 2–22 Cervical vertebrae. Note wide angle of the atlas and progressive increase in size of the remaining vertebra to C.7.

along the occipital bone. Avulsion of fibers in this area is a source of occipital headache, and the scarring may implicate cutaneous nerve branches like the lesser occipital.

CERVICAL VERTEBRAE

The cervical vertebral bodies are relatively fragile and considerably smaller than those in the lumbar region. The interbody space and the discs are also much smaller. The fragility must be borne in mind when carrying out surgical procedures like bone grafts because it is much easier to split a cervical vertebral body than a lumbar vertebrae (Fig. 2–22).

Four articulating mechanisms are related to each vertebra, one more than in the lumbar region.

Interbody Mechanism

The structure is similar to the lumbar region, with a well defined cartilaginous plate, anulus fibrosus, and nucleus pulposus. Fine nerve fibrils from the adjacent spinal nerves ramify in the anulus and the posterior longitudinal ligament, but these have not been identified as reaching the nuclear pulp (Fig. 2–23).

Apophyseal Joints

In the lower segment of the cervical spine, C.3 to C.7, there are small pairs of synovial

apophyseal joint

Lushka joint

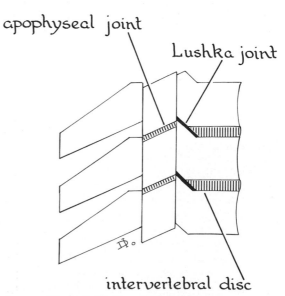

intervertebral disc

Figure 2–23 Interbody mechanism.

articulations. These have concave-convex rather than straight plane surfaces. This allows both flexion and extension as well as a forward and backward gliding motion. Well defined capsules with synovial lining can be identified; branches of the adjacent spinal nerves innervate these capsules (Fig. 2–24).

Joints of Luschka

Joint-like spaces or clefts at the anterior angles of the bodies on the superior surfaces have been identified (Fig. 2–25). Considerable variation in the size and shape of these articulations from one individual to another has been encountered.

The position and configuration of these articulations are such that they have a tendency to prevent anterior slipping of the bodies on each other and, hence, are subject to distortion and osteophyte formation. Their intimate relationship to the intervertebral foramen is a source of mechanical encroachment; spurs which develop at their edges, may affect the nerve root in the canal.

POSTERIOR SPINOUS PROCESSES

No true joint mechanism exists between the spinous processes, but there are well defined interspinous ligaments; a superficial one which is quite heavy contributes to the ligamentum nuchae. In some pathological states, impingement of one spinous process on the other occurs, and a bursa may be found in between the tips. The tips of the spinous processes also participate in other pathological processes such as clay shoveler's fracture and extension-flexion injuries resulting from

the "whiplash" mechanism. (See Chapter 12.)

Muscles of the Posterior Aspect

The musculature in the posterior neck and shoulder region has many clinical applications. Heavy groups of muscles extend from the occiput to the shoulder girdle, connecting the head to chest and extremity. A superficial layer consisting of the trapezius is identified, beneath which is a layer composed of the levator scapulae, rhomboid minor and rhomboid major from above downward and attached to the vertebral border of the scapula. Beneath this layer lie the splenius capitis in the center and the sternomastoid laterally; beneath the splenius is the semispinalis capitis and then the layer of small muscles (Fig. 2–26).

Under the rhomboids is a layer consisting of the serratus posterior, superior and inferior. The digitations of this muscle pass from the spines to the ribs. Beneath this muscle layer is the thoracolumbar fascia; the layer is quite thin superiorly, extends laterally from the spinous processes to the angles of the ribs, and inferiorly passes deep to the serratus posterior and blends with the latissimus dorsi.

The deepest or fifth layer, which is the erector spinae and consists of spinalis, longissimus and iliocostalis in the thoracic region, extends upward and splits into three columns, only the middle one of which reaches the skull. The sixth layer is the semispinalis and is termed the transversus spinalis group of muscles. The suboccipital muscles lie beneath this sixth layer.

Figure 2–24 Apophyseal joints.

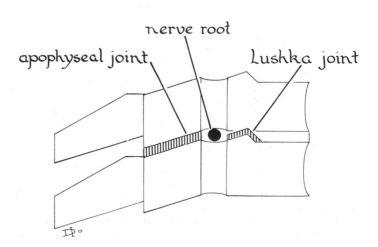

Luschka joints

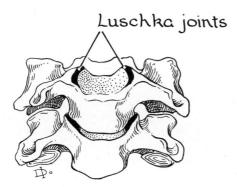

Figure 2–25 Luschka joints.

THE SUBOCCIPITAL REGION

The base of the skull is formed by a nearly straight line extending from one mastoid process to the other. The superior nuchal line curves laterally from the external occipital protuberance and extends to the mastoid process, dividing it into a smooth upper and a rough lower part. Below the superior nuchal line are attached the heavy neck muscles. The contents of the suboccipital region are the layers of muscles of which the semispinalis capitis forms the posterior wall. The muscle is pierced by the greater occipital and third occipital nerves (Fig. 2–27). Frequently a branch appears below the superior nuchal line and extends upward, piercing the galea above tke superior nuchal line. The occipital artery follows a similar course. It arises in the region of the inferior nuchal area below the transverse process of the atlas; farther down a branch of the third occipital nerve pierces the semispinalis and ascends

near the midline. Beneath the last layer of muscles is a vertebral venous plexus.

The floor of the suboccipital triangle is formed by the posterior arch of the atlas. From it the posterior atlanto-occipital membrane passes to the margin of the foramen magnum above and to the laminae of the axis below. Branches of the suboccipital nerve and C.2 pass through this membrane.

The transverse and sigmoid sinuses extend intracranially from just above the external occipital protuberance or in a curving fashion to a point about three quarters of an inch behind the external auditory meatus, going to a point in front of the mastoid process and below the external meatus to join the internal jugular vein.

THE SCAPULA AND ITS BED

In the center of the posterior aspect of this region lies the scapula. The upper eight ribs, at the point at which they are curved as an arch, form the track on which the scapula swings. When this is looked at from above, the scapula is curved to fit the chest wall (Fig. 2–28). It has a sharpened medial or vertebral border digging into the overlying muscle layers (Fig. 2–29).

In contrast, the lateral border is rounded and strong. Important muscles are related to the scapula. The serratus anterior is attached underneath and along the medial edge so that, as it contracts, the scapula swings, as it were, or tends to come away from the rib cage. The spinati fill the grooves above and below the spine and, on top of these,

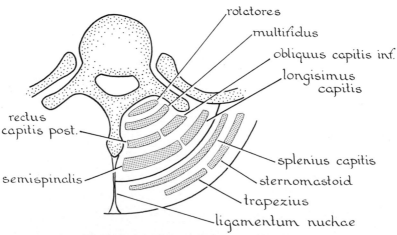

Figure 2–26 Muscles of the posterior region.

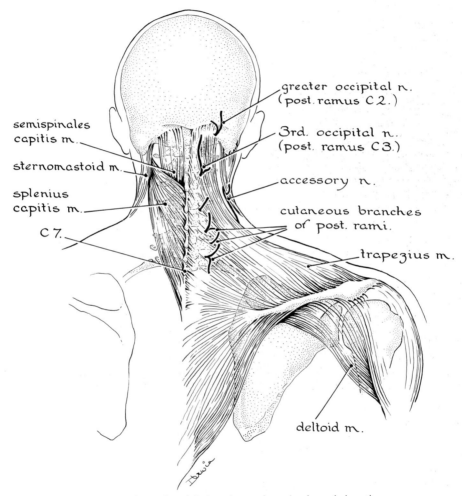

Figure 2–27 Suboccipital region and cervicothoracic junction.

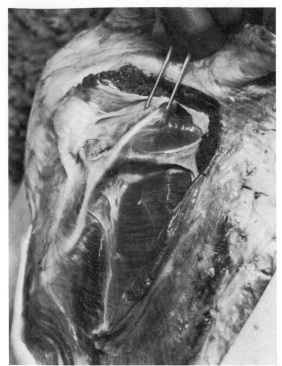

Figure 2-28 Dissection of the bed of the scapula.

there is a broad quilt of the trapezius. At the top is attached the levator scapulae, and this represents the deep layer of connection of the scapula with the neck. The inferior angle of the scapula is blunt, rough and strong for attachments from teres major, rhomboids and serratus anterior.

TRAPEZIUS MUSCLE SYSTEM

When viewed from the back, the sloping line of the shoulder is formed by the upper border of the trapezius. This muscle is really a system of muscles, providing a powerful suspensory apparatus for the whole shoulder girdle. It has the most extensive origin of any muscle in the body, extending from the skull all the way down to the lumbar region. The attachments in the cervical area are to the spinous processes and all along the top of the spine of the scapula.

In its medial attachment it contributes to the ligamentum nuchae and, through this, is attached to the cervical spine. The attachments of the trapezius in the cervical area and to the spine of the scapula are important. The muscle has two strong attachments, one to the neck and the other to the spine of the scapula so that both ends of the huge

muscle system have a mobile anchorage. When the cervical spine is bent and the shoulder is used at the same time in an act such as reaching, pull is applied simultaneously in opposite directions, so that some of the fibers may give way, producing a typical "kink" in the neck.

The trapezius holds the shoulder back and up, thereby forming a suspensory strut for the pendulum swing of the arm and hand (Fig. 2–30). It has been described as a postural muscle since the upper fibers contribute a constant tension, helping to keep the trunk erect. The nerve supply of the muscle is also important. The accessory nerve supplies it and reaches it by crossing the posterior triangle of the neck, where it is the highest nerve in the triangle, lying quite superficially (Fig. 2–38). Lymph glands in the supraclavicular area are often involved in pathological processes and lie scattered along the path of the accessory nerve. Hence, the nerve may be involved in disease of these glands, or it may be injured in the surgical procedures like a simple biopsy done under local anesthetic.

When the trapezius is paralyzed, the normal sloping neck line changes to a sharp angular one and the point at the shoulder drops downward and forward. The nerve dips under the upper and anterior margin of the trapezius at a point 1 to 2 inches above the clavicle. It sticks to the deep surface of the muscle, running at right angles to the fibers down to the lower end. The nerve may be easily exposed just as it crosses the upper border of the scapula by gently spreading the trapezius fibers. Higher up it may be exposed as it emerges from beneath the sternomastoid approximately at the junction of the upper third and distal two thirds of the anterior border of the posterior triangle.

The accessory nerve supplying the trapezius has a further important function. Since

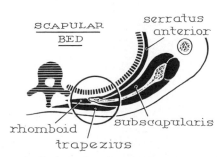

Figure 2-29 Muscle relations of the medial border of the scapula.

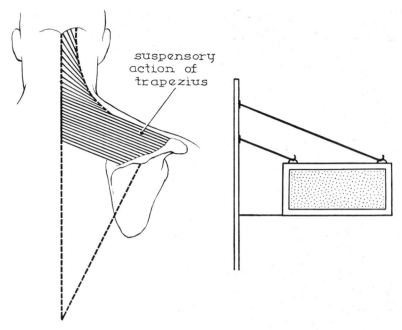

Figure 2–30 Suspensory action of the trapezius.

it arises from cranial and upper cervical sources, it is rarely disturbed in common traction injuries which damage the brachial plexus. Serious plexus injuries involving C.5 and C.6 leave the shoulder paralyzed so that the arm cannot be properly abducted. The one remaining muscle usually uninvolved which can contribute to abduction is the trapezius since it still has an intact nerve supply. Various operations, making use of this fact, change the distal attachment of the trapezius so that it acts direcly on the upper end of the humerus either by simple transfer of the tendon or by transfer of the tendon along with a piece of the acromion. (See Chapter XIV). In this fashion, a degree of abduction can be supplied to the shoulder girdle as a whole by this unparalyzed muscle.

QUADRILATERAL SPACE

In this posterior shoulder region a further area of surgical importance may be demarcated in the quadrilateral space. This is bounded above by the inferior aspect of the glenohumeral joint, the neck of scapula, the capsule and the head of the humerus. The long head of the triceps and the teres majors crisscross, forming the lower border (Fig. 2–31). Branches of the posterior cord, axil-

lary, posterior humeral circumflex and radial nerves are related to the shoulder joint at this point. The circumflex nerve and vessels pass through the space closely related to the upper bony margins. The radial nerve branches of the axillary extend to the triceps not far from the bony structures; an extensive collection of small veins accompanies these nerves.

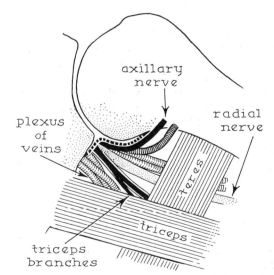

Figure 2–31 Relations and contents of the quadrilateral space.

THE CLAVICLE

The collar bone is the strut of the shoulder girdle. It is subcutaneous along its entire length but is crossed by structures of some importance, the supraclavicular nerves. The whole bone may be exposed on the superior surface but, as a rule, the middle half is the zone of surgical importance.

On palpation the clavicle has a distinct -S shape. In most people it is possible to grasp the bone at either end and manipulate it. This is a help in diagnosing suspected fractures since crepitus can be produced easily. The subcutaneous portion also aids in providing purchase for the manipulative reduction of fracture deformities.

The double curve of the clavicle has given rise to its name, which is from *clavis* (key). In cross section the lateral curve is somewhat flat, whereas the medial one is decidedly tubular. The alterations in shape in cross section account for localization of many of the fractures to the middle third (Fig. 2–32). The clavicle acts as a shock absorber in the transmission of force from both the hand and the lateral aspect of the shoulder to the center of the body; this makes the junction zone of the two curves a weak spot, and it may give way.

The greater strength of the tubular medial third provides rugged protection for the subclavian vessels which run directly beneath. Standard positions for x-rays are necessary to prevent a distorted appearance because of the curvature.

Muscle and ligament attachments are re-sponsible for the typical deformities of certain fractures at the different sites. At the extreme lateral end there is little displacement because the coracoclavicular ligament holds the clavicle down. Medial to this ligament, the fracture ends are more freely displaced, the lateral one being pulled down by the pectoralis major and the medial one up by the sternomastoid.

THE SUSPENSORY LIGAMENT OR CORACOCLAVICULAR MECHANISM

The whole upper extremity is suspended by a strong ligament extending from the coracoid to the undersurface of the clavicle. The coracoclavicular ligament serves as a joint mechanism, producing a fulcrum near the lateral end of the clavicle so the girdle can swing on it. Anatomically the coracoclavicular ligament consists of two parts, but functionally it is a single ligament (Fig. 2–33). The posterior and medial fibers are in a cone-shaped group extending from the clavicle to an apex on the medial aspect of the coronoid.

The anterior and lateral fibers are in a box-shaped group (trapezoid) and extend forward and laterally from the coronoid attachment. The direction of these fibers is such that they resist downward and inward slipping of the scapula, with the clavicle holding the arm out like a signpost.

Normally the ligament may be stretched enough to allow the clavicle to sit up on the acromion without rupturing completely. Stretching sometimes loosens the periosteum, initiating calcification which spreads along the ligaments and is quite visible in the x-rays. In severe grades of acromioclavicular dislocation (Grade 3), the ligaments may be torn and surgical repair is then required. The ligament is exposed through a vertical superior incision just medial to the acromioclavicular joint. Care is needed to avoid damage to the neurovascular bundle, which runs just below the coracoid process. The direction of the ligaments in suspending the scapula serves to protect the scapula from riding medially.

CORACOID PROCESS AND PECTORALIS MINOR

The coracoid process, a thumb-like projection from the neck of the scapula, consti-

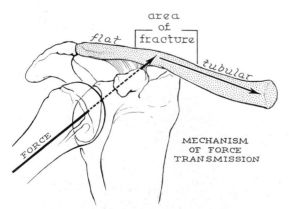

Figure 2–32 Fracture zone of the clavicle, resulting from the bony configuration and the common mechanism of force transmission.

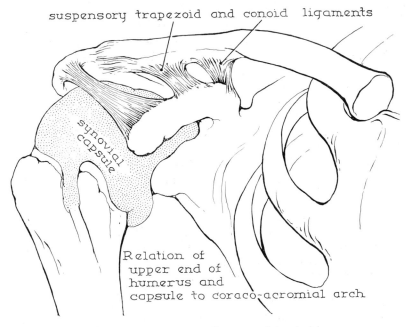

suspensory trapezoid and conoid ligaments

synovial capsule

Relation of upper end of humerus and capsule to coraco-acromial arch

Figure 2–33 Suspensory ligament of the clavicle.

tutes an important bony landmark just below the lateral edge of the clavicle. Important structures are attached to the coracoid and the great vessels run beneath it.

Attached to the tip and extending toward the chest wall is the pectoralis minor; this is a short, thick muscle arising from the third, fourth and fifth ribs and, occasionally, the second, third and fourth ribs. The great vessels and nerves at the upper limb pass under the pectoralis minor on their way to the arm. By pressing just below the coracoid, it is possible to feel pulsation of the subclavian artery and to compress it against the chest wall (Fig. 2–34). Abnormalities related to the coracoid and the pectoralis minor may compress the neurovascular bundle at this site. As the subclavian artery and the brachial plexus branches stream out from under the clavicle, they are enveloped in a sleeve of clavipectoral fascia and proceed distally in the cervico-axillary canal. The fascial covering at its upper part blends with the costocoracoid ligament, which is all that remains of a primitive extensive process which is seen in reptiles (Fig. 1–5). Sometimes the edge of the costocoracoid membrane is thickened and contains remnants of cartilage. Tightening or thickening of this structure presses the underlying bundle.

The cervico-axillary canal is roofed by the clavicle, subclavius, clavipectoral fascia,

pectoralis minor and, finally, more fascia which blends with the axillary fold.

In extreme extension and lateral rotation of the arm, traction force compressing the bundle against the head of the humerus can

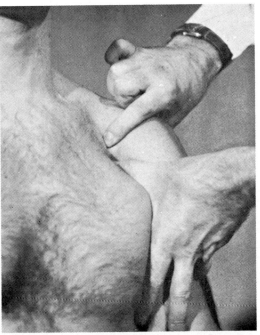

Figure 2–34 Coracoid process with neurovascular bundle just beneath it being compressed against the chest wall.

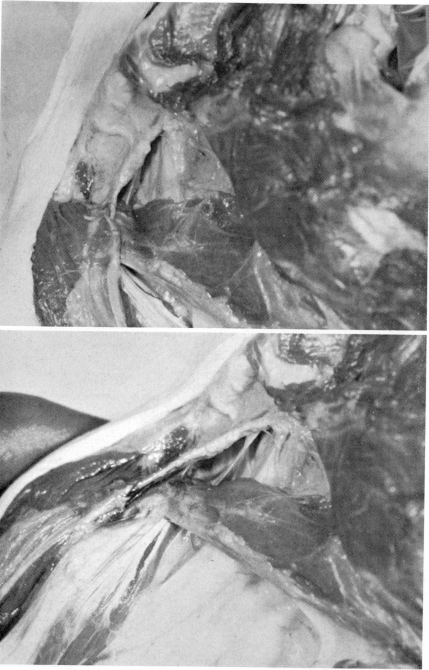

Figure 2–35   Relations of the pectoralis minor and neurovascular bundle.

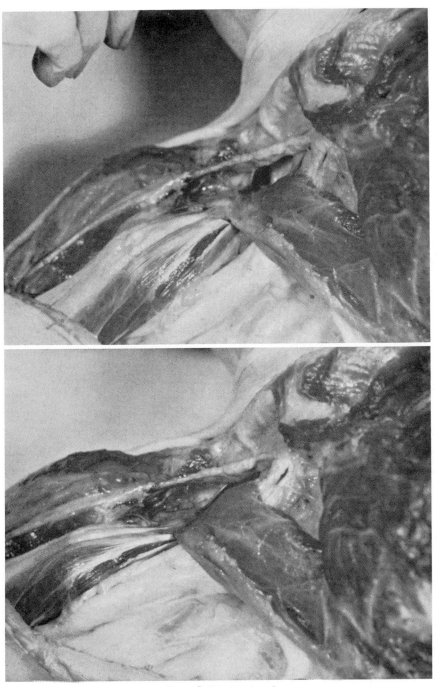

Figure 2–35 *Continued.*

be seen. This is the position that is assumed in sleep and is a frequent cause of unpleasant radiating numbness. In some instances, relief from such symptoms is obtained by transecting the pectoralis minor close to the coracoid process (Fig. 2–35).

THE STERNOCLAVICULAR JOINT

The sternoclavicular joint is exposed through a transverse incision about 3 inches in length at the medial end of the clavicle (Fig. 2–36). The anterior aspect of the joint is covered by capsule with which the fibers of the sternomastoid muscle blend. Behind the joint there is a thick pad of muscle fibers (with contributions from the sternohyoid and the sternothyroid) which serves to cushion the posterior aspect, protecting the great vessels which course beneath.

The medial end of the clavicle is rounded and bulbous and articulates in a shallow socket with the sternum (Fig. 2–37). About half the medial end of the clavicle rides above the slanting sternal notch. Instability or a tendency to medial dislocation is favored by this configuration.

Inside the joint there is a thick articular disc or check ligament attached from the top of the clavicle around the medial end to a point on the sternum beneath it; force applied to the lateral aspect of the shoulder and transmitted along the clavicle is snubbed or checked by the action and attachment of this ligament. The margins blend front and back with the capsular extension, strengthening the attachment of the central cartilaginous disc.

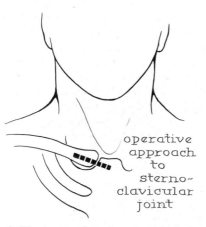

Figure 2–36 Approach to the sternoclavicular joint.

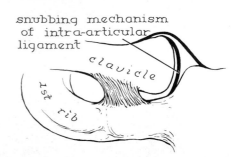

Figure 2–37 Sternoclavicular joint and ligaments.

The intra-articular disc may be torn or damaged, leading to an internal derangement of the joint somewhat similar to meniscus injuries in the knee. Dislocation of the sternoclavicular joint, acute or chronic, is a not infrequent injury in sports because of the heavy body contact force applied to the lateral aspect of the shoulder girdle. A short, square ligament, the costoclavicular, contributes stability to the end of the clavicle. It is attached to the inferior ¾ inch of the medial end and runs downward and medially to the cartilage of the first rib. This ligament is also ruptured in complete sternoclavicular dislocation. In conjunction with the intra-articular disc these ligaments are strong stabilizers of this extremely mobile joint.

ANATOMY OF THE SUPRACLAVICULAR REGION

Surgically this is an important area because operations on the supraclavicular portion of the brachial plexus are performed through this zone, as are procedures for resection of a cervical rib and transection of the scalene muscles (Fig. 2–38). The most useful approach to this region is vertical incision which extends obliquely downward from just above the middle of the posterior border of the sternomastoid to meet the clavicle at the junction of the outer third and the inner two thirds. A layer of platysma is incised, exposing the deep fascia covering the posterior triangle. At the apex of the triangle the accessory nerve may be seen coursing across beneath the fascia. At about the same level on the medial aspect some lymph glands may be encountered, and at this point a leash of cutaneous nerves is present. From a focal point here, the great auricular and lesser occipital nerves proceed upward and

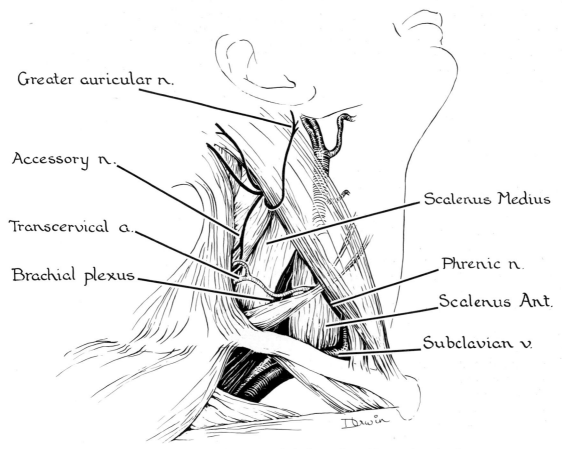

Greater auricular n.

Accessory n.

Transcervical a.

Brachial plexus

Scalenus Medius

Phrenic n.

Scalenus Ant.

Subclavian v.

Figure 2–38   Anatomy of the supraclavicular region and posterior triangle.

backward, while branches of the supra-clavicular nerves extend downward and distally.

In proceeding from above downward beneath the cervical fascia, branches of the brachial plexus, specifically trunks C.5, C.6 and C.7, can be palpated. The highest branch arising from the upper trunk is the supra-scapular nerve. Roots of C.5 and C.6 blend to form the upper trunk, extending to the level of the clavicle. The C.7 root proceeds as the middle trunk behind the clavicle. Along the medial border of the supraclavicu-lar posterior triangle, the medial side of the sternomastoid can be retracted, bringing into view the scalenus anticus. The phrenic nerve runs down the anterior aspect of this muscle. Coursing across the triangle about a finger's breadth above the clavicle is the omohyoid muscle, and just below this and deep to the deep fascia are the transverse cervical vessels. The external jugular vein lies at the inner aspect, extending up over the sterno-mastoid.

NERVE SUPPLY OF THE SHOULDER REGION

An understanding of the nerve supply to this area is extremely helpful in interpreting many clinical states. Characteristic pain patterns can be recognized implicating the shoulder-neck zone, the shoulder area proper or the shoulder plus peripheral parts. These are mediated through different nerve pathways. The cutaneous supply differs from that of the deep structures and, there-fore, the superficial and deep zones have different segmental connections. Anatomical-ly the nerve supply is most important in planning surgical procedures (Fig. 2–38).

CUTANEOUS SUPPLY

The supraclavicular area, the acromion, the upper half of the deltoid and the intra-clavicular zone are supplied by the supra-clavicular nerves. These arise from cervical

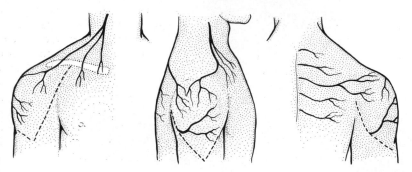

Figure 2–39 Cutaneous nerve supply of the shoulder region.

roots C.3 and C.4 and run beneath the platysma across the supraclavicular triangle, ending by passing over the clavicle. Occasionally a single branch will pierce the lateral third of the clavicle. The distribution of these nerves is important surgically since transverse incisions will cut them, frequently leaving painful subcutaneous neuromata. The nerves also frequently become involved in scar tissue and, since they are superficial, are subject to pressure irritation.

The sensory supply below the point of the shoulder, is from the circumflex nerve, giving to the arm an upper lateral cutaneous branch which winds around to the front.

The posterior aspect of the shoulder is supplied by cutaneous branches from the posterior rami of cervical and thoracic nerves piercing the muscle layers (Fig. 2–39). These branches are accompanied by small vessels and come through apertures in the musculo-

tendinous zone through which small herniations of fatty tissue also may occur.

One set of branches becomes cutaneous not far from the cervical posterior spinous processes while, more laterally, another network not quite so large reaches the skin at a point midway between the spines and the axillary border.

NERVE SUPPLY OF THE SHOULDER JOINT PROPER

The shoulder joint has a profuse nerve supply arising from nearby main nerve trunks. Medullary and nonmedullary fibers are distributed from these to ligaments, capsule and synovium. After piercing the capsule, the branches form a plexus, producing a profuse branching network to the synovium. When the shoulder joint is probed under local anesthesia, painful reactions are

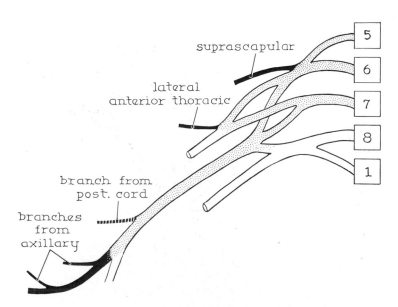

Figure 2–40 Source of shoulder innervation.

recorded from stimulation of ligament and capsule. These are diffuse and not well localized. Needle punctures in the synovium, however, produce a sharp localizing element. If the articular surface is scratched, no definite sensation is felt.

The anatomical law of innervation is that any main trunk crossing a joint may contribute a branch to the articular structures. Branches reach the shoulder joint from suprascapular, musculocutaneous, axillary and subscapular nerves. In addition, the musculocutaneous nerve and posterior cord of the plexus may give short branches. There is considerable reciprocal distribution; for example, if the branch from the axillary nerve is large, or there are several branches, the twig from the musculocutaneous nerve may be missing or very small. Since the supply arises from many sources, it is difficult to carry out a complete denervation of this joint. The branches are reasonably large but are not consistently located, and many of them follow the small vessels into the periarticular structures, which further hampers peripheral denervation. The branches are derived from spinal segments C.4 to C.7, but largely from C.5, C.6 and C.7, with the most constant contributions coming from C.5 and C.6 (Fig. 2–40).

NERVE SUPPLY OF THE ANTERIOR ASPECT

Axillary, subscapular and musculocutaneous nerves supply the anterior portion of the joint. The branch of the musculocutane-

ous nerve arises near the top and may not be constant. The main supply comes from the axillary nerve, which usually contributes two branches, an upper and a lower. One of these sends a twig to the bicipital sulcus region. The subscapular nerve is a source of further supply, and the branch from this nerve reaches the joint by penetrating the subscapularis muscle. Occasionally the branch will come directly from the posterior cord. Reciprocal distribution is common, so that there may be a large branch from the posterior cord and one not quite so big from the axillary nerve (Fig. 2–41).

NERVE SUPPLY OF THE SUPERIOR ASPECT

The superior aspect is supplied by suprascapular, axillary and musculocutaneous branches and, occasionally, a branch from the anterior lateral thoracic nerve. The most constant supply is a branch from the suprascapular nerve arising in the supraspinous fossa which curves around from the back, extending to the region of the coracoid and coraco-acromial ligament. Another branch is distributed to the posterior aspect. A twig from the anterolateral anterior thoracic nerve frequently supplies the coracoclavicular joint, accompanying the branch from the thoraco-acromial artery. This twig may continue onward to the capsule of the shoulder joint. The axillary and musculocutaneous supplies overlap on the top and at the front.

Figure 2–41 Anterior supply of the shoulder joint. A plexus is formed with twigs reaching the synovium from the large branches of the area.

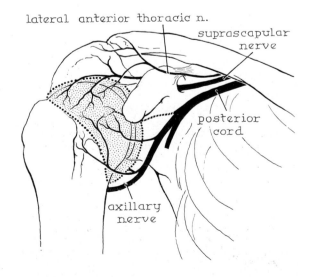

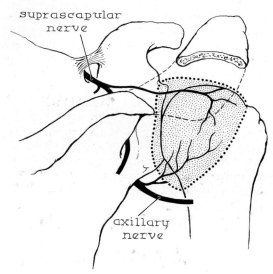

Figure 2–42 Innervation of superior and posterior aspects of the shoulder capsule.

NERVE SUPPLY OF THE POSTERIOR ASPECT

The posterior region is supplied by branches from the suprascapular and axillary nerves (Fig. 2–42). The former contribution arises near the top, and further branches reach the joint after piercing the supraspinatous tendon near the musculotendinous junction.

The branch from the axillary nerve curves around from the inferior aspect.

REFERENCES

Compere, E. L.: Origin, Anatomy, Physiology and Pathology of the Intervertebral Disc. Instructional course lecture of the American Academy of Orthopedic Surgery. St. Louis, The C. V. Mosby Co., Vol. XVII, 1961.

DePalma, A. F.: Surgical anatomy of the rotator cuff and the natural history of degenerative periarthritis. Surg. Clin. N. Amer. *43*:1507–1520, 1963.

DePalma, A. F.: Surgical anatomy of acromioclavicular and sternoclavicular joints. Surg. Clin. N. Amer. *43*: 1541–1550, 1963.

DePalma, A. F., Collery, G., and Bennett, G. A.: Variational Anatomy and Degenerative Lesions of the Shoulder Joint. Instructional course lectures of the American Academy of Orthopedic Surgeons. Vol. VI, 1949, pp. 255–281.

Ferlic, D. C.: The nerve supply of the cervical intervertebral disc in man. Bull. Hopkins Hosp. *113*:347–351, 1963.

Fielding, J. W.: Normal and selected abnormal motion of the cervical spine from the second cervical vertebra to the seventh cervical vertebra based on cineroentgenography. J. Bone Joint Surg. *46A*:1779, 1964.

Francis, C. C.: Dimensions of the cervical vertebrae. Anat. Rec. *122*:603, 1935.

Freedman, L., et al.: Adduction of the arm in the scapular plane: Scapular and glenohumeral movements. A roentgenographic study. J. Bone Joint Surg. (Amer) *48*:1503–1510, 1966.

Gardner, E.: Innervation of the shoulder joint. Anat. Rec. *102*:1–18, 1948.

Grant, J. C.: A Method of Anatomy. Baltimore, The Williams & Wilkins Co., 1940.

Grant, J. C. B.: An Atlas of Anatomy. Baltimore, The Williams & Wilkins Co., 1943.

Hadley, L. A.: The convertebral articulations and cervical foramen encroachment. J. Bone Joint Surg. *39A*:910, 1957.

Harris, R. S., and Jones, D. M.: The arterial supply to the adult cervical vertebral bodies. J. Bone Joint Surg. *38B*:922, 1956.

Malinsky, J.: The ontogenetic development of nerve terminations in the intervertebral disc of man. Acta Anat. *38*:96–113, 1959.

Moseley, H. F., et al.: The arterial pattern of the rotator cuff of the shoulder. J. Bone Joint Surg. (Brit) *45*: 780–789, 1963.

Mulligan, J. H.: The innervation of the ligaments attached to the bodies of the vertebrae. J. Anat. *91*(4): 455, 1957.

Overton, L. M., and Grossman, J. W.: Anatomical variations in the articulation between the second and third cervical vertebrae. J. Bone Joint Surg. *34A*:155, 1952.

Orogino, C., Sherman, M. S., and Schechter, D.: Lushka's joint—a degenerative phenomenon. J. Bone Joint Surg. *42A*:853, 1960.

Piganiol, G., et al.: Anatomical and radiologic research on the non-posterior approach to cervical discovertebral compression. Neurochirurgie *11*:338–343, 1965.

Ranson, S. W., and Clark, S. L.: The Anatomy of the Nervous System. 10th ed. Philadelphia, W. B. Saunders Company, 1959.

Robinson, R. A., and Southwick, W. O.: Surgical Approaches to the Cervical Spine. Instructional course lecture of the American Academy of Orthopedic Surgeons. St. Louis, The C. V. Mosby Co., Vol. XVII, 1960, pp. 299–330.

Roofe, R. P.: Innervation of the annulus fibrosus and posterior longitudinal ligament at the fourth and fifth lumbar level. Arch. Neurol. Psychiat. *44*:100–103, 1940.

Rothman, R. H., et al.: The vascular anatomy of the rotator cuff. Clin. Orthop. *41*:176–186, 1965.

Sabotta, McM.: Atlas of Human Anatomy. New York, G. E. Stechert & Co., 1932.

Sahadevan, M. G., et al.: The anatomical basis of cervical spondylosis. J. Indian Med. Ass. *46*:594–596, 1966.

Scapinelli, R. J.: Sesamoid bones in the ligamentum nuchae of man. Anatomy *97*:417–422, 1963.

Singleton, M. C.: Functional anatomy of the shoulder. Phys. Ther. *46*:1043–1051, 1966.

Southwick, W. O., and Keggi, K.: The normal cervical spine. J. Bone Joint Surg. *46A*:1767, 1964.

Stilwell, D. P.: The nerve supply of the vertebral column and its associated structures in the monkey. Anat. Rec. *125*:139, 1956.

Tsukada, A.: Nerve endings in intervertebral discs. Mitt. Med. Akad. Kioto *24*:1057–1091 and 1172–1174, 1938; *25*:1–29 and 207–209, 1939.

Turnbull, I. M., et al.: Blood supply of cervical spinal cord in man. A microangiographic cadaver study. J. Neurosurg. *24*:951–965, 1966.

Wiedhopf, H.: On spondylolisthesis in the cervical region. Beitr. Orthop. Trauma *12*:694–696, 1965.

Chapter III

APPLIED PHYSIOLOGY OF THE SHOULDER AND NECK

The shoulder is a system of joints, and many movements of this system implicate the neck. Completely independent action is possible, but not independent simultaneous action. Primary functions can be identified in both these areas, and a natural synchrony may be defined supplementing these. The shoulder exists so that our hands can be used to greatest advantage; the neck is so built that we can use the vital properties of our special senses to greatest advantage.

PRINCIPLES OF SHOULDER FUNCTION

Three primary functions can be identified in the shoulder; suspension of the upper limb, fixation for motion, and provision of a fulcrum for the extremity.

SUSPENSORY ACTION

Suspension is accomplished by the clavicle acting as a strut snubbed at its inner end in the sternoclavicular joint and with powerful suspensory muscles holding it upward and backward close to the neck. Strong ligaments and muscles, in turn, hang humerus and scapula to the clavicle. The suspensory mechanism is both static and dynamic and is under constant stress because of the pull of gravity. The suspensory muscles include, in order of importance, trapezius, sternomastoid and levator scapulae. The trapezius is really a muscle system since four separate parts are identifiable, each producing a different motion. The whole muscle, acting as a unit, braces the shoulder backward. The upper fibers shrug the shoulder upward and help to suspend the girdle, performing an important static role. At the opposite end, that is, in the neck insertion, they also have a static function, contributing to the balance and support of the head on the shoulders. The upper and central fibers, in their attachment to the acromion, pull the whole shoulder girdle upward and inward, i.e., as in breast stroke or in the recovery portion of the crawl stroke in swimming. The lower portions of the muscle contribute to circumduction of the arm by clamping the scapula to the chest wall so that it cannot rotate or slip sideways. In this fashion, along with the serratus anterior, a fixed point is provided for contraction of the deltoid to lift the arm level (Fig. 3–1).

When the trapezius is paralyzed, the two important functions missing are the lack of upward pull on the shoulder girdle, which leaves a sense of dragging or increased weight felt by the patient in the shoulder, and the firm base, from which constant action of the deltoid is lost because the scapula slips and is not clamped steadily to the chest. The result is that a hunching type of girdle motion results, limiting the upward excursion markedly and weakening the action of the deltoid.

Sternomastoid

The sternomastoid is commonly referred to as a "breathing muscle" because of the role it assumes in labored respiration. However, it performs an important shoulder-neck function. The clavicular portion assists in elevation of the clavicle, acting from above. The whole muscle acting from below and in unison with its fellow on the opposite side, flexes the neck forward strongly. Acting from above, the muscle rotates the head and neck to the opposite side. It is the distortion of this latter action that is the basis for the clinical state of congenital torticollis.

Levator Scapulae

The levator scapulae, although a much smaller muscle than the sternomastoid, is

an important suspensory mechanism; it contributes support to the scapula in standing and assists in elevating the scapula. It is composed of purely parallel fibers with a tendinous insertion into the scapula. Because of its attenuated and parallel structure, it is easily involved in postural strain of a chronic nature and is a prime site for the development of "trigger" zones of scar formation in habitual round-shoulderedness.

Arm Suspension

The link below the clavicle which holds the arm up has two important segments: one, a heavy ligament, the suspensory or coracoclavicular ligament; and the other, the powerful deltoid muscle. When either of these is lost, which happens from rupture of the ligament or paralysis of the deltoid, the humerus and scapula slip downward and forward; eventually sufficient slack develops that pressure on the neurovascular bundle becomes clinically apparent.

Deltoid Muscle

The deltoid is one of the most beautiful muscles in the body. It has a multipinnate structure with fibers so arranged that a powerful diagonal pull can be produced. This mechanism allows a large number of fibers to contract, but focuses tremendous force at a single point. The anterior and posterior portions are composed of parallel fibers to facilitate range in the acts of flexion and extension. The middle portion contributes most significantly to the act of abduc-

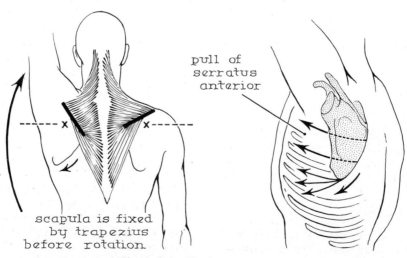

Figure 3–1 Fixation mechanism.

tion. After the scapula has been fixed and the head of the humerus snubbed by the cuff mechanism, the deltoid lifts the arm outward and upward. In this motion it contracts as soon as the scapula is steady and continues to lift the arm outward and upward on its base in the glenoid. The middle fibers initiate the motion and, as the arm is lifted higher, the anterior and posterior parts reinforce this action.

The deltoid may be used as an example of the parallelogram of forces. The resultant of two forces acting at an angle to each other can be computed by drawing a diagram, with arrows representing magnitude and direction. The diagonal of this parallelogram represents the resultant of the two forces (Fig. 3–2A). In pitching a ball, the deltoid acts to control movement of the upper arm during the preparatory backward swing and also to control the forward swing during the delivery.

The deltoid combines with other muscles, particularly the pectoralis major, in the powerful follow-through of the pitching action. Similar acts, like punching, syncronize these two muscles to produce a powerful stroke also. In extension of the arm the posterior fibers of the deltoid are strongly supported by the teres group so that the deltoid and the two teres muscles synchronize in the extensor action as, for example, in the back swing of the golf stroke.

When the deltoid is paralyzed, abduction of the arm is markedly weakened or completely lost. If the rotator cuff is intact, sometimes abduction can still be accomplished through powerful assistance from the biceps in front and the triceps behind. Occasionally, advantage of this synchrony is taken in performing an operation for deltoid paralysis. Under these circumstances, biceps and triceps tendon transfer may assist abduction, in which case the rotator cuff replaces the central portion of the deltoid.

Suspensory Ligament

The conoid and trapezoid ligaments have a powerful hold on the scapula, uniting it to the clavicular strut. The round portion of this ligament, the conoid element, has short thick fibers going in an almost straight direction. The trapezoid element acts more as a check rein, preventing forward tilting of the scapula and at the same time contributing some upward pull.

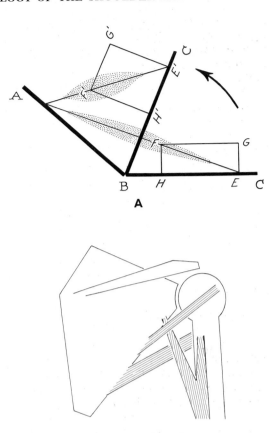

A

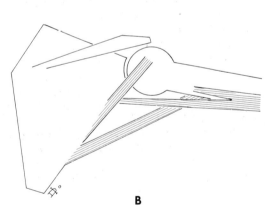

B

Figure 3–2 *A*, Deltoid action system compared to parallelogram of forces. *B*, Scissor protective action of the long muscles inferior to the joint.

STABILITY AND FIXATION

The arm lever is useless unless it has a fixed base. This contribution largely comes from the layers of flat muscles piled one on top another and attached to all surfaces of the scapula.

Paralytic disorders implicating these muscles come into clinical focus by evincing weakness in the fixating mechanism. The serratus anterior, when paralyzed, allows the scapula to swing backward and lose its attachment to the chest. The trapezius allows the scapula to spin like a pinwheel, again contributing a loss of fixation.

MOBILITY OF THE SHOULDER

The most mobile segment of the body results from the configuration of the bony parts and the mechanically advantageous attachment of the multiple powerful muscles. The shallow socket and ball head favor frictionless spinning, and the main joint has four accessory articulating zones which compliment and enhance its action. Shoulder motion, therefore, can be fully appreciated only by understanding both the main and the accessory zone phases.

Mechanics of the Glenohumeral Joint

Most of the movement of the shoulder occurs between the head of the humerus and the glenoid fossa. Suspension and stabilization of the whole girdle are designed to enhance this action. It functions as a machine of the third class, with the head as fulcrum, the arm, forearm and hand as mass, and force applied between these. The point of practical importance in this mechanism is the retention of stability in the face of the wide range of motion that is favored by the shape of the smooth ball in the shallow socket.

In the stabilization action there are two elements: The ball needs to be kept closely applied to the surface of the socket and in such a fashion that it is not allowed to slip or lose position when powerful force is applied (Fig. 3–2*B*). Secondly, the socket needs to be strengthened to withstand the tremendous pull that can be applied as the arm flails forward with the hand as a weight, such as occurs in the follow-through action of pitching. In this action, maintenance of the head of the humerus in the shallow socket depends largely on the support of the soft parts.

Prevention of Slipping of the Head. When the arm is hanging at the side, the direction of the pull of the most powerful elevator, the deltoid, is almost parallel to the long axis of the humerus (Fig. 3–3). Contraction of the deltoid alone jumps the head vertically upward in a slippery socket. Unless this jumping tendency is offset, any attempt at abduction will result in irritation of the whole girdle instead of the smooth swing of the humerus in the glenoid.

Prevention of Dislocation of the Head. Powerful abduction and external rotation favor slipping of the head of the humerus from the socket. When some further force is applied, as in a fall, the head of the humerus may slip out of its fixed place in the joint. Normally the firm attachment of a snug casing or capsule all around the glenoid saucer prevents this. When the capsule is lax or insecurely attached, greater freedom of the head results and it may more easily be wrenched from the socket. The antero-inferior zone, the weak area, is normally protected by the subscapularis tendon. The act of recurrent dislocation can be prevented by limiting the range of external rotation or by reattaching a lax capsule snugly to the rim of the glenoid. Both these principles are the basis for operations for recurrent dislocation of the shoulder.

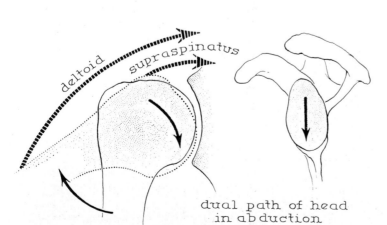

Figure 3–3 Supraspinatus snubbing mechanism for the humeral head.

A further arc of motion involves the head of the humerus in that it follows a vertical linear course in its act of full rotation to complete the arc of circumduction.

The fulcrum of the head in the glenoid is a linear line rather than a stationary point (Fig. 3–3). The greater length of the glenoid in the vertical axis deliberately accommodates this movement of the head. Rotation of the humerus on its long axis is easily accommodated by the saucer-like shape of the glenoid, enhanced and deepened by the labrum. When there are abnormalities in the relationship of the head of the humerus to the glenoid, that is, should the head be retroverted, greater external rotation is required to bring the head of the humerus into proper alignment in the glenoid. The converse of this is of clinical significance because it is felt that in the condition of recurrent congenital posterior dislocation of the shoulder, a state of retroversion of the head of the humerus exists and, as the arm hangs at the side, the face of the humerus is twisted somewhat posteriorly. Under these circumstances simple forward flexion of the arm will then move the face of the humerus posteriorly to an abnormal degree and will favor posterior luxation without continuing approximation of the head to the glenoid in the normal fashion.

Mechanics of the Rotator Cuff. The group comprised of the supraspinatus, infraspinatus and teres minor muscles constitutes one of the most important muscle systems in the body and contributes vitally to shoulder action. The insertions of these muscles blend into a single tendon through which the action of all is directed. In analyzing cuff function it is useful to study the contributions of superior, posterior and anterior parts.

SUPERIOR PORTION OF THE CUFF. The superior portion of the cuff is made up largely of the supraspinatus, which controls this zone by applying tension through a short lever inserted into the top of the humerus. As the muscle contracts it pulls or depresses the head, causing it to slip downward slightly in the glenoid. In this way the stage is set for the application of force through a longer lever by the powerful deltoid. The stabilization by the cuff produces a steady fulcrum, allowing the deltoid to act to its greatest efficiency (Fig. 3–4).

POSTERIOR PORTION OF THE CUFF. The infraspinatus largely controls this segment, with some contribution from the teres minor. It is a bulky muscle with a much larger cross section than the supraspinatus and, consequently, it exerts more force. The fleshy fibers extend well up into the capsule, and

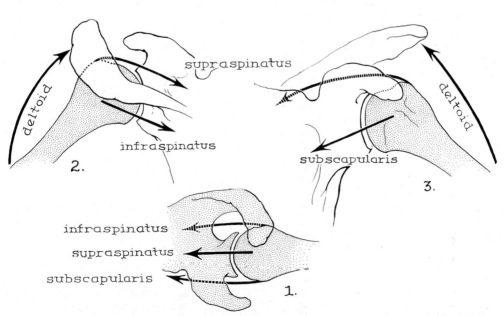

Figure 3–4 Action of cuff muscles in abduction. (1) Supraspinatus steadies head from above. (2) Infraspinatus depresses the head because of the direction of its pull. (3) Subscapularis steadies the head in front and parallels the action of the infraspinatus. Combination of these actions allows deltoid to swing arm up on a steady fulcrum.

the line of pull is almost vertically downward. In this position it can also act as an extensor in the horizontal plane or initiate external rotation of the head of the humerus. The combination of depression, extension and external rotation is the vital contribution to swinging the greater tuberosity underneath the overhanging coraco-acromial arch during the act of abduction and circumduction (Fig. 3–4). When there is interference with this mechanism, as in rupture or degeneration, circumduction may be obstructed because the head of the humerus then jams on the overhanging arch. The external rotation action of the muscle requires fixation of the scapula by the flat muscles such as the rhomboids. The teres minor enhances the arc of the infraspinatus in most of these phases.

ANTERIOR PORTION OF THE CUFF. The subscapularis controls this portion through a broad flat muscle and tendon which is intimately adherent to the capsule anteriorly and inferiorly. It acts as an internal rotator and adductor. At the same time it exerts a downward tension, depressing the head of the humerus and aiding the snubbing action of supra- and infraspinatus (Fig. 3–4).

In addition to its rotator contribution, the subscapularis has an important static function; it acts as a "live" ligament, helping to maintain the head of the humerus in the glenoid. If the attachment of the subscapularis to the scapula becomes lax, strong muscle force may then favor slipping of the head of the humerus out of the capsule antero-inferiorly. All the rotator muscles act through a common tendon which is constantly under tension on the top, at the back and at the front; such a role favors wear and tear damage. Once a weak point or tear develops, enlargement of the defect is favored because of the constant directional pull. Such a complication leads to a further irritation from the head of the humerus, which exerts abnormal upward pressure. In turn, more wear is favored and a vicious cycle develops.

Mechanics of the Sternoclavicular Joint

The medial end of the clavicle fits into the sternal notch, serving as an anchor for the swinging strut of the upper extremity. Movement occurs at this joint through all phases of circumduction and in many other shoulder acts. The clavicle tips upward and downward from front to back and rotates on its long axis (Fig. 2–37). The vertical movement of the clavicle is through an arc of about 35 degrees in active abduction, most of which occurs during the first half, or 90 degrees. Maximum use of this excursion is made in such actions as shrugging or lifting the point of the shoulder up to the ear.

The clavicle rotates on its long axis, particularly in the upper arc of flexion, but it also moves in circumduction. As the arm is lifted from the side, the clavicle rolls upward and backward; as it is brought down, it rolls downward and forward. This can easily be verified by palpating the inner curve of the clavicle. Along the inner aspect the clavicle is a rugged pipe-like structure with a pronounced anterior curve. As it rotates on its long axis, this stout zone still serves as a protector for the neurovascular bundle which runs beneath. The curve allows the protecting "pipe" always to swing free of the underlying vessels. In flexion and extension of the shoulder such as occurs in punching, the clavicle moves backward and forward in a horizontal plane, and the tip at the acromial end sweeps through an arc of 35 degrees.

In addition to the motion which occurs at this joint, two further important physiological observations may be made. The ligament which divides the sternoclavicular joint snubs the clavicle into position at the medial end, pulling on it from the top downward. When force is transmitted along the clavicle, as in a fall, the bulbous sternal end is buffered by this tough intra-articular ligament and its attachment in such a fashion that it prevents the clavicle from jumping out of the socket (Fig. 2–37). When there is recurrent injury, damage to the intra-articular ligament produces an internal derangement of the sternoclavicular joint.

Mechanics of the Acromioclavicular Joint

The importance of the acromioclavicular joint in shoulder action has not received proper attention. Motion occurs at this joint in nearly all movements of the shoulder. The surfaces, when viewed from above, are crescentic so that the acromion swings in an arc around the clavicle to accommodate for strong flexion and extension, such as occurs in the striking movement. The action that takes place at this joint in circumducting the

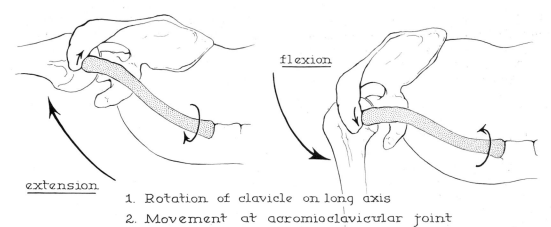

flexion

extension

1. Rotation of clavicle on long axis
2. Movement at acromioclavicular joint

Figure 3–5 Rotation of the clavicle involves both acromioclavicular and sternoclavicular joints.

arm is important. During the early part of the second 90 degrees of circumduction, the acromion hinges on the clavicle, but this does not start until the arm reaches a right angle. The joint is used extensively beyond this point. This is the basis for the clinical observation that pain arising out of acromioclavicular disorder is usually not appreciated until the patient has lifted his arm almost 90 degrees. Pain that develops before this point is reached is not likely to be based in the acromioclavicular joint (Fig. 3–5).

A further function of extreme importance of the acromioclavicular joint is that it substitutes for a phase of abduction when rotation of the head of the humerus in the glenoid is interfered with. In those patients in whom glenohumeral disturbance from any source has produced some interference with rotation, attempted compensation is developed by more motion taking place at the acromioclavicular joint or at an earlier than normal phase in the swing. In other words, once the head of the humerus is locked and can no longer rotate externally, abduction girdle action shifts from this fulcrum to the acromioclavicular joint and movement starts earlier than usual in this joint.

The result of this compensatory mechanism is that irritation of the acromioclavicular joint develops, and wear and tear changes progress at a greater rate than is normal. Once the rotation at the glenohumeral joint has been restored to a more normal level, the acromioclavicular joint does not contribute so extensively. The important corollary of this is that, artificially, one may obtain more abductive power. The acromioclavicular joint is loosened and its obstruction is

decreased by doing a resection of either the medial aspect of the acromion or the lateral aspect of the clavicle, leaving greater play at this joint so that its powers of compensation are greater than under normal circumstances. Clinical advantage is frequently taken of this physiological arrangement in arthrodesis of the shoulder or in acromioclavicular arthroplasty in certain standard shoulder exposures when primary disease implicates the acromioclavicular joint (Fig. 3–6).

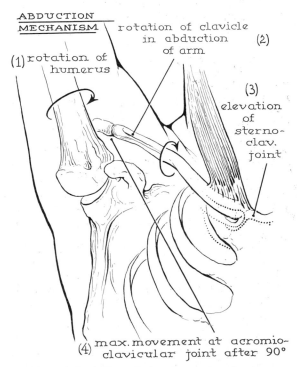

ABDUCTION MECHANISM

rotation of clavicle in abduction of arm (2)

(1) rotation of humerus

(3) elevation of sterno-clav. joint

(4) max. movement at acromio-clavicular joint after 90°

Figure 3–6 Action of glenohumeral and accessory joints in abduction of the arm.

Mechanics of the Scapulothoracic Mechanism

The contribution of the scapula to shoulder function is one of the most ingenious mechanisms in the body. It acts as a base or platform for the upper extremity and yet takes part in movement of the whole girdle in addition to enhancing motion at the glenohumeral joint. Movements made possible by the scapulothoracic mechanism are abduction, adduction, elevation, depression and rotation. All these are accomplished by the shifting of the flat scapula on the chest wall. The same bed is used constantly, so that any irregularities of this zone that arise from constant or excessive wear and tear will come into clinical focus as discomfort or pain reflected in this region (Fig. 3–7).

Abduction or Lateral Movement of the Scapula. The scapula moves around the chest wall a distance of 3 to 4 inches, reaching a maximum as the arm is flexed across the chest. This act is accomplished by the pectoralis minor, serratus anterior and, to a slight degree, pectoralis major. The excursion follows a curved course on the chest from just behind the posterior angle of the ribs around to the front. The significant clinical corollary is that weakness of the serratus anterior seriously interferes with this action. Atony of the fixator muscles of the scapula or general muscle laxity favors the shifting of the scapula laterally, with a consequent increase in the interscapular dimension, which may be seen in some cases of chronic postural disturbance.

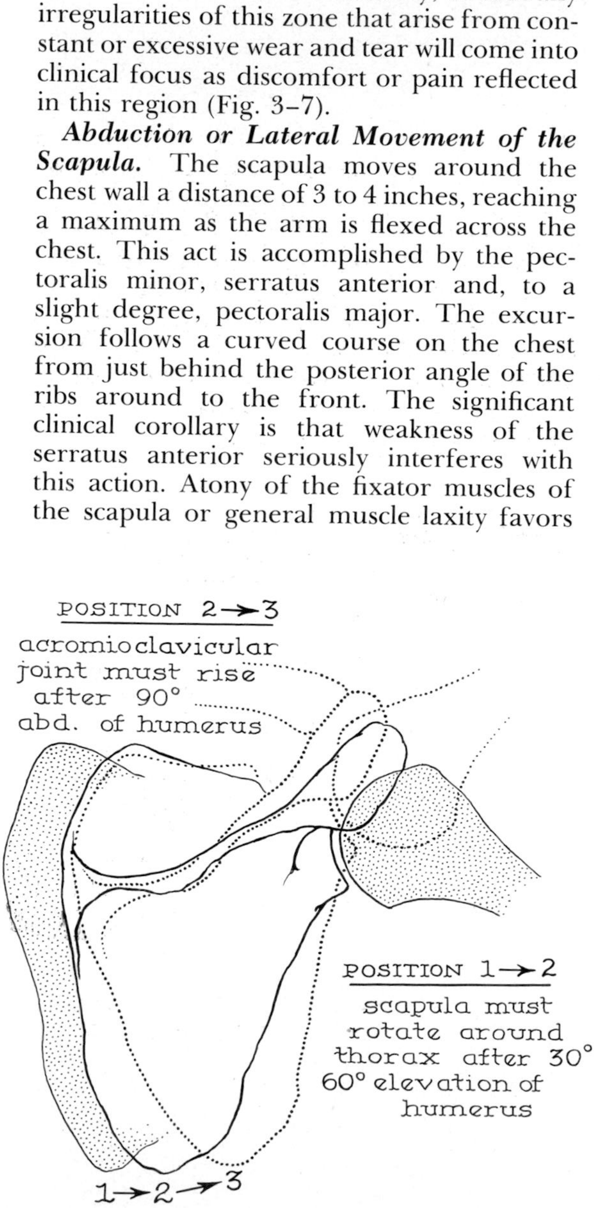

Adduction or Medial Movement of the Scapula. One scapula may be moved toward its fellow from the resting position, stopping just lateral to the line of the posterior spinous processes. As this occurs the tissue and muscle between the two scapulae tend to be bunched and folded together, resisting the action. During this motion the scapula shifts over the prominent posterior curve of the ribs, moving a distance of 1½ to 2 inches. This act of adduction is accomplished by the trapezius and rhomboids exerting pull on the medial border and spine of the scapula. Soft tissue related to the medial border and base of the spine is a frequent site of posttraumatic and degenerative changes because of the repeated abnormal creasing and folding of these structures, resulting in shoulder-neck discomfort.

In states of muscle atony and postural disturbance the scapulae slide sideways on the chest, increasing the range of adduction and, consequently, the stress or strain on the rhomboids and trapezius. In many instances this common postural fault can be remedied by muscle training to improve the power and tone in these suspensory muscles.

Elevation of the Scapula. The scapula is lifted up on the chest in such movements as shrugging the shoulder. It rides up roughly 2 inches, shifting a little laterally in its course. This motion is accomplished by the levator scapulae and the upper segment of the trapezius. During the shrugging action, motion also occurs at the sternoclavicular joint at the front to allow the shift of the whole girdle.

Depression of the Scapula. The point of the shoulder may be lowered actively, but only a small portion of this is due to movement of the scapula on the chest. It shifts downward about half an inch because of downward rotation rather than true depression. The lower fibers of the serratus anterior, assisted by pectoralis minor and subclavius, accomplish this maneuver (Fig. 3–4).

In addition to excursion in vertical and horizontal planes, the scapula rotates on itself like a pinwheel clamped to the chest. The center of the wheel is just below the middle of the spine. This action of rotation is necessary in raising and lowering the arm. During the first 30 degrees of circumduction the scapula is fixed, but at this point it starts to tilt upward so that the base of the

POSITION 2→3

acromioclavicular joint must rise after 90° abd. of humerus

POSITION 1→2

scapula must rotate around thorax after 30° 60° elevation of humerus

1→2→3

Figure 3–7 Rotation of the scapula in its bed on the chest wall.

glenoid is able to follow the excursion of the head of the humerus. From this level to the completion of the arc of elevation the scapula rotates roughly 60 degrees (Fig. 3–7). This maneuver is accomplished by the serratus anterior and the trapezius. The return to the normal position results from the pull of the levator scapulae, rhomboids and pectoralis minor and is assisted by gravity.

Physiology of Specific Shoulder Movement

Shoulder motion is interpreted in terms of excursion of the arm from the body and is recorded according to the anatomical planes. For practical purposes, however, the action of lifting the arm, regardless of the plane, is the vital function because rotation of the body or rotation of the trunk then converts what is a simple lift into flexion or abduction, depending upon the position the body has assumed. The universal multiplane action of the shoulder itself is an indication of the fettering concept of rigid anatomical plane interpretation. The summation of shoulder motion is reached in circumduction, which is a magnificent example of integrated joint action and muscle control. Most of the movement occurs at the glenohumeral joint, but this is appreciably enhanced by contributions from the sternoclavicular, acromioclavicular and scapulothoracic mechanisms. An understanding of shoulder movement comprises a study of all these joints and the principal muscles.

Elevation of the Arm from the Side, or Abduction. Lifting the arm from the side of the body, up over the head, is a complex procedure (Fig. 3–8). The normal range is 180 degrees and is accomplished largely at the glenohumeral joint, but all the axillary joints contribute. The muscles chiefly concerned are the trapezius, the serratus anterior, the deltoid and the rotator cuff group.

In this motion the base of the arm lever is first steadied to allow the hoisting machinery to operate. This maneuver is accomplished by the trapezius and serratus, which clamp the scapula to the chest wall. In observing a shoulder from the back in the motion of

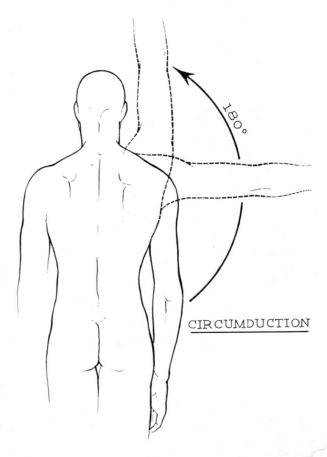

Figure 3–8 Circumduction.

CIRCUMDUCTION

abduction, the first thing that happens (and so quickly that it may be missed) is a trembling or waving of the inferior angle of the scapula, indicating the clamping action to the chest by serratus and trapezius. After this base is solid, the muscles directly acting on the humerus come into play. Snubbing of the slippery head of the humerus is accomplished by the supraspinatus and infraspinatus, and after the head of the humerus is steady, the stage is set for the application of full contraction of the deltoid, which swings the arm up on its way (Fig. 3–9). The snubbing by the cuff group and the grasping elevation of the deltoid are applied simultaneously.

Some overlap in action between the cuff and the deltoid can sometimes be enhanced so that one can produce the result of both. For example, the arm with a paralyzed or damaged supraspinatus can be abducted by the deltoid but, in most instances the rhythm will be faulty and the range limited. Similarly, when the deltoid is paralyzed or absent the arm can sometimes be abducted by extremely forceful action of an intact cuff enhanced by accessory muscles like the biceps.

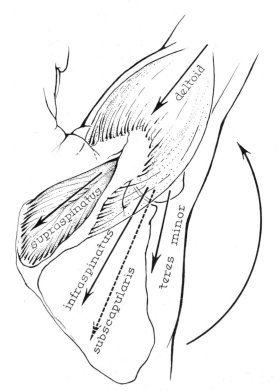

Figure 3–9 Muscle action in abduction of the shoulder.

The movement of circumduction starts at the glenohumeral joint, but movement occurs at the accessory articulations also. During the second 45 degrees of elevation, movement at the sternoclavicular joint reaches a maximum and falls off during the second 90 degrees. For every 10 degrees elevation of the arm to a right angle, there are 4 degrees of elevation at the sternoclavicular joint, as estimated by Abbott, Inman and Saunders (Fig. 3–10). The second 90 degrees of elevation is accomplished at the glenohumeral joint aided by contributions from the acromioclavicular and scapulothoracic joints. As the humerus reaches 90 degrees in the glenoid, obstruction is encountered in the overhanging bony ligamentous coraco-acromial arch. This is overcome by the humerus rotating externally on its long acis, which allows the greater tuberosity to slip underneath the bony ligamentous obstruction (Fig. 3–11). Disturbance of this mechanism is frequent and occurs early in many shoulder disorders.

It may readily be seen that any pathological process which mars the efficiency of the external rotators prevents the head from moving out of the way of the obstructing overhang, and impingement may occur. Similarly, decrease in the space beneath the arch due to a thickened bursa, ragged capsule or high riding humeral head will be a source of derangement. When this is the case, discomfort develops just before the arm reaches 90 degrees because it is at this point that the obstruction would be encountered. When pain on motion is experienced later in the range, the source of the discomfort is likely to be in an accessory area such as the acromioclavicular joint, because this is the mechanism on which stress is then focused (Fig. 3–11).

Once the head of the humerus has rotated under the overhanging arch, the scapula and humerus swing upward and outward aided by 20 degree movement at the acromioclavicular joint. Maximum motion at the acromioclavicular joint takes place in the second 90 degrees, so that pain experienced during this range of movement is highly suggestive of acromioclavicular derangement. During the whole phase the scapula rotates on the chest wall around the thoracic cage. In this maneuver the trapezius fixes the scapula and the rotation is supplied by the powerful serratus anterior pulling on the inferior angle of the scapula.

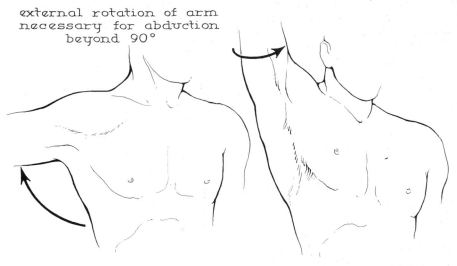

Figure 3–10   Unlocking action of external rotation permits full circumduction.

Lowering the Arm to the Side, or Adduction.   From 180 degree circumduction the arm may be pulled down to the side and, at the end of the excursion, carried behind the back 5 to 10 degrees further. This action takes place with the assistance of gravity and, when resistance is added, the latissimus dorsi, teres major and pectoralis major are the motors. As the arm descends from 180 degree circumduction, the clavicle rotates downward on its long axis. The scapula moves on the chest wall during the middle 90 degrees, starting at 45 degrees from the top and stopping 45 degrees from the bottom. Motion is largely at the glenohumeral joint, with the head of the humerus rotating internally and following a linear arc from the bottom to the top of the glenoid, reversing the route taken on abduction.

The latissimus dorsi, pectoralis major and teres major complete adduction. Should the head of the humerus be somewhat fixed in the glenoid, such as occurs from shortening of structures on the superior aspect, there is interference with the normal glenohumeral rhythm and a more girdle-like motion results. In the act of pitching, when great force is used, stress falls on the structures at the back of the joint, which at the end of the delivery act in a braking fashion. The long head of the triceps and teres major support the joint, but the maximum stress falls on the triceps because of its strong contraction from extension of the elbow. Repetitive stress

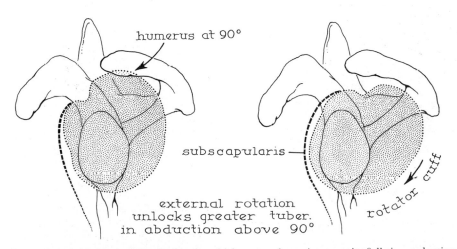

Figure 3–11   Diagram of mechanism by which external rotation permits full circumduction.

in this fashion is the explanation for some instances of chronic disability in baseball pitchers (Fig. 3–12).

Forward Motion, or Flexion. The arm may be brought forward 110 degrees at the shoulder and carried on up to 180 degrees in circumduction flexion. In this movement the head of the humerus does not encounter the same obstruction from the coraco-acromial arch that occurs in abduction. The scapula is fixed to the chest initially and then moves forward around the chest wall during the second 90 degrees of elevation, ending up farther in front than during the motion of abduction (Fig. 3–13).

Flexion is accomplished by the anterior deltoid, pectoralis major, coraco brachialis and biceps. Some pathological processes other than adhesive capsulitis and glenohumeral arthritis interfere with flexion. When it is limited, the defect is not noticeable because scapulothoracic or girdle action with spine flexion substitutes extensively to permit many acts like forward reaching and bending (Fig. 3–14).

Backward Movement, or Extension. The arm may be swung backward at the shoulder behind the line of the body for 30 degrees. In this action the clavicle rotates downward a little on its long axis and moves backward with the sternoclavicular joint as the fulcrum. The scapula shifts backward and tilts up a little on the chest wall. Extension is accomplished by the posterior deltoid, latissimus, teres major and minor, infraspinatus and triceps. Adhesive joint disorders and arthritis in the glenohumeral joint interfere with extension. The motion of placing the hand behind the back is initiated by extension and completed by internal rotation. Both these movements are hampered considerably by any freezing or constricting process implicating the capsule or periarticular structures. As is the case in adduction, the act of extension can be aided by gravity, so its loss is not a serious defect (Fig. 3–13).

External Rotation. From the midposition, with the arm at the side or abducted horizontally, the shoulder may be externally rotated almost 90 degrees. Nearly all this movement occurs at the glenohumeral joint (Fig. 3–15). When the arm is at the side this action is accomplished by the infraspinatus, teres minor and posterior deltoid. When the arm is horizontal the supraspinatus also contributes. External rotation is a most important movement, and when it is lost, shoulder action is seriously compromised. Disturbances such as rupture of the rotator cuff weaken external rotation so that, as the arm is abducted, the greater tuberosity cannot be rotated under the coraco-acromial arch, and this obstruction means that further elevation is blocked. Constant attention is paid to maintaining the strength and efficiency of the external rotators in shoulder disorders (Fig. 3–16).

Internal Rotation. The arm may be

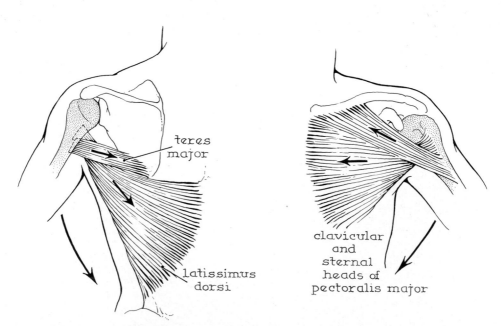

teres major

latissimus dorsi

clavicular and sternal heads of pectoralis major

Figure 3–12 Muscle action in adduction of the arm.

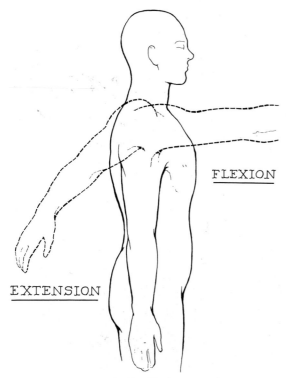

Figure 3-13 Flexion-extension.

turned inward a little more than 90 degrees in both horizontal and vertical planes. This movement occurs chiefly at the glenohumeral joint and is powered by subscapularis, pectoralis major, latissimus dorsi and teres major (Fig. 3-17). It is a powerful action which synchronizes with adduction, as in striking a blow. It is interfered with chiefly in paralytic deformities or when there is a fixed internal rotation deformity such as may be encountered in poliomyelitis in children. In the latter condition internal rotation starts at 45 degrees, or almost with the arm in the line of the chest. This means that when the arm is swung behind the back, it may be taken a further 45 degrees beyond the normal range. When this occurs, the elbow is flexed in front of the body and it strikes the chest below the neck and the hand cannot be brought to the mouth as in eating. Children overcome this deficiency by flexing the neck, but it is most inconvenient.

Fixed internal rotation deformity may be corrected by freeing the contracted structures about the shoulder or by doing a rotation osteotomy of the humerus. (See Chapter I.) The degree of fixed internal rotation is also significant in the condition of recurrent congenital posterior dislocation of the shoulder. When there is an abnormal retroversion of the head of the humerus, the simple act of flexion favors luxation of the head of the humerus posteriorly.

PHYSIOLOGY OF INTEGRATED SHOULDER MOVEMENTS

Everyday activities are made up of acts such as lifting, holding, pushing, turning and shoving. It is in such common and accepted motions that clinical disorders are presented, rather than in terms of normal anatomical planes. These are combined pattern motions with contributions from many parts of the shoulder complex. In-

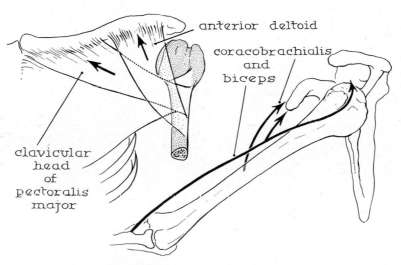

Figure 3-14 Muscle action in flexion.

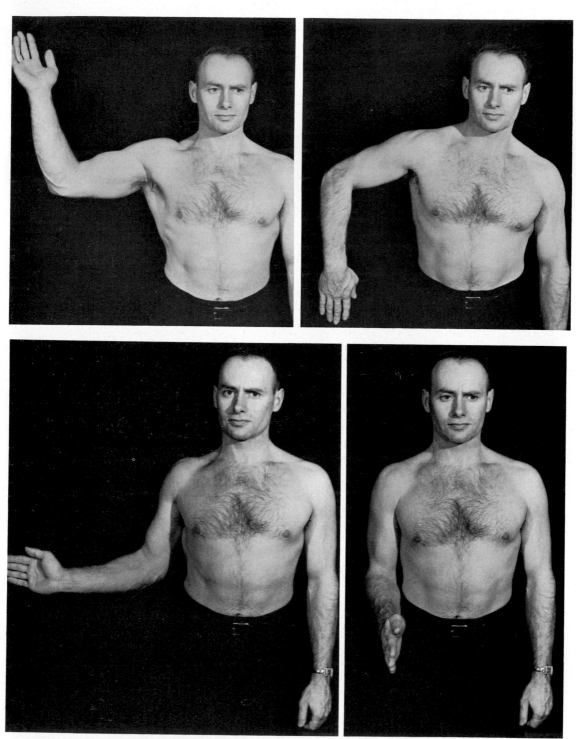

Figure 3–15 Internal and external rotation range in two planes.

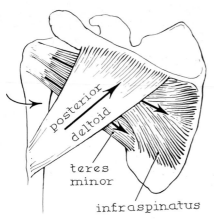

Figure 3-16 Muscle action in external rotation.

dividual joint and muscle contribution may be analyzed in these acts to aid localization and understanding of injury and disease. Consideration must also be given to the part played by the elbow and hand in shoulder function. Shoulders are used unconsciously in actions of hand, wrist and elbow. Injury or disease may hamper normal action of any one of these so that increased replacement effort is sought from the shoulder. For example, loss of rotatory range, as in an arthrodesis of wrist or elbow, unconsciously results in increased rotation at the shoulder. Weakness or disorder of one muscle group evokes replacement effort in another as, for example, the hunching motion of the shoulder by the trapezius which follows attempted abduction as a replacement in paralysis of the deltoid. Scrutiny of these purposeful patterns is of the greatest help in understanding disability in this region.

SHOULDER ACTION IN LIFTING AND CARRYING

Lifting is one of the commonest everyday activities and is accomplished largely below the level of the shoulder at bench level or close to the height of the hip. The contribution of the shoulder is to anchor the upper extremity so that the lifting force may be applied (Fig. 3-18). The lift should be made as close to the body as possible to bring the resistance close to the fulcrum of motion. Most objects are carried in front of the body so that the serratus, trapezius and pectoralis major fix the scapula while the biceps and anterior portion of the deltoid pull the humerus forward. As the object is grasped by the fingers, as much as possible of the hand and arm should be placed beneath the weight. In this way the lever arm from the shoulder is shortened and power is increased. As the object is lifted after the grasp is secure, the level is swung backward by the infraspinatus, latissimus dorsi, triceps and teres muscles. When the shoulder is stiff at both the glenohumeral and scapulothoracic joints, the use of the hoisting machinery is seriously hampered. It means that the fulcrum moves from shoulder to elbow. The hand then has a grossly limited field of action and objects can be lifted only in one narrow plane. When rotation is lost, more strain is placed on the rotators in the forearm; since the arm cannot be abducted, the only range of mediolateral excursion is through movement at the wrist.

The scapulothoracic mechanism is a vital accessory joint and assumes increased sig-

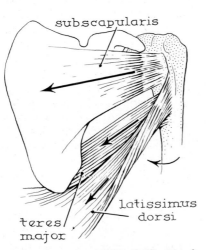

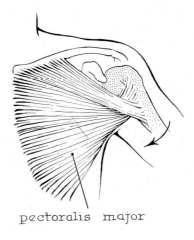

Figure 3-17 Muscle action in internal rotation.

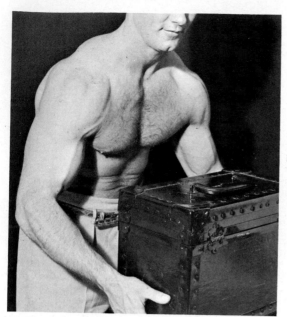

Figure 3–18   Muscle action in lifting and carrying.

nificance if the glenohumeral joint is stiff. Under these conditions it compensates in such movements as lifting, carrying and reaching. After 90 degrees of abduction, much of the normal movement is at the scapulothoracic and sternoclavicular joints and less occurs at the glenohumeral joint.

SHOULDER ACTION IN FALLING

So many injuries occur as a result of falls that more attention should be paid to the mechanism of this action. It has been estimated that over 20 per cent of industrial accidents are due to falls or slips. In a fall the upper extremity is used involuntarily for protection and, depending upon the position and force of the impact, various segments are damaged. Any strong strut transmits force until a weak point or the end is reached; a weak strut gives way quickly. Consequently, in strong, young extremities, force is more apt to reach the base of the arm in a fall than in the elderly group, where the first point of impact, such as the wrist, may give way and be fractured with the dissipation of the force.

The strength of the strut also favors the use of natural resilience in the region of the joints. The wrist, elbow and shoulder buffer the fall so that, by the time the clavicle is reached, the force may be insufficient to break bone. Many factors contribute to the effect of falls on the shoulder, but for practical purposes two principles may be recognized. In the indirect application of the force, the position of the arm as the strut conducting the force to the shoulder is extremely important, whereas in direct contact the level or point of application of the force controls the damage. Four common positions of the arm may be recognized in falls: with the arm at the side, with the arm partly abducted, with the arm fully abducted, and with the arm extended. Resulting damage to the shoulder varies with each of these positions (Fig. 3–19).

Adduction Falls.   In this injury the dropping of the body takes place so suddenly that adduction is barely started and is still incomplete when force is taken on the hand as the body falls. In this action the head of the humerus is shoved up against the coracoacromial arch so that the brunt is taken superiorly and anteriorly rather than at the glenoid buttress. This results in force applied and possible damage to the cuff, the acromion and the biceps mechanisms rather than to the clavicle or the scapula (Fig. 3–19).

Abduction Falls.   When the tumble is a little less sudden, the patient is able to get the arm farther from the side for protection so that force is transmitted through the arm to the scapula and clavicle. Injury to these two bones occurs more frequently (Fig. 3–19).

Full Abduction Falls.   When the arm is fully abducted and externally rotated, as occurs in headlong tumbles, maximum force is applied to the antero-inferior capsule. The head may be wrenched from the socket because the major impact evades the glenoid and a dislocation can occur. When weight is transmitted to the head in the fully abducted, externally rotated position, the force may be sufficient to indent the posterosuperior quadrant of the head of the humerus on the glenoid much the way a ping-pong ball is creased, which is the mechanism of formation of the defect in the humerus head in recurrent dislocation of the shoulder (Fig. 3–19).

Falls in Extension.   When a person falls backward the arm is involuntarily extended behind the body for protection so that the head of the humerus dips forward from under the coraco-acromial arch. Major stress then falls at the front on the capsule and soft tissues, such as the biceps tendon, which can be ruptured in this act (Fig. 3–19).

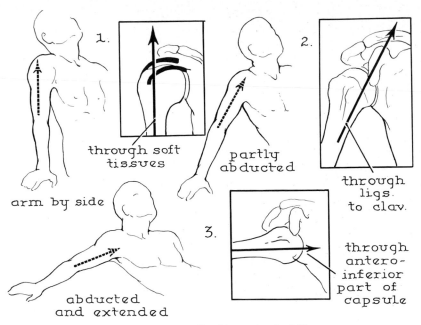

1. through soft tissues

arm by side

2. partly abducted

through ligs. to clav.

3. abducted and extended

through antero-inferior part of capsule

Figure 3–19 Shoulder action in falling.

SHOULDER ACTION IN THROWING AND PUSHING

Throwing is one of the most beautifully coordinated acts which the body produces. It really starts in the lower extremities, which provide the body with a base for the flinging action of the arm. The shoulder and upper arm act like the handle of a whip, with the shoulder drawing the arm backward in preparation for a forceful forward fling of forearm and hand. The scapula is clamped to the chest by the trapezius and serratus to form a firm base for the arm lever. At the same time, scapula and chest are elevated a little on the throwing side. The backward thrust of the arm is accomplished by posterior deltoid, latissimus and infraspinatus. After this phase, the pectoralis major and the deltoid fling the humerus forward. The action of the pectoralis muscles is enhanced by the backward swing of the arm, which puts them on the stretch in a position for powerful contraction. The humerus, like the handle of the whip, flails the hand and forearm forward at the end of the lever in the follow-through motion. In this action from trunk to fingertip, the speed of movement is continually increased as momentum passes from the heavy body region to the lighter hand section. The shoulder and heavy upper arm contribute momentum as well to this throwing action (Figs. 3–20 and 3–21).

Sometimes the shoulder is watched as an indication of arm action; in baseball, for example, a runner on first base may judge from the movement of the shoulder the direction in which the next throw from the pitcher is likely to go. The triceps is important in throwing because it extends the forearm powerfully and contributes support to the inferior aspect of the shoulder posteriorly (Fig. 3–2).

ACTION OF SHOULDER REGION IN STANDING, SITTING AND LYING

The shoulder participates in the accepted and little thought about activities of standing, sitting and lying. Disorders arise in this region that are directly attributable to faulty function.

Standing. Structures in the shoulder-neck region are important in balancing and supporting the head. Normally the head erect position is accomplished unconsciously by the configuration of the bones, the ligaments and muscle action. The extensor muscle group, trapezius and erector spinae, are the muscles most concerned. These have been labeled postural muscles because of the continuous involuntary contractile tension they contribute. Normally this is at a subclinical level, but when extra strain, fatigue or injury is added, the delicate balance is altered,

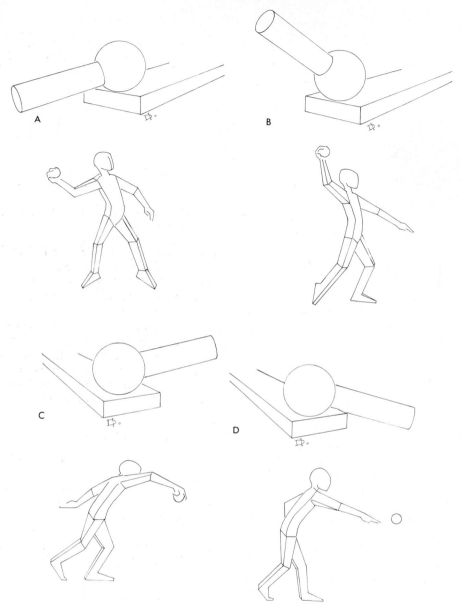

Figure 3–20 Shoulder action in throwing. *A,* Wind-up. *B,* Delivery. *C,* Follow-through. *D,* Breaking.

initiating increased effort which then impinges as a conscious act or discomfort. Prolonged standing, faulty stance and poor muscle development increase the stretch stimulants to the postural muscle group. The slouched position with slumped shoulders seen in tall thin individuals is an example. Poor postural habits followed in the occupation may similarly lead to increased strain.

Sitting. The action in sitting differs from standing, and stress on the shoulder zone is greater. In prolonged activities such as working, irritation may develop in these muscles. Since our work is kept at the front of the body so that our hands and eyes may be used, the natural tendency is toward bending forward. In sitting with attention forward, the balancing and compensatory action of the normal lumbar lordosis of standing is lost; consequently, there is a constant flexion of the spine until the cervical region is reached. At this point, since all the flexion angle must be compensated, maximum mus-

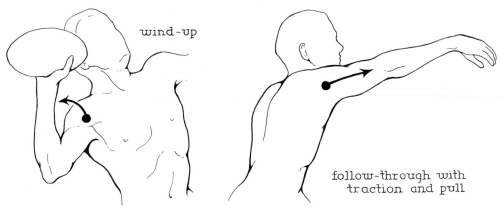

Figure 3–21 Shoulder action in passing. Greater stability is required in this act because of the pushing element in the throw.

cle pull is applied from the cervical thoracic junction upward. This strains suspensory muscles like the trapezius and may initiate discomfort. All good sitting postures emphasize the straight position of the spine so that the balancing factor may be used to ease the burden on these suspensory muscles. A further irritant is constant use of shoulder muscles in the sitting position. This is particularly stressing if the shoulder action required is at a right angle or shoulder level. In most instances, however, the shoulder is used at bench level well below this position, and the intrinsic muscles escape constant strain.

Lying. The horizontal position relaxes all regions, the extensor postural zones in particular. Resting on the back allows the shoulders to drop into a neutral position, with head and neck similarly at rest. Extensor muscles are relaxed by firm body support and a pillow of normal height. Sagging body support flexes the spine, and a hard thick pillow further stretches muscles, particularly in the neck-shoulder zone. This type of irritation is avoided by use of a firm bed and a relatively soft pillow. Other horizontal positions may exert abnormal stress on the shoulder region. The neurovascular bundle may be compressed by lying on the side with the arm under the body. Sleeping with the arm in the abducted and externally rotated position may stretch nerves and vessels, leading to the typical tingling discomfort in the hand and fingers.

NECK FUNCTION

Our necks are used to control the position of the head and so enhance the scope of our vital senses. Special functions may be identified in different segments of the cervical spine. The composite acts are so well synchronized that it is difficult to appreciate the specialization (Fig. 3–22).

Radiographic studies underline the segmental action of the neck. Rotation through 120 degrees occurs at the atlanto-occipital joint. This appears as a composite act of the neck, but actually the upper segment accomplishes the action almost exclusively.

PHYSIOLOGY OF THE NECK

The neck supports, moves and transmits. In identifying these functions, emphasis has been placed on useful or applied physiology rather than on an academic dissection of precise properties. In interpreting the function of the neck, many anatomical features require consideration because of significant contributions to its action.

Supporting Mechanism

Certain precise properties may be singled out as contributing to the function of support. These include the pattern of bone configuration, the intervertebral discs and the ligaments.

Bone Configuration. The function of supporting the head is made possible by the shape and structure of the cervical spine. It consists of an apical tower on which is perched an expanded base gripping the head. The shape of the cervical segments is such that they are stacked one on top of the other like a pile of movable chairs. This produces a series of intermingling locks contributing individual fulcra and, at the same time, maintaining great stability. The vertebral

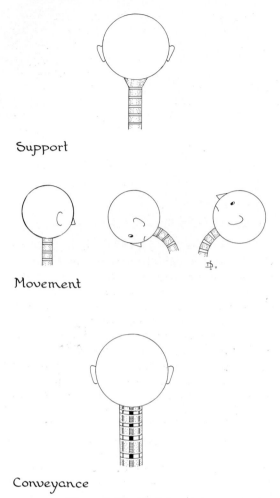

Support

Movement

Conveyance

Figure 3–22 Neck function.

bodies when viewed from the front are an inverted V with the lateral edge formed by the Luschka articulations at the apex of the lateral mass. When viewed from the side the vertebra is also an inverted V, with the body sloping downward and forward and the spine downward and backward from a central apex. (See Figure 2–22.) This double V configuration contributes both stability and mobility. Such a mechanism locks the spine, except in flexion. Rotation is limited; lateral bending is a composite tilt without significant shift.

A further specialized mechanism of support is contributed by allowing the upper segment to rotate freely while holding the head of the vertebra on the lower segment, which can either stay rigid or move with the upper segment as is needed. There results a complex of motion-on-motion segments, each of which has specialized stabilizing mechanisms.

Interbody Discs. The stability of one vertebral body on the other is largely the result of the compound structure of the intervertebral discs. The annulus contributes approximately half of the mass of the inter-body substance. Its layers follow a reinforced criss-cross pattern which tightens the hold on the contiguous bodies and also prevents the escape of nuclear material. The fibers extend directly down into the vertebral body, there being no layer of cartilage intervening in this arc. This attachment is so firm that it favors spur formation as a result of traction rather than central rupture unless unusual stress is applied. The annulus is strongly supported anteriorly by the anterior longitudinal ligament, but posteriorly this support is less. This configuration along with the flexion stress and vertical compression force favors posterior rather than anterior herniation of the nucleus. (See Figure 2–23.)

Cracks may occur in the annulus, the weak point for bulging or extrusion of the nucleus. The annulus is a powerful check ring for motion of one vertebral body on the other. In the mobile areas of cervical and lumbar spine, a constant gliding action at many levels is a composite contributor to flexion, extension, rotation and lateral bending. The annulus has significant control in all these actions.

Ligaments. Considerable support is obtained from ligaments in the neck and they play a relatively more important role in this area than elsewhere. The anterior longitudinal ligament on the front of the vertebral bodies limits extension and interbody gliding. It is firmly attached at the level of the annulus rather than at the center of the vertebral body. Several layers can be identified in shingle arrangement. This overlapping arrangement contributes strength, but the anchoring mechanism favors spur formation at the edge of the vertebral bodies.

The interspinous ligaments of the neck are amalgamated into a specialized ligamentous bow posteriorly, extending from the external occipital protuberance to the tip of the spinous process of C.7. This arrangement favors stress, being focused at the top or the bottom of the cervical spine. Avulsion of the C.7 spinous process is seen much more frequently than in any other of the cervical spines. Similarly, pain in the suboccipital region from tendon bone junction stress will be experienced much more at this level than in the central portion of the cervical region.

Motion

Many factors contribute to the mobility of the cervical spine. Loss of outrigging ribs, relatively thick discs and absence of laminar overlap all favor mobility. Two basic acts can be demarcated: the rotation of the head and neck; and flexion, extension and excursion. Separate mechanisms largely subserve these functions, and extremely specialized elements make them possible.

Rotation of the Head and Neck. The act is a composite one, with the rotation of the head for seeing and hearing being the vital maneuver. The neck turns in this process also, but it is a minor means to an important end. The cervical spine has a specialized upper segment consisting of occiput, atlas and axis that make it possible to rotate the head and neck and yet maintain vertical stability.

Head rotation occurs principally at the atlantoaxial joint. The atlas holds the head and rotates it on the odontoid as a pivot. The excursion is about 30 degrees to each side and is principally restricted by the short stout check ligaments that reach from the lateral tip of the odontoid to the inner side of the condyles of the occipital bone. Further excursion of rotation is then contributed by the cervical spine. (See Figure 2–24.)

The total act receives a contribution from the lower five cervical vertebrae. The configuration of the apophyseal joints, with an upward and medial angulation of the superior facet, favors a rotatory motion as the spine is angled laterally. Gliding at the interbody level occurs to assist this rotatory act.

Rotation is checked by the articular capsules of occipito-atlantal and atlantoaxial joints, the powerful odontoid check ligaments, the capsules of the lower cervical apophyseal joints, the Luschka joints and the interbody annulus mechanism (Fig. 2–24).

Flexion-Extension. Free flexion and extension occurs in both upper and lower units. Nodding of the head results from tilting of the occiput on the atlas. The condyles of the occiput are elongated convex ovals that ride in concave ovals of the atlas. The direction of fixation is forward and medially, which allows some long axis slipping as well as simple tilt but favors security. Two capsular and strong anterior and posterior atlanto-occipital ligaments and the locking of the superior atlas facets in the condylar fossae of the occipital bone check this motion.

Main extension and flexion excursion is made possible by the configuration of the articular facets at the lower five cervical vertebrae. The joints are angled at 45 degrees so that when a gliding element is added, the forward and backward motions, some rotatory effect results. The total range is 80 to 90 degrees, with flexion normally allowing the chin to reach the chest and, in extension, the occiput to come close to the shoulder line. The most mobile area is centered at the C.5, C.6 level.

Transmission (Function of Conveyance)

Vital structures are conveyed by the cervical spine, including the spinal cord, the cervical nerve roots and the vertebral artery. Anatomical design aids this function profoundly, and investigations show that pathological states may cause serious interference.

Spinal Cord. From the foramen magnum to the cervicothoracic junction the cord runs through a triangular section framework of the vertebral arches. It is suspended in cerebrospinal fluid and protected by the pia-arachnoid and the dura mater. The dura of the brain is thicker and has two layers. The outer layer becomes continuous with the periosteum at the foramen magnum; it is the inner layer that continues as the spinal dura.

There is sufficient room for movement of the cord so that, under some circumstances, dislocation of the atlas on the axis has been reported without serious cord damage. Less mobility is present at the level somewhat lower. Angulation at the lower border of the axis or a fracture dislocation at this level is likely to crush the cord easily, as has been demonstrated in the "hangman's" fracture.

Cervical Nerve Roots. Eight pairs of spinal nerves spring from the cord in the cervical region. They arise as anterior and posterior divisions; in each instance several filaments unite to form two bundles each before reaching the foramen and then coalescing into the spinal root. The sheath of the dura becomes continuous with the perineurium of the roots, forming a strong sleeve. The nerve root rests on the groove in the transverse process, the edge of which forms the usual fulcrum in brachial plexus avulsion.

Rupture of the root sleeve can be identified by contrast studies and, in some instances, is indicative of extensive root damage. However, such a conclusion cannot be made in all cases, because loss of continuity of the sleeve does not necessarily indicate complete rupture of the contents. Nor does avulsion at one level necessarily mean complete avulsion at another. An even application of the avulsing force is rare. The author has repeatedly observed incomplete root avulsion at operation when there has been some loss of continuity of the root sleeve.

The nerve supply of the foraminal area comes from the small meningeal branch which arises from the common spinal nerve after it exits from the foramen and then re-enters the foramen, reaching ligaments, blood vessels and cord coverings.

Progressive angulation of the roots occurs from above downward so that the course of seventh and eighth roots from the cord is more oblique than of C.3 and C.4. The roots arise opposite the vertebral body, but in descending a greater portion of the root will become related to the interbody level as one progresses from C.2 to C.8,7. For this reason a lower cervical spine disc herniation may implicate two roots more easily than at the higher levels.

Some observers (Abdulla, Bay) have identified motion of the cord within the vertebral canal and suggest that this may focus stress more acutely in some pathological states. The fact that the nerve roots progress in obliquity from above downward also influences this observation.

Vertebral Artery. The blood supply of vital neck structures, including bony spine, spinal cord, nerve roots, coverings and posterior cranial fossa and cerebral visual cortex, is derived from the vertebral arteries. The tortuous course they take and the susceptibility of their intimate coverings to structural change has placed them in a vulnerable position. In most instances the protective mechanism is amazingly adequate. However, when changes within the vessels such as atheromatous cracks develop, circulation may be compromised or temporarily obstructed.

The artery is intimately related to the joints of Luschka medially and the apophyseal joint posterolaterally, so that osteophyte formation at either site may encroach on its usual course. The efficiency of the vertebral artery system is related to the anastomosis with the circle of Willis from the internal carotid system. A weak point in one area may influence the other.

Contrast studies have been used to show that head and neck motion, principally rota-tion, may alter flow in the vertebral artery. Thus, Hutchinson and Yates have reported that pathological changes in the vertebral artery may favor ischemia. The flow between C.2 and C.6 may be followed on the same side to which the head and neck is turned and to the opposite vessel at the point the artery twists over the arch of the atlas. Changes in such a mechanism could explain transient attacks of a vertigo attributed to vertebrovascular ischemia (Fig. 12–5*B*).

PAIN PATHWAYS IN THE SHOULDER-NECK REGION

Pain is the important symptom of disease in the shoulder-neck region. The derangement of any component of this broad area may initiate it. There are patterns indicative of specific disorders that can be recognized, but in a broader sense there is a special distribution in certain ailments that also can be an aid in classifying the diseases of the region. Most disorders of this region can be identified from their pain distribution pattern: some disorders lead to purely neck discomfort; others clearly implicate the shoulder and neck; the third group are those implicating the shoulder joint proper; and the last group develops shoulder plus radiating pain. These broad clinical subdivisions also have an anatomical and physiological basis (Fig. 3–23).

Pain is a sensation impinging on consciousness as an impression of discomfort. A complex mechanism mediates it, but the parts of practical importance are the receptors and conductors of the sensation (Fig. 3–24). The receptors are bare nerve endings arising from sensory branches in the area. Special endings are not required to record the pain. They are imbedded in skin, fascia, muscle, tendon, ligament, periosteum, bone, joint capsule and synovium. They are much more abundant in the skin than in the deeper structures. Terminals of the same nerve branch extend to skin and periosteum, fascia or synovium. Branches divide and interlace so that the pain-receiving mechanism should be visualized as a network rather than as an individual fiber.

In addition to the bare terminals, more complicated arrangements are recognized in muscle, tendon and fascia. This is to be expected since muscle, for example, has special properties such as lengthening and shortening which require more specialized

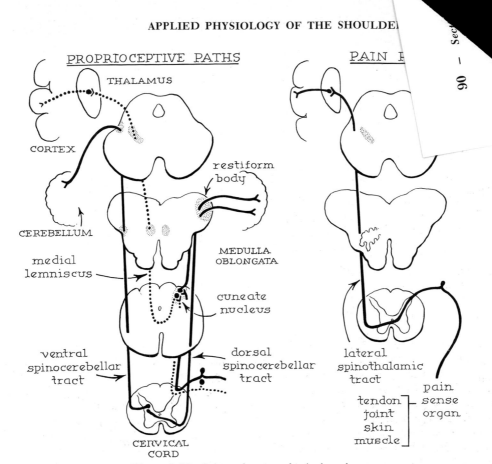

Figure 3–23 Pain pathways and spinal cord.

interpretation. Receptors record changes resulting from trauma, inflammation, degeneration, abnormal use, paralysis and many other irritants. Direct force stimulates nerve endings by pressure; so does the edema of inflammation. Stretch stimuli similarly arise from swelling and edema. Nerve endings also react to abuse such as scarring or roughening.

The segment for conducting pain extends from the nerve endings to the spinal cord. After supplying a given zone extending from skin to bone, the branch joins a peripheral nerve and so reaches the spinal cord.

In the spinal cord sensory pain fibers cross to the opposite side of the cord and ascend to the brain in this position. The sensation of pain is really a synthesized product and has a multiple origin. Pressure, stretching, cutting and compression are various combinations that may be interpreted as discomfort and recorded as pain. It remains for the sensation of localization and specific relationship to add qualifying specific properties. Keeping in mind common clinical syndromes, it is possible to classify the pain

mechanisms about the shoulder, which assists in identifying the pathological sources. Not all clinical conditions conform to a precise pattern but the majority do and, in the remainder, an understanding of the basic pain mechanism will be helpful.

PAIN MECHANISMS OF NECK AND SHOULDER-NECK DISORDERS

The sensation of neck pain enters by way of posterior rami of the cervical spinal nerves. The posterior rami, which are involved because they supply so much of the posterior soft tissues, divide into medial and lateral branches. The medial branches supply the skin and superficial layers, reaching the surface close to the cervical posterior spines or a little more laterally. The lateral branches supply the muscles such as the erector spinae. This means that irritation in this muscle group due to tension, stretching or bruising will be recorded in the same skin area.

The mechanism of pain from muscle deserves special attention. Bare sensory nerve

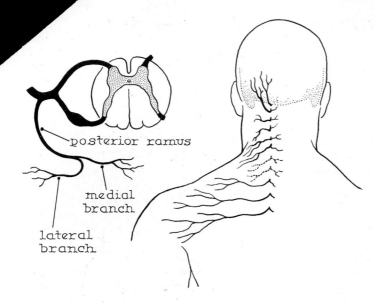

Figure 3–24 Innervation of shoulder and neck.

endings are in muscle and are abundant at a point close to the muscle insertions. They also infiltrate aponeurosis close to bone attachments. They are irritated by trauma and the reactive edema of injury. Repeated and extensive injuries stimulate fibrosis, and the endings become involved in the scar. Many cutaneous branches pierce the trapezius zone in particular at the root of the neck and are susceptible to irritation in extension-flexion injuries.

The posterior neck muscles are involved permanently in postural disorders. Constant stretching resulting from a slumped posture, sloped shoulders and spreading scapulae

evokes a dragging, aching type of pain. Specialized sensory nerve endings in muscle, tendon and fascia are particularly susceptible to stretch stimuli. Between muscle fibers there are spindle-shaped endings responding to passive pinching or stretching. These are not susceptible once the muscle begins to contract actively. This physiological explanation explains the frequently noted fact that pain in such ailments disappears once the muscles are used actively. These receptors have a low threshold and are acutely responsive to tension changes. There are other endings concerned with the total tension of the muscle which come into play in strong active

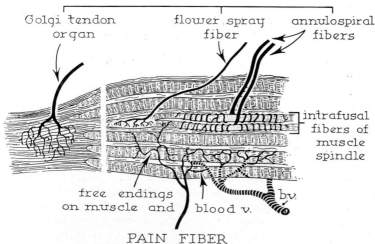

Figure 3–25 Postural pain mechanism.

PROPRIOCEPTORS

Golgi tendon organ   flower spray fiber   annulospiral fibers

intrafusal fibers of muscle spindle

free endings on muscle and   blood v.   b.v.

PAIN FIBER

POSTURAL PAIN MECHANISM

movements in contrast to the chronic but largely postural stimuli (Fig. 3–25).

Pain from muscle lesions has a diffuse quality which has been studied exhaustively by Kelogran. Injected noxious agents produce local pain but, in addition, discomfort is experienced at a distance in structures with the same segmental nerve supply. This is a logical explanation of the pain syndrome in disorders like fibrositis. Muscle spasm is also a contributor to the pain of purely muscular disorders. Irritation produces a tension response in the muscle, but there is an overreaction, with the spasm element persisting after the local irritation has subsided.

Referred Pain in Shoulder-Neck Disorders

The shoulder-neck area is a frequent site for pain referred from disorders occurring at a distance. Two important mechanisms are involved.

Disturbances of Emotion and Tension. The areas of the back of the neck and the root of the neck contain powerful suspensory muscles involved in support and balance of the head and also in suspension of the shoulder. These muscles function involuntarily. Disorders occurring apart from the area, for example, sinusitis, migraine headache or emotional tension, may lead to pain recorded in the shoulder-neck region. The mechanism of this pain has been investigated by Simmons-Day, Goodal and Wolfe, who have demonstrated that it is due to sustained, prolonged contraction of the powerful posterior muscles. For example, the injection of an irritating solution into the temporal muscle produces headache because of sustained contraction of the neck muscles

which splint the head region and so produces secondary neck-shoulder discomfort. A similar mechanism operates in lesions like persistent periodic headache or migraine, accounting for some of the shoulder-neck discomfort commonly seen in somewhat neurotic women.

Distant Lesions. The mechanism of pain referred to the shoulder and the root of the neck from intrathoracic and upper abdominal lesions has long been used as a classic example of referred pain. The undersurface of the diaphragm is supplied by the phrenic nerve derived from cervical segments 3, 4 and 5. These same segments innervate the cutaneous sensation in the neck-shoulder area so that processes irritating the undersurface of the diaphragm may be interpreted as pain in the neck-shoulder zone. Stimuli arising from the diaphragm reach the cord and are interpreted in the cutaneous supply of the same segments (Fig. 3–26).

Central lesions reflect pain into the neck and root of the neck; lesions to the center of the diaphragm cause discomfort between the neck and shoulder; and irritations near the lateral aspect are reflected at the point or tip of the shoulder. The pain is a dull ache, purely localized. Sometimes this sensation lasts after the primary and distant pathology have been controlled, suggesting the overlap for reinforcement mechanism of the internuncial pool within the spinal cord.

Local Anesthetic Action on the Pain Mechanism

The effective relief of pain from the injection of local anesthetic agents has been soundly established clinically. The pain is

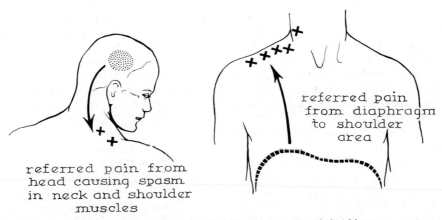

referred pain from head causing spasm in neck and shoulder muscles

referred pain from diaphragm to shoulder area

Figure 3–26 Paths of referred pain to neck and shoulder.

relieved directly at the irritating site, as is discomfort in more distant parts. This wide relief of pain has not been completely explained, but an analysis of the pain components and their cause throws some light on it.

The immediate effect of the anesthetic is to numb the nerve endings most insulted by the injury or irritating focus. This results in cessation of pain stimuli in the local region and also stops interpretation of the referred elements which is contributing to the diffuse nature of the pain. Muscle spasm also is decreased because of the lessening of tension stimuli on the special muscle spindle endings. Some of these endings have been shown to adapt very rapidly, particularly those identified with the fascial sheath of muscle, so that when pain stimuli have been interrupted, such as a pinching stimulus from a sensory organ, it is no longer admitted and the muscle is released from spasm. It has also been suggested that the innervation of certain endings in series as opposed to parallel is an explanation for the more widespread effect added to a purely local response. The combination of relief of local pain, referred pain and pain from the spasm accounts for the broad relief obtained from application of a local anesthetic.

PAIN MECHANISM IN PREDOMINANT SHOULDER DISORDERS

Two areas are to be considered in discussing pain caused by joint disorders. The way in which pain and joint disease is recorded, and analysis of the distribution of this record in the area.

Articular Pain Mechanism

Major nerve trunks passing a joint may send sensory twigs to articular and periarticular structures. Periosteum, tendon insertions and ligament attachments are copiously innervated. Nerve endings in these are particularly susceptible to stretch stimuli and have a threshold higher than the postural mechanism so that some definitely abnormal movement is required to irritate them. Pain and subluxations, for example, are common irritants that initiate pain through such a mechanism. The pain is localized to the joint area, but that is distinctly related when the more intimate joint covering or capsule or synovium has been involved.

Branches from the same nerves, in this

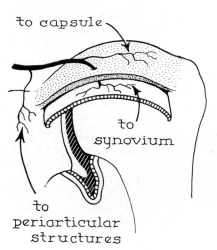

Figure 3-27 Intimate joint innervation.

case axillary, suprascapular, subscapular and musculocutaneous, reach the capsule and synovium as a fine network. The capsule is particularly well supplied, and twigs extend to the synovium along with minute blood vessels. The capsular supply pinpoints intimate joint disorder; the periarticular contribution has a less definite localization (Fig. 3–27).

Cutaneous Interpretation of Shoulder Joint Pain

Much discomfort from shoulder joint disease occurs apart from the obvious joint site over the upper end of the humerus. The site of the shoulder, the insertion of the deltoid, the medial aspect of the arm, the back of the deltoid and the immediately adjacent root of neck zone are examples. These parts record a dull aching type of pain different from the sharp, acute, articular sensation. Pain in the deltoid insertion is explained by the concentration of sensory endings of the muscle toward the insertion zones. The deltoid fibers converge to a highly packed point, concentrating sensory endings in a small zone, and more pain is experienced here than from the body of the muscle when any process irritates the muscle.

Clinical and experimental observations by Inman and Saunders further elucidate the less well localized aching pain. In mapping out the innervation of bone muscle and periosteum and relating it to spinal segments they found that this did not necessarily correspond closely with the cutaneous patterns of the same segments. This helps to explain pain patterns not adequately answered by the cutaneous distribution of peripheral nerve.

MECHANISMS OF RADIATING PAIN

Radiating pain is a common symptom, but in this discussion it is used to denote discomfort extending well beyond the shoulder into the forearm, hand and fingers. Many patients describe initial and moderate shoulder pain but quickly add the radiating element, indicating that this dominates the picture. Two distinct sources of such discomfort may be recognized, one neural and one vascular; they depend upon the type of disease involved.

Radiating Pain of Neural Origin

The common example of this type of pain is that due to herniation of a cervical intervertebral disc or some common nerve root syndrome. The sharp, lancinating, intermittent pain from the shoulder down to the base of the thumb, for example, is due to nerve root compression. The sensory root supplies an area of skin or dermatome and also a group of deep structures—muscles, tendons and bone. The superficial and deep patterns do not correspond accurately, so that the cutaneous discomfort is recorded in one area and deep, less well localized pain is interpreted in a slightly different zone (Fig. 3–28). The nerve roots most frequently involved in this process are C.6 and C.7. In the diagram it will be seen that much of the sensation of shoulder musculature is derived from C.6, and the skin distribution of the same root is along the forearm to the base of the thumb. This is one explanation of the deep shoulder discomfort encountered in some lesions. The distribution of the branches of the posterior division of these two roots is largely to muscle at the root of the neck—semispinalis, for example—and there is very little cutaneous supply. This favors the production of a deep postural type of muscular pain in this zone. The pain distributed like an electrical shock down the arm is due to compression of the cervical root. Maximum discomfort from this mechanism is then experienced in the zone of autonomous sensory supply.

Radiating Pain of Vascular Origin

A form of radiating discomfort that has a predominantly vascular etiology can be identified. In many disorders of the shoulder the great vessels may be implicated, with compression, traction, or both, initiating pain. The usual pattern is aching discomfort followed by a feeling of fullness in the finger; a prickly tingling occurs in the fingertip followed by numbness of the ends, with the sensation progressing proximally. Shortly there is stiffness and weakness in the fingers and hand which may progress to a total insensitivity and paralysis involving forearm and radius. Such numbness, weakness and tingling are familiar to anyone who has slept on his outstretched arm. These symptoms result from arterial and venous obstruction. The sense of fullness is due to venous stasis; the tingling results from the ischemia and paralysis; and then follows severe nerve ischemia. The distribution of the pain does not conform to peripheral nerve supply and starts at the tip of the finger.

Considerable work has been done by Wright in establishing a vascular basis for such pain. Observations on a group of patients showed that in 97 per cent alteration of the radial pulse was present in the involved side. Serious and prolonged defects result in loss of nerve function due to the ischemia.

Pain Pathways. The distribution of pain of vascular origin does not conform to the peripheral nerve supply (Fig. 3–29). Experimentally, nerve conduction fails after compression for 20 to 30 minutes, with the anoxia from the ischemia apparently being the source of pain. For some time it has been observed that ligation of vessels such as main arteries does not produce extensive pain. This has been explained by Lewis, who suggests that the pain arises from the muscles rather than the vessels. In Raynaud's disease the worst pain is associated with trophic disturbances; this tingling is due to deficient nutrition, which also accounts for the trophic ulceration. Usually it is the relief of ischemia that produces maximal pain, a sudden rush of warm blood into the extremity, similar to putting a cold hand under a hot water tap.

The recognition of this type of pain and understanding of its origin is important. The principal clinical components are an aching pain in the shoulder, arm and forearm with a feeling of numbness in the fingers or the

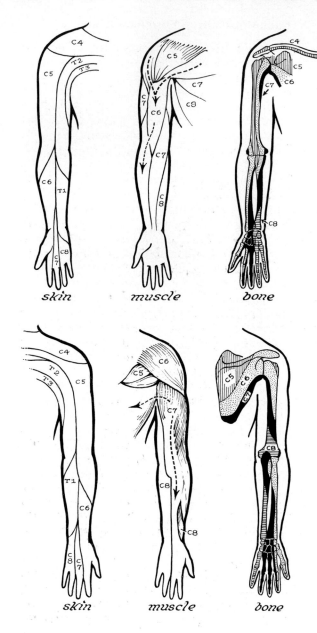

skin   muscle   bone

skin   muscle   bone

Figure 3–28 Comparison of segmental innervation of superficial and deep structures.

whole hand. The hand often feels quite limp. This phase is followed by tingling at the fingertips; then a feeling of burning or a prickly sensation develops in the proximal part of the fingers and the forearm. The cramp-like ache leaves and the extremity comes to life when the circulation is restored. Discomfort follows a different pattern from that of nerve damage and leaves a more diffuse impression harder to localize. Such authorities as Lewis and Lourish have written extensively on the etiology and mechanism of this pain. Out of the mass of discussions certain principles may be ac-

cepted; many have a practical and pathological basis but are less clearly established physiologically. From the standpoint of diagnosis and treatment of conditions producing this discomfort, the present explanation is useful, but more physiological research is needed to clarify the issues.

The main cause of this pain has been laid to irritation of the vascular bundle, which produces the peripheral alterations. In turn, sensory nerve endings are irritated, producing the pain. Vasoconstriction appears as a basic irritant in initiating the syndrome, but this action alone does not produce all the

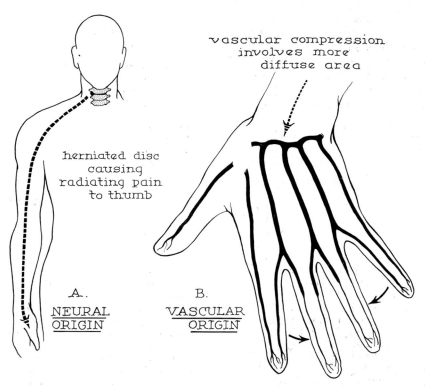

Figure 3-29   Neural versus vascular pain distribution.

peripheral pain. Vasoconstriction interferes with the local metabolic processes, which leads to stimulation of sensory endings. This occurs in the distribution of the vessels and, therefore, differs considerably from the peripheral nerve pattern.

Clinically, involvement of the central fingers or the whole hand rather than ulnar or median distribution is characteristic. Vascular etiology accounts for the difficulty in defining the painful region, for the intermittence and for the continuance of the discomfort. Pain follows the vascular distribution rather than peripheral nerve pathways.

The intermittent mechanism that irritates the nerve endings is controversial. Altered nutrition has been suggested as the cause of peripheral vasoconstriction and metabolic upset. The tingling which occurs in pernicious anemia is an example. The imbalance between vasoconstriction and vasodilation may also be a basic irritant. If the vasomotor upset has been established for some time, structural changes may be expected such as trophic ulceration, altered nail growth and shiny skin. This is not nearly so common as the more transient pain disturbances.

The trophic changes seen in nerve in-

juries have a vasomotor basis also but belong, like Raynaud's disease, to a group of serious disturbances. The cramp-like pain of which such patients complain occurs when activity is superimposed on the vasoconstriction; it is a further manifestation of muscular instability. This cramp-like pain becomes a feature in some disorders involving clavipectoral compression. Writer's cramp is a classic example. Many of these patients are engaged in occupations such as accounting and develop these symptoms because of the strain and tension caused by prolonged holding of the writing position, which favors mild vascular compression.

The precise etiology of vascular pain probably is related to the innervation of the minute vascular elements. Vasoconstriction has been the commonest explanation, and the reaction which ensues following injection of an artery has been used as support for this theory. In this procedure, spasm occurs and is followed by acute pain and then deeper pain which arises, according to Leriche, from the area of the vessels of distribution. It may be mediated by other factors, but the pars affecta is vascular rather than neural and comes from the whole distal territory of the vessel that has been stimulated. Nerve endings in the vasomotor elements are probably highly susceptible to the slightest change in circulation, and these are reflected immediately to the conducting pathways. Possibly some balancing action by the vasomotor nerves after the extremity is congested plays a part. The suggested sequence is obstruction, which leads to distention, which leads to vasoconstriction; nutritional changes follow, producing the pain. In Leriche's concept these physiological changes later become structural, initiating increased sympathetic upset.

REFERENCES

Bakey, L., et al.: Surgical treatment of vertebral artery insufficiency caused by cervical spondylosis. J. Neurosurg. *23*:596–602, 1965.

Cattell, H. S., et al.: Pseudosubluxation and other normal variations in the cervical spine in children. A study of one hundred and sixty children. J. Bone Joint Surg. *47A*:1295–1309, 1965.

Codman, E. A.: The Shoulder. Boston, published by author, 1934.

Colachis, S. C. Jr., et al.: Radiographic studies of cervical spine motion in normal subjects: Flexion and hyperextension. Arch Phys. Med. *46*:753–760, 1965.

Engen, T. J., et al.: Method of kinematic study of normal upper extremity movements. Arch. Phys. Med. *49*:9–12, 1968.

Goldie, I.: Calcified deposits in the shoulder joint produced by calciphylaxis and their inhibition by triamcinolone. An experimental model. Bull. Soc. Int. Chir. *24*:91–96, 1965.

Hohl, M., and Baker, H. R.: The atlanto-axial joint. Roentgenographic and anatomical study of normal and abnormal motion. J. Bone Joint Surg. *46A*:1739, 1964.

Hohl, M.: Normal motions in the upper portion of the cervical spine. An instructional course lecture of the American Academy of Orthopedic Surgeons. J. Bone Joint Surg. *46A*:1777, 1964.

Inman, V. T., and Saunders, J. B. de C.M.: Referred pain from skeletal structures J. Nerv. Ment. Dis. *99*:660, 1944.

Jung, A., et al.: The auricular disorders of unco-vertebral cervical arthrosis. Their treatment by uncusectomy and decompression of the vertebral artery in 15 cases. Ann. Chir *20*:181–194, 1966.

Leriche, R., and Jung, A.: Les calcifications sousdeltoidiennes de l'épaule, Rev. O'Orthop., *20*:289, 1933.

Lysell, E.: Motion in the cervical spine. An experimental study on autopsy specimens. Acta Orthop. Scand. Suppl. 123, 1969.

Markhashov, A. M.: Variations in the arterial blood supply of the spine. Vestn. Khir. Grekov. *94*:64–74, 1965.

Morehouse, L. E., and Cooper, J. M.: Kinesiology. St. Louis, The C. V. Mosby Co., 1950.

Munro, D.: The factors that govern the stability of the spine. Paraplegia *3*:219–228, 1966.

Popelianskii, I.: On the topographo-anatomical relationship between crescent processes of the cervical vertebrae and the vertebral artery in man. Arc. Anat. *48*:50–55, 1965.

Selye, H.: The experimental production of calcified deposits in the rotator cuff. Surg. Clin. N. Amer. *43*:1483–1488, 1963.

Southwick, W. O., and Keggi, K.: The normal cervical spine. J. Bone Joint Surg. *46A*:1767, 1964.

Wrete, M.: Sensory pathways from shoulder joint. J. Neurosurg. *6*:351, 1949.

Section
II

INVESTIGATION
AND DIAGNOSIS

Chapter IV

INVESTIGATION OF DISEASES AND INJURIES IN THE SHOULDER AND NECK

Many phases of management of shoulder and neck problems have improved, but nothing as yet has appeared to take the place of a proper history and meticulous physical examination in the identification of any of these disorders. As more is learned about the lesions in this region, even greater emphasis needs to be placed on these fundamentals of investigation. A formula or system is extremely helpful in sorting out these conditions, and the author has suggested that emphasis be placed on the precise delineation of the pattern of pain or discomfort of which the patient complains. The large number of injuries which fall into the suggested groups highlights the need also to carefully evaluate the mechanism of injury as it may have been applied to either the neck or the shoulder region. The physical examination follows accepted routines, but again a systematic assessment with accurate recording of the findings is essential if records are to be helpful both in the treatment period and for final assessment. Whenever possible, full use should be made of the special forms of advanced investigation with special x-ray studies, laboratory examination and electromyographic assessment. The more scrutiny given many of these lesions, the more useful do certain special aids appear.

THE HISTORY TAKING APPROACH TO CLASSIFICATION OF NECK AND SHOULDER DISORDERS

The presenting symptom in the majority of shoulder and neck problems is some form of pain. If this symptom is assessed carefully it may be a useful indicator for separation of the condition into one of the large groups, and then may be scrutinized more closely. Much can be gained from this approach, but it requires some practice to elicit the maximum amount of information from the patient.

PAIN PATTERNS

Specific pain patterns can be singled out that are suggestive of a general group of disorders. This should be elicited first and, when an individual category has been suggested, leading questions may be asked to more closely define one of the lesions in that group.

One group of patients will talk only of pain and stiffness in the neck that does not extend downward. Sometimes, however, there is extension of pain to the base of the skull or an accompanying headache. Such patterns probably indicate purely neck de-

rangements. Another group may talk of neck and shoulder pain and implicate the angle between the shoulder and the neck. Such a pattern is typical of another discrete collection. The commonest pattern involves the shoulder joint proper. With a considerable degree of certainty patients suffering from these lesions know the source of their discomfort and indicate it in typical fashion. A final characteristic pain pattern includes the shoulder, but tends to concentrate immediately on extension of the pain below the elbow to the hand and fingers.

Thus, the initial step in assessing the source of pain is to obtain a picture of the course and the pattern the pain follows; this primary sorting allows a minute inspection for the likely entity in a given group.

PAIN QUALITY

Differences in the intensity and quality of the pain can be recognized and are significant. Neck lesions tend to produce a chronic grumbling type of discomfort, and patients frequently try to avoid discomfort by holding the neck in one position. Patients with a postural type of pain rarely suffer any acute episodes. In contrast, patients with calcified tendinitis are subject to acutely disabling attacks alternating with a chronic discomfort of much less severity. Lesions with a neural background incorporate a sharp, extensive lancinating property and present intermittently.

EFFECT OF MOTION ON PAIN

Motion plays an important part in the discomfort that people experience from lesions in this whole region. Neck motion typically incites pain from disorders localized in this region, so that when patients have learned that pain is prevented by keeping the neck still, they often assume a characteristic attitude. Shoulder-neck disorders which implicate much of the suspensory mechanism to the girdle frequently are relieved by rest and aggravated by prolonged standing. Lifting the arm in abduction or flexion or attempting to get it above the shoulder typically triggers pain resulting from glenohumeral disorders. If the pain is not experienced until the shoulder is above a right angle but is still localized to this area, the acromioclavicular joint is implicated. Bending the head and

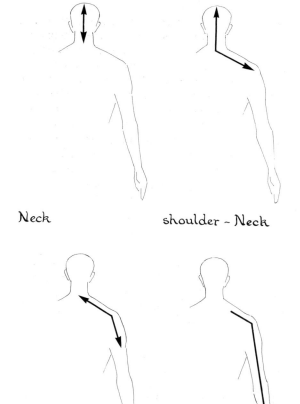

Neck   shoulder - Neck

Shoulder

Shoulder- radiating

Figure 4-1 Diagram of regional pain patterns.

neck toward the side of the pain are notorious irritants of the cervical root syndromes caused by extruded discs. Similarly, passive motion of the head and neck away from the side of the pain tends to aggravate scalene disorders.

INFLUENCE OF POSTURE AND OCCUPATION ON PAIN

Many complaints involving this region may be related to disorders of posture relevant to the upright position. Assumption of the vertical position has placed a load on this area not experienced in the lower animal forms. The neck balances the head and also supports it. The shoulder girdle is a suspensory mechanism, with heavy muscles and ligaments contributing to this suspension. The same structures participate in maintaining the balance of the head and controlling the neck, so that a constant interplay of use is focused on these elements. Normally balance is obtained, so that the effort required by one zone does not jeopardize the needs of the other. When the balance is disturbed, however, increased effort, particularly muscular, is called for and gradually impinges as a conscious process in the form of a postural pain (Fig. 4–2).

Severe deformity is not necessary to produce this complaint. The forward bent neck, slumped shoulder, drooping chest and protruding abdomen are the classic picture of poor posture. Just as this has been recognized as a contributor to low back pain, it should be appreciated that the same mechanism operates in relation to the cervicothoracic junction.

Further characteristics of this pain may be identified, such as the relief obtained by recumbency. Fatigue comes on usually toward the end of the day or with the approach of the maximum workload during the day. Often it is necessary to question the patient precisely in this regard, because the unsupported or slumped position at work, or a cramped position during sleep, may be intimately related to the patient's disorder.

Influence of Occupation

The patient complaining of discomfort in the shoulder-neck region should be questioned precisely regarding his occupation. Those who work long hours with the arms in an overhead position, like painters or decorators, may experience discomfort only in this position, but find it is relieved when they work at a lower level. Draftsmen may have persistent neck discomfort during working hours or toward the end of their working years, an effect which would be further aggravated by assumption of a cramped position in sleeping. Baseball pitchers may notice a twinge of pain at the end of the delivery of the ball, whereas golfers may notice it during the back swing. Patients with short stature develop numbness and tingling after they have been working at unaccustomed above-shoulder level for some time. These relationships are significant not only from the standpoint of diagnosis but also in clinical management (Fig. 4–3).

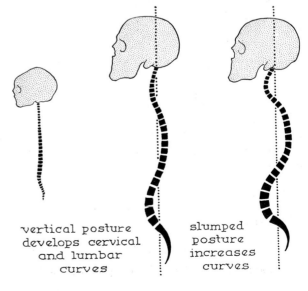

Figure 4–2 Foundation for postural shoulder-neck pain.

vertical posture develops cervical and lumbar curves

slumped posture increases curves

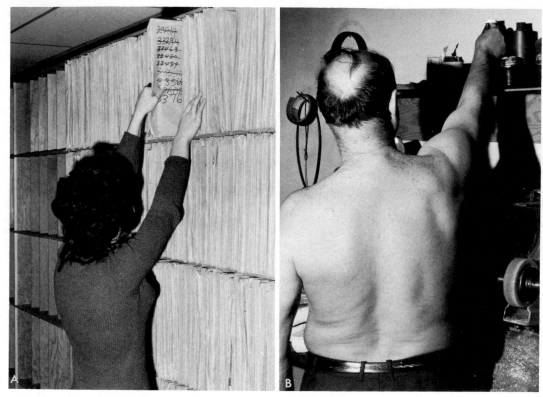

Figure 4–3   Influence of occupation.

RELATIONSHIP OF INJURY TO SHOULDER AND NECK DISORDERS

Determination of the manner in which an injury has occurred is extremely important in investigation of injuries of the neck and shoulder. A limitless variation of forces may be applied to this region; the patterns are compounded by the extensive mobility of the neck and shoulder system alone and in combination. These properties are in direct contrast to lower limb injuries, where the factor of stability plays such as important part and gives a structural sturdiness that repels or modifies many injuries. The upper limbs with their flexibility and resiliency, more often than not escape damage to the bony structures, but the soft tissues are involved with greater frequency. More careful assessment is required to identify this type of lesion.

The shoulder-neck is an exposed region, particularly in industry. Falling objects and blows from above strike this unprotected zone easily. The natural protective act of the workman in fleeing a falling object is to bend the neck forward and expose the pos-

terior upper portion of the back and shoulder region (Fig. 4–4).

In many instances the precise positioning of the arm and neck and their relationship to one another are particularly significant. It matters a great deal whether the brunt of the force falls in such a way that the body falls backward and is protected by an extended arm, or whether it falls forward and is protected by an outstretched arm. The position of the neck at the moment of impact in automobile accidents profoundly affects the distribution and severity of the damage. Similarly, the position of the neck when the brachial plexus is jeopardized by projectile tumbles is extremely important.

Many illustrative examples may be selected: A patient experiences a sudden pain in the shoulder that came on while he was lifting the hood of his car; it is due to the sudden twist of the joint into external rotation and involves the bicipital mechanism. A middle-aged workman who falls on his outstretched hand and, upon getting up, experiences sudden pain in the shoulder and inability to lift the arm from the side has probably ruptured his cuff. However, he may not feel that a description of these events is significant unless the examiner questions him specifically.

Sometimes there is no good history of injury, the patient being unable to remember a specific episode associated with the onset of discomfort. Questioning, then, should be directed toward the possibility that repetitive minor or less severe trauma is the cause of symptoms. Such repeated stress is less obvious but is common to many workmen such as bricklayers, pneumatic tool users or machinists who consistently work with some irritating movement or constantly lift objects in front of them. Housewives who iron clothes with great force transmit that force to the shoulder capsule; similarly, hod carriers sustain a constant downward traction force on the point of the shoulder. The significant injury may result from a routine act, and inquiry should be made as to how frequently this act is repeated.

Some indication of the severity of the reaction from the injury should be documented also. Was the patient able to carry on at his work, or did he have to stop? Did the pain become apparent the day following injury and become so severe that he could not carry on? Did the discomfort become so great that it was necessary for him to change his occupation completely.

PAIN THRESHOLDS

The tolerance of individuals to discomfort is an obvious variable. This is often more easily assessed in industrial accidents than in civilian cases. For the most part, patients put up with considerable discomfort before seeking help, but this may not always be so.

Functional disturbances with emotional overlay are often found in the shoulder-neck area. The chronic disorders of degenerative neck lesions and soft tissue shoulder irritants frequently are a basis for prolonged complaints, with little apparent structural change to justify them. For the most part, adequate reason can be found for chronic complaints, but sometimes overemphasis is encountered; this also can largely be identified by careful history taking. Psychiatrists can now conduct a scientific study of pain, using not only clinical assessment but also

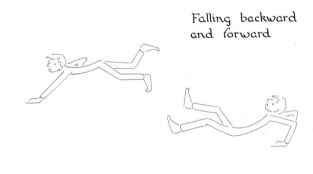

Falling backward and forward

Figure 4–4 Influence of mechanism of injury; example, cuff tears.

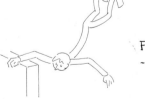

Falling with arm fixed - preventing rotation

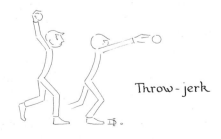

Throw-jerk

an examination under anesthesia. In many cases this type of assessment is extremely helpful, but it should still be coordinated with all the other findings.

GENERAL HEALTH

Significant information may be obtained by inquiring into the general health, previous injuries or illnesses, and possible associated complaints. The age of the patient is significant. Up to 30 years of age, the usual impairments in this region are associated with some form of injury or obvious developmental deformity. In the range of 30 to 60 years, during the period of greatest productivity, occupational disorders are more prominent; toward the end of this period the effects of degeneration are superimposed. From 60 years on the acute incident resulting from less serious trauma is prominent, but to this must be added frequent disorders of the systemic state. No investigation is complete without a thorough examination of the patient.

EXAMINATION OF THE NECK AND SHOULDER

So many disorders implicate both the neck and shoulder that it is good practice to automatically assess both when complaints implicate either.

EXAMINATION OF THE NECK

On external inspection the contour and general proportions are automatically noted. Considerable variation in the length of the neck occurs, the long giraffe-like development contrasting sharply with the short, thick-set variety. Both have propensities for certain cervical disorders. Specific assessment of the neck is best carried out from the back. Palpation identifies tender areas and

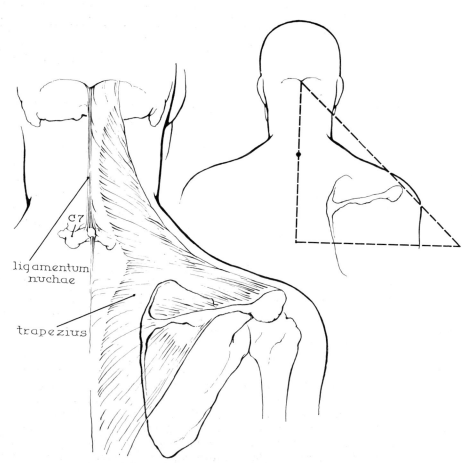

ligamentum nuchae

trapezius

Figure 4–5 Surface markings from the back.

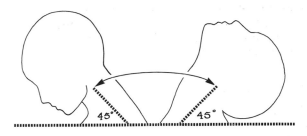

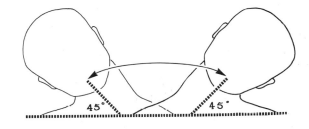

Figure 4–6 Diagram of range of neck motion. Combination of flexion-extension, lateral bending and rotation.

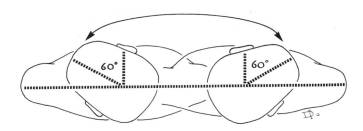

their relationship to bony points. Palpate the central posterior spines up and down, looking for tenderness, crepitus or abnormal mobility, or altered contour. Palpate the paraspinal zones seeking tender points, spastic zones or trigger points in the muscle and hypersensitivity of the transverse processes. Atrophy of the cervical erector spinae is automatically noted, as is any spasm, resistance or increased muscle tension as the area is palpated. The slope of the shoulder margin from the back is significant. The right angle configuration may be accentuated, as, for example, in trapezius paralysis, or it may have a decided apical sloping pattern suggestive of postural atony.

The principle in examining this area is to start in the middle and extend to the sides, assessing the consistency, tension, strength and action of the heavy suspensory muscles on each side (Fig. 4–5). The suboccipital zone is assessed for tender areas, too. Sensitive zones related to the attachment of the muscles to the skull are particularly important. Motion of the cervical spine is estimated actively and passively. There are special in-

struments designed to measure neck motion accurately; these are protractors fitted to a head band.

Normally the range of extension and flexion of the neck is 90 degrees, and this is evidenced by the patient's being able to touch the chin to the chest and the back of the head to the region of the first thoracic spinous process. Side to side or lateral bending is a little less than 90 degrees in combination (Fig. 4–6).

The front of the neck should also be examined. The boundaries of the posterior triangle of the neck are defined with the trapezius posteriorly and the sternomastoid anteriorly. Streaming through the middle of this triangle are the trunks of the brachial plexus, which can be felt 2 to 3 inches above the clavicle if the head and neck are tilted gently to the opposite side (Fig. 4–7). Just above the medial third of the clavicle, the subclavian pulse is identified by pressing firmly at the border of the sternomastoid. Medial to it and superiorly, the carotid artery can be palpated. This sequence of palpation leads the hand naturally to the sterno-

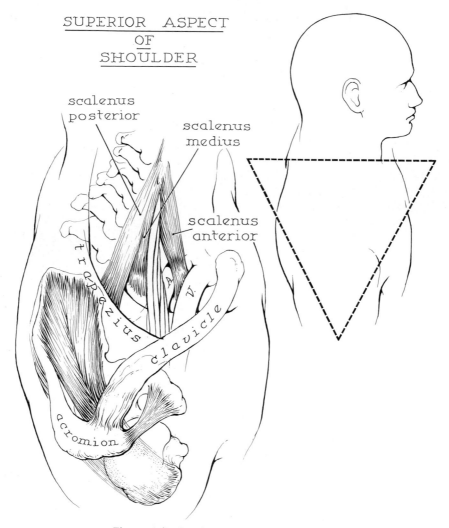

SUPERIOR ASPECT
OF
SHOULDER

Figure 4–7 Landmarks of neck from the top.

cleidomastoid muscle, which should be tested in the relaxed and tense positions. The clavicular attachment is felt and its anchorage to the mastoid process is assessed.

In the midline the act of swallowing should be assessed. The scalene point is identified 1 inch above and medial to the sternal end of the clavicle; pressure here will identify a cervical rib when it is present.

EXAMINATION OF THE SHOULDER SYSTEM

The shoulder is really a system of joints, of which the glenohumeral mechanism is but one entity in the center of four satellite articulations (Fig. 4–8).

General Impression of the Area. One automatically notes the general body pos-

ture related to shoulder girdle — whether it is slumped, erect or curved. The body build is also obvious. A short, squat, thick-necked workman contrasts markedly with a tall, thin, frail woman. The relationship of the shoulder girdle to the chest should be particularly noted. The erect, well-muscled laborer contrasts with the relaxed, slumping teen-ager or frail housewife with chin down, shoulders forward, scapulae spread and chest flattened. After these observations on general body habitus, attention is turned to the shoulder region proper.

The patient may walk into the office holding the affected extremity rigidly to the side, making use of the hand by moving it from the elbow. Such a posture is usually typical of acute glenohumeral involvement. Important observations can be made as the patient takes off his clothing or attempts to undo a blouse or remove a shirt. The clothes may have been completely removed without evoking complaint, and yet on examination there is voluntary limitation of movement.

After these observations on automatic or spontaneous shoulder movement, specific ranges of motion and critical areas are assessed. The patient should be asked to do the best he can to lift the arm in forward flexion, backward into extension, then to abduction and, finally, into circumduction if this is feasible. He should shrug the shoulder in an attempt to touch his ear; brace the shoulder backward; bend the neck forward, backward, laterally; and rotate the chin. Any arcs of pain evinced by this performance should be examined more carefully.

Abduction and Circumduction. This is the arc of shoulder motion most significantly impaired in many shoulder disorders. Typically, when the glenohumeral mechanism is disturbed, a girdle type of motion develops; this is best seen from the back. In this maneuver, the normal effortless swing of the arm upward or sideways is replaced by a hunching of the shoulder. The scapula and humerus move as if glued together and the arm moves slowly and weakly to less than the midpoint of the normal range (Fig. 4–9).

Frequently efforts to further elevate the extremity are accompanied by a tilt of the head and the neck to the opposite side (Fig. 4–10). A few more degrees of abduction are added by this maneuver, but this results from movement of the shoulder girdle as a whole and not further abduction at the glenohumeral joint. In recent injuries to the rotator cuff, a catching sensation is appreciated by the patient; as the arm comes to below a right angle, abduction and external rotation produce a momentary catching spasm. As the head of the humerus dips under the coraco-acromial arch, this pain from impingement increases. In long-standing injuries or in extensive full-thick-

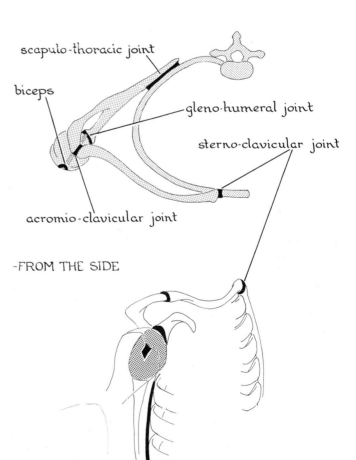

Figure 4–8 Diagram of shoulder system from above and from the side.

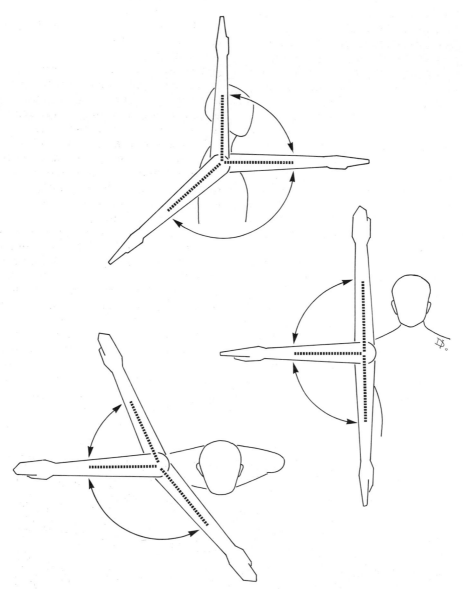

Figure 4–9 Normal range of shoulder motions.

ness cuff defects, further abduction is not feasible and further attempts at motion implicate the whole girdle, indicating a disrupted pattern (Fig. 4–11).

In contrast, patients with acromioclavicular disturbances most often experience discomfort after the arm is abducted to a right angle and, characteristically, no difficulty is encountered in reaching this point. If the patient is then asked to rotate the arm across the chest at a right angle, the discomfort is accentuated.

Passive Motion. Passive motion and assisted active motion should also be carefully assessed. This examination is best carried out with the patient sitting sideways on the chair and the examiner standing behind or at the side. He grasps the flexed elbow, placing his other hand over the shoulder (Fig. 4–12). Forward movement, backward movement and rotation are then tested, with the humeral head being palpated by the opposite hand. If voluntary motion has demonstrated a painful arc, this is left to the last and the arm is gently abducted and rotated into the painful zone. The palpating hand notes the movement of the head of the humerus and automatically feels the scapula also. In this fashion the typical frozen shoulder can be demonstrated. Laxity of the head of the humerus in the capsule is assessed by placing the thumb over the head of the front and using the fingers to grip the posterior part of the head of the humerus. With the examining hand in this position, pressure by the thumb can shove the head backward and forward with a springing action.

Assessment of excursion of the head of the humerus in the glenoid is extremely important in disturbances such as recurrent subluxation. The movement is also vitally important in examining for anterior or posterior recurrent dislocation. When the capsule is particularly lax posteriorly but the head cannot be shoved too far forward, it is strongly suggestive of a posterior recurrent subluxation.

Tenderness over the upper end of the humerus is identified by firm pressure, usually by pulling the arm into slight extension so that more of the upper surface of the cuff is exposed in front of the acromion. Crepitus is looked for when the head of the humerus is rotated under the examining finger. In some instances firm pressure through the deltoid will give the suggestion of subjacent defects in the cuff; as the humerus is rotated under the examining finger, the roughened zone may become more apparent. Snapping or clicking sounds related to shoulder movement are often apparent. When the clicking sensation is related to passive rotation of the head of the humerus, it is the subacromial bursa or adjacent zone of the rotator cuff which is at fault. When the clicking sound can be produced only by the patient's moving the arm himself in rotation, there often is an element of anterior prominence of the head of the humerus accompanying it which is highly suggestive of a subluxing joint. A clicking sensation that can be traced

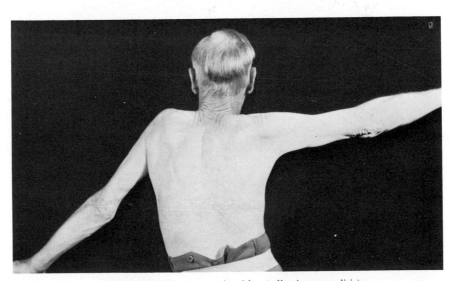

Figure 4–10 Frozen shoulder (adhesive capsulitis).

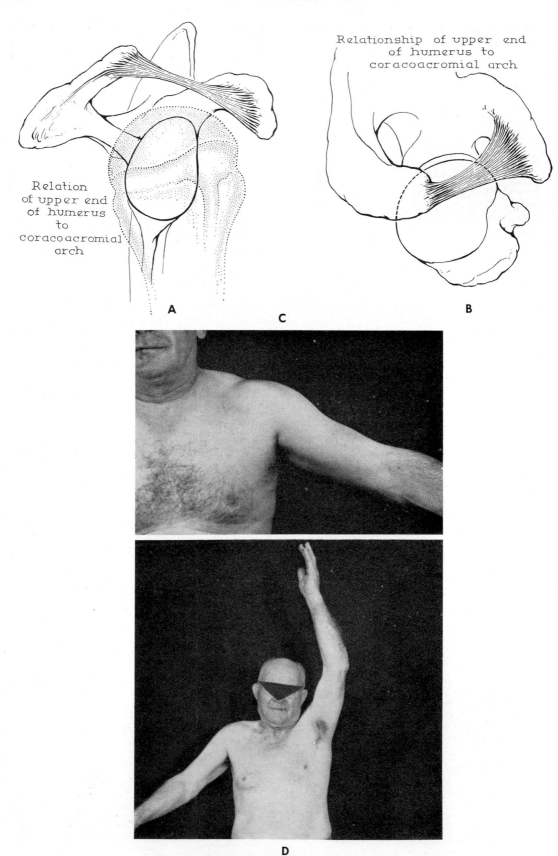

Figure 4–11 Point of impingement.

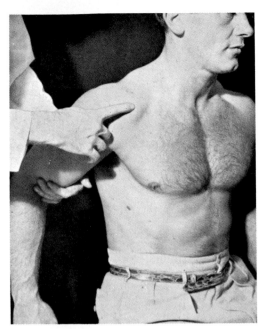

Figure 4–12 Examination of upper end of the humerus.

to the acromioclavicular joint, which is also painful on palpation, may be produced by abduction above a right angle; this suggests internal derangement of the acromioclavicular joint, subluxation or osteochondritis. The most obvious example of snapping shoulder results from luxation of the long head of the biceps, which often presents a loud snap as the shoulder is rotated internally and externally with the arm at a right angle.

Bicipital Area

Careful study should always be made of this area in shoulder disorders. The initial assessment is carried out by the examiner's identifying the bicipital groove between the two tuberosities, with the examining finger digging through the anterior aspect of the deltoid as the opposite arm passively rotates the head of the humerus. Tenderness in this region is noted, as is crepitus. A maneuver of particular importance is lifting the arm at the side and palpating the bicipital groove with one hand while the other passively rotates it upward and downward. It is in such a maneuver that luxation or dislocation from the groove of the long head of the biceps can best be identified. This often occurs with a definite clicking sensation (Fig. 4–13).

Various tests for the continuity and function of the long head of the biceps have been developed. This tendon really has a somewhat stationary or steadying effect on the head of the humerus in that the humerus moves on the tendon, rather than the tendon contracting and moving on the humerus. Roughening of the groove in which the tendon lies, or a fraying of the fibers of the tendon, can sometimes be identified by having the patient flex the elbow and supinate the forearm against resistance. However, this maneuver is not always reliable. Function of the tendon is also tested by resistance against forward flexion of the shoulder; when the long head is ruptured, considerable weakness in this act can be demonstrated if function is compared with the opposite side.

Acromioclavicular Joint

An often overlooked but clinically important area lies at the lateral end of the clavicle. The acromioclavicular joint is a constantly used and abused accessory articulation of the glenohumeral mechanism. It should always be carefully examined (Fig. 4–14). Any abnormal configuration such as enlargement or malalignment should be noted.

The joint line is felt by pressing up on the

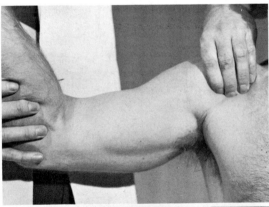

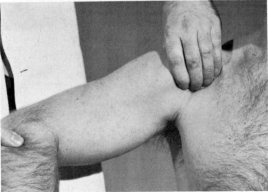

Figure 4–13 Examination of biceps apparatus.

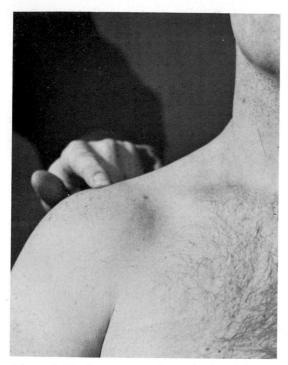

Figure 4–14 Examination of acromioclavicular joint.

elbow with the arm at the side and the palpating finger over the lateral end of the clavicle. The patient should be checked for any complaint of pain referred to this area when the humerus is abducted without rotation. Pain should also be tested for by passively pushing the arm across the chest at the horizontal level; pain during this maneuver is highly typical of acromioclavicular disorders. Crepitus or luxation can often be felt on any of these maneuvers. Force applied across the body is focused on the acromioclavicular joint, and the sideways compression will be resisted by this compound strut of acromion and clavicle. In this fashion, luxation of the clavicle above the acromion may occur.

In flexion of the arm the scapula rotates around the outer end of the clavicle; in young patients considerable anteroposterior play can be demonstrated after certain injuries. This is best evaluated by shoving the acromion forward with one hand and steadying the clavicle with the opposite hand so that this anteroposterior luxation is reproduced. As this act is carried out, discrepancy in the level of the outer end of the clavicle with the articulating zone of the acromion will sometimes become apparent and is suggestive of recurrent subluxation.

Scapulocostal Mechanism

The scapula, its bed and its coverings play a part in many common pathological states of this region. Both neck and shoulder structures are intimately integrated. The important structures are soft tissues such as heavy muscles and thick ligaments. The scapula swings on an arched track over the upper eight ribs. The thin vertebral body border insinuates between the layers like a blunt probe. Muscle root attachments of the rhomboids and serratus creep onto this border, and if these elements become frayed, a palpable crepitus develops. In assessing this region the medial border of the scapula is palpated with the flat of the hand as the arm is moved actively and passively from the side. The area at the base of the spine of the scapula is assessed in particular during this maneuver (Fig. 4–15).

The rhythm of the scapula should be observed because it is an indicator of proper glenohumeral function. If it is obviously distorted, as in cuff tears, a typical girdle or shrugging rhythm replaces the normal well anchored swing of the arm. In paralytic lesions, such as involvement of the accessory or long thoracic nerves, fixation of the scapula is markedly deranged so that the posterior border swings free, pointing laterally in the former condition and almost directly backward in the latter.

The trapezius is an extremely important muscle in neck-shoulder action; it may be implicated in derangements of either neck or shoulder because it works on both levers. Function of this strong accessory muscle may be assessed by palpation of the medial attachment, the ligamentum nuchae and the

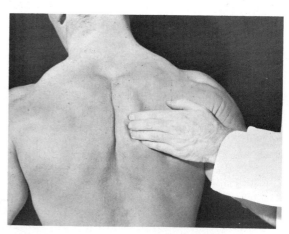

Figure 4–15 Scapulocostal mechanism.

posterior cervical spinous processes (Fig. 4–16). Trigger points in this attachment to the spine of the scapula and posterior spinous processes are identified. Deformity of the upper medial border of the scapula and, in particular, curling of the edge produces a particularly coarse grating. This noise or snapping effect is accentuated by the thoracic cage, which then acts as a sounding box, perceptibly increasing the audibility.

Sternoclavicular Joint

Abnormalities of the sternoclavicular joint are easily overlooked. Sometimes the soft tissue padding conceals deformity of the sternoclavicular area, so it is a zone that should be included in the routine investigation of the shoulder system. This zone should be assessed particularly in any shoulder with restriction of motion. Arthritic processes commonly enlarge and roughen the medial end. The medial end of the condyle should be palpated by digging the fingers in the sternoclavicular junction, grasping the bone and directly testing its mobility. Comparison should be made with the contours of the opposite side, because it is extremely rare that both sides are involved in a pathological process at the same time (Fig. 4–17).

The common distortion is one in which the medial end of the clavicle rides above the sternal notch. It often has a bulbous enlargement, and this may project posteriorly and superiorly. After injury the whole medial end may be riding medially out of the notch in the sternum.

Important structures adjacent to the

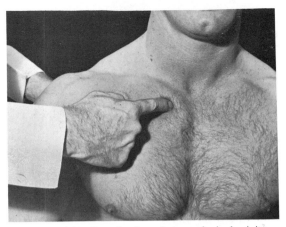

Figure 4–17   Examination of sternoclavicular joint.

sternoclavicular joint should also be assessed: the attachment of sternocleidomastoid, carotid pulsation, subclavian pulsation and, finally, the scalene point above and just lateral to the sternoclavicular articulation. Sometimes inspection of the joint from the front does not show the distortion and it is necessary to look at the chest from the side or obliquely to detect the anterior displacement of the medial end of the clavicle.

Testing Motor Power

Assessment of innervation of the main muscles about the shoulder should be an integral part of the investigation, particularly in injuries. Special equipment is not essential since simple clinical assessment by palpation and muscle tensing can localize most significant defects. Some important muscles can be singled out for particular attention, and examination thereof should be part of the routine of assessment of this region.

Trapezius. The trapezius forms the sloping angle of the shoulder and contributes significantly to the stability of the whole upper limb. Paralysis is not uncommon and can easily be missed on simple external inspection because of the filling in by the soft tissues. Suspicion of the lesion should be aroused by alteration in the contour at the back of the shoulder. The normal sloping angle is lost and is replaced by a much sharper right angle appearance. Often the patient himself has noticed the flattening of the shoulder blade. The patient is asked to lift the point of the shoulder to touch his ear, and one examining hand acts as resistance on the point of the shoulder and the

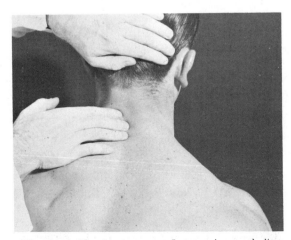

Figure 4–16   Assessment of trapezius and ligamentum nuchae.

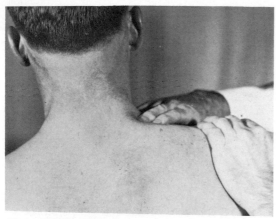

Figure 4–18 Testing for motor power in trapezius.

other hand palpates the suspensory fibers (Fig. 4–18).

Serratus Anterior. Weakness or paralysis of this muscle seriously hampers rotatory control of the scapula and loosens the fixation of the scapula to the chest. The muscle is tested by exerting pressure with the forward placed arm, at the same time palpating the medial border for posterior displacement (Fig. 4–19).

Deltoid. The state of this important muscle is automatically assessed on inspection, and atrophy is usually quite apparent; however, paralysis of part or all of it can be overlooked. It is tested by palpating the fibers with one hand as the arm abducts against resistance from the other. The anterior por-

tion is tested by resisting forward flexion and the posterior part by resisting extension. The muscle fibers must be palpated and tested against resistance since abduction is possible by accessory muscles, and loss of this action alone is not a reliable index of the deltoid function (Fig. 4–20).

Latissimus Dorsi. One of the least commonly involved muscles in the upper limb is the latissimus dorsi. It is tested by the examiner's holding the arm under the elbow and having the patient press down toward the side; with the opposite hand the examiner palpates the broad tendon as it crosses the posterior axilla (Fig. 4–21).

Spinati. Particular attention should be given to the supra- and infraspinati. Atrophy and loss of substance are easily noted on inspection. Specific contraction of these muscles is obtained by having the arm at the side palm forward and performing internal and external rotation of the glenohumeral joint (Fig. 4–22).

Pectoral. Some injuries, particularly those involving the brachial plexus, may implicate these muscles; their assessment may be important. They are tested for resistance to adduction and forward flexion at the glenohumeral joint, with the opposite hand of the examiner palpating the muscle fibers (Fig. 4–23).

Sternomastoid. The sternomastoid is often an important structure both from the standpoint of a landmark and for its contribution to abnormalities of structure and function in this region. The muscle is investigated by palpating the sternal attachment with one hand, applying resistance to tilting of the chin in the opposite direction with the opposite hand. The muscle is palpated along its length from the clavicular attachment to the tip of the mastoid process. Assessment of the continuity of its substance is particularly important in children because scarring and fibrous contracture produce the typical wry neck deformity and eventual facial asymmetry (Fig. 4–24).

Testing for Sensory Defects

Disturbances in sensation are much less common in the shoulder region than are alterations in muscle innervation. The supraclavicular nerves are sometimes injured in incisions made parallel to the clavicle. These may leave tender scars with embedded neuromata producing an unpleasant radiating

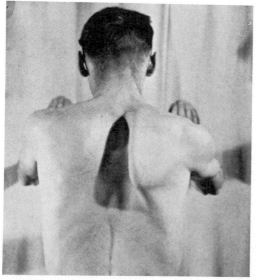

Figure 4–19 Testing for power in serratus anterior.

A

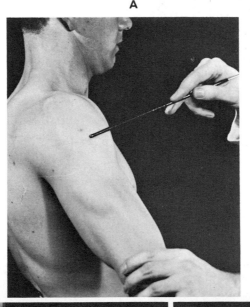

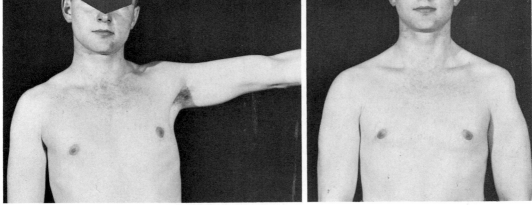

B

Figure 4–20 *A*, Proper method of testing deltoid. *B*, Assessing abduction alone is insufficient. Accessory muscles may give a degree of abduction when deltoid is paralyzed as above.

burning type of pain. Touch appreciation is diminished below the incision and patients complain of the unpleasant burning sensation. The neuromata can be palpated in the scar. Injuries in the region of the posterior triangle may implicate the great auricular and lesser occipital nerves. Radiating pain extending up to the ear or behind the ear, sometimes related to the mastoid process, may result. Some superficial diminution of light touch in these areas can be identified.

Paralysis of the posterior circumflex nerve or the axillary trunk leaves an area of hypesthesia over the lateral border of the deltoid about 2 inches below the acromion. Response to touch and pinprick should be assessed in this area in injuries such as anterior dislocation of the shoulder. When there is any suggestion of plexus involvement, sensation in the hand should be assessed. Alteration in appreciation of touch along the lateral border of the forearm is suggestive of lateral cord involvement; involvement of the median distribution implicates the medial cord; and hypesthesia along the fifth finger implicates the ulnar and medial cord also.

Electrical Investigation. Assessment of muscle action by electrical means has assumed a progressively significant role. The frequent implication of nerves in this area makes this study particularly important. Several separate entities may require assessment: investigation of muscles in cases of nerve involvement; testing muscle function apart from nerve damage; and investigation of patients suspected of malingering.

INVESTIGATION OF NERVE INJURIES. The response of muscle substance to electrical

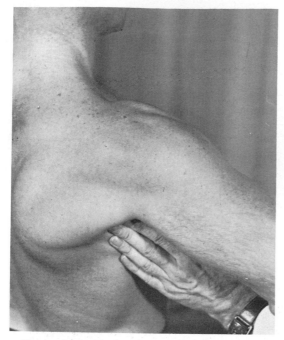

Figure 4–21 Testing the latissimus dorsi action.

stimulation varies according to the type of current used and the site to which this current is applied. Indirect faradic or induced current elicits a muscle response only when it is applied at the point of entrance of the motor nerve into a given muscle. It is dependent on the connection of that nerve to the muscle being intact and undamaged. If the physical state of the conducting nerve is altered as a result of cutting or crushing, there will be no conduction of the current to the muscle and no response in the muscle. Such loss of response to a faradic, induced or interrupted current is highly suggestive of significant damage to the nerve supply. When the nerve has been repaired and regeneration has occurred the response will return, but, peculiarly enough, voluntary power can sometimes be demonstrated before the faradic response develops.

The assessment with a direct or galvanic current is on quite a different basis. This type of current stimulates muscle substance directly so that it may be applied at any point, and a reaction of the muscle will occur as long as there are muscle fibers present with sufficient health to contract. When degeneration of the fiber substance has occurred or denervation has been present for so long that the muscle substance is replaced by fatty tissue, no response can be obtained. Persistent loss of response to direct or galvanic current connotes serious nerve and muscle damage. In some instances, however, if the direct current is applied repeatedly, after a period of days, or sometimes weeks, some reaction can be obtained from the muscle. When both faradic and galvanic response have been lost, there is no longer any functioning nerve or muscle.

MUSCLE ASSESSMENT IN CASES OTHER THAN NERVE INJURIES. Electrical stimulation is a help in assessing the continuity of various muscles apart from paralytic disorders. If stimulation to a given muscle results in contraction and movement similar to the usual voluntary pattern, the attachments are likely

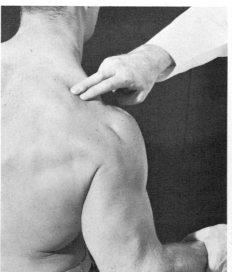
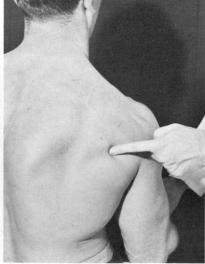

Figure 4–22 Testing spinalis muscles.

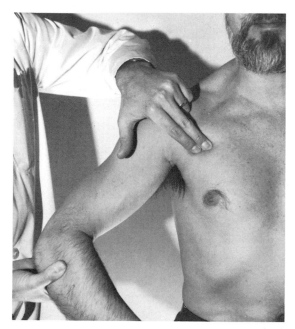

Figure 4-23 Testing pectorals.

intact. When normal movement is not initiated or is very weak, some alteration of the muscle attachments may be suspected. For example, the biceps may be stimulated and, normally, no pain in the region of the long head is experienced; if pain develops on stimulation, it occurs apart from movement of the shoulder so that specific discrete action of the biceps must then be responsible for the

pain since other capsular structures are not implicated. Such a response is suggestive of bicipital disorder. The muscles about the shoulder which commonly may need such electrical testing are trapezius, deltoid, pectoralis, biceps and spinati.

Trapezius. Accessory nerve injuries are not uncommon and result in trapezius paralysis. In assessing the response in this muscle the examiner should be careful not to confuse contraction of the rhomboids or levator scapulae as action of the trapezius. The motor point for faradic testing is just below the lateral fold along the upper border where the accessory nerve dips into the muscle.

Deltoid. Electrical stimulation and assessment of the deltoid is often needed since it is the most frequently paralyzed muscle about the shoulder. The motor point for faradic stimulation lies at the back at the midpoint of the posterior border where the posterior circumflex branch enters the muscle. Galvanic or direct current assessment may be carried out at any point in the muscle.

Biceps. Paralysis of the biceps is not common, but it may be helpful sometimes to stimulate contraction in the muscle to assess its reaction and its relationship to other tissues. Isolated action of this muscle is helpful in diagnosing bicipital disorders. The motor point for faradic stimulation lies about 2 inches below the coracoid, with the electrode being placed under the edge of the medial border of the deltoid.

EXAMINATION FOR MALINGERING. Some patients are encountered in whom one suspects that the responses have an element of voluntary restraint or the patient is deliberately refractory. Gross malingering is rare, but reluctance in certain movements, particularly when the patient is involved in negotiations, is not uncommon. Under these circumstances it is most helpful to use an electric current to stimulate muscle response. A faradic current is used and it is often possible to produce a greater range of motion than the patient will present on a voluntary basis. Sometimes the method has a decidedly beneficial effect on the patient also. In some instances the patient is encouraged by seeing the given muscle work, or the examination so conclusively exposes his refractoriness that this attitude is abandoned.

ELECTROMYOGRAPHY. Precise assessment of minute muscle changes can now be done with the electromyograph, and this means of assessment now constitutes a most accurate

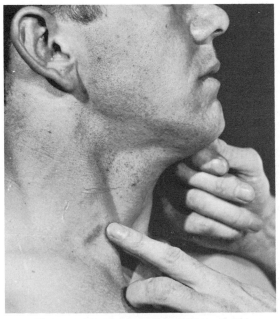

Figure 4-24 Testing sternocleidomastoid.

examination. The principle of the electromyograph is magnification of the small electrical changes that occur in muscle when it contracts; these are recorded on a cathode ray oscillograph for study. The apparatus exists of a preamplifier, an oscilloscope, a speaker and a camera. Permanent records are possible with the use of a camera, but the study comprises both visual and auditory assessment of the electrical response (Fig. 4–25).

In normal muscle at rest no electrical potentials can be recorded, but when it contracts, minute potentials or motor unit action potentials are produced of sufficient strength and duration that they can be recorded on the oscillograph. The pattern which these changes produce is very much like that of a typical electrocardiograph record. Since voluntary contraction is under voluntary control, these potentials are produced by a voluntary action. Paralyzed muscle, on the other hand, has a completely different electrical pattern, there being no motor unit action potential possible; instead there are much smaller uncontrolled action potentials which are known as fibrillation action potentials. Normal MUAP's present a broad deflection in contrast with the small FAP's. When the nerve supply or muscle is damaged, fibrillation develops and replaces the normal motor unit action potential picture. As the muscle starts to recover, a form of motor unit action potential called a nascent potential gradually develops, replacing the fibrillation changes. This examination is extremely useful in diagnosing nerve injuries and also in assessing the stage of recovery after a nerve has been repaired. It is feasible to record electrical changes with the oscilloscope at a much earlier date than by any other form of investigation in assessing regeneration following repair.

In addition to aiding in investigation and prognosis of nerve injuries the apparatus is useful in investing many other neurological disorders. Nerve root lesions, muscular dystrophies and all similar related disturbances can be assessed. The apparatus has also been extremely useful in the investigation of the physiology and action of different muscles in the patterns of limb motion. In the shoulder, for example, abduction has long been thought to be dependent upon the supraspinatus, but electromyographic studies show conclusively that the instant abduction is started, the deltoid contracts too, so that this movement results from a combined and coordinated effort of both muscles.

Technique of Electromyographic Investigation. Electromyographic investigation is neither painful nor time-consuming. The apparatus in common use is shown in Figure 4–25. If many examinations are being done, a screened room is preferable to eliminate interference, but this is not essential. For examination of the shoulder the patient sits on a stool close to the machine, and a ground electrode is applied to the forearm. Two electrodes are used in relation to the muscle

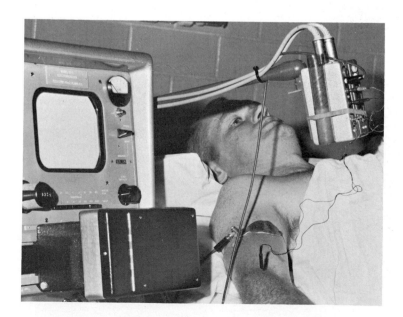

Figure 4–25 Electromyograph. Cathode screen, camera recording and multiple electrodes.

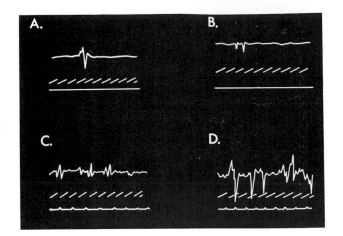

Figure 4–26 Electromyographic tracings. *A,* Normal motor unit action potentials. *B,* Fibrillation action potentials. *C,* Nascent units. *D,* Normal interference pattern.

being examined, a ground surface metal electrode and a needle electrode inserted directly into the muscle. The skin electrode is strapped over the muscle to be examined. Good contact is obtained by use of electrode jelly. The skin directly over the muscle is prepared with iodine, and the needle is inserted into the muscle belly. No anesthetic is required, and the maneuver is not significantly painful. The electrodes are connected to the recording units and the amplifier. The patient is asked to move the extremity as he would in making the deltoid contract; if the muscle is working normally, a staccato sound is produced, with broad deflections characteristic of motor unit action potentials. If the muscle is paralyzed, no such staccato sound is produced and the normal pattern is replaced by the fine uncontrolled fibrillation action potentials. Frequently, as the needle is inserted into muscle, there is an outburst of fibrillation action potentials even in unparalyzed muscle, but this is a normal reaction to the needle insertion and quickly subsides (Fig. 4–26).

Nerve Conduction Study. An exceedingly useful further assessment in the form of nerve conduction studies can be carried out with the electromyographic apparatus. In this examination the needle electrode is inserted at a point in the nerve. The time that the impulse takes to travel between the two fixed points can be recorded and the speed of conduction then calculated.

Radiological Investigation. Good x-rays are an essential part of any complete shoulder-neck investigation.

NECK. Much greater attention has been focused on the neck because of the great increase in neck injuries in automobile accidents. So important have proper x-ray studies become that all injuries, even of a minor nature, should be x-rayed. The routine for injuries is much more intricate than for elective investigation, but a systematic plan should be established so that a standard of comparison can be made. The routine for neck injuries should include anteroposterior, lateral and oblique views of the cervical spine. Lateral views in flexion and extension should also be done. The open mouth view of the odontoid process should be made.

Study of Routine X-rays

1. Anteroposterior views. In this view general alignment of the vertebral bodies can be assessed, but the presence or absence of anomalies such as cervical ribs is particularly apparent. A fracture of the vertebral body will appear as a tilting of one body on the other (Fig. 4–27, *A*).

2. Lateral views. Fracture or dislocation will be apparent from crushing of the bodies or alteration in alignment (Fig. 4–27, *B*).

3. Oblique views. Any suggestion of degenerative changes will be apparent, as will any derangement of the posterior spinous processes. Chip fractures of the anterior margin of the vertebral bodies will be identified in these views but should not be confused with anatomical variations such as intercalary bone or epiphyseal disturbances of growth.

Fractures of the posterior spinous processes are sometimes confused with extra centers of ossification of the tip of the spinous process. Similarly, calcification in the ligamentum nuchae will be apparent in this view.

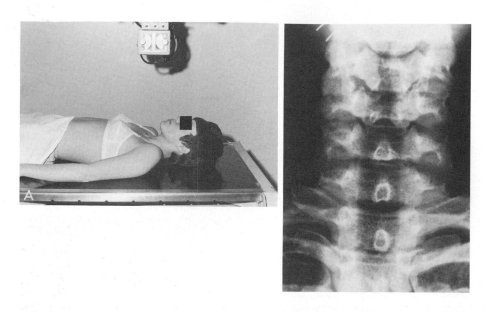

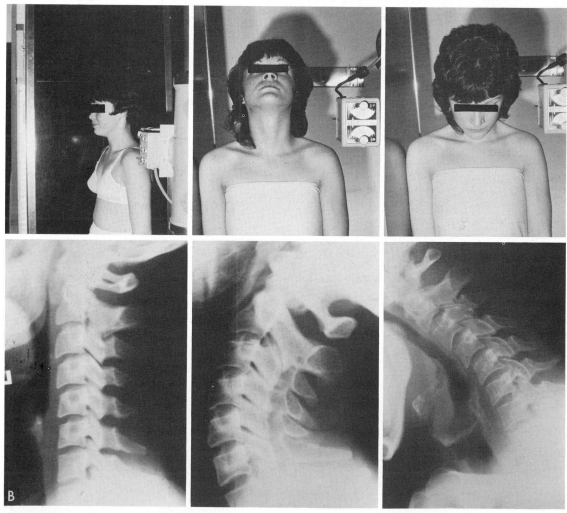

Figure 4-27 Routine cervical spine films. *A*, Anteroposterior; *B*, Lateral straight, lateral extension, and lateral flexion.

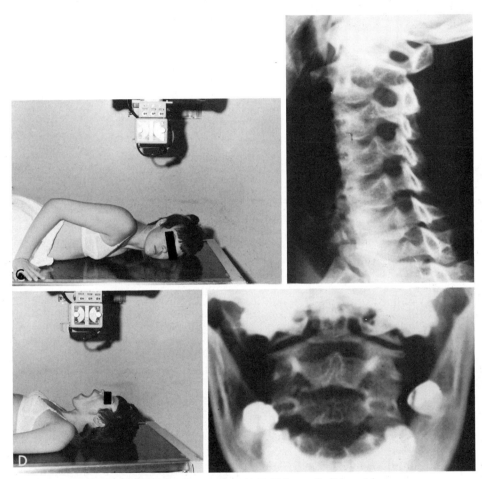

Figure 4–27 *(Continued.) C*, Oblique: *D*, Odontoid.

4. Flexion-extension lateral views. These views are taken particularly to identify luxation of the vertebral bodies or articular facets. Fractures of the posterior arch or laminae are visible in the lateral views also. The open mouth view of the odontoid process allows study for fracture, congenital anomaly or any abnormal position of the lateral mass, as in occipito-atlantal subluxation (Fig. 4–27, *B*).

MYELOGRAPHY. A cervical myelogram is exceedingly useful in identifying space-taking lesions involving the cord, in identifying foci of extradural pressure and also in assessing the relationship of the sleeve prolongation of the cervical roots in plexus injuries (Fig. 4–28).

The dye is inserted in the lower lumbar region and the patient tilted so that it will run into the cervical zone. The examination is carried out by the radiologist in the usual fashion (Fig. 4–29).

A block of the column of dye is highly indicative of a space-taking lesion such as a cord tumor, but this can also be found in myelopathy due to spondylosis. Indentations of the dye are frequent findings and are suggestive of extradural nerve root pressure from degenerative or traumatic processes.

Studies have been done on the anteroposterior diameter of the normal cervical canal. Narrowing of the canal by osteophytes can be calculated from the established measurements. Various observers have assessed the anteroposterior diameter of the spinal canal; from C.2 to C.7, the average is 20 to 17 mm, with variations occurring at the level of C.3 or C.4 from 23 to 12 mm, according to Wolf and his associates. Cord compression has been estimated as probable if the diameter is 10 mm or less when the head is in the vertical or central position. Compression is also possible when the minimum diameter is 10 to 13 mm, but if the diameter is greater than 13 mm it is unlikely that the cord is compressed.

Atlantoaxial Articulation. Recent attention to this area has uncovered a greater number of derangements than was previously appreciated (Fig. 4–30). Subluxation of the atlas on the axis, in particular, has come in for careful scrutiny. Two millimeters has been accepted as the usual distance between the odontoid and the posterior portion of the anterior arch of the atlas. Subluxation has been suggested when an excursion of 3 or more ml can be established.

The Apophyseal Joints. Derangement of these articulations, particularly as a result of degenerative changes, is now recognized as a cause of neck disorder and, sometimes, a radiating type of pain. As a rule the joints in the upper segment are more frequently involved. These joints are best demonstrated by a facet view or what is sometimes called an off-lateral view (Fig. 4–28). This is a view

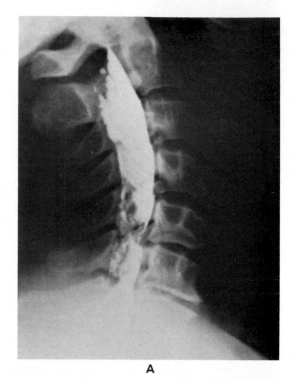

A

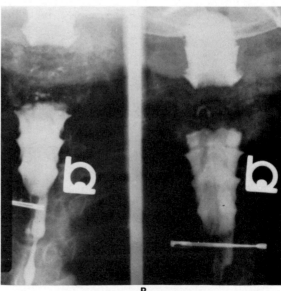

B

Figure 4–28 *A*, Cervical myelogram in herniated disc. *B*, Cervical myelogram in complete block with cervical cord pressure.

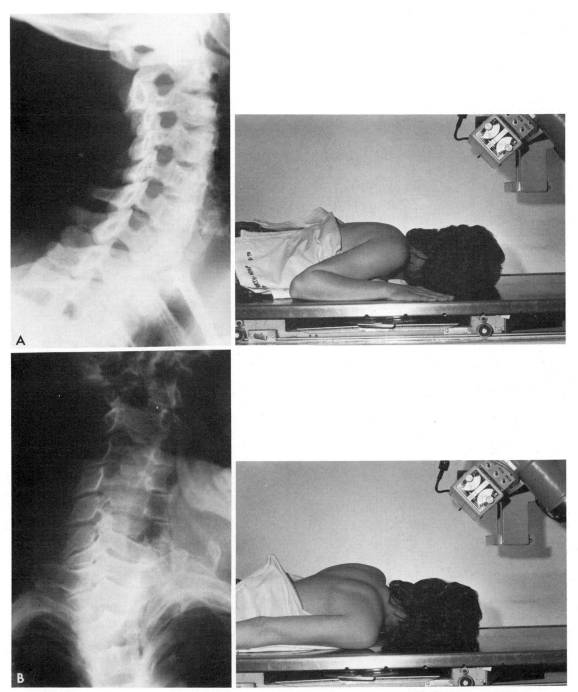

Figure 4–29   Special cervical films to show uncinate processes. *A*, Facet view. Patient is in prone oblique position with tube tilted 18 degrees candal. *B*, Pillar view. Patient as in *A*, but more tilt to tube.

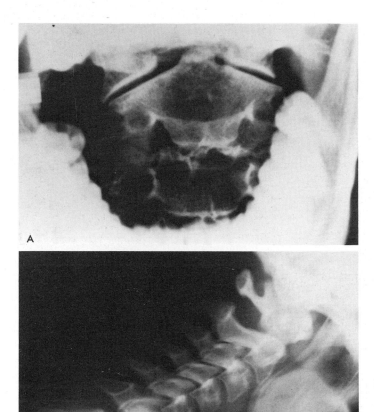

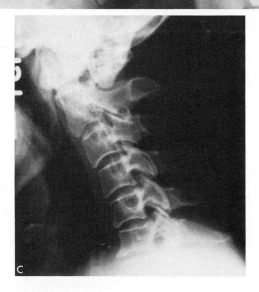

Figure 4–30 X-rays of atlantoaxial joints. *A*, showing luxation; *B*, extension; *C*, flexion.

made at about 12 degrees rotation from the true lateral position. So that the individual sides may be identified, the views should be done from both right and left lateral aspects.

RADIOLOGICAL TECHNIQUE IN SHOULDER INJURIES. Some principles of the use of x-rays should be kept in mind. All recent injuries should be x-rayed, and the procedures should be carried out with a minimum of disturbance yet with sufficient views being taken so that no defect is overlooked.

Careful handling of fresh injuries allows enough study to be done to demonstrate major disorders, but it is not always essential to follow a precise or usual routine. The x-ray is an important record in all legal cases, serving as protection for both patient and doctor. Wet or poorly made films are no basis on which to express an opinion regarding minor changes; it is preferable to await clear dry films. Often a magnifying glass picks up changes which might otherwise be overlooked. Most clinicians are familiar with normal anatomical variations, but alterations of age and developmental abnormalities must also be kept in mind; the radiologist is best able to assess these.

X-rays should always be made after reduction of a dislocation or a fracture; this is particularly important for the shoulder area. Periodic x-rays are needed to assess healing and position, and a final plate should be done before the patient is discharged.

Technique in Recent Injuries. Positioning and manipulation may be so painful to patients with recent injuries that some compromise is necessary in following the usual routine. In most instances an anteroposterior view and a lateral view through the chest would be sufficient to demonstrate fractures and dislocations. The anteroposterior view is done most comfortably with the patient in the sitting position and his body rotated until the scapula is parallel with the plate. The central ray is directed parallel and caudal to the acromion. Lateral views are also essential; a view through the chest outlines the upper end of the humerus and the relationship to the glenoid (Fig. 4–31). This is done with the patient sitting. The plate is placed at the injured side, the injured shoulder is depressed, the opposite one is elevated and the body is rotated to throw the spine image posteriorly. The central ray is directed through the neck of the humerus angled 30 degrees cranially.

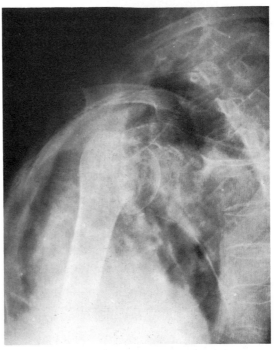

Figure 4–31 Lateral view through the chest in recent shoulder injuries.

Technique in Elective Cases. Standard views of the shoulder yield much information. Anteroposterior views in neutral, internal and external rotation should be done as well as a lateral or superoinferior view (Fig. 4–32).

Changes of significance include cortical eburnation, cystic areas, eroded zones, small detached flakes, roughening of the cartilage, narrowing of joint space, calcification in the subacromial area, and unusually high position of the head of the humerus in the glenoid. Special views are required to show the acromioclavicular joint well and for demonstration of the bicipital groove and the scapulocostal region and thoracic inlet.

Anteroposterior View. Demonstration of the subacromial zone without overlap of the head of the humerus is essential in this view. This is accomplished by placing the shoulder flat against the x-ray table and angling the tube caudally so that the central beam is parallel to the acromion.

Frequently this view is done incorrectly, producing a picture in which both subacromial and glenohumeral relations are indistinct because of overlapping. The first correction required is to be sure that the shoulder is flat against the x-ray table. This outlines the glenohumeral joint space more clearly. The second adjustment required is to angle the

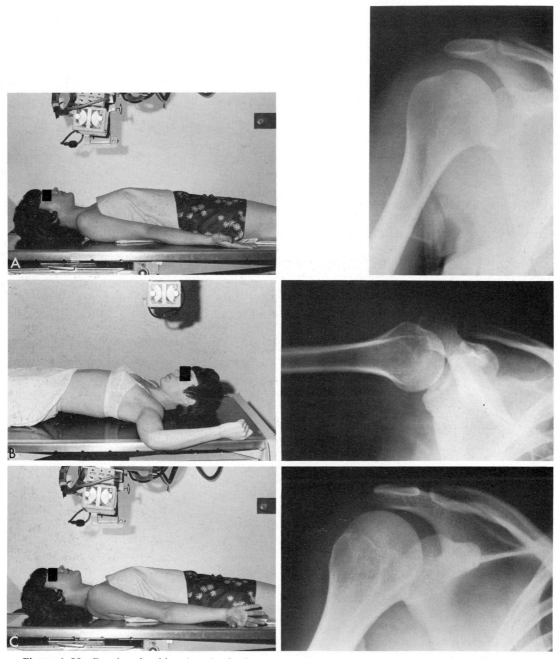

Figure 4–32   Routine shoulder views in elective cases. *A*, anteroposterior; *B*, lateral; *C*, internal rotation.

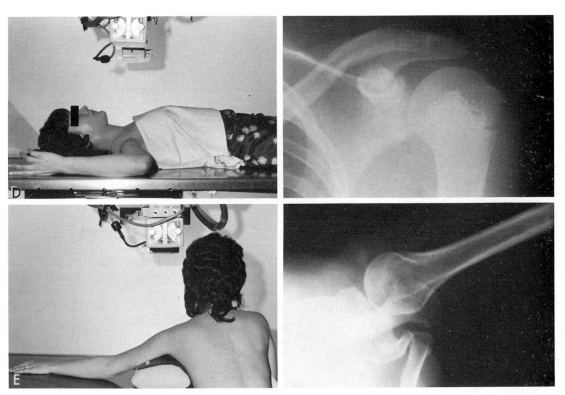

Figure 4–32 *(Continued.)* *D*, internal rotation; *E*, superoinferior.

tube caudally so that the central beam is parallel to the acromion. The subacromial space is then seen clearly. This technique of correct anteroposterior assessment is particularly important in carrying out contrast studies.

Internal Rotation. The patient is supine when this view is taken, with the shoulder against the table and the hand in full internal rotation. This throws into relief the supraspinatus and teres minor insertions, and the greater tuberosity overlaps the glenoid. In those instances in which there is a defect from recurrent anterior dislocation, this is a view that brings out the notch or defect on the posterior aspect of the articular surface of the glenoid. It is formed by this area of the head of the humerus resting on the anterior margin of the glenoid. It comes into view in the upper quadrant when the humerus is fully rotated internally.

External Rotation. This is taken with the patient supine and the hand fully rotated externally. The lesser tuberosity then forms the lateral margin of the film. The subscapularis attachment is shown at this point.

Lateral View. The patient is placed in the sitting position with the tube in the axilla and the plate steadied by the patient on the top of the shoulder. This provides a good lateral view, and the same position gives a superoinferior view.

Acromioclavicular Joint. Routine anteroposterior and superoinferior views show this articulation, but to demonstrate subluxation, weights are held in each hand and the x-rays are taken with the patient in the standing position. The film holder is placed behind the patient and the central ray is directed toward the sternal notch, thereby affording a means of comparing the two sides (Fig. 4–33).

Scapular Bed. Demonstration of the median border of the scapula in profile is required in scapulocostal lesions and fractures of the scapula. This is obtained by the patient's pulling the arm well across the front of the body so that the medial border moves away from the chest. The scapula is then outlined as it stands away from the chest margin (Fig. 4–34).

Clavicle. Examination of the scapula should be made so that the lateral end and the acromioclavicular joint are shown. A posteroanterior view is preferable so that the bone is closer to the film; the central ray is directed perpendicular to the clavicle.

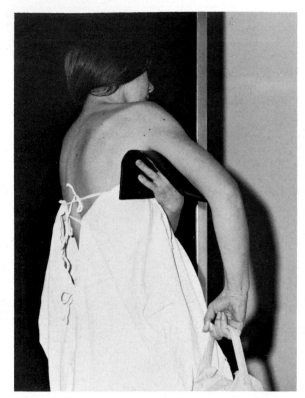

Figure 4–33 Technique for demonstration of acromioclavicular subluxation.

Views in two planes are required to show some fractures in this region: one at 20 degrees caudal, and a second at 45 degrees cranial.

Bicipital Lesions. The outline of the bicipital groove is obtained by taking a view from below upward, with the plate placed over the top of the shoulder and the hand in slight external rotation (Fig. 4–35).

Thoracic Inlet. The relation of scapula, clavicle, neck and chest are important in assessing neurovascular radiating problems. The contour of the first rib is best outlined by a posterior projection; a superoinferior view beamed toward the root of the neck is needed to demonstrate encroachment on the inside of the inlet. The lateral view as outlined with a tube angled slightly is sufficient.

SPECIAL POINTS IN INTERPRETATION OF X-RAYS. The epiphysis of the upper end of the humerus does not close until the age of 20; before this time it can be mistaken for a fracture. The epiphyseal junction has a wavy uniform line in contrast to the sharp or acutely angled line of a fracture. Comparison with the opposite side clarifies the situation

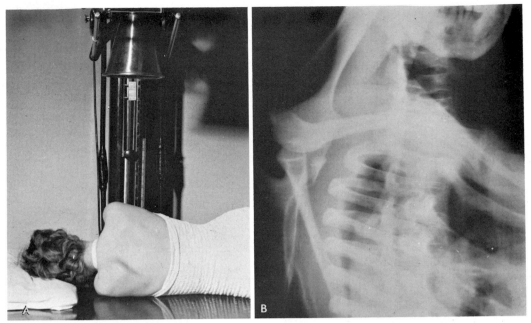

Figure 4–34   Technique for demonstration of medial border of scapula.

when a similar line on the uninjured side is identified. Impacted fractures in elderly people may be difficult to interpret, but suspicion is aroused by a little heaping up or irregularity of the cortex on the lateral side or some angulation of the glenoid face which is unusual. In dislocations, lateral views or views through the chest are essential since a posterior dislocation, in particular, may be missed.

Chip fractures of the greater tuberosity are sometimes difficult to separate from calcium deposits. The fracture is sharply outlined, with cortex on one side, whereas the calcium deposit tends to be more flattened and has a homogenous consistency. An extremely small calcium deposit may sometimes be interpreted as a fleck of bone or vice versa. Multiple views are necessary to adequately outline calcium deposits.

Clavicle. Abnormalities of the acromio-clavicular joint are frequently overlooked, since there is considerable variation in what are apparently normal joints. The medial end of the clavicle is often bulbous. The angle of the joint line varies, and irregularities similar to arthritic changes are frequent. Careful demonstration of the joint, particu-

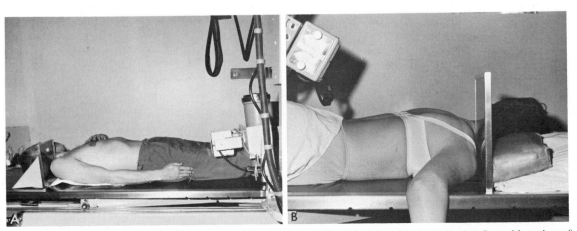

Figure 4–35   Special shoulder views: *A,* bicipital groove; *B,* axillary view. Used in investigation for subluxation of the shoulder.

larly on the anteroposterior view, is necessary to identify many of the changes. Fractures of the outer end of the clavicle may be missed if this aspect is not carefully depicted.

The curve of the shaft of the clavicle is exaggerated in some views and displacement may be distorted. Views at right angles should be done for clearer interpretation of the displacement.

Scapula. Persistent epiphyseal lines may be mistaken for fractures at the tip of the acromion or at the end of the coracoid. Similar changes in the upper half of the glenoid and the lower angle of the scapula may be erroneously interpreted. In both instances comparison with the opposite side is the clue to the change. In some instances there are markings along the axillary border which are vascular markings; these may be interpreted as a pathological change, but again comparison with the opposite side is helpful. A difficult view to obtain is that of the vertebral border, particularly the upper angle, in investigation of scapulocostal disturbances and also when looking for the cause of a snapping scapula.

Video Studies. The development of the television screen and image intensifier has introduced a new tool for investigating joint disorders. In the case of the shoulder it is particularly helpful to have motion studies done in cases of suspected subluxation or dislocation. The examination can be carried out by the radiologist, but it is wise for the surgeon to view the initial examination at the same time. The video screen produces a tape which is a permanent record and can be reviewed, but it is extremely helpful to corrolate any clinical changes with the video study. In cases of possible subluxing of humerus it is particularly helpful to carry out passive manipulation of the shoulder under the video screen and to observe the degree of subluxation anteriorly and posteriorly. In cases of recurrent posterior subluxation, the diagnosis may only become apparent with such investigation.

Similarly, in young adults or teen-agers, this examination may make quite clear a diagnosis of subluxating shoulder which in the past has been overlooked. The patient is asked to take his arm through the range of motion which habitually produces the clicking painful change in the shoulder; as a rule, the examiner can see the tendency toward anterior luxation of the head of the humerus in the glenoid.

Arthrography of the Shoulder. Contrast studies have become extremely valuable in identifying internal derangements of the shoulder. No other method of investigation, clinical or special, identifies cuff tears with as much certainty as does arthrography. In addition to its usefulness as a diagnostic tool, it is now of value in assessing the solidity of cuff repairs and in assessing recurrent dislocation problems, subluxation of the shoulder, capsulitis, frozen shoulder and ruptures of the biceps, all of which may be identified by quite distinctive patterns.

In addition to full thickness tears, it is possible to identify partial tears, and some localization of the position of a tear and its extent may be deduced.

TECHNIQUE OF ARTHROGRAPHY. The procedure is carried out in the x-ray department and is usually performed by the radiologist, but in many instances the surgeon carries out the injection of the dye. A quickly absorbed watery solution such as Diodrast is used. The author's preference is to make the injection from the posterior aspect so that any minute leak of dye will not produce an artifact which may be confused with true disease. Nearly all the pathological changes are at the front and superior aspect, so it is particularly desirable not to have artifacts produced in this zone. When the injection is done from the back, the radiologist may outline the joint contour for the injection, or, in a blind fashion, a point selected 1 inch below and 1 inch medial to the angle of the spine of the scapula.

The area is prepared and draped and the surgeon, wearing gloves, uses a number 20 or 21 extra long needle or one of lumbar puncture length. The point of entrance is infiltrated with 5 to 10 cc of 2 per cent Novocain. The needle is directed upward and a little laterally, seeking the angle between the head of the humerus and the glenoid in the upper portion of the joint. Often it is possible to feel the needle slip over the head of the humerus through the capsule into the joint. Should the needle strike bone, it is gently moved from this site to another until this resistance is missed and the needle enters the joint. When it is felt that the needle is correctly placed, 1 cc of Diodrast is injected; this is checked by the fluoroscope or on the video screen. The indication that the dye is in the joint comes from the production of a crescentric line, with the dye outlining the inferior approach and following the head of

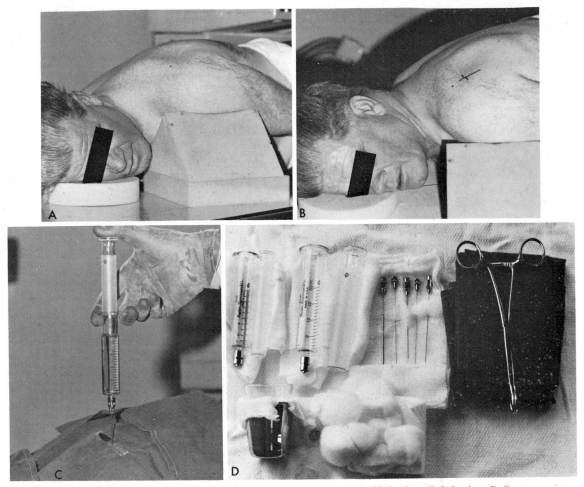

Figure 4–36   Technique of arthrography. *A*, Position. *B*, Point of injection. *C*, Injection. *D*, Set-up.

the humerus. If this has been obtained, a further 8 to 10 cc is injected.

Should it not be possible to enter the joint directly between the head of the humerus and the glenoid, an alternative technique is to insert the needle until it meets the resistance of the head of the humerus and then draw back 1 or 2 mm and make the trial injection. If the dye forms a crescentric outline, the remainder of the dye is inserted without shifting the point of the needle.

The needle is withdrawn and pictures are taken immediately. The shoulder is massaged at the back and in the axilla, and the humerus is rotated so that the dye is spread throughout the joint. The procedure may be done with the patient lying on his face on the x-ray table. If preferred, the sitting position may be used and the injection carried out with the aid of the video screen. Injection of the dye may occasionally

be painful, in which case some local anesthetic may be added as the injection is completed. It is not necessary to remove the dye, because this type of contrast medium is quickly absorbed. No ill effects have been

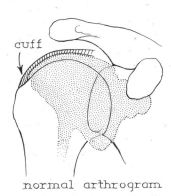

Figure 4–37 Configuration of dye pattern in a normal arthrogram.

encountered from carrying out this procedure. Some local pain may persist for a short time, but since the dye is quickly absorbed it does not last significantly.

INDICATIONS FOR CONTRAST STUDIES. Arthrography is of the greatest help in identifying full-thickness tears of the cuff. When the tear is present, the dye escapes from the joint through the slit into the subacromial area, producing a very characteristic picture. With this method it is possible to demonstrate the lesion much earlier, leading to early repair and superior results. In bicipital lesions, frozen shoulder and recurrent dislocation, the arthrogram patterns are also definite and conform with the disorder found at operation. It is particularly helpful in problem cases such as dislocations with signs suggestive of cuff damage. Arthrography will demonstrate clearly a lesion of the cuff which might otherwise be overlooked.

NORMAL ARTHROGRAM. Practice in injecting the joint is helpful. The needle used must be of sufficient length and stiff enough to be controlled and guided accurately.

The dye inside the joint outlines a quite constant pattern. A central or body area of the joint may be identified, and over the greater tuberosity a thin line of dye extending to the attachment of the rotator cuff can be identified (Fig. 4–37). The bicipital sheath can be seen, with the dye extending between the greater and lesser tuberosities; there is also extension of the dye into the subscapular recess (Fig. 4–38). Occasionally at the posterior aspect, if the dye is inserted in the muscle substance, it will travel along the fibers of the supraspinatus and may be seen tracking transversely following the line of the fibers, making it quite easy to depict this artifact.

CUFF TEARS. When there is a defect in the capsule the dye escapes and lies in an irregular pool under the acromion or extends all through the joint in an irregular fashion. It is often possible to identify the point of leakage of the dye in tears that are not too extensive, and the position of the full-thickness defect is then apparent. If the dye has extended throughout the joint in a quite haphazard fashion, it is extremely suggestive of a massive tear, because there has been no retaining capsular structure to give any normal outline to dye distribution (Fig. 4–39).

BICIPITAL LESIONS. In some instances, distortion of the bicipital appartus can be

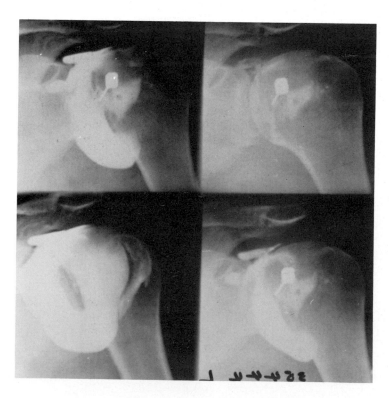

Figure 4–38 Stages in dye insertion. *A*, Tear-drop configuration indicating that the dye is properly placed in the joint. *B*, Progressive covering of head and filling of the capsule. *C*, Injection completed. Note clear subacromial area, bicipital extension, body of the joint and the subscapularis bursa. *D*, Complete filling of the joint.

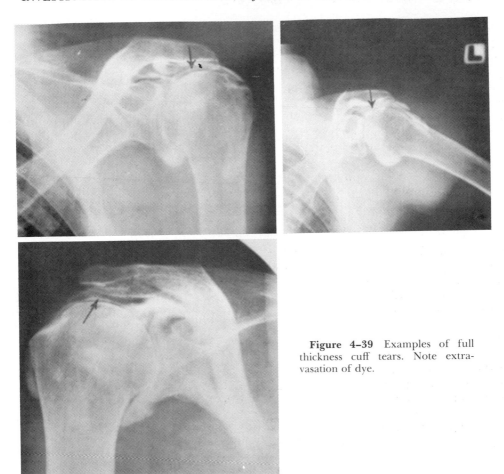

Figure 4–39 Examples of full thickness cuff tears. Note extravasation of dye.

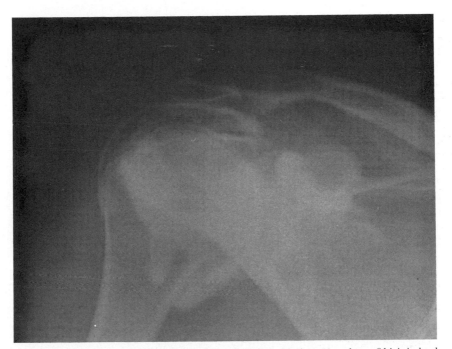

Figure 4–40 Bicipital deformity. Arthrogram in bicipital lesion. Note loss of bicipital tube.

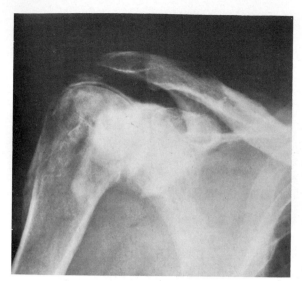

Figure 4-41 Arthrogram in frozen shoulder.

identified by the leak of dye anteriorly and the loss of a clear-cut bicipital tunnel (Fig. 4-40).

FROZEN SHOULDER. Frozen shoulder presents a very characteristic picture in the arthrogram. The normal, rounded capsule outline is replaced by a squat, square, contracted patch. The subacromial space is increased and this is of diagnostic importance. The redundant fold at the inferior portion of the joint is completely obliterated. Normally this hangs down like a pleat, but in adhesive capsulitis it is obliterated (Fig. 4-41).

SUBSCAPULARIS RUPTURE. A distinctive configuration of dye leak occurs when the subscapularis has been torn completely. In contrast to other full-thickness ruptures, the subacromial space is quite clear, but the dye escapes downward and medially so that the normal contour of the inferior aspect is completely lost. Frequently the dye does not fill the body of the joint or the bicipital mechanism either, since it leaks directly through the subscapularis defect. The picture is extremely typical and cannot be misinterpreted (Fig. 4-42).

RECURRENT DISLOCATION AND RECURRENT SUBLUXATION. The ballooning of the subscapular recess is grossly increased and the line of dye in the region of the neck of the scapula extends much farther medially than normal, indicating a lax capsule (Fig. 4-43).

PARTIAL CUFF TEARS. A study of the upper line of dye over the head of the hu-

merus sometimes demonstrates a thin prolongation upward, somewhat like the change that is seen in a barium meal outlining a duodenal ulcer. Such a defect may be somewhat square, but more often it is triangular because of seepage of the dye through a partial tear into the interstices of the cuff, though not all the way through into the subacromial space (Fig. 4-44).

ARTHROGRAPHY OF THE ACROMIOCLAVICULAR JOINT. In some instances it is desirable to carry out contrast studies of this joint also (Fig. 4-45). The technique involves use of a fine hypodermic needle. After injection of 1 or 2 cc of Novocain into the joint, it is entered posteriorly and superiorly by allowing the needle to slide along the edge of the acromion and gradually be led into the joint. The approach is a little from the back rather than the top because the angle of the joint is sometimes oblique rather than directly vertical, and it is difficult to hit the joint line if the approach is directly from the top. Two cubic centimeters of dye is usually all that can be injected into the joint.

RESULTS OF ARTHROGRAPHY. In some 1000 contrast studies no ill effects have been encountered. When a shoulder joint is opened the day following a contrast study, there may be slight injection of the synovium and a little extra watery fluid may be present, but there are no other changes to be detected.

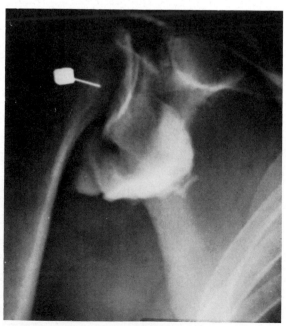

Figure 4-42 Arthrogram in ruptured subscapularis.

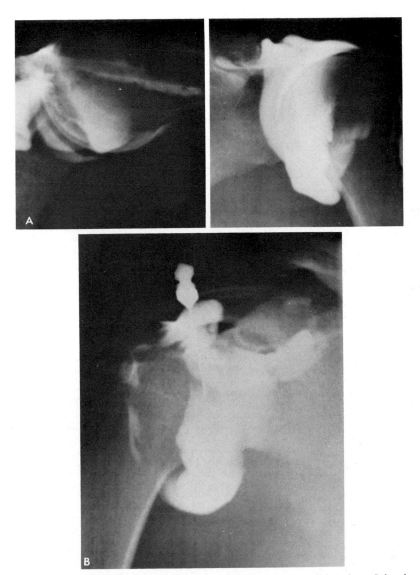

Figure 4–43 Arthrogram of recurrent subluxation and recurrent dislocation of the shoulder.

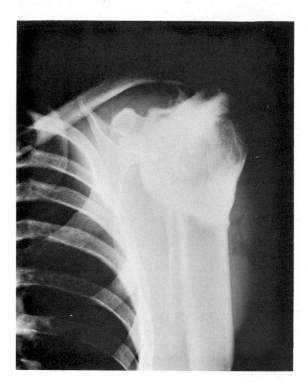

Figure 4–44 Arthrogram in partial-thickness tear of cuff.

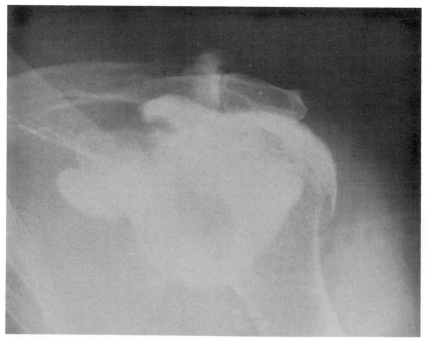

Figure 4–45 Arthrogram of acromioclavicular joint. Geyser effect in cuff tear.

In many instances not even this amount of change occurs.

In some 500 patients in whom cuff tears were suspected, full-thickness tears were found in all but three instances in which the arthrogram had suggested there would be one. In the three remaining patients a partial tear was found and it was felt that, following the arthrogram, some sealing off had been done or that the limiting remnant was so thin that the dye seeped through.

The same degree of accuracy is feasible in other disorders such as frozen shoulder, bicipital lesions and glenohumeral subluxations, all of which are identified with extreme accuracy by the arthrogram.

The arthrogram is helpful also in identifying an intact capsule and sometimes aids in identifying an internal derangement such as a tear of the minute meniscus.

REFERENCES

Brailsford, J.: Radiographic findings in 347 painful shoulders. Brit. Med. J. *1*:290, 1929.

Cloward, R. B.: Cervical discography. Ann. Surg. *150*: 1052–1053, 1959.

Gassel, M. M.: A test of nerve conduction to muscles of the shoulder girdle as an aid in the diagnosis of proximal neurogenic and muscular disease. J. Neurol. *27*:200–205, 1964.

Hagen, D. E.: Introduction to the pillar projection of the cervical spine Radiol. Techn. *35*:239–242, 1964.

Holt, E. P., Jr.: Fallacy of cervical discography. Report of 50 cases in normal subjects. J.A.M.A. *188*:799–801, 1964.

Smith, G. W., and Nichols, P., Jr.: The technique of cervical discography. Radiology *68*:718–720, 1957.

Wilson, P. D.: The painful shoulder. Brit. Med. J., *11*: 1261, 1939.

Chapter V

DIFFERENTIAL DIAGNOSIS OF LESIONS IN THE SHOULDER AND NECK REGION

Together the neck and shoulder represent the most mobile region of the body. The shoulder also provides stabilization of an appendage. Passing through this mobile zone, and partly encased in the stabilizing structures, is the neurovascular bundle (Fig. 5–1).

These features of stability, mobility, innervation and vascularization give rise to distinctive pain patterns that are the principal disorders of this region.

Two principles are to be followed in differentiating the complaints. The pathological problems are best interpreted by a clinical classification rather than a purely anatomical one. Consideration must be given to the multiple parts within the area that can give rise to similar general clinical pictures, but which on more minute inspection produce specific signs.

For clinical purposes the shoulder should be regarded as a region and not as a single joint. Many patients are referred as having shoulder problems when the cause of their discomfort really arises elsewhere; the neck, root of neck, interscapular, scapular, clavicular, axillary and pectoral zones must always be examined as well. The shoulder joint itself is an articular system with important auxiliary articulations, and sternoclavicular, acromioclavicular, coracoclavicular, bicipital and scapulothoracic mechanisms belong to this system also (Fig. 5–2). Occasional implication of the shoulder by disease in the heart, the chest, the abdomen or the breast must also be considered. Once this broad scope of origin of shoulder distress is appreciated, organization and classification are simplified.

The patient's story is the starting point for

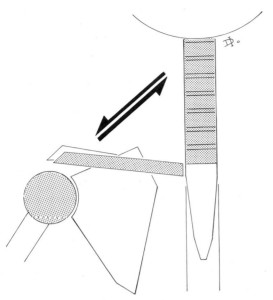

Figure 5–1 The shoulder-neck aggregate—two mobile segments suspending a limb supporting a head and containing major neurovascular systems.

investigation. To be of greatest use, a plan for differential diagnosis should be based on a study of the common symptoms. Every practitioner has a particular routine or system that he follows automatically when confronted with a problem in a given area. Pain is the common complaint of shoulder and neck disability, and the author has found that an analysis of the pain pattern is an extremely useful guide to the differential diagnosis and classification of a specific disorder. Neck pain alone, shoulder-neck pain, predominant shoulder pain, and shoulder plus radiating symptoms constitute the dominant patterns which may be recognized. Most ailments involving the shoulder and neck will fall into one of these groups (Fig. 5–3). In some patients with longstanding problems there may be an overlapping of symptoms that obscures the exact cause. However, there will still be an overriding picture, and careful search will usually reveal this discrete pattern.

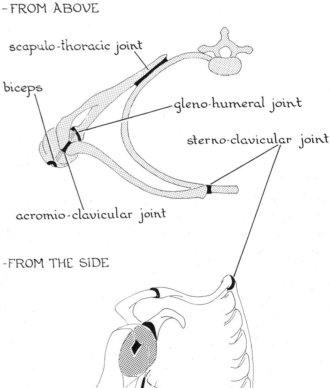

THE SHOULDER SYSTEM
-FROM ABOVE

scapulo-thoracic joint

biceps

gleno-humeral joint

sterno-clavicular joint

acromio-clavicular joint

Figure 5–2 Shoulder system of joints.

-FROM THE SIDE

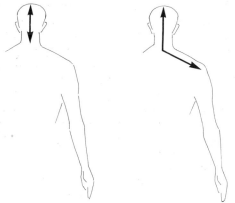

Neck   Neck - shoulder junction

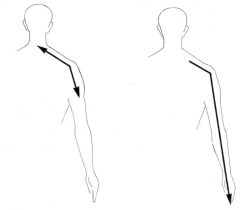

Shoulder - root of neck

Neck to finger

Figure 5-3   Pain patterns of shoulder-neck disease.

In the ensuing discussion an effort is made to follow a clinical grouping of problems that will lead to a definitive diagnosis rather than an assumption. Such a classification is not merely clinical, because the pain pattern characteristic of each group has an individual underlying anatomical and physiological basis.

Purely localized neck or suboccipital pain is mediated through branches of the posterior primary rami of spinal nerves and cervical plexus. Shoulder-neck pain often arises from disease in the posterior scapular, interscapular and suspensory muscle area, and is also mediated through posterior spinal nerve branches. Localized shoulder pain is most commonly caused by shoulder joint disease and is recorded from branches of the brachial plexus extending to this joint. Shoulder pain plus radiating symptoms

results from nerve root or vascular irritation and, hence, follows a quite different pathway. We shall present the distinctive features of the groups and list the common disorders of each group. For example, the shoulder-neck complaints caused by postural disorders and fibrositis differ vastly from those of bicipital and cuff injuries, which represent pathological states of the shoulder joint proper. Similarly, the pain pattern from an extruded disc as an example of shoulder plus radiating pain is quite different from the pain distribution in acromioclavicular arthritis. In each group there are disorders which are somewhat alike, and the distinguishing features of these similar disorders will be compared in tables. More detailed considerations with appropriate treatment of all these conditions and of rare disorders have been included in later chapters. Oversimplification has a tendency to foster a false sense of security, but it is felt that the average physician can make good use of a planned approach if, at the same time, he recognizes the limitations of such a procedure.

LOCALIZED NECK DISORDERS

SUBOCCIPITAL ARTHRITIS

Recent work has focused new interest on many phases of neck disorders and it has become apparent that this is a not infrequent pathological state (Fig. 5–4). The atlantooccipital and atlantoaxial joints may show degenerative changes that frequently have

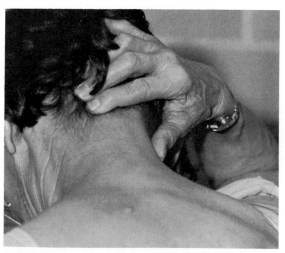

Figure 5–4   Characteristic attitude of patients emphasizing neck pain.

originated in trauma. Pain results from movement of the head rather than the neck. The complaint is often somewhat diffusely suboccipital. Interference with rotation or pain on slight flexion and extension of the head without much neck movement is characteristic. Frequently the pain is identified early in the neck bending process, before the lower vertebral bodies have contributed to the movement. Tenderness is localized in the suboccipital area, usually on both sides of the midline rather than directly in the center. A frequent accompaniment of this disorder is tendinitis of the erector spinae attachment in the suboccipital zone. Nearly always this has a traumatic origin.

STERNOMASTOID TENDINITIS

A frequently overlooked cause of suboccipital pain is derangement of the musculotendinous junction over the mastoid process. Patients with this problem have high neck pain, do not particularly relate it to rotation, but have an aching sensation a little more laterally than the suboccipital regions. It is more often found unilaterally, maximum tenderness being localized over the distal mastoid process. Occasionally, calcified streaks in the sternomastoid can be made out. Sometimes the sternomastoid appears somewhat atrophic in the zone of its mastoid fixation.

ARTHRITIS OF THE CERVICAL SPINE

By middle age most cervical spines show some evidence of degenerative wear and tear or osteoarthritis. Few patients have discomfort from these changes unless there is superimposed on them some irritating factor such as injury, increased strain or debilitating disease. When the disturbance passes beyond normal bounds, aching pain in the posterior neck-shoulder area can develop. This is related to neck movement and is influenced very little by shoulder use. After it has been present for some little time there is frequently an extension of the discomfort from the root of the neck out toward the tips of the shoulders. A sense of stiffness develops and the patient is reluctant to move the neck. It is at this point that the disc disorder may be confused with other abnormalities of the shoulder region. Spur formation on the anterior margin of vertebral bodies C.4–C.5 and C.5–C.6 is a normal finding

after the age of 40 or 50. However, this fact should not be accepted as an explanation of all shoulder-neck disorders; more extensive search of the region should be made to explain any persistent pain. Of special significance is the involvement of the articular facets, narrowing of joint space, lipping and spicule formation of the intervertebral foramina. When this process progresses so that the nerve roots are compressed, radiating pain is added to the local shoulder-neck discomfort.

The condition is well defined by the type of pain, the absence of muscle disturbance, the relation to cervical motion and the changes evident in x-rays. It may be confused with rheumatoid arthritis, but the latter is usually part of a much more extensive general disturbance. There is little difficulty in differentiating it from Strümpell-Marie disease.

ACUTE NECK KINKS

Neck pain is often encountered following an acute spasm crick in the neck. It has a sudden onset, and the maximum discomfort is felt in the angle between the neck and the shoulder. It is related mostly but not entirely to neck movement, since only some movements initiate the discomfort. There is little or no relation to movement of the arm. Muscular soreness is acute. There is local muscle spasm, particularly in the trapezius, cervical erector spinae and rhomboids or combinations of these. As a rule, a history of sudden onset or injury is present. Only one side of the neck is involved and there is no radiation to the shoulder tip or beyond.

ACUTE POSTERIOR SPRAIN

Local posterior neck pain is predominant, and the condition frequently develops after sleeping in a cramped position, from strain on the neck or arm, or as a result of reaching and twisting actions. Sometimes after the first golf drive or tennis game of a new season, the neck is seized with a sudden spasm. The sudden onset, soreness at the root of the neck, spasm of the posterior muscles and relation to the neck motion are the diagnostic features.

"STOP-LIGHT" SPRAIN

This topic is covered fully in the section on injuries but is mentioned at this point for completeness. Aching pain in the neck, with radiation across the back to the shoulder zone, develops from tearing and partial rupture of the ligamentum nuchae. This distribution develops after a moderately severe flexion, or sometimes after several similar episodes of less severity. There is initiated a chronic discomfort interrupted by acute exacerbations. Sometimes there is complete subsidence of discomfort for a matter of months. On examination crepitus is present in the midline of the neck and is related to the posterior spinous processes. The lower area of the neck is most frequently involved. Sometimes calcification can be seen in the ligament in relation to the tips at the posterior spinous processes. The history of injury (usually an automobile accident), localized neck tenderness, crepitus in the ligament, occasional calcification and an aching type of neck pain not particularly related to shoulder motion form the basis for diagnosis of this entity.

ACUTE POSTERIOR NECK PAIN

Attention is called to the sudden onset of generalized posterior neck pain developing quite apart from trauma. There are serious systemic disturbances which may be ushered in by this type of discomfort. The progress of these diseases usually makes the diagnosis obvious, but it is in the early stages that recognition may be most vital. Posterior neck pain occurs in meningitis, in premonitory cerebrovascular disease, in poliomyelitis, as a prodrome to certain acute infectious anthemata like scarlet fever and, occasionally, in tetanus and pneumonia. The pain is similar in all these conditions, being intensified by flexion, and the neck is held stiffly. It is accompanied by the signs of a generalized systemic febrile process, anorexia and lassitude. A stiff neck accompanied by pain should always receive careful attention, particularly when it occurs in children. In cerebrovascular disease neck and occipital pain is sometimes a premonitory symptom of a more serious intracranial disturbance.

PURELY NECK DISORDERS

Certain neck disorders, most of which are not confused with the shoulder, occasionally have some bearing on the neck-shoulder area. Conditions in the root of the neck are more liable to produce pain extend-

ing out toward the shoulder than are anterior neck lesions.

Acute Infection of the Pharynx. Acute sore throat from tonsillitis or laryngitis produces a characteristic picture of difficulty in swallowing, anterior neck pain and some fever. Tenderness is present in the neck under the angle of the jaw. Progress of the infection to peritonsillar abscess or retropharyngeal abscess results in more diffuse neck discomfort, with stiffening as a result of muscle splinting and limitation of motion. Such a process can become so extensive as to result in atlantoaxial subluxation. The diagnosis of these acute throat conditions is straightforward and not likely to be confused with neck-shoulder disorders, but the possibility of cervical spine complications should be kept in mind.

Lymphadenitis of the Neck and Shoulder. The lymphatic system may be involved in a local infection or as part of a generalized lymphadenopathy concentrated in the cervical region. This may result in pain in the neck-shoulder area. Infections of the mouth, teeth, tongue, lips and face may produce enlargement of anterior and lateral cervical glands, with local pain and soreness. The posterior cervical and auricular glands are involved in scalp and ear infections and also in measles and chickenpox. The lymphatic enlargement caused by Hodgkin's disease, tuberculosis, metastatic carcinoma, and other diseases may produce some local pain, but it is rarely progressive and does not reach significant proportions unless there is secondary infection. Otolaryngologists report an elongated styloid process may produce pain along the course of the glossopharyngeal nerve, and this may implicate the neck-shoulder area.

CONGENITAL AND DEVELOPMENTAL ABNORMALITIES OF THE NECK

There are two uncommon disorders which produce swelling in the neck that may result in generalized pain, with extension to the root of the neck region.

Thyroglossal Cyst. This is a congenital abnormality resulting in a midline swelling above the thyroid gland. It usually appears in younger patients. The protuberance moves with swallowing or with movements of the tongue. These features clearly identify the disturbance.

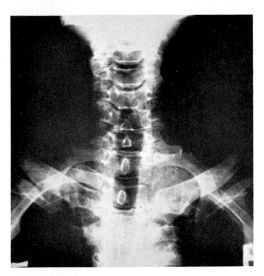

Figure 5–5 Pulmonary sulcus tumor producing shoulder-neck pain (Pancoast's syndrome).

Lateral Cervical Cysts. A further disturbance of childhood or early adult life has been identified as lateral cervical cysts. These appear as swellings at the side of the neck and may lie as far distal as the clavicle. Both thyroglossal and lateral cervical cysts may become infected, resulting in swelling, pain and restriction of neck motion.

OTHER UNCOMMON CONDITIONS

Local neck pain results from laryngeal disturbances also. Papillomata, carcinoma, tuberculosis, syphilis and impacted foreign bodies can all produce neck pain, but the history and findings are quite characteristic.

Referred Pain. Distant disease processes may affect the root of the neck and upper shoulder area. This does not happen often but must be kept in mind when neck pain develops in patients with cardiac disease, pulmonary sulcus tumor (Fig. 5–5), duodenal ulcer and acute cholecystitis, all of which may irritate the inferior aspect of the diaphragm and refer symptoms to the neck-shoulder zone.

Local Conditions. Disturbances of the superficial structures, such as skin and hair follicles, are also causes of local neck and shoulder-neck pain. The existence of such disorders as hair follicle infections and carbuncles is obvious.

CONDITIONS PRODUCING NECK PLUS SHOULDER PAIN

There is a well defined group of disorders giving rise to a pain pattern that almost equally implicates neck and shoulders, particularly the zone between the cervical spine and the glenohumeral joint proper (Fig. 5–6). These patients indicate that pain centers in the posterior aspect of the neck-shoulder zone, and their characteristic reaction is to wrap the hand over the sloping shoulder-neck interval, digging the fingers in posteriorly. The pain has an aching, gnawing quality that seems to encompass the whole

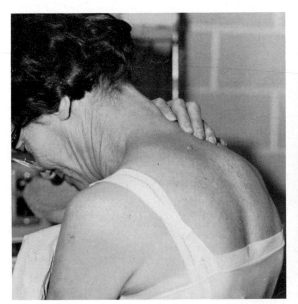
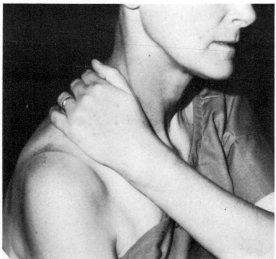

Figure 5–6 Attitude of shoulder-neck pain sufferers.

region. Localization is sometimes difficult, and tender areas are hard to find. Sharp tingling pain, stabbing shocks and electric-like radiation are not commonly part of the picture. A history of injury is not common either, and the only significant episodes appear relatively minor. Since this area contains largely muscle and fibrous tissue, the common ailments are fibrositis, neck-shoulder kinks, musculoligamentous injuries, postural disturbances and their sequelae, and scapulothoracic disorders.

POSTURAL DISTURBANCES

Keeping the head up and supporting the upper extremities in the erect position is a constant unconscious burden. When some alteration in balance occurs, or there is an added constant strain or general muscular laxity, keeping the head erect becomes an effort and discomfort is experienced. Postural disturbances are a common cause of neck-shoulder discomfort. The suspensory function of the neck-shoulder group of muscles, with the girdle suspended like a sign from the cervical spine as a post, is naturally susceptible to derangement. The rounded shoulder, slumped posture and asthenic development predispose to persistent aching shoulder pain. In some instances these patients appear to have an unusually long neck. Usually both sides are involved, but the master hand side has the predominant discomfort. Aching shoulders and neck are common in overworked and undernourished females. Faulty occupational posture without underlying structural abnormalities is also a frequent cause. This persistent somewhat diffuse complaint must be differentiated from other more severe shoulder disorders which result in somewhat similar discomfort.

FIBROSITIS

A common source of shoulder-neck pain is the large group of musculotendinous disorders labeled "fibrositis." In these there is a gradual onset of aching, gnawing shoulder pain, indicated by the patient's putting the palm between the neck and shoulder in characteristic fashion. These disorders are allied to postural disturbances and often develop as a sequela to habitual or occupational shoulder strain.

The complaints arising from this disorder are definite as to area but indefinite as to precise localization. The usual patient is a poorly nourished, thin, introspective female who complains of persistent aching shoulder pain. No severe trauma is associated, as a rule, but there is a gradual "building up of tension or pressure" in the posterior neck-shoulder area. Palpation discloses thickening or nodular thickening in the suspensory muscles such as trapezius, cervical, erector spinae, levator scapulae and rhomboids. The muscles have a dry, stringy feel, and areas of soft crepitus may be felt. Small nodules or areas of thickening are common at points of strain or fulcra of muscle action. The area at the base of the spine of the scapula is a very common site. From this general zone pain radiates up the back of the neck or out to the shoulder points. Occipital headache is frequently associated; occasionally the pain reaches the upper part of the arm, but it is always poorly localized. No acute distress is associated with either shoulder or neck action, but a vague soreness is experienced with activities of both. When the lesions are long standing, more distant radiation may occur, but examination will disclose the characteristic trigger points localized to the neck-shoulder interval. In the acute phase whole segments of muscles are prominent or in spasm. The prominence and tension persist, even in the relaxed position.

Muscles are best assessed for spasm in the relaxed position with the patient lying on his face. The texture and consistency of a given area are compared with the patient in this position and then standing.

SCAPULOTHORACIC DISTURBANCES

The posterior scapula-chest region is a common, long neglected source of shoulder-neck discomfort. The scapula glides and turns on the chest constantly with every motion of the shoulder. Irregularities in the bed on which it moves or disturbances in its contour interfere with the normal, smooth course. The interscapular muscles are constantly bunched and folded together by movements of both upper extremities.

Various degrees of this scapulothoracic or scapulocostal syndrome may be recognized. In the least severe there is persistent posterior shoulder pain related to scapular movement. Palpation discloses tender points all along the vertebral border of the scapula. The area related to the upper angle is commonly disturbed by stringy thickening of the muscles. The "snapping" scapula belongs in this group. In this syndrome there is a loud snapping sound in certain phases of scapular movement. It is produced by a dog-eared infolding of the upper vertebral border. The sharp edge bumps over the chest wall, producing pain and a diagnostic, palpable, reverberating sound.

Scapulothoracic lesions are distinguished from other disorders of the neck-shoulder group by the localization of the pain and tenderness and the definite relation to scapular movement.

NEUROLOGICAL DISTURBANCES

Neurological disturbances should be kept in mind in investigating shoulder-neck pain. Significant lesions are more apt to be manifested as a general girdle weakness rather than as loss of a single precise action. The pain has a vague, diffuse quality described by the patient as a feeling of heaviness involving the neck-shoulder area. It may have a dragging quality that is particularly noticeable, for example, when wearing a heavy overcoat or carrying a weight on the shoulder. Such a complaint should suggest shoulder girdle weakness; careful search will often show thinning and weakness of some of the major muscles or muscle groups about the shoulder.

Paralytic disorders that implicate the suspensory muscles, whether they be peripheral nerve lesions or systemic disorders, may come into clinical focus with shoulder pain; syringomyelia, accessory nerve paralysis, and long thoracic nerve paralysis may produce this type of discomfort. Physical examination will identify these different sources, and more intricate electrical assessment will confirm the diagnosis.

Trapezius Paralysis. Involvement of the accessory nerve, with paralysis of the trapezius, may follow many shoulder injuries, but one of the more common origins is the excision of a gland in the posterior triangle for biopsy purposes. Paralysis of the trapezius allows the shoulder to droop, and the patient complains of the characteristic dragging, aching pain.

Serratus Anterior Paralysis. A similar complaint may also be elicited in patients with serratus anterior paralysis. An example of this is presented in a patient who developed pressure injury to the long thoracic nerve of Bell as a result of wearing a tightly fitting body cast. The patient was in a shoulder spica for a fracture of the opposite arm and lay heavily on the uninvolved side. Pressure from the edge of the plaster produced serratus palsy.

Deltoid Paralysis. Trauma in the posteroinferior aspect of the shoulder other than dislocation or fracture may produce damage to the axillary nerve. The history of a blow on the back that compresses the arm or penetrates the posterior axillary area and is followed by shoulder weakness makes the diagnosis obvious.

Progressive Muscular Atrophy and Allied Lesions. The complaint of weakness and vague shoulder-neck pain may develop very gradually and spread to both shoulders. One should keep in mind the somewhat rare but serious neuromuscular disorders such as progressive muscular atrophy. The diagnosis is usually obvious but may be overlooked. An example is presented of a patient who had been operated on elsewhere for acromioclavicular disturbance, but who had a clear-cut progressive atrophy of a scapulohumeral type.

LESIONS WITH DOMINANT SHOULDER PAIN

Among patients complaining of all types of shoulder discomfort, the largest group are those who specifically localize pain to the shoulder region proper. These patients omit neck and radiating complaints, concentrating on shoulder discomfort. Most of the acute shoulder disabilities belong in this group. The discomfort is localized clearly and quickly, with the patient grasping the point of the shoulder with the hand of the good side (Fig. 5–7). The patient will usually have learned that movement of the shoulder influences the pain more than any other act. The neck and hand may be implicated in longstanding disorders, but the shoulder complaint is the initial and predominant one. In general, those in the more active age bracket are the ones afflicted. Once started, the pain has a persistent aching quality that is sharply aggravated by shoulder movement and is often most bothersome at night. Progressive limitation of shoulder movement accompanies the pain. A history of trauma is usually prevalent in this group.

On examination, points of maximum

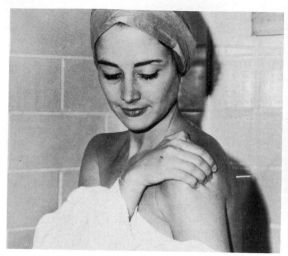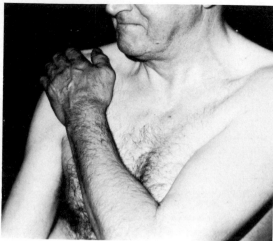

Figure 5-7 "Shoulder grasp" typical of patients with disorders of the shoulder joint proper.

tenderness can be identified in the shoulder joint. Shoulder movement, particularly abduction and rotation, is hampered. Not only can general limitation of movement be recognized, but there are specific zones of limitation which can be identified as typical of specific disorders. For example, the arc of tuberosity impingement, which occurs just as the greater tuberosity begins to come into contact with the coraco-acromial arch, is characteristic of cuff lesions, whereas the limitation of acromioclavicular disease starts after the arm has been abducted to a right angle. When the disorders have been present for some time, muscle atrophy occurs and is especially obvious in the supra- and infraspinati. The malady may have a fulminating course, such as is seen in calcified tendinitis, or it may progress slowly as in degenerative tendinitis. Both these conditions, if untreated, may result in adhesive capsulitis or the so-called frozen shoulder.

The terms bursitis, subacromial bursitis, subdeltoid bursitis and frozen shoulder have been used commonly in the past to describe most of the disorders in this group. The terms do not demarcate the diseases sufficiently clearly and are not descriptive of the underlying pathology. Peritonitis is recognized as a result of many lesions occurring in the abdominal cavity but is rarely a primary diagnosis. In the same way, the generalized term bursitis should be replaced by a more accurate description of the lesions present. Abdominal adhesions used to be a common diagnosis just as frozen shoulder is today. Too many conditions have been loosely lumped together under this heading,

and a more specific indication of the underlying pathology signifying the true cause is preferable. Careful attention to the investigation and examination of this group of shoulder disorders facilitates treatment tremendously. Most of the shoulder disorders which are helped by surgery are found in this group. The conditions comprising this group include degenerative tendinitis of the rotator cuff, tendinitis with calcification, tears of the rotator cuff, bicipital lesions, acromioclavicular arthritis, adhesive capsulitis. There are less common conditions also that may be included in this category, including osteoarthritis, infectious arthritis, metabolic arthritis and certain neurological disturbances. Neoplastic changes of the upper end of the humerus and the adjacent zone of the glenoid also fall into this group.

Finally, there is a group of conditions which refer pain to the tip of the shoulder or adjacent area which may have their origin in the neck, chest, heart or biliary tree. The duodenal ulcer is a classic example of a condition occasionally referring pain to the top of the shoulder.

DEGENERATIVE TENDINITIS

The basic cause of most shoulder disorders is wear and tear degeneration in the rotator cuff, of which various degrees, phases and complications may be encountered. The typical case of degenerative tendinitis is encountered in a middle-aged patient who complains of localized shoulder pain with a painful "arc of impingement" on abduction, starting at 75 degrees, reaching a maximum before 90 degrees and disappearing as the shoulder passes under the overhanging arch. Tenderness is present over the upper end of the humerus or at the lateral side of the head over the tuberosity. The location of the point of maximum tenderness is in contrast to bicipital lesions, in which the maximum point lies anteriorly in relation to the bicipital groove.

Aching pain at night is an outstanding characteristic. Later in the disease a typical girdle type of rhythm develops on abduction, in which the normally free swing of abduction is replaced by a hunching movement and the scapula and humerus move together as one unit. The range is grossly limited. A history of relatively minor injury may be associated, but most often the process is gradual until the night pain, stiffness and limitation of movement force the patient to seek attention. Older laborers and housewives are typical subjects. X-rays may be quite negative but should be studied carefully for minute changes in the head of the humerus, such as sclerosis, eburnation, minute cyst formation or small detached flakes. A diagnostic injection of Novocain decreases the pain and usually increases the movement. An arthrogram demonstrates an intact capsule, although sometimes the capsule is irregular and thinned.

The history and findings as just outlined quickly indicate the diagnosis. The pain is related to arm movement and not to the neck. It may extend to the deltoid insertion area, but there is no significant radiation down the arm as there is in root lesions. The disease may be confused with calcified tendinitis, minor tears of the rotator cuff and bicipital lesions. The calcified lesion is usually encountered in a younger age group, may present a much more acute picture and x-ray examination will show the calcareous deposits. Degenerative tendinitis of the cuff is differentiated from bicipital lesions by (1) the type of pain, which is not related to movements of the biceps tendon, and (2) the point of tenderness, which is diffuse or related to the greater tuberosity and not to the bicipital groove. Tears of the cuff may be difficult to distinguish from degenerative tendinitis, but in these there is a history of injury and the sudden onset of more acute distress following the injury. Cuff tears present with a more constant progressive course and with more weakness and more limitation of movement. The arthrogram shows a

typical defect. Fibrositis and musculofascial disturbances of the suspensory muscle group may also be confused with degenerative tendinitis. These conditions produce neck-shoulder pain with discomfort related to the cervical spine. The points of tenderness are in the posterior group of muscles, and manipulation of these points reproduces the discomfort. Degenerative tendinitis should not be confused with the typical root syndrome of protruded discs or with the radiating pain pattern of compression of the neurovascular bundle.

TENDINITIS WITH CALCIFICATION

The most painful disorder of shoulder disease is acute tendinitis with calcification. It presents a distinctive picture of a relatively young patient with acute shoulder pain of sudden onset which rapidly increases in severity. There is exquisite tenderness over the upper end of the humerus and often swelling and enlargement of the shoulder. Agonizing pain may be experienced on the slightest movement. X-ray examination shows the calcified deposits, which are diagnostic. This condition may be so fulminating that an acute infectious arthritis of the shoulder may be suspected; however, the history and x-ray are distinctive, and it is not easily confused with other disorders. Occasionally a chip fracture of the tuberosity may be confusing or the calcified deposit may be interpreted as a detached piece, but there are distinctive x-ray findings which separate these two conditions. The chip is corticated and sharp, and a corresponding defect in the head of the humerus may be seen. The deposit tends to be narrower, flatter and further separated from the bone.

TEARS OF THE ROTATOR CUFF

A familiar and significant picture is presented by the middle-aged workman who falls, taking his weight on the arm or shoulder. Sharp, sudden pain occurs and the arm feels limp and powerless. Under these circumstances, when there has obviously been no fracture or dislocation, a tear of the rotator cuff should be suspected. If there is also persistent shoulder pain and inability to raise the arm or hold it after it has been abducted for him, the diagnosis is confirmed. Further investigation will show a point of tenderness on the anterolateral aspect of the head of the humerus. Sometimes in thin patients a ridge or definite depression can be felt, indicating the separation of the sinews. Later, atrophy of the supra- and infraspinati occurs. Electrical stimulation shows appropriate innervation, but stimulation of the muscle bellies has no effect on the upper end of the humerus. An arthrogram shows distortion of the normal capsule contour and a leak of dye into the subacromial area in the region of the greater tuberosity. Plain x-rays also suggest that the head is riding higher than normal as related to the glenoid.

Massive tears are easily diagnosed, but difficulty arises in picking out less severe lesions such as partial ruptures or concealed tears. In these the history and age group are likely to be the same, but the local signs are not so definite and the pain is not so severe. After the injury there is weakness, which may pass off, and later some loss of power of abduction is apparent, and a normal range is not attained. The effort at abduction is accompanied by typical hunching of the shoulder, in which the point is elevated as the arm stays dependent. Crepitus is present, and often a snapping or catching sensation that can be felt by the patient and the examiner occurs as the humeral head reaches the coraco-acromial arch. The injury is partially disabling; it is helped but not corrected by the usual conservative measures.

When such a picture persists for a matter of weeks without subsidence of pain or increase in movement, more damage to the cuff must be postulated than simple bruising or degeneration. The arthrogram is of considerable help; any leak of the dye into the subacromial space will be indicative of a defect in the cuff. This lesion is most often mislabeled a simple bursitis. If the injury is neglected, these patients remain disabled or end with a frozen shoulder and adhesive capsulitis. The history of injury, persistent disability and no relief by the normal measures separate this condition from degenerative tendinitis and calcified tendinitis. There is no related neck pain or radiating discomfort, which keeps the disorder in the group with predominant shoulder discomfort.

BICIPITAL LESIONS

The role of the biceps mechanism as a cause of common shoulder disabilities has not generally been appreciated. The course taken by the long head of the biceps through a narrow tunnel and over a mobile joint makes it susceptible to wear and tear changes such as those that occur in the rotator cuff. Injury and degeneration of the biceps produce shoulder pain, local tenderness, limitation of movement and a specific pain pattern on certain tests. Flexion and supination of the forearm against resistance initiate pain localized to the front of the shoulder and down the inside of the arm along the biceps tendon. The position of the point of maximum tenderness is characteristic in that it lies over the bicipital groove at the top or along the tendon at the front. Flexion and supination may spring the biceps tendon from the groove when the arm is externally rotated, and the patient will localize the pain to the area that is tender on palpation. Injury, as a rule, brings the disorder into clinical focus.

When the general signs and symptoms indicative of this lesion have been appreciated, further consideration and examination will identify several different types. The common derangements are bicipital tendinitis, rupture of the biceps tendon and rupture of the intertubercular fibers. Any alteration in the smooth relation of the tendon to the tendon sheath or to the groove may produce the typical syndrome. The test of flexion and supination against resistance is significant but may not always be positive. A localized snapping sensation in the region of the biceps groove and abnormal mobility of the tendon, particularly with the arm abducted and externally rotated, is diagnostic of rupture of the transverse humeral fibers. Frequently patients with bicipital injuries assume a characteristic posture. They have learned that much pain is avoided if the arm is kept close to the side, so they tend to use the forearm, moving it at the elbow but keeping the arm close to the chest.

Tendinitis or tenosynovitis produces definite tenderness along the tendon and sometimes a creaking sensation in the tender zone along the groove. Rupture of the long head leaves the typical shortened muscle belly with gross weakness on flexion of the elbow. Avulsion of the intertubercular fibers leaves a lax tendon which snaps, accompanied by pain, particularly on abduction and external rotation. Laxity of the tendon can be demonstrated best in the abducted and internally rotated position, in which the tendon may be slipped from side to side in the groove.

These lesions are most often confused with rotator cuff disorders, either tendinitis or partial rupture. It should be possible to differentiate bicipital lesions from these. The point of maximum tenderness is over the biceps tendon, at the front, and is related to the bicipital groove in distinction to the cuff lesion, in which the sore point is over the tuberosity on the lateral or anterolateral aspect. Ruptured cuff lesions do not have a lax or snapping biceps or shortened relaxed muscle belly. Separating a simple rotator tendinitis from bicipital tendinitis is more difficult; the best guide is the site of maximum tenderness and pain on flexion against resistance.

ACROMIOCLAVICULAR ARTHRITIS

Disturbances of the acromioclavicular joint produce localized shoulder pain. Sometimes they are overlooked or confused with the more common rotator cuff and bicipital lesions. When the acromioclavicular joint is involved, the point of maximum tenderness is on the upper aspect of the shoulder, directly over the articulation. There is pain related to shoulder movement, particularly abduction, and it occurs in a particular segment of the circumduction arc, after 90 degrees. This is in contrast to cuff lesions, in which the pain starts before the tuberosity reaches the acromion, usually at 60 to 70 degrees. Some patients will volunteer the information that the arm can be lifted to shoulder level and that it is after this point is reached that they have the discomfort. Other characteristic findings in acromioclavicular arthritis are enlargement of the lateral end of the clavicle and cracking or grating sensation on manipulation.

X-rays show a narrowing of joint space and roughening or erosion of the lateral end of the clavicle, which clinch the diagnosis. A suspected joint should always be compared with the opposite side, particularly when the contour seems a little abnormal. It is not uncommon to have both ends of the clavicle a little large or unusually prominent without producing symptoms. When the point of tenderness, the zone of pain and x-ray changes have been demonstrated, there is little difficulty in distinguishing acromio-clavicular arthritis from glenohumeral arthritis and cuff or bicipital lesions.

ADHESIVE CAPSULITIS OF THE SHOULDER (PERIARTICULAR ARTHRITIS, FROZEN SHOULDER, ETC.)

There remains a large group of disorders that have predominant shoulder pain and obvious local shoulder signs. These have been lumped together loosely as frozen shoulder. Any of the lesions that have previously been described—rotator cuff tendinitis, bicipital lesions, acromioclavicular arthritis, cuff tears, and so forth—may end in typical frozen shoulder. This term describes a sign or symptom complex which, instead of being a separate etiological entity itself, results from diverse pathologies. Too many disorders have been labeled frozen shoulder without identification of the true underlying cause. Frozen shoulder arises most commonly as a reaction to the process of degeneration in the rotator cuff or bicipital mechanisms. Degeneration in the cuff results from impairment of blood supply or constant snubbing action of the tendon against the acromion, favoring a general wear and tear process. A similar situation exists in the action of the biceps tendon from constant wear and tear in the groove and over the articular surface. Cuff tears produce pain as the arm is used, as does acromioclavicular arthritis, and the patient learns to avoid the pain by keeping the arm at the side. This favors adhesions and contraction of the redundant capsule and synovial folds on the inferior aspect of the joint. When the capsule becomes stuck, with the folds glued together, gross limitation of movement results. The disorder may be initiated by disease at a distance, such as injury to the forearm and hand, for example, but the process is the same, with constriction and eventual gluing together of the normally free synovial capsular surfaces (Neviaser, 1945).

There remain a small group of cases, usually among women of menopausal age, in which it is difficult to unearth the primary cause. In the majority of these patients this process arises as a result of some other disturbance, so that the thickening and adhesive action in cuff and capsule are a secondary and not a primary lesion. There is no mistaking the characteristic picture, with atrophy, gross limitation of movement and the hunching girdle action.

Comparison of Degenerative Tendinitis, Rupture of Cuff and Bicipital Lesions

The greatest difficulty in differential diagnosis of the disorders with predominant shoulder pain occurs in separating degenerative tendinitis, rupture of the cuff and bicipital lesions. The points of importance in the diagnosis are in Table 5–1. Most of the time, by careful physical examination and history, the diagnosis can be made accurately, but considerable help can be obtained from electrical investigation, careful x-ray study, certain special tests, Novocain injection and arthrography.

Many cases of degenerative tendinitis have been overlooked because sufficiently careful x-ray examination has not been carried out. Minute changes in the head of the humerus, such as detached flakes, cystic formation and sclerosis of the tuberosity, are significant but can be completely overlooked in a routine investigation. In ruptures of the rotator cuff, the massive tear is straightforward, but minor tears are harder to demonstrate. Small tears and degenerative lesions are both improved by local anesthetic infiltration, but in the case of cuff tears, weakness and pain persist; a degenerative lesion runs a less progressive course and may retain some improvement after injection.

In suspected bicipital lesions the point of tenderness is well around to the front in relation to the groove and is not over the lateral aspect. There is pain and weakness on supination and flexion of forearm against resistance. Tenderness often follows the long head of the biceps down the arm, and slipping of the long head in the groove is a diagnostic finding. Many are not familiar with the use of electrical stimulation as a diagnostic aid, but it has a very definite place in investigation of shoulder problems. Stimulation of the biceps without using the arm produces pain in bicipital lesions. Stimulation of the supra- and infraspinatus has little effect on the humerus when the cuff is torn. In persistent lesions the arthrogram is extremely helpful in diagnosis and will usually help to differentiate cuff tears from other lesions.

LESS COMMON CONDITIONS

Posttraumatic and Osteoarthritis. These conditions do not occur frequently and, when they do, are not likely to be confused with the preceding disorders. Posttraumatic and osteoarthritis have characteristic x-ray findings and there is no question of pain and discomfort arising from shoulder movement. Muscle weakness is not prominent. There are no specifically localized painful arcs of movement. Posttraumatic arthritis has the obvious history of injury. Osteoarthritis occurs in the older age group; the x-rays are characteristic.

Acute Infectious Arthritis. This lesion is also uncommon. It is easily recognized by the signs and symptoms of an acute inflammatory process, with acute local tenderness and limitation of movement. There is a febrile systemic disturbance also. The only lesion which may be confused with this disorder is acute tendinitis with calcification and, under these circumstances, the x-ray examination is diagnostic.

Metabolic Arthritis. This is a very rare lesion usually encountered only in conjunction with involvement of other joints in the body by the same process. It also may be confused with degenerative tendinitis with calcification, but a test therapeutic dose of colchicum usually settles the issue.

Neurological Disturbances. Paralytic disorders that implicate the suspensory muscles, whether they be peripheral nerve lesions or systemic disorders, may come into clinical focus with shoulder pain. Thus, syringomyelia, accessory nerve paralysis or long thoracic nerve paralysis may produce this type of discomfort. Physical examination will identify the source, and more intricate electrical assessment will confirm the diagnosis.

Neoplasms. Neoplasms of humerus, scapula and clavicle frequently produce localized shoulder pain that is sometimes related to shoulder movement. There is very little neck pain, and radiating symptoms are rare until the advanced stage. The pain has a characteristic persistent, boring quality that is unrelieved by rest or the supported position. The problem has a progressive quality, becoming less and less susceptible to relief from mild analgesics. When this progressive picture is presented and is completely unrelieved by simple measures, it is suggestive of serious disorder.

Table 5-1 Comparison of Common Lesions Producing Localized Shoulder Pain

Lesion	History of Injury	Mechanism of Injury	Pain	Tenderness	Muscle Weakness	Persistence of Symptoms	Electrical Stimulation	X-rays	Special Test	Local Anesthetic Injection
Degenerative tendinitis	Not prominent, occasionally repeated minor trauma	Minor incident	Night pain prominent, shoulder to deltoid insertion to elbow in later stages	Over head of humerus, lateral to acromion	Not prominent	Gradual development; may be remissions	Normal response or very little alteration	Important. Detached flakes; sclerosis; cystic formation		Decreases pain; good active movement possible
Rupture of cuff	More severe episode, usually in workmen over 50 years of age	Major episode, usually a fall on the outstretched arm or a direct blow	Local shoulder	Head of humerus, lateral aspect, sometimes with sulcus palpable	Prominent	Persistent and progressive	Poor response	Little change in routine films usually, but arthrograms are diagnostic	Inability to maintain abduction	Improvement in active power very little and not sustained
Bicipital lesions	Usually a recent episode	Often sudden extension of elbow when lifting, or a fall backward with the arm and hand behind the body as protection	Shoulder plus radiation along biceps tendon	Medially or anteromedially along bicipital groove and along biceps tendon	Bicipital weakness	Protective movements develop	Frequently reproduces the pain	Special views of tuberosity may show osteophytes	Supination against resistance of the flexed forearm produces pain	Infiltration of the bicipital area produces relief

Referred Pain. Disturbances apart from the shoulder may give rise to pain which is appreciated in this general area. Referred pain is often difficult to localize, sometimes occurring at the root of the neck, in the neck-shoulder angle, at the point of the shoulder, or in the upper arm. Superior pulmonary sulcus tumor, cardiovascular lesions, gastric and biliary lesions, subdiaphragmatic disease and metastatic lesions may all produce pain in the general shoulder zone. As a rule, signs and symptoms belonging to the primary disturbance become apparent before the referred sensation is paramount.

Neck Lesions. Disturbances in the neck frequently refer pain to the shoulder, as has been previously pointed out. However, investigation will show that the neck is implicated much more than the shoulder. Spinal cord lesions, disc lesions and arthritis of the cervical spine may refer pain to the shoulder, but the pain has a poorly localized quality, shoulder action is not involved and examination does not demonstrate significant local points of tenderness. In addition, there are the other spinal signs and symptoms not present in disorders of the shoulder proper.

LESIONS CAUSING SHOULDER PLUS RADIATING PAIN

Perhaps the most perplexing group of conditions are those affecting patients who talk of shoulder discomfort but immediately complain of extension of the pain below the elbow or as far as the hand (Fig. 5–8). Extension of pain to the deltoid insertion is quite routine in the glenohumeral or clearly defined shoulder proper group, but there exist other disorders that clearly implicate the extremity far beyond this region and often tend to emphasize the more distal zones. These patients present themselves as having shoulder problems, but in the next breath they talk about pain in the arm, forearm, hand and fingers. When questioned they tend to concentrate on the radiating discomfort and say less about the shoulder. Frequently, the discomfort has been experienced in the shoulder area for a short while in the beginning and then radiating discomfort has set in later and persists as the most disturbing element. There has been a tendency to lump together many entities of this group under transiently popular terms, such as scalenus anticus or cervical rib syndromes,

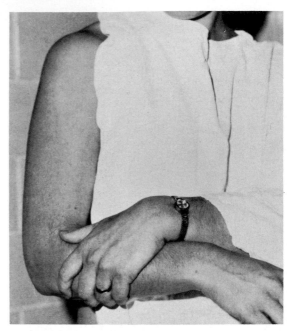

Figure 5–8 Patients with radiating shoulder pain implicate the shoulder but emphasize peripheral distribution.

without delving into the possibility of other causes. Investigation shows there are many lesions in this group, but two fundamental causes may be recognized: a group of conditions with a dominant neural background, and a further distinct group with a vascular or neurovascular association.

Certain qualities of radiating pain should be demarcated. There is a pain pattern from the posterior shoulder or scapular zone which flits to the back of the elbow and then to the back of the hand. Most often the back of the hand and fingers are involved, and the patient usually cannot identify a precise peripheral distribution. Such a pattern most often stems from soft tissue disturbances such as the fibrositic lesions in the shoulder-neck angle and, as a rule, can be identified by these properties. Sometimes the distribution of the pain specifically involves the little finger, but when it does, it usually affects the posterior surface rather than the whole digit. Characteristically, pain due to such soft tissue disturbances is dispersed by activity and aggravated by inactivity. In contrast, pain of neural origin is quite different, comprising a tingling shock-like sensation that is usually alleviated by rest. Vascular pain, in turn, differs from both these modalities in that it contributes a feeling of fullness to the hand, and the whole hand is usually implicated rather than one or two fingers. Frequently there is a persistent postural or positional irritant, and motion rapidly diffuses the pain.

CERVICAL ROOT SYNDROME (EXTRUDED INTERVERTEBRAL DISC, INTRAFORAMINAL NERVE ROOT COMPRESSION, SPONDYLOSIS, CORD TUMORS)

Irritation of a cervical nerve root produces discomfort in the shoulder area and usually characteristic radiating pain. The root syndrome results from many conditions, including spinal cord tumors, extruded intervertebral discs, alterations in the bony contour of intervertebral foramina, compression fractures, and so forth. Ultimately radiating pain is prominent in these conditions. It often starts in the neck, extends to the shoulder and later is more obvious in the forearm, hand and fingers. It shortly assumes a sharp or shooting quality and is aggravated by neck movement, coughing, sneezing and jarring. After the nerve root pattern has been recognized, the individual lesion may be sorted out.

Tumors of the cervical cord and nerve roots are not common but should be suspected when there is a gradual onset of neck pain that persists quite unrelieved by rest and the usual conservative measures. Pain which is not alleviated by rest should always be carefully assessed. When the lesion has been present for some little time, other signs and symptoms appear that are suggestive of cord or root compression. Lower motor and sensory neuron signs appear in the upper extremity, whereas the legs show signs of upper motor neuron irritation in the form of increased tone, upgoing toe, clonus, and so forth. Total protein in the spinal fluid is increased in cord tumors and lesions with space-taking proportions. The myelogram and Queckenstedt test are diagnostic.

Root disturbance from disc irritation has some of the same local and radiating pain characteristics, but these are not so severe or intractable as in the case of tumors. Movement of the neck aggravates the pain. Flexion to the involved side increases the pain, whereas tilting the head away from that side decreases the discomfort. The common sensory and pain patterns travel to the base of the thumb when C.6 is involved and to the index finger in involvement of C.7. The

biceps jerk is disturbed in the former and the triceps altered in the latter. Increased spinal fluid protein is commonly found, but is not nearly so high as in the case of tumor. The myelogram indicates a notch defect or space-taking abnormality. Symptoms from disturbances at the C.5–C.6 level are by far the commonest.

Bony abnormalities of the intervertebral foramen, such as arthritic lipping encroaching on the nerve root space, produce root symptoms also more frequently than previously realized. This disturbance has a more chronic course and is usually preceded by considerable neck and neck-shoulder discomfort before radiating symptoms develop. They are not nearly so clear-cut as in tumors or disc irritations, and frank motor and sensory signs are not so common. The pain is not aggravated nearly so much by bending to the same side or relieved by bending to the opposite side. Jugular compression does not reproduce the radiating pain, as is the case in tumors and root disturbances. Oblique x-ray studies of the intervertebral foramina must be done to show bony encroachment on the intervertebral foramen. Lipping of the vertebral bodies alone is not enough to substantiate this diagnosis since this often occurs without producing significant clinical signs and symptoms.

CERVICAL RIB AND SCALENE SYNDROME

Further out from spinal cord the nerve roots are grouped into trunks and cords and become intimately associated with the vascular bundle to the arm. The union takes place above the clavicle at a point where an additional cervical rib or a tight scalenus anterior muscle may partially block the combined neurovascular bundle.

Compression of this bundle results in radiating discomfort and shoulder pain. The character of the radiation changes, however, from a pure, well defined, neural pattern to a broad, more vague discomfort because of the vascular association. The general properties of both these conditions should be appreciated first; the individual characteristics typical of rib and muscle disorders will be defined later. Both conditions produce aching neck-shoulder pain, a feeling of numbness and tingling going down the arm to the fingers. The inner aspect of forearm and hand is the site usually involved, as compared with the outer aspect of thumb and index finger in the common cervical root lesions. The tingling frequently involves all the fingers, producing a sense of fullness in the hand. If motor and sensory signs develop, they involve the ulnar supply most often because of pressure on the medial cord of the plexus. The small muscles of the hand are involved, but either median or ulnar groups are singled out. This distribution of atrophy following a definite peripheral nerve pattern is in contrast to progressive muscular atrophy, in which there is generalized involvement not following a specific pattern.

Shoulder and arm movement are not particularly involved in either cervical rib or scalenus anticus disorders. Points of tenderness and soreness may be identified in the supraclavicular region, away from the shoulder area proper and lying above the clavicle. When neck pain is present it tends to be at the front, in contrast to the posterior discomfort of fibrositis and postural disorders.

Cervical ribs may be present and not cause symptoms, but when they are the cause, symptoms occur in early adult life and, frequently, in both arms. Sometimes the ribs are palpable, or a tight band can be felt extending from the side of the neck across the posterior triangle to the first rib. X-ray is very helpful in diagnosis of this problem. Sometimes bands can be suspected when there is an unusually long transverse process of C.7 without definite rib formation; or a longer than normal process in an apical neck may be enough to irritate the lower cord.

The scalene syndrome is quite similar to the cervical rib disturbance but has distinguishing features. It is more commonly encountered on one side only and occurs in a somewhat older age group than cervical rib. Investigation of the scalenus anterior itself usually demonstrates local signs and symptoms. On pressure the muscle is tender, and deep pressure reproduces the radiating discomfort. Injection of the muscle relieves the local pain and decreases radiating signs. Extension of the neck commonly reproduces or increases the pain, and sometimes the radial pulse can be shut off by this maneuver. Both cervical rib and scalene syndromes differ from root lesions resulting from disc irritation. The type of pain is more diffuse with the vascular component added, and there is more frequent involvement of the inside of forearm and hand compared with the outside in root lesions. Compression flexion to the side of disturbance increases pain in extruded discs but decreases it when the scalenus anticus is the neurovascular constricting agent. Further differentiating signs are the stiff neck, x-ray changes in the cervical spine and positive myelogram obtained in root lesions. Atrophy of the small muscles involves the ulnar group chiefly in cervical rib in distinction to the index and thenar group in discs. The predominant vascular basis of the radiating pain resulting in diffuse hand discomfort differs from the more localized, sharp type of radiation in root lesions.

CLAVIPECTORAL COMPRESSION SYNDROMES

There is a further group of disorders manifesting shoulder and radiating symptoms that do not belong in the cervical root or scalenus cervical rib classes. They resemble the latter because the findings suggest a vascular or neurovascular etiology; many have been erroneously called scalene or cervical rib lesions. In this group there are further distinguishing features separating several entities. The complete etiology and pathology have not yet been firmly established so that clinical attributes are largely relied upon for classification.

The symptoms common to the group as a whole are paresthesias or numbness and tingling in the hand and fingers that develops after vague shoulder discomfort. The peripheral portion of the extremity, forearm, hand and fingers, quickly becomes the seat of the prominent discomfort and the shoulder symptoms fade. The paresthesias follow no well defined distribution and the pattern is indistinct, particularly as compared with the pain or numbness of peripheral nerve lesions. Frequently both sides are involved. The vascular contribution is manifested by coldness, cyanotic hue and crampy pain on effort. Writer's cramp is an example. Many of the symptoms and disorders have a striking relation to the position of the arm or the head. The abducted position of the arm at work or at rest is a potent irritant in many instances.

The fundamental pathology common to the group appears to be stretch and compression of the neurovascular bundle, at some point in its periclavicular, not clavicular, course. This possibility above the clavicle has been acknowledged in cervical rib and scalene lesions, but it has not been recognized that a similar disturbance may arise behind and below the clavicle as well. Pressure on the neurovascular bundle along the cervico-axillary canal may develop directly behind the clavicle, below the clavicle or behind the pectoralis minor. The bundle lies on a firm bed along its entire course, but the structures on top of it move in three separate zones. Superiorly, the clavicle rolls up and down and may pinch the vessels or the first rib. Lower down, the costocoracoid membrane, as a remnant of the precoracoid of primitive forms, may tighten on the bundle through its connections with the enveloping fascia. Still more distally, the sharp edge of the pectoralis minor may become the compressing force or fulcrum. A soft bundle on a hard bed is easily crushed by these structures. Several special types of compression may be recognized: costoclavicular, postural and hyperabduction. All of these conditions are to be differentiated from the carpal tunnel syndrome in which there is no shoulder involvement and numbness and tingling are clearly confined to median nerve distribution.

Costoclavicular Neurovascular Compression

The neurovascular bundle in entering the axillary canal runs through a narrow cleft beneath the clavicle and on top of the first rib. This is a slit-like aperture with the subclavius muscle arching across it, sometimes with a sharp, fusiform lower margin. Alterations and abnormalities in this cleft can compress the neurovascular bundle. Since the vein is the most medial structure running into the arm and lies in the narrowest part of the cleft, it bears the brunt of any narrowing that develops. Abnormalities, fractures, and dislocations of the medial third of the clavicle or fractures of first rib followed by excess callus formation can constrict this space. The resulting symptoms are a sense of fullness in hand and fingers and an aching, crampy pain in the forearm and hand. Vague shoulder or shoulder-arm discomfort may be mentioned, but the radiating pain is emphasized. The hand may be swollen intermittently, and sometimes superficial veins about the shoulder are engorged. There is no limitation of shoulder movement, which contrasts with the shoulder-hand syndrome

in which gross shoulder immobilization is prominent and there are hand symptoms. The radiating discomfort has the typical diffuse vascular pattern not localized to nerve root or peripheral nerve distribution.

In addition to those patients with obvious abnormality of rib and clavicle, some develop this disturbance from a sagging shoulder girdle and atonic musculature. Normally it is difficult to encroach upon the neurovascular bundle beneath the clavicle, but it is conceivable that some sagging occurs, and when some tension in the bundle and enveloping sheath is added, the vessels may be compressed.

This costoclavicular group can be separated from scalene and cervical rib disturbances by several findings. There is no relation to cervical spine movements and no scalene or supraclavicular tenderness. The x-rays are different since no cervical rib is present. Arterial symptoms are not prominent, and most of the disturbances appear to be the result of venous obstruction. Costoclavicular compression can be differentiated from postural compression by the absence of any significant relation to body position, either at work or when sleeping. It is also clearly differentiated from hyperabduction compression by the lack of significant relation to shoulder movement.

Postural Compression and Sleep Syndromes

There is a large group of patients manifesting the general signs and symptoms of neurovascular compression which have a definite relation to the position of the body, the neck and the arm. The two common types of this disorder are associated with occupational posture and with sleep habits. These patients have vague shoulder pain but they are much more concerned with a feeling of pins and needles, unpleasant numbness or a feeling of the hand going asleep on one or both sides. Tingling is felt in the fingertips, but it is a spasmodic discomfort not continually present. There are no motor or sensory signs, but a light subjective hypesthesia is present in several fingers when the tingling is present.

The key to these disorders is their relation to posture changes, either occupational or nocturnal. Some patients have just assumed a new occupation in which the use of the arms has increased. It will be noted that some activity or position, such as lifting heavy paper rolls in the slumped position or constant stretching and lifting at shoulder level or above, is the irritant and sets off the numbness and tingling. Most of these patients are in the young, active group. The cardinal finding is that the majority of the symptoms can be reproduced by compression of the vascular bundle as it passes below the coracoid process.

The other postural disturbances are the nocturnal dysesthesias. Patients with this problem complain of pain in the shoulder and numbness and tingling in arm and hand. The hand "goes to sleep" or "goes dead," and they have to shake it to bring back the feeling. The patients usually do not notice that the resting or sleeping posture is the aggravating or initiating factor; they volunteer that the disturbance is frequent at night but have not related the sleeping position to their symptoms. When the condition is of long standing, relatively little compression or irritation sets off the reaction. As in the previous group, the discomfort is reproduced by subcoracoid pressure. Often the radial pulse of these patients is obliterated by abduction and external rotation a little more easily than normal. Various positions may be responsible, such as lying on the arm and shoulder or sleeping with arm abducted and externally rotated. Sometimes no disturbing sleeping position is apparent, but use of a new mattress, a different pillow or a shorter bed has altered the usual posture and alleviated the problem. When the syndrome is appreciated and its relationship to sleep is apparent, it is not confused with other conditions.

Hyperabduction Syndrome

Wright has labeled a further group of compression problems as the hyperabduction syndrome. Patients with this disorder are usually young males of short, stocky stature who work long hours with the arms held above shoulder level. Shoulder pain and finger paresthesias develop. In some instances the discomfort appears without extreme abduction. Some people are more prone than others to develop these symptoms; they are separated from the rest by the definite history, their youth and the characteristically easy obliteration of pulse on abduction.

SHOULDER-HAND SYNDROMES

The shoulder and hand are associated in a common symptoms complex, the lesion being a reflex sympathetic dystrophy in which painful contracture of the hand and the fingers develops with or following some shoulder disorder. Usually this is a secondary development and the primary cause lies in the shoulder as a sequel to trauma to the upper extremity or in lesions in the heart, the chest, the neck or the nervous system. This syndrome is easily differentiated from other causes of shoulder plus radiating discomfort. The dystrophic changes in hand and fingers are typical, stiffness and limitation of movement rather than pain being the manifestation. The fingers are reddened, moist and swollen. There are no sensory disturbances, and there is no relation to posture or activity. Contracture of hand and fingers may be severe enough to resemble Dupuytren's contracture. The hand disability often overshadows the shoulder stiffness.

CARPAL TUNNEL SYNDROMES

Tingling discomfort in the fingers and numbness and clumsiness in use may develop from compression of the median nerve at the wrist. Such lesions are sometimes confused with the many entities in the shoulder plus radiating pain disorders. They may be separated from fibrositic and vascular disturbances because, typically, it is a precise median nerve distribution that is involved; this means that the pain is usually on the opposite side of the hand. The real problem is differentiating a cervical root disturbance at the C.5–C.6 level from these carpal tunnel syndromes. The history of neck pain, neck stiffness, cervical x-ray changes, reproduction of the pain on vertical compression of the neck or neck bending, the intermittent character of the pain, the less clearly demarcated sensory changes and the less likelihood of atrophy will aid definitive diagnosis.

In the carpal tunnel syndrome, as a rule, the signs and symptoms are clearly localized to the median nerve distribution in the hand. The pain and sensitivity implicate the anterior aspect predominantly. Occasionally discomfort extends up the forearm because of a severe nerve compression in the tunnel, but this pain has quite different qualities from that caused by nerve root compression in the cervical region. The special investigation of particular help in differentiating these two lesions is electromyographic examination. In the carpal tunnel syndrome the changes obviously involve the thenar eminence; in the cervical root disturbance changes may be found as high as the posterior cervical musculature as a result of involvement of the posterior spinal nerve. Alterations in other parts of the limb well above the carpal zone may also be detected. Nerve conduction studies serve to further differentiate the two states.

REFERENCES

Bozyk, Z.: Shoulder-hand syndrome in patients with antecedent myocardial infarctions. Rheumatologia (Warsz.) 6:103–106, 1968.

Cinquegranao, D.: Chronic cervical radiculitis and its relationship to "chronic bursitis." Amer. J. Phys. Med. 47:23–30, 1968.

Coventry, M. B.: Problems of painful shoulder. J.A.M.A. 151(No. 3.):177–185, 1953.

Engelman, R. M.: Shoulder pain as a presenting complaint in upper lobe bronchogenic carcinoma: Report of 21 cases. Conn. Med. 30:273–276, 1966.

Finke, J.: Neurologic differential diagnosis: The lower cervical region. Deutsch. Med. Wschr. 90:1912–1917, 1965.

Gascon, J.: A current problem: Diagnosis of the shoulder pain syndrome. Un. Med. Canada 94:463–469, 1965.

Gligore, V., et al.: Shoulder pain as a manifestation of visceral disease. Deutsch. Gesundh. 20:956–960, 1965.

Heck, C. V.: Hoarseness and painful deglutition due to massive cervical exostoses. Surg. Gynec. Obstet. 102:657–660, 1956.

Kapoor, S. C., et al.: Cervical spondylosis simulating cardiac pain. Indian J. Chest Dis. 8:25–28, 1966.

King, J., Jr., and Holmes, G.: The diagnosis and treatment of four hundred and five painful shoulders. J.A.M.A. 89:1956, 1927.

Kosina, W., et al.: Neurological disorders and radiological diagnosis of developmental abnormalities of the cervical spine. Rheumatologia (Warsz.) 3:135–145, 1965.

McRae, D. L.: The cervical spine and neurologic disease. Radiol. Clin. N. Amer. 4:145–158, 1966.

Neviaser, J. S.: Adhesive capsulitis of the shoulder; study of pathological findings in periarthritis of the shoulder. J. Bone Jt. Surg. 27:211–222, 1945.

Neviaser, J. S.: Musculoskeletal disorders of the shoulder region causing cervicobrachial pain: Differential diagnosis and treatment. Surg. Clin. N. Amer. 43:1703–1714, 1963.

Ott, V. R., et al.: Differential diagnosis of ankylosing spinal disease. Arch. Phys. Ther. (Leipzig) 17:141–148, 1965.

Pichler, E.: Cervical headache. Landarzt 41:1553–1560, 1965.

Scoville, W. B., et al.: Lateral rupture of cervical intervertebral discs. Postgrad. Med. 39:174–180, 1966.

Sharp, J.: The differential diagnosis of ankylosing spondylitis. Proc. Roy. Soc. Med. 59:453–455, 1966.

Smith, G. W., and Robinson, R. A.: The treatment of certain cervical spine disorders by anterior removal of the intervertebral disc and interbody fusion. J. Bone Joint Surg. 40A:607–624, 1958.

Wright, I. S.: Neurovascular syndrome produced by hyperabduction of the arms. Amer. Heart J. 29:1, 1945.

Wright, I. S.: Vascular Diseases in Clinical Practice. Chicago, Year Book Medical Publishers, Inc., 1948.

Section

III

CLINICAL SYNDROMES

Chapter VI

LESIONS PRODUCING NECK PAIN ALONE OR PREDOMINANTLY

Much attention is now focused on cervical spine disorders. The symptoms arising from diseases in this area initially implicate the local zone, but some progress to produce radiating discomfort also. This chapter will consider those states dominantly manifested by local neck symptoms and signs.

ATLANTO-OCCIPITAL AND ATLANTOAXIAL ARTHRITIS

These joints have powerful protecting ligaments and are rarely implicated before middle life unless injuries have occurred. Wear and tear changes may lead to articular irregularities, but commonly they are much less frequent than in the lower cervical spine. Limitation of head rotation or head flexion and extension in contrast to altered neck action is the common finding. Pain extends laterally and to the suboccipital zone rather than down the neck posteriorly. Local tenderness is present, and points of maximum sensitivity on either side in the suboccipital region can be identified (Fig. 6–1).

Treatment. In the acute arthritic phase treatment is by immobilization in a Plexiglass cervical collar during waking hours and by a soft cervical collar or small pillow at night. Traction is not routinely effective except for its contribution to immobilization of the region. Sedatives and phenylbutazone (if tolerated) are administered routinely. Once acute signs and symptoms have abated, physiotherapy, including massage, short wave diathermy and gentle assisted active motion is introduced. The collar is gradually discarded over a 10- to 12-week period, but proper sleeping posture is maintained indefinitely.

STERNOMASTOID TENDINITIS

The attachment of the upper end of the powerful sternomastoid muscle to the skull is sometimes the seat of tendon-bone junction disturbances such as may be encountered in similar anatomical situations elsewhere in the body. The patient is conscious of local pain that sometimes implicates the ear and

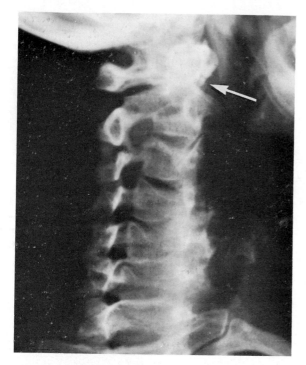

neck slightly to the opposite side because of the tension or spasm in the muscle. Active motion to the opposite side evokes pain related to the mastoid zone. In some instances there is a history of trauma to the neck or a period of unaccustomed stress from prolonged lying, reading or similar activities. In many instances no antecedent trauma is recalled (Fig. 6–2).

X-ray examination will sometimes identify changes in the form of a calcified deposit.

Treatment. In the acute stage local anesthetic infiltration and the injection of a steroid preparation are helpful. This is followed by a period of immobilization in a cervical collar; with subsidence of the acute symptoms, a program of physiotherapy is initiated. Medication, usually some form of phenylbutazone and a light sedative, is required also.

ACUTE CERVICAL SPRAINS

Sudden onset of a painful kink in the neck is sometimes encountered in a somewhat younger age group. The usual story is a sudden twisting trauma implicating the central lateral portion of the neck. These are

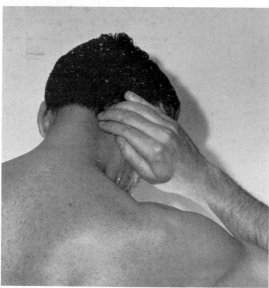

Figure 6–1 Atlantoaxial arthritis. *A*, X-ray showing area of involvement; *B*, point of tenderness.

often extends on one side up the back of the head. It almost never involves both sides at the same time. On examination a somewhat tight or spastic sternomastoid may be identified, and tenderness well localized to the tip of the mastoid process and adjacent zone of sternomastoid attachment is present. The patient has a tendency to tilt the head and

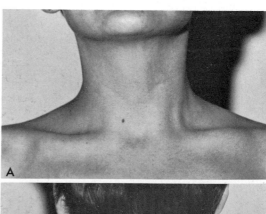
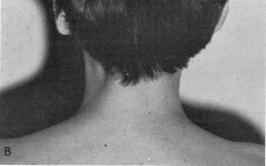

Figure 6–2 Sternomastoid tendinitis. Note that the sternomastoid muscle stands out in both back and front.

adequately treated by sedation, light traction and muscle relaxants.

OSTEOARTHRITIS

Degenerative changes in the cervical spine are found almost universally after the age of 50 (Fig. 6–3). They are clearly seen in x-ray studies and all too frequently are interpreted as the causative agent for neck and shoulder pain. Discomfort does not arise from these changes nearly so often as it does from some of the soft tissue disturbances which have previously been described. As a rule, symptoms arise only when some added disturbance, such as trauma, increased strain, continuous postural effort or progressive debilitation, is superimposed.

Cardinal Signs and Symptoms. Aching pain in shoulder and neck that is associated with activity and relieved by rest is the commonest complaint. Stiffness, soreness and pain frequently begin in the morning and increase during the day. The patient tends to keep the neck straight, moves it stiffly and is apprehensive of turning it to the side. Turning the head as one is backing a car out of a garage may be an irritant.

Treatment. Acute exacerbations of pain are treated by immobilization in an appropriate cervical collar followed by physiotherapy that is accompanied by adequate systemic medication (Fig. 6–4). Medication includes such anti-inflammatory drugs as may be tolerated by the patient, muscle relaxants and light sedatives. The collar is not worn indefinitely since a period of six to eight weeks is usually sufficient for subsidence of the acute irritation. Following this, progressive increase in active motion can be started. The collar is kept available for use during periods of occupational or working distress or further acute exacerbations.

"STOP-LIGHT" SPRAIN

This entity has been fully covered in the section on injuries.

RHEUMATOID AND STRÜMPELL-MARIE ARTHRITIS

Acute pain that causes gross restriction of neck bending and a poker stiff spine develop when the cervical region is involved in these processes. The symptoms are largely local, in contrast to some states of osteoarthritis in which radiating pain commonly develops. Ankylosing spondylitis almost always involves the cervical spine, producing gross restriction of motion and considerable deformity. The atlanto-occipital joint may be spared, so that the patient retains some rotatory motion, but extensive restriction remains. The complications that may occur as a result of the extreme rigidity can be serious. Subluxation of the cervical spine at the atlanto-axial joint or fractures in the midcervical region are a frequent occurrence (Fig. 6–5).

Treatment. During the acute arthritic phase, systemic measures such as indocin, phenylbutazone alone or in combination with a steroid like prednisone, may be used, depending upon the response and tolerance of the patient. The neck should be supported to prevent forward flexion, which contributes to the tendency of flexion contracture. Physiotherapy is important to preserve even a small amount of motion at any of the joints and should be started as soon as the control of pain will allow. Because of the severity of the late complications and luxation and dislocation, immediate reduction and immobilization are required until stability is restored. Cord damage is easily sustained; fatalities

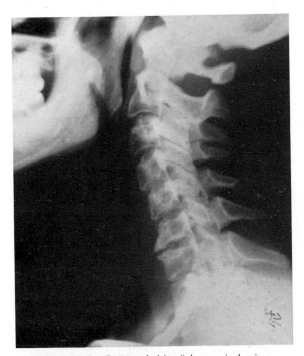

Figure 6–3 Osteoarthritis of the cervical spine.

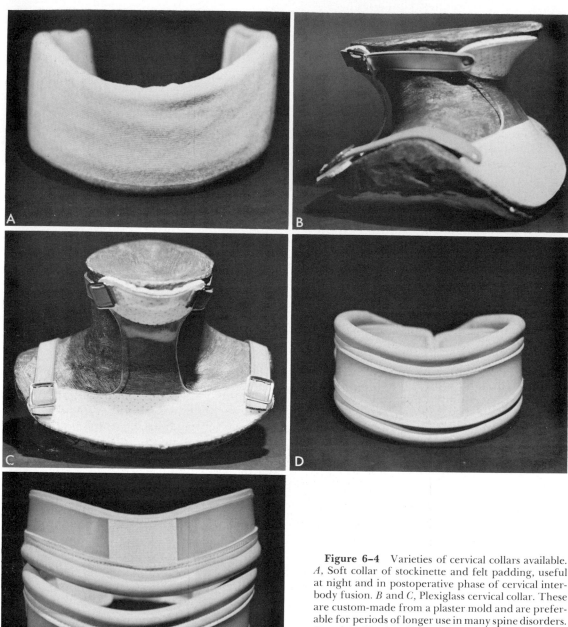

Figure 6-4 Varieties of cervical collars available. *A*, Soft collar of stockinette and felt padding, useful at night and in postoperative phase of cervical interbody fusion. *B* and *C*, Plexiglass cervical collar. These are custom-made from a plaster mold and are preferable for periods of longer use in many spine disorders. *D* and *E*, Plastic collars of commercial manufacture useful in injuries and chronic neck pain.

are not uncommon if much force is involved in the process of subluxation. Various degrees of hemiplegia may ensue and require skeletal traction in ice tongs or the application of a halo brace.

When immediate reduction is carried out, the ligaments and associated traumatic reaction may provide sufficiently firm control. In many instances when the luxation is once initiated it becomes chronic, and some form of occipitovertebral stabilization is required. Cregan has pioneered an approach to this difficult problem. In some instances simple posterior stabilization by bone grafts

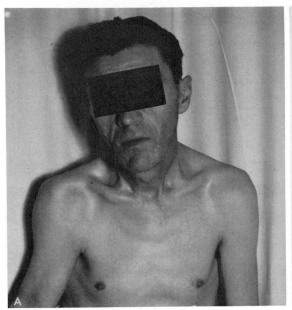
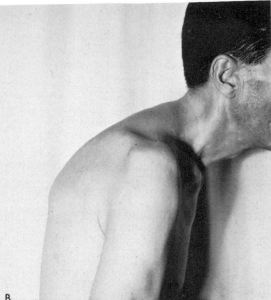

Figure 6-5 Ankylosing spondylitis.

in the usual fashion suffices. In others more intricate measures are needed and require use of special plates that attach the cervical spine to the suboccipital region. Occasionally fixation is obtained by insertion of a heavy screw at the point of coalescense of bony ridges of the occiput; this is used for fixation to the cervical spine, maintaining the head erect.

ACUTE INJURIES OF THE NECK AND SUBOCCIPITAL REGION

These have been fully considered in the section on injuries.

TORTICOLLIS

The disturbance of wry neck may be congenital, developmental or spasmodic.

CONGENITAL TORTICOLLIS

The accepted explanation of this birth deformity is that a derangement of the anatomy of the sternocleidomastoid occurs as a result of intrauterine malposition, leading to a degree of ischemia that involves the muscle. In most instances delivery of the fetus has been difficult or has been a breech birth. Initially the disturbance is limited to the sternocleidomastoid muscle, but as growth progresses, asymmetry of the face and jaws characteristically appears. A hard swelling is identified in the sternomastoid at birth or within the first two weeks afterward; this may gradually increase in size, leading to shortening and contracture of the sternomastoid muscle.

Examination of the involved muscle shows a replacement by fibrous tissue over a distance of approximately an inch.

Treatment. In many instances early recognition provides an opportunity for conservative treatment of this disturbance. In some cases this is governed by the extent of the lesion. When there is extensive shortening and an obvious considerable zone of fibrosis in the muscle, operative measures are mandatory. The conservative treatment consists of daily stretching of the muscle; this is initiated in the physiotherapy department but subsequently carried out by the mother after proper instruction and observation.

OPERATIVE TECHNIQUE. A transverse incision 2 inches in length is made just below the sternal end of the clavicle. Dissection is carried through the platysma and deep fascia over the sternomastoid by gentle elevation of the skin incision. The attachment of the sternomastoid is identified and elevated and a Luer clamp is used to carefully dissect it posteriorly. The sternal and clavicular segments are severed.

In some instances there is a contracture of the scalenus anticus muscle also; should this appear, at the time of division of the sternomastoid by careful resection, the phrenic nerve is retracted medially and the scalenus anticus is divided. In this maneuver care should be taken to avoid damage to the brachial plexus and the C.5-C.6 roots. The fibrotic process may extend through to the scalenus anticus, making dissection difficult. It is preferable to identify the C.5-C.6 roots and retract them prior to carrying out resection, because occasionally these roots lie directly in the substance of the scalenus anticus and may be damaged as this muscle is cut.

Following operation, a pressure dressing and firm collar are applied. In the severer cases cervical traction is required, and in all instances a program of physiotherapy with manual stretching and corrective exercises is initiated. The exercises are continued for a period of at least six months.

DEVELOPMENTAL TORTICOLLIS

Other causes of torticollis have been identified as spontaneous subluxation of the cervical spine, platybasia and anomalies of the cervical spine. Correction of the primary deformity is required to control the wry neck appearance. In adults a mild cervical bony deformity leads to associated shortening of the sternomastoid, and under these circumstances, resection of the distal end should be

carried out in the same fashion as for the congenital lesion.

SPASMODIC TORTICOLLIS

A particularly disturbing entity may be encountered in the later years of life in the form of spasmodic torticollis. This can be a true paralytic lesion, but sometimes is a hysterical process (Fig. 6–6).

Structural Spasmodic Torticollis

A clinical state in which the patient is subject to recurrent uncontrolled spasms of the sternomastoid and adjacent muscles, producing repeated rotatory motions of the head and neck, may be identified. In some instances there is a mild underlying congenital deformity of the cervical spine or a tendency toward shortening of the sternomastoid, but the condition can occur without any such predisposing cause. These patients are usually in midadult life and note the gradual onset of this uncontrollable spasm. In many instances it would appear that this starts as a tick or habit spasm; nervous stimuli or stress of situational circumstances force the patient to adopt this habit of twisting and turning the head and neck to one side. It nearly always implicates the muscle on the master arm side; a right-handed patient typically turns his head and neck to the left. He is always able to bring it back to the midline and apparently bring the spasm under control, only to have it recur. A distinct tendency for stress and nervous reac-

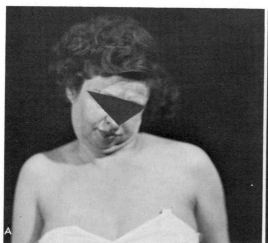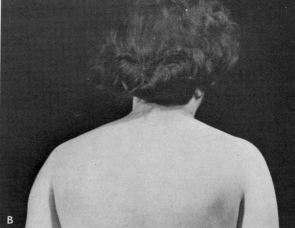

Figure 6–6   Recurrent torticollis.

tion to initiate this state has been postulated, but examples have been seen of muscle contraction as a result of pure neural stimulation. Examination often demonstrates slight tenderness related to the attachment of the sternomastoid either at the clavicle or the mastoid area, but this is not extensive. Electromyographic studies show a normal muscle subject to what appears as involuntary contractions that produce the head and neck turning.

Treatment. In many instances the patient is helped by the application of a light cervical collar, preferably of Plexiglass. This can be made in such a way that the control of the chin by a small lip on the edge of the splint prevents the head and neck from turning to the side. There is a tendency for the condition to worsen with the passage of time, and those patients not adequately controlled by the application of a brace sometimes require surgery.

SURGICAL TREATMENT. In at least half of the patients with spasmodic torticollis relief is obtained from a tenotomy of the involved sternomastoid. However, this does not eradicate the tick completely, and it may be necessary to avulse the nerve supply to these muscles. This is accomplished by making an incision along the posterior border of the sternomastoid muscle in its midportion, elevating the muscle and retracting it. The accessory nerve is identified at the level of the hyoid bone, passing beneath the muscle as the highest structure in the posterior triangle. A branch from the accessory to the muscle can be identified and this is severed. The upper portion of the sternomastoid also receives several branches directly from roots C.3 and C.4; these can be identified in the proximal portion of the wound, related to the anterior border. They can usually be felt by sweeping the finger beneath the muscle, but this must be done with care to avoid injuring the carotid sheath structures. In most patients it is desirable to section the attachment of the muscle to the clavicle as well as carry out the denervation. Sometimes considerable tension in the scalenus anticus is encountered, and this muscle should be severed also in the manner just described. True spasmodic torticollis is difficult to control, and even after a period of splinting followed by surgery, patients continue to show this rotatory habit. However, many are significantly helped if not completely cured by the surgery.

Neurectomy. In some instances the spastic state is so well established that more extensive measures than simple sternomastoid tenotomy will obviously be required. McKenzie has made a fundamental contribution to this problem by developing the operation of neurectomy for these intractable states.

The operation consists of a posterior laminectomy and exposure of the roots of the spinal accessory nerve and the anterior roots of the first, second and third cervical nerves. These are divided bilaterally intradurally. The accessory nerve is divided on one side in the neck, preserving the trapezius. Postoperatively the patient is kept in a Plexiglass collar to maintain the neutral position. In some instances, in spite of the extensive resection of the neural elements, some degree of deformity remains. Under these circumstances patients sometimes need to be fitted with a Plexiglass neck and chin guard that prevents the head and neck from turning to the involved side; the collar may need to be worn almost as a permanent splint.

In some instances an element of hysteria is present, and it is principally in these states that the continued use of the splint may be required.

Hysterical Torticollis

A large number of patients with a spasmodic type of torticollis are encountered in whom the disturbance is purely hysterical or psychological. Many sources have been identified in this relationship, and by and large they are situational factors that produce anxiety and depression, leading to a frank spastic tick. They differ from the preceding group in that the twisting is completely voluntary. Although the spasms may appear to be on an involuntary basis for a given period, almost all patients can be shown to have intervals in which the spasm does not develop with the same continuity.

Should there be any suspicion of such an etiology, the proper procedure is to arrange for a neuropsychiatric assessment; otherwise, the lesion may prove most difficult to control. Usually identification of the antecedent factors will help to control this type of torticollis. Rarely, if the habit spasm has been present for a long time, there is some shortening of the involved muscle and it may be necessary to carry out a tenotomy. Sometimes tenotomy supplemented by psychotherapy is the most effective program.

OCCIPITAL NEURODYNIA

A group of superficial disorders can be identified that mainly implicate soft tissue and which involve the branches of the cervical plexus, producing suboccipital and lateral occipital pain. The discomfort involves one side of the neck posteriorly and may extend to the region of the mastoid process or to the front of the ear. The posterior primary divisions of the upper four nerves are distributed to the scalp and neck in this region. From the first cervical nerve arises the suboccipital nerve, which supplies the muscles of the suboccipital triangle. The lesser occipital nerve is derived from C.2 and C.3 and supplies the skin over the lateral occipital zone of the scalp, reaching to the mastoid process and upper medial portion of the oracle. This nerve is not infrequently involved in traumatic episodes, implicating the erector spinae, as has been described in the discussion of whiplash lesions (Fig. 6–7). Tendinitis of the erector spinae attachment in this region can also implicate this nerve in precisely the same fashion. In addition to

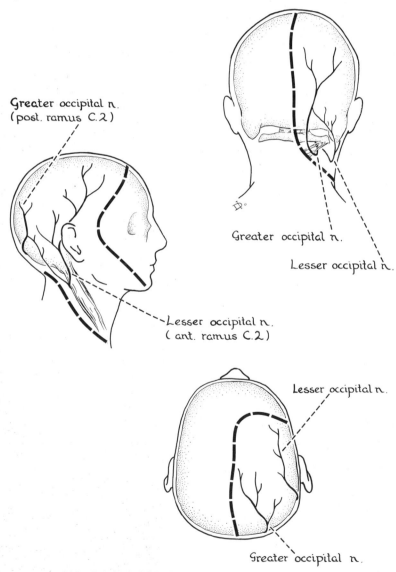

Greater occipital n.
(post. ramus C.2)

Greater occipital n.

Lesser occipital n.

Lesser occipital n.
(ant. ramus C.2)

Lesser occipital n.

Greater occipital n.

Figure 6–7 Distribution of greater occipital nerve.

the distribution of pain following this pattern, the patients complain of local tenderness; manipulation of the area characteristically reproduces their discomfort. Frequently it can be relieved by local anesthetic injection. In some instances a small amount of absolute alcohol is added, producing a solution of 20 per cent. One cubic centimeter of absolute alcohol plus 4 cc of a 2 per cent anesthetic solution injected into the trigger area is often effective in relieving these symptoms.

CONGENITAL ANOMALIES

Cervical scoliosis resulting from hemivertebra predisposes to foraminal lipping. Congenital torticollis may eventually lead to bony structural changes, producing foraminal osteophyte formation.

Less common congenital anomalies such as occipito-atlanto fusion have a tendency to distort the normal mechanics of the cervical spine; abnormal stress when focused at the C.1-C.2 level may distort odontoid and tuberal internal wall of atlas relations, encroaching upon the cord. In occipitalization of the atlas, the odontoid lies within the foramen magnum, favoring basilar impression and consequent cord pressure (Figs. 6–8, 6–9 and 6–10).

DISC PROTRUSIONS

The process of disc aging includes a fibrosis and progressive dehydration leading to a decrease in disc substance and a diminution of interbody space and possible bulging of the annulus fibrosis. These changes involve the vertebral foramen, but the effects more deeply implicate the angle accessory joints of Luschka and the apophyseal joints which, in turn, then involve the nerve root foramen.

Frank rupture of the cervical annulus with disc protrusion producing major pressure on the cervical cord is uncommon but can occur as a result of severe trauma which then may be of sufficient severity to damage the bony structure, producing a fracture or fracture dislocation. Much more frequently, however, this trauma is dissipated in such a fashion that it produces a more lateral extrusion of the disc, with nerve root foraminal encroachment rather than spinal canal encroachment.

ROOT FORAMINOSIS

Encroachment on the nerve root foramen, particularly at the levels of C.5 and C.6 is a much more frequently encountered disorder than spinal cord foraminosis. Changes of age, trauma and metabolism can be more intently focused on the nerve root area than on the spinal cord zone.

The resulting picture of typical nerve root involvement is mild neck discomfort and rotary head and neck restriction accompanied by intermittent and gradually persisting attacks of numbness, and tingling implicating the forearm and hand. A sensation of intermittent needlelike pain extending to the fingertips is a typical development. The pa-

Figure 6–8

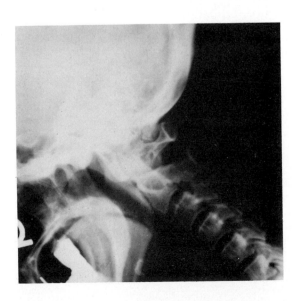

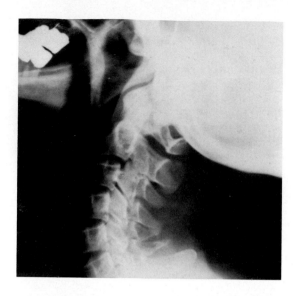

Figure 6–9

tient quickly learns that it is the attitude of the cervical spine that profoundly affects this. Bending the head and neck to the side may initiate or increase the radiating discomfort, whereas vertebral stretching or tilting to the opposite side tends to diminish it.

The pathology, clinical course and treatment of nerve root syndrome developing from this entity and associated entities have been extensively considered in Chapter IX.

VERTEBRAL ARTERY FORAMINOSIS

Recognition of the significance of vertebral spondylosis has led to the study of possible involvement of the vertebral artery by a

precisely similar condition. It has become apparent that obstruction of the vertebral artery produces signs and symptoms typical of this development.

The symptoms result from distortion of the vertebrobasilar system and may take the form of headaches and intermittent dizzy spells, progressing in some instances to more profound "blackouts." In some instances rotation or extension of the head and neck may compress the artery, precipitating one of these attacks.

As is the case with the cervical osteophytosis elsewhere, involvement of the transverse foramen may be correspondingly extensive with the general process but yet not present symptoms at all suggestive of vascular impairment. In most instances it is probable that an additional irritant or other changes

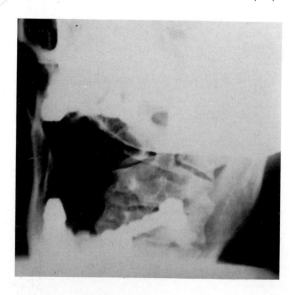

Figure 6–10

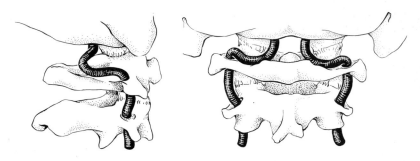

Vertebral artery - head A.P.

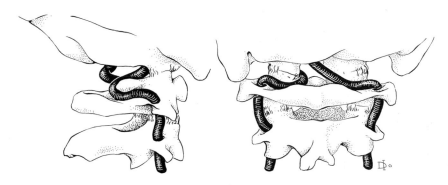

Vertebral artery - head rotated

Figure 6-11

are necessary to bring the vascular syndrome into clinical focus.

Atheromatous changes in the vertebral artery have been identified and may play a more important role than the foraminal pressure alone. However, the combination of mild foraminosis along with the atheromatous change may constitute significant stenosis leading to clinical changes. Arteriography has aided a great deal in the identification of these lesions and should be carried out when this pathological state is suspected.

Two zones of physiological distortion of the vertebral artery have been identified: As the artery enters the neck through the foramen of the transverse process of C.6 it may be compressed in some individuals by turning of the head and neck forcibly to the opposite direction. Rotation of the head and neck may alter the flow through the vertebral artery on the side to which the head is turned (Fig. 6-11). Secondly, the blood flow is altered in turning the head and neck at the point where the artery starts toward the cerebrum as it passes through the trans-

verse process of the atlas. The development of artheromatous plaques in the vertebral artery is then a further element favoring stenosis or diminution of the arterial flow at these sources when there are osteophytes present. The clinical pictures develop most noticeably when the patient turns the head and neck forcibly to one side. In the same way it may be anticipated that torsion-trauma could initiate such symptoms under these conditions.

Decompression of the vertebral artery has been reported by Verbiest and is best performed by the anterolateral approach.

REFERENCES

Bleck, E. F.: Arthritis of the CI-C2 intervertebral facets. GP *33*:94–95, 1966.

Dandy, W. E.: An operation for the treatment of spasmodic torticollis. Arch. Surg. *20*:1021, 1930.

Eynolds, G. G., et al.: Electromyographic evaluation of patients with post-traumatic cervical pain. Arch. Phys. Med. *49*:170–172, 1968.

Fierro, D., et al.: On the significance of calcifications and limited ossifications of the posterior cervical ligament. Minerva Radiol. *11*:157–165, 1966.

Harris, P.: Plastic foam neck support. Brit. Med. J. *2*:1004, 1966.

Hulbert, K. F.: Congenital torticollis. J. Bone Joint Surg. *32B*:50, 1950.

Javid, H.: Vascular injuries of the neck. Clin. Orthop. *28*:70–78, 1963.

Kovacs, A.: Subluxation and deformation of the cervical apophyseal joints. Contribution to the aetiology of headache. Acta Radiol. *43*:1–16, 1955.

Krout, R. M., et al.: Role of anterior cervical muscles in production of neck pain. Arch. Phys. Med. *47*:603–611, 1966.

Middleton, D. S.: The pathology of congenital torticollis. Brit. J. Surg. *18*:188, 1930.

Pearson, R. W.: Head and neck pain. J. Maine Med. Ass. *57*:264–266, 1966.

Pichler, E.: Cervical headache. Landarzt *41*:1553–1560, 1965.

Raney, A. A., and Raney, R. B.: Headache, a common symptom of cervical disc lesions. Arch. Neurol. *59*:603, 1948.

Roy, L. P., et al.: Some aspects of cervical spondylosis. Un. Med. Canada *95*:734–740, 1966.

Wiberg, G.: Back pain in relation to the nerve supply of the intervertebral disc. Acta Orthop. Scand. *19*:211, 1949.

Chapter VII

LESIONS PRODUCING NECK PLUS SHOULDER PAIN

It is possible to delineate a well defined group of disorders that are ushered in by pain that implicates both shoulder and neck. They stem from abnormalities between the shoulder blades in the suspensory area and at the angle made by the neck and shoulder. The general region of the scapula is also implicated. These areas are closely linked embryologically, and congenital defects in one part are often accompanied by malformations in another. When this area is accepted as a region, signs and symptoms can be recognized that are specific of disorders emanating from this zone. Patients often complain of discomfort in the shoulder joint when what they really mean is the area at the root of the neck or about the scapula.

The components of this forequarter are largely soft tissue, muscle, fascia, tendon and ligament. They are plastered on bones which serve as a scaffolding and as anchors for tendon insertion. The region is the important center of two extremely mobile segments, the cervical spine above and the shoulder proper below. Some of the muscles, the trapezius, for example, can act on both segments at the same time. The specific function of the area is twofold: to support

and hold the head and the neck, and also to suspend and power the shoulder girdle. These acts involve a constant postural musculoligamentous movement; at the same time the structures integrate powerful dynamic forces applied to both moving segments. The shoulder-neck zone may be compared with the lumbosacral region, and many similarities can be identified (Fig. 7–1). Cervicothoracic and lumbosacral zones are at the bottom of ribless, mobile zones of the spine. Broad flat muscles connect the mobile spinal segments to the adjacent appendages, the arm in one case and the leg in the other. These muscles cross a large universal type joint in each case, so that they are subject to the demands of a universal articulation as well as the demands arising from their static postural contribution. There is a long, thin set of muscles, the erector spinae, that is common to both areas. Involvement of the tendinous attachment of this postural mechanism at its lower end has been accepted and, in the same way, one would expect to find disorders implicating its superior attachment.

When the structural function and the components of these two regions are appre-

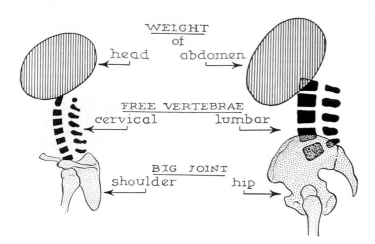

Figure 7–1 Comparison of cervical and lumbar regions as to postural strain and major joint influences.

ciated, susceptibility to postural disorders, muscle strains, fibrositis, ligamentous injuries, as well as referred symptoms from the large mobile joint can be anticipated. The pain from disorders in this region has a distinctive pattern and quality. It is usually described as an ache rather than a pain. It has a constant gnawing quality; changes in posture affect it; chronicity is common; and patients have trouble identifying the source precisely, tending to implicate the whole region (Fig. 7–2). Radiation of pain beyond this zone is not prominent but occasionally the discomfort pattern will extend to the upper third of the arm, although this aspect is not emphasized in the presentation of the complaints.

POSTURAL DISORDERS

Standing and working in the upright position has been accomplished in man by adaptation of front and back appendages for special purposes. The forearm has increased its mobility, whereas the rear limb has developed greater balance and stability. This means that in the vertical position the head and shoulder need to be balanced and constantly supported. Support is provided by the spine and balancing is controlled by the paraspinal musculature. The upper limb is suspended as a strut, extending like the beam on a sign post (Fig. 7–3). In contrast to the lumbosacral area, fewer congenital anomalies mar this transition zone, but the vastly increased and varied action of the neck and limb create a whole new set of stresses. The discomfort rarely radiates beyond the point of the shoulder. In longstanding cases, the pain may be a little more diffuse, but questioning discloses a quite specific pattern.

SIGNS AND SYMPTOMS

Certain physical types may be recognized as being predisposed to this type of stress. Shoulder slope shows considerable variation, from a slanting apical type at one end of the

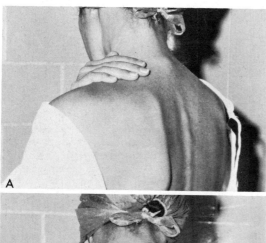

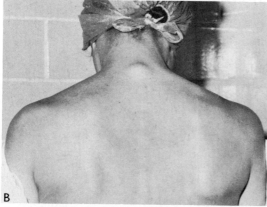

Figure 7–2 The typical indication of shoulder-neck pain of soft tissue postural stress. Frequent sufferers are thinly upholstered females with flaring scapulae.

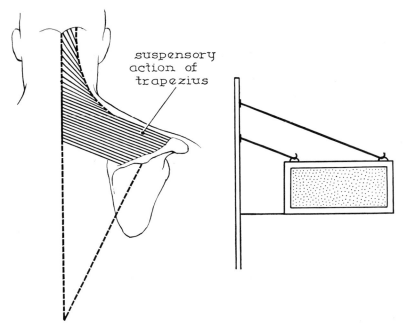

Figure 7–3 "Sign-posts" suspension of upper extremity at shoulder-neck angle.

scale to a stout, thick-set appearance at the opposite extreme (Fig. 7–4). Similarly, rib contour alters shoulder suspension; the very round form favors scapular separation and the medial borders tend to flare, whereas the angular type has much more firmly placed flaring shoulder blades.

People working long hours in a slumped over position develop a pain that usually comes on after some hours of retaining this unbalanced position. If this continues, less and less strain is necessary to provoke the ache. Periodically patients straighten and stretch their necks and brace their shoulders to relieve the ache. After a while this exercise is less effective, and gradually a persistent ache develops and extends from the neck outward. It is also common after acute illnesses, or following sudden assumption of a new working position or new habits in sleeping. The use of a new thick, hard pillow, for example, often favors the onset of this disorder.

Tailors have long known the importance of the shoulder proportions in the proper draping of coats. They recognize a point at the side of the neck, between the shoulder and midline, as the balance point (Fig. 7–5). If this area is fitted properly, the rest of the coat automatically tends to hang well. It is

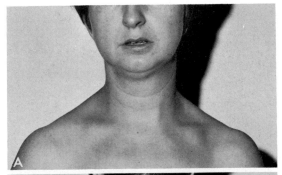

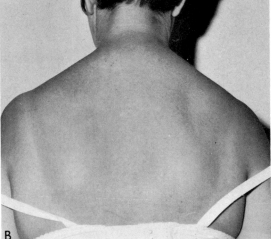

Figure 7–4 Apical shoulder configuration favors shoulder-neck and soft tissue strain.

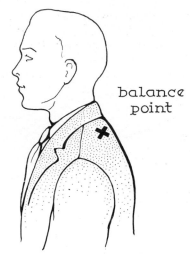

Figure 7-5 The tailor's balance point. If this area is well fitted the coat hangs properly.

arthritis of the spine the complete freezing of the spine tilts the head forward and the patient complains of occipital and cervical pain as well as shoulder-neck discomfort. The hyperflexion of rheumatoid arthritis is also characteristic; in compensation, thoracic epiphysitis produces hyperextension of the cervical spine.

This is the general picture; it may be complicated by an acute episode of sudden twisting, stretching or other trauma that acts as the proverbial straw breaking the camel's back, initiating diffuse pain in the whole region. Examination shows some prominence of muscles as a result of spasm, and movement of the cervical spine brings on pain. Arm action may cause an aching sensation that extends up the side of the neck.

ETIOLOGY AND PATHOLOGY

Postural abnormalities have long been accepted as a frequent cause of low back pain, but they have been less well recognized as the cause in the shoulder-neck area. However, this region serves as a base for two mobile segments and two weighted pendula, and the major supporting and suspensory strain is focused at the root of the neck and between the shoulder blades. It is reasonable to anticipate reaction in this zone to chronic strain, such as may be produced by abnormal posture. The supporting base is stationary, while the moveable segments of the neck and arm shift, exerting stress on the supporting

rare for any two shoulders to be maintained at the same level, and the tailor frequently calls this to a customer's attention. Usually the right shoulder is lower in right-handed individuals. The position of the scapula in relation to the chest wall and to the arm shows considerable variation, as has been pointed out by Kendall. Normally the scapulae should be flat against the chest, without the angle or medial border being unduly prominent. A round back widens the space between the scapulae, and the medial border tends to flare. Scoliosis of all degrees may reflect disturbances in the cervical spine, favoring postural neck pain. In rheumatoid

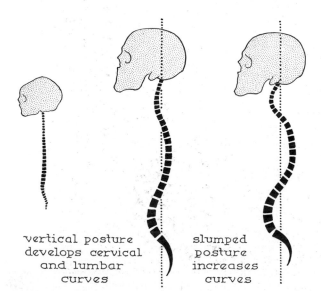

Figure 7-6 Cervical and lumbar curves developed from assumption of erect stature. Some posture exaggerates these curves, increasing the stress and retaining soft parts.

vertical posture develops cervical and lumbar curves

slumped posture increases curves

soft parts. Weakness and stretching of the suspensory muscles then may occur.

When the imbalanced position becomes so well entrenched that it is habit, there may be an alteration of the normal weight-bearing axis of the spine so that weight, instead of being transmitted through the vertebral bodies, tends to exert pressure on the apophyseal joints posteriorly (Fig. 7–6). Uneven joint wear and tear then follow. When persistent malalignment occurs, uneven pressure is increased and the mechanical fault is followed by another one consisting of bony overgrowth as the reaction to anterior longitudinal ligament strain. This results in limitation of movement and stiffness in the uncorrected position. Distortion of bony alignment produces uneven ligamentous and muscular pull, which again is reflected as pain. When some acute episode is added to this disturbed posture mechanism, overstimulation of the muscles occurs, resulting in prolonged muscle contracture, recognized clinically as muscle spasm. Kendall has pointed out that associated weakness and laxity of the suspensory group is followed

by shortening and contracture of the antagonists. Further deformity develops, adding a chronic fixating element; the rounded chest with sagging scapulae allows fixation by the front muscles like the pectorals, and the whole process ends in a much more stable deformity.

TREATMENT

Correction of Obvious Postural Faults. The abnormal posture which produces these symptoms may be a living habit, an occupational habit or an established structural change (Fig. 7–7). Instruction for correction is given when faulty posture in standing, sitting or lying is apparent. This involves examining the body as a whole, since the primary fault may well lie away from the neck-shoulder zone; for example, a short leg, exaggerated lumbar lordosis, weak abdominal muscles or poor foot stance with abnormal weight-bearing patterns.

When occupational habits are the cause, efforts are made to adjust the factors that can be improved in a given situation. For exam-

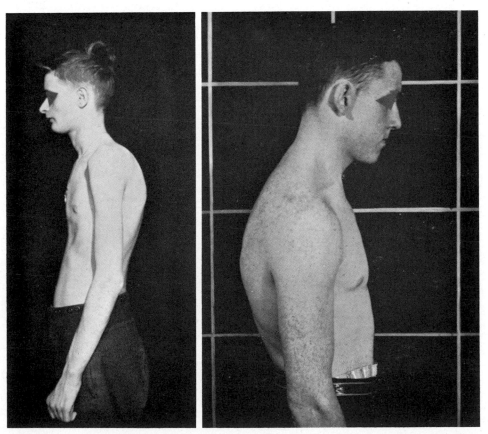

Figure 7–7 Structural changes featuring slumped shoulder posture and shoulder-neck pain.

ple, the patient's chair may need to be changed to a different height, the desk level may need to be altered, the bench size and level may need to be changed, tools should be changed from one arm to the other, or a mechanical hoist may need to be provided to decrease lifting strains. No two patients will have the same irritant or same response. Employers should be encouraged to make such common sense adjustments as the physiques of their employees might suggest. A tall man working at a below-waist level and a short man working at above-shoulder level are prime candidates for postural pain.

In some cases obvious structural abnormalities such as scoliosis, congenital elevation of the scapulae or ankylosis of the neck can be recognized and treated accordingly.

Muscle Therapy. Instruction should be given to the patient to help him to improve power and tone of the suspensory shoulder-neck muscles. Exercises of the trapezius are emphasized particularly. A good trapezius exercise is to place the back against the wall and extend the arm backward to touch the wall. Keeping the back straight and staying pressed against the wall, lift the arms forward. Contractures or shortening in antagonists like the pectorals or latissimus dorsi are treated by stretching exercises such as lying prone and lifting the arms up over the head until they touch the floor above.

Supports and Braces. Exercises must be stressed as the way to develop a good lifting support. However, some patients need more than this, and exercises without correction of the postural faults may not be enough.

SHOULDER BRACE. A useful canvas support consists of two straps fitted in a circle through which the arms are passed, and which cross diagonally at the back and are fastened by a circular belt around the waist. This brace pulls the shoulder backward as in the ordinary figure-of-eight shoulder application.

High Back Support. A Taylor type of brace may be necessary in some kyphotics, with or without the shoulder attachment added. The brace is worn during the daytime but is discarded at night.

Lumbar Support. In some instances the prime fault may lie lower down in the lumbar region, as for example when there is a much exaggerated lumbosacral lordosis which must be compensated by an inordinate thoracic kyphosis. A good lumbar brace which flattens the lumbar spine is often effective.

Brassieres. Heavy breasts are a common cause of aching shoulders. When there is excessive weight, the breast should be held up by strong brassieres or supports with bone reinforcement incorporated in a body support. Often the use of a strapless type

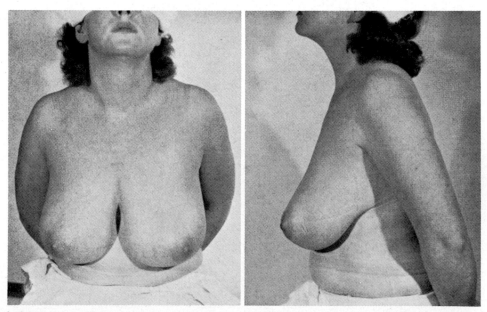

Figure 7–8 Heavy pendulous breasts poorly supported with narrow brassiere straps may cause shoulder-neck pain. Note the pressure mark from the too-narrow shoulder strap.

bra is beneficial. Sometimes it is necessary to add additional shoulder straps or to widen them to avoid small straps digging in across the top of the shoulders (Fig. 7–8).

None of these supports are suggested to be worn as a permanent fixture. The maximum effort should be toward improving the tone and balance of the muscles so that support is not necessary. A support is an aid to correction, relieving the strain in the early periods, but should be discarded unless there has been extensive structural change or muscle paralysis.

Physiotherapy Measures. Heat, massage and radiation therapy are used in certain instances, but prolonged courses are not recommended. The acute episode of muscle strain on top of a postural abnormality is helped by the application of heat followed by massage of the spastic zone. Infrared heat and deep massage are used to stretch contracted groups such as the pectorals.

GENERAL MEASURES. Often these problems are of a chronic nature and require lengthy treatment, so that persistence on the part of the patient and patience on the part of the doctor are required. Many of these sufferers have a listless, unaggressive makeup and constant encouragement is necessary. The general body nutrition needs to be improved with a well balanced diet or a food supplement such as concentrated protein. This should be coupled with a proper general exercise program.

FIBROSITIS OF THE SHOULDER-NECK REGION

Fibrositis is a term used to describe a disturbance in soft tissues which produces pain localized frequently to the posterior shoulder-neck region, a feeling of stiffness in the shoulders, often a sensation of weakness and limitation of movement of the shoulder. The areas most frequently involved usually are related to some moving part under repeated stress. Soft tissues such as fascia, muscles, tendons, ligaments or the fibrous supporting elements of these tissues almost anywhere in the body may be involved, but the two zones most frequently afflicted are the shoulder-neck area and the lumbosacral region. In the former it constitutes one of the commonest sources of discomfort. Mechanical factors associated with the assumption of the upright posture are a potent predisposing element. Nutritional and constitutional factors ag-

gravate any predisposition. Repeated minor trauma or microtraumas commonly initiate the syndrome but it may also be started by more major episodes. Probably all of us have some degree of this lesion involving either or both of the usual areas.

SIGNS AND SYMPTOMS

Women between 30 and 50 years are the most frequent sufferers. They present themselves complaining of aching pain between the shoulder blades extending out to the shoulder tip. Often they are thinly upholstered and appear to have a somewhat low pain threshold. Fatigue, worry, lowered resistance, chronic illness and undernourishment are common irritants. In many patients socioeconomic or psychic disturbances also occur. The disorder may be influenced, for example, by a sudden increase of strain and stress in frail young mothers. Poorly adjusted women in the menopausal age with a generally less rugged constitution are also frequent sufferers.

The pain is indicated in characteristic fashion by the patient's wrapping her hand around the shoulder-neck angle between the shoulder and the neck (Fig. 7–2). The patient describes a sense of pressure building up at the back of the neck and extending to the shoulder. This is accompanied by aching pain between the shoulder blades. Often the patient has developed characteristic movements which initially relieve the pain, but as the discomfort persists it is harder and harder to obtain relief by these movements. The patient frequently illustrates how the pain may come on by working her shoulder blades backward and forward, producing a soft crepitant sound. The discomfort is worse in the morning or following any period of inactivity. It seems to improve as the muscles are used, when the extremity is warm, or after the patient has been up and about for an hour or so. It is typically aggravated by dampness, drafts and cold. The patient may be unable to pinpoint the precise focus of maximum pain, describing a diffuse ache which is referred to the whole trapezius supraspinatus region. The pain has a constant dragging quality. It may occur in bouts and be followed by spontaneous intermissions of weeks or months. When some new stress or strain is added, either physical or emotional, the discomfort recurs or flares up. As a rule, the pain has been present for months or years without assuming incapacitating proportions until some new incident precipitates the whole symptom complex.

On examination the patient is usually thin and of poor muscular development. The painful area is pointed out as lying at the root of the neck posteriorly between this area and the shoulder or in between the shoulder blades. In acute cases, spasm of the suspensory muscles can be identified. Tenderness will involve the whole muscle, but palpation will identify certain painful trigger zones (Fig. 7–9). In longstanding cases the muscles have a definite stringy feeling and appear atonic. Deep pressure at the trigger points is exquisitely uncomfortable, and firm manipulation of these areas reproduces the whole distribution of the patient's discomfort (Fig. 7–10). Usually there is no real limitation of neck or shoulder movement, but forward and backward movement of the neck may be uncomfortable, as may manipulation of the shoulder girdle so that the scapula moves backward and forward.

ETIOLOGY AND PATHOLOGY

No one agent has been identified as the cause of this disturbance. Chronic strain, repeated minute trauma, occupational stress, heredity, focal infection and even some infective agents have been presented as the cause. The term fibrositis conveys the suggestion

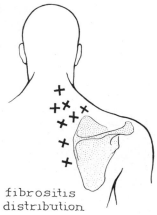

fibrositis distribution

Figure 7–10 Distribution of common trigger areas in fibrositis.

of inflammation, but this is misleading because the process is not a true inflammatory reaction as we commonly interpret the term. It appears much more like a reaction in musculotendinous tissue which may occur anywhere as a result of chronic strain, poor posture or repeated occupational irritation. Movement has some relation since it is in the mobile areas of neck, shoulder and lumbar region that the disturbances are most commonly found. The remainder of the trunk and the long muscles of the arm and leg are almost never involved, possibly because they are not subject to persistent postural stress.

Thickening in the muscles is encountered and is related to the points of maximum tenderness. Sometimes this is a fairly well demarcated nodule, but more often it is a diffuse fullness without clear-cut margins and may not seem to be the same area of muscle that is palpated each time. When a definite nodule is present, excision will show it to be composed of fibrofatty or fibrous tissue which has replaced muscle fiber. Sometimes only a little infiltrating fibrosis with atrophy of adjacent muscle fibers is identified. When exploration of these dense areas in muscles shows little pathological change it may be because the spasms in the muscles represent an early stage before structural change has occurred. It seems logical to accept the term "fibrositic lesion" as the guise of a musculofascial reaction to many irritants and to anticipate differences in the lesion corresponding to varying phases of the process. In some instances the nodule consists of a fibrofatty herniation through the superficial fascia.

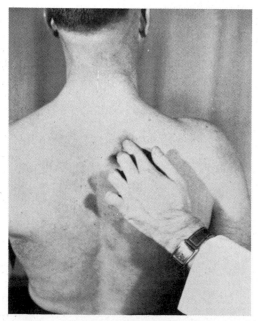

Figure 7–9 Demonstration of typical fibrositic tender point.

Copeman and Ackerman have investigated these lesions carefully and have contributed the most significant and logical explanation of the symptoms developing in this process. They plotted the distribution of the deep fat deposit in the commonly involved zones and found that they coincided with the areas most frequently producing the nodular fibrositic lesions. It was concluded that deficiencies in the fascia favored herniation of fat lobules through them and that these became strangulated or devitalized by the constricting fibers. Deficiencies in the fascia occur constantly at the points of perforation of the neurovascular bundles, thus providing a route for escape of subjacent fat (Fig. 7–11). The fibrofatty herniation irritates adjacent tissue, edema occurs, pressure nerve endings are irritated and pain is recorded. Such areas, being subject to osmotic changes, might be influenced by atmospheric weather changes. This would serve to explain the acuteness of symptoms with variations of the weather which is so characteristic of this lesion.

TREATMENT OF FIBROSITIS

Keeping in mind what we know of the pathology of this condition, the principles are to provide sufficient relief locally so that the patient can continue to keep the part mobile and the muscles active. When muscle spasm and tenderness are controlled, muscle activity then limits further acute pain.

Injection Therapy. The most satisfactory treatment to date is local injection of the trigger zones or nodules with an anesthetic solution such as procaine (Novocain). This therapy has become an effective tool therapeutically and diagnostically and deserves some special mention. The approach to the patient and the technique of this simple procedure merit consideration.

PREPARATION OF THE PATIENT. Injection therapy can usually be carried out as an office procedure. Usually the patient is not expecting to have such treatment, so that proper explanation will help him to accept a somewhat unpleasant procedure. Many patients dislike the sight of a long needle,

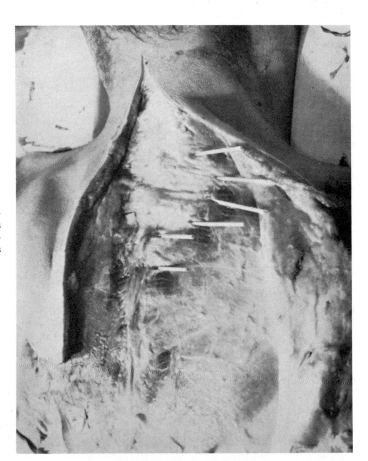

Figure 7–11 Dissection showing the neurovascular foramina in the musculotendinous zone of the posterior neck region. The openings are potential sites for minute hernias as well as scar tissue formation.

and for some this alone is most upsetting. The procedure is explained; the purpose and need are outlined; the amount of discomfort that may be anticipated is indicated; and the likely results are stated. This prepares the patient and increases confidence. When this is a therapeutic procedure, it is wise to err on the side of conservatism in predicting or anticipating the duration of relief. It can be explained that it is hard to assess individual reactions since these vary. In the same way the tissue reaction, the size of the lesion, and so forth, also vary from patient to patient. The patient may be reassured that no harm will come from the procedure.

SOLUTIONS AND REACTIONS. Inquiry is made regarding any sensitivity to local anesthetic injections and any other allergic responses of which the patient is aware. Serious reactions are uncommon, and most patients have had some experience with local anesthetic injection, for example, during dental procedures. A small amount of the anesthetic is injected initially and a few minutes are allowed to pass before more extensive infiltration is made. The author uses 2 per cent procaine (Novocain) without adrenalin and 5 to 10 cc. is injected. A solution of 1 per cent strength is usually not quite strong enough, but it may be used if it is anticipated that a large amount may be needed. The physician should use a local anesthetic preparation with which he is familiar. As new and longer acting local preparations appear, improved solutions may become available. Addition of a spreading agent such as hyaluronidase is sometimes helpful. When this is used the field affected is enlarged, but relief may not last so long. For some longstanding, well localized lesions absolute alcohol may be added to the preparation, 1 cc. per 5 cc. of anesthetic. This is effective when a small, deep trigger point can be defined. The initial reaction is a little painful, but the relief lasts much longer; only a small amount of alcohol is needed.

TECHNIQUE. Use a sharp 22- or 23-gauge needle of ordinary intramuscular length. Occasionally a long needle is necessary for more obese subjects. Hypodermic size can be used in the skin but this is not long enough to reach the muscle planes. In some cases the injection can be carried out with the patient sitting, but it is preferable to have the patient lying face down on the table with the arms lying by the side. Once the patient is steady and comfortable, the trigger zone is identified and the skin is prepared with iodine or alcohol. After the cutaneous wheal is raised, the needle continues toward the deep site, injecting only a little anesthetic. Once the pain and radiating discomfort have been reproduced by needling the trigger region, the bulk of the solution is injected. The needle is withdrawn a little, and the tissue about the acute zone is infiltrated also.

PHYSIOLOGY OF LOCAL ANESTHETIC ACTION. Relief from local anesthetic injection has been looked upon somewhat credulously. There can be no question of its effectiveness, so that the explanation of the precise mechanism becomes less important. One of the most effective remedies for gout, colchicum, has been used by the medical profession for years without any clear understanding of its mechanism of action. Yet it is prescribed without hesitation. Local anesthetic numbs sensory endings, and with the cessation of pain stimuli muscle spasm is decreased. This explains both the local and more distant relief that is obtained. Once the cycle is severed, it does not recur until the old or a new irritant is applied. It is common to find new areas of tenderness in the same general region after initial injection but these are definitely away from the primary focus. If desired, these may be injected at the initial treatment or taken care of later.

REACTIONS TO LOCAL ANESTHETIC. This is a safe procedure and significant complications are rare. Some people are sensitive to such agents as procaine and inquiry should be made before massive infiltration is carried out. Others have ill effects from the pressor substance rather than the anesthetic agent. Probably this is a more common source of reaction than sensitivity to the anesthetic. Reactions vary from a little giddiness to slight diplopia or a feeling of faintness and lassitude. Pentothal has been described as the ideal antidote.

Explanation of the Lesion to the Patient. The general nature of this disturbance should be explained to the patient; building up the confidence of the patient in the doctor goes a long way in curing the malady. Some of these patients apparently have a somewhat lower pain threshold than normal or are subject to situational anxieties or have some functional overlay. However, it rarely helps to bluntly tell them that this is the main cause of their upset. Muscle spasm, painful nodules and constant palpable trigger points cannot be imagined. They may be but a part of the whole picture, but our responsibility clearly is to alleviate such problems if we can. Situational or functional irritants may be diagnosed later and may subsequently be dealt with as may be necessary.

Physiotherapy. Good physiotherapy helps these patients significantly also. Fibrositis is a painful state, with considerable muscle spasm, particularly in the trapezius and spinati. Expert massage should supplement injection therapy when the acute pain from trigger points has been controlled. Introductory heat followed by massage is applied daily or every other day for a week to ten days, depending upon the patient's response. Diathermy is not recommended for these lesions because it favors stretching and stringiness of muscle fibers at the musculotendinous junction and may act as an irritant.

Postural Instruction. Instruction in proper posture and an adequate exercise program are helpful adjuncts also. Obvious postural faults such as slumped shoulders and sagging or spreading scapulae should be corrected. Groups of weak muscles should be strengthened by specific exercises. Often the isometric type of exercise is most beneficial. Active movement is most important in conjunction with all the local remedies. Muscle contraction favors absorption of reactive edema after injection. Massage prevents recurrence and extension of the fibroblastic reaction. The muscle fibers are so often thin and atrophic that active movement is the only way of increasing muscle and fiber length. The exercise regimen should expand to include resistance exercises. The active movement routine differs from that used in articular and periarticular disturbances such as supra- and intraspinatus tendinitis. In the latter, mobility of the joint is needed and must be carefully protected. In fibrositic lesions the joint and periarticular zones are comparably uninvolved so that attention is directed toward the muscular elements.

Home Remedies. Certain simple home remedies are helpful, such as soaking in a hot tub or using a relatively inexpensive heat lamp or bulb. The painful areas may be massaged after they have been suitably warmed.

FOCAL INFECTION

On general principles any obvious foci of infection, such as diseased tonsils, should be treated particularly if symptoms persist. This is not to suggest a wholesale extraction of teeth, gallbladder or appendix, but infected tonsils, teeth, ears or antra should receive prompt attention.

PROGRESS OF THE LESION

Chronicity characterizes this disturbance and exacerbations are frequent, but may be months apart. A typical manifestation is an almost total lack in increase of severity of the lesion, unless special irritants such as recurring injury are added. Future attacks are prevented by avoiding the obvious irritants, like fatigue, poor posture, poor sleeping habits and unprotected exposure to cold. Frail individuals should wear warm clothing; wool is better than flannel because moisture is absorbed rather than retained close to the skin. Keeping the general health at a high level and keeping free of unnecessary stress are also deterrents.

MUSCULOLIGAMENTOUS INJURIES AT THE SHOULDER-NECK REGION

These injuries are common and important and have been considered in the section on trauma.

OSTEOARTHRITIS OF THE CERVICAL SPINE

Degenerative changes in the cervical spine are found almost universally after the age of 50 years. They are clearly seen in x-ray studies and all too frequently are interpreted as the causative agent for neck and shoulder pain. Discomfort does not arise from these changes nearly so often as it does from some of the soft tissue disturbances which have been described. As a rule, symptoms arise only when some added disturbances such as trauma, increased strain, continuous postural effort or progressive debilitation are superimposed.

CARDINAL SIGNS AND SYMPTOMS

Aching pain in the shoulder-neck area associated with neck movement and relieved by rest is the commonest complaint. Stiffness, soreness and pain begin in the morning and increase with the day's activity. This is in contradistinction to many of the soft tissue disturbances which are improved by exercise and are at their worst when the patient is getting out of bed in the morning. The pain may radiate to the base of the skull and up the back of the head. Patients soon learn that neck movement aggravates the discomfort, and the neck is kept still to bring relief. The maximum discomfort is appreciated in the area between the neck and the shoulder; patients rarely talk about the discomfort as being precisely confined to the neck.

On examination some tenderness may be identified in the paravertebral, cervical musculature. Movement of the spine aggravates the discomfort, and frequently there is limitation of motion. Principally it is side-to-side bending that is restricted, or turning of the head and neck to one side along with extending the neck such as one does in backing a car out of a driveway. None of the symptoms may be present until the patient experiences a sudden jarring incident such as may occur in the abrupt stopping of a car or a fall. The head is flicked forward suddenly, and pain in the shoulder-neck area and adjacent root of the neck develops.

ETIOLOGY AND PATHOLOGY

In the embryo the spinal column has a uniform curvature with a concavity directed forward to accommodate the viscera. In the thoracic and sacral regions this curvature persists, but compensatory curves in the opposite direction develop in the cervical and lumbar zones. At about the end of the third month the cervical spine develops anterior convexity as a result of the addition of the weight of the head. The cervical and lumbar zones are free of the outrigging support of the rib elements so that they remain the most mobile segments of the vertebral column. The function of extra mobility is aided by abundant turgid disc tissue between the vertebral bodies. The combination of weight-bearing mobility and lack of stabilization favors accumulation of strain in these zones. Inevitably, structural changes reflect this wear and tear process. In the cervical spine they are seen first and most often in the region of the anterior bodies of C.5–C.6 as marginal lipping and thinning of the interspace. The pathological picture is one of degeneration with repair. The process of degeneration starts in the intevertebral disc, leading to a loss in the normal rubbery re-

silience. This favors increased strain on the retaining annulus and short intervertebral fibers of the anterior longitudinal ligament. Stretching and loosening initiates peripheral periosteal reaction at the rim which extends into the ligament fibers, producing the typical marginal osteophytes. The development of osteophytes is frequent at the small accessory articulations or joints of Lushka.

The aging process is common to all spines, and most of the time no clinical sequelae develop. When trauma, debilitation, systemic devitalization or postural stress are added, the reaction comes into clinical focus.

When the normal balance is upset anteriorly, the small apophyseal joints are subjected to stress posteriorly (Fig. 7–12). This disturbs their planes of movement, alters surface contacts and increases the strain on capsular and articular ligaments. Unequal and poorly balanced movement then sets the stage for roughening and erosion of the cartilage. Articular cartilage is not very rugged, and poor nutrition results in inadequate repair. As joint spaces become thin, the normal mechanics are further altered and this unresolved cycle just keeps on. When the small joints reach the stage of marginal lipping, loss of joint space and thickened inelastic capsules, movement decreases and pain increases. Such is the usual process that eventually produces neck and shoulder discomfort. The changes may progress so that osteophyte formation, narrowing of the intervertebral space, disc bulging and articular subluxation gradually encroach on the intervertebral foramen. When this occurs radiating discomfort and root compression are frequently added to the local pain. Apart from injury, these changes produce local discomfort as a rule. They may progress, but when this happens new peripheral signs and symptoms appear just as lumbosacral discomfort can be followed by the development of typical radiating sciatica.

TREATMENT

(1) Rest is imperative; immobilization in a light cervical collar during the acute period often helps. (2) Frequently cervical traction applied judiciously without excessive weight is beneficial. If the traction is irritating to the lesion, it should be discontinued. (3) Pain should be relieved by adequate sedation. (4) After an acute attack has come under con-

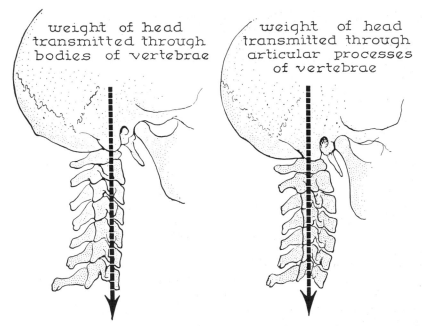

weight of head transmitted through bodies of vertebrae

weight of head transmitted through articular processes of vertebrae

Figure 7–12 As forward curve increases, greater stress falls on the apophyseal joints posteriorly, favoring degenerative changes.

trol, if there are weakened muscle zones, these should be strengthened. (5) Discomfort at night is often relieved by the use of a special contour pillow which supports the neck and prevents sleeping in a twisted position. (6) If the pain is disabling the cervical collar should be worn constantly during the day and replaced by a light fabric collar at night. (7) Development of radiating pain is best controlled by repeated cervical traction. In some instances, operative measures are required and these have been considered in the chapter Neurological Disturbances.

SCAPULOTHORACIC LESIONS

As our concept of shoulder disturbances enlarges it becomes apparent that the region of the shoulder blade is a frequent source of disorders producing typical shoulder-neck discomfort, a region that has often been overlooked as a source of significant pain. The focal point of origin of these lesions is the medial border of the scapula. The scapula slides, swings and rotates constantly on a bed of ribs covered with flat thin muscles (Fig. 7–13). Roughening of this bed or the contiguous surfaces of the scapula disturbs the normal smooth action, producing discomfort. Irregularities of the vertebral border, chest injuries, fractures of the ribs and muscle tears are all a source of abnormal friction during the shoulder blade excursion. Poor muscle development and sagging faulty posture contribute also. These disorders as a group are labeled scapulothoracic or scapulocostal lesions. The general underlying derangement is in the relation of the scapula to the chest, but several distinct entities may be recognized.

SCAPULOCOSTAL TENDINITIS

Scapulocostal tendinitis is a relatively mild but quite frequent ailment developing in this region. It is ushered in by a complaint of dragging aching shoulder discomfort or nagging shoulder pain that seems to come from between the shoulder blades. Patients indicate the zone of maximum distress as being related to the inner border of the shoulder blades and often cannot quite reach around to the back to precisely identify the sore spot. This discomfort has a tendency to build up with progressive use of the shoulder during the day. Certain precise chest skeletal configurations contribute to the stress on the muscles in the area, such as round chest, which favors sagging shoulder blades and stretching of the suspending muscles. This type of constant muscle stress initiates a dragging type pain.

The patients become aware that it is the motion of the shoulder blades which aggravates the discomfort and they avoid this

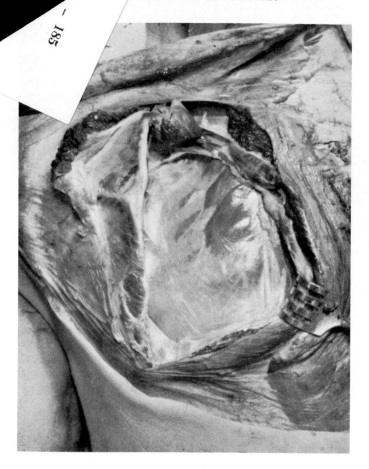

Figure 7–13 Dissection showing medial border of scapula and scapular bed.

irritation by keeping the arm at the side and develop a tendency to hunch the shoulder forward and around the chest. On examination definite tender points, principally related to the medial border of the scapula but also in the area of muscles between the border and the midline, can be identified. A grating sensation is imparted when these zones are palpated. The commonest area is the region opposite the base of the spine in thinly upholstered asthenic individuals. The inferior angle of the scapula is frequently involved also. Manipulation of these trigger zones reproduces the discomfort, which permeates the shoulder-neck region. Firm palpation identifies the trigger points, but the surrounding musculature has a stringy atonic feeling.

While this is partly a postural disturbance, the localizing properties set it apart from purely postural disorders. The primary source is assumption of the upright position, with the greater range of swing of the scapula which then develops. The scapula rotates like a pinwheel as well as swinging backward and forward around the chest. The vertebral border is a sharp blade that cuts into soft tissue if it does not fit smoothly into the proper layer. (See Figure 7–13.) Fraying of muscle fibers and minute ruptures occur from constant wear. Weakness and atony favor the process, and zones of fibrous scar tissue then develop.

Treatment of Scapulothoracic Disturbances

Injection of Trigger Points. The tender areas in the region of the base of the spine of the scapula should be freely infiltrated with a 2 per cent local anesthetic such as procaine (Novocain) or a similar solution. No adrenaline should be used. In some instances repeated injections are necessary; in chronic cases it may be helpful to add 0.5 ml. of absolute alcohol to a solution of 5 ml. of local anesthetic and inject this directly into the trigger area. At the same time postural faults should be corrected and instruction given in proper shoulder-neck exercises.

SNAPPING SCAPULAE

A similar yet quite different form of this disorder may be identified in a group of elderly patients, with the derangement being identified more properly as a "snapping scapula." The feature of this disorder is a distinct thump or snapping sound occurring as the scapula is moved across the back of the chest. Patients with this abnormality learn how to produce the sound, which is characteristic and may be the most prominent presenting complaint. It is a more severe grade of the previous disturbance in that bony alteration interferes with the normal swing of the shoulder blade. Commonly this is a spur in the region of the superior angle, but it may occur at any point along the vertebral border of the scapula. The corner of the superior angle may be turned down dog-ear fashion, forming a sharp beak that scrapes across the scapular bed as the scapula is swung. At other times bony lipping of the vertebral body or irregularities from fractured ribs produce a similar type of derangement.

The noise which is so characteristic of this disorder can be heard distinctly; the chest acts as a resonance box, magnifying the sound. By palpation it is sometimes difficult to localize the precise source of the sound. It appears to come from the front top or back, and it is not until the flat of the hand palpates the vertebral border of the scapula that the true origin may be identified (Fig. 7–14). Occupations requiring forceful repeated shoulder action favor development of this lesion. Swinging a heavy axe, for example, pulls strongly on the anchoring

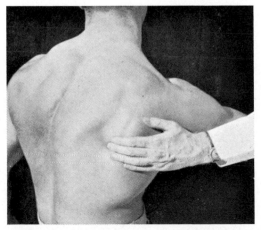

Figure 7–14 Palpating trigger areas along the medial border of the scapula.

tissues of the scapula. Minute periosteal tears favor osteophyte formation, and gradually a spur forms at this site. Special x-rays can be taken that demonstrate a curling of the medial border or a small beak-like process close to the angle of the scapula (Fig. 7–15). A severe form of this disorder results from the growth of an osteoma or osteochondroma, usually near the inferior border of the scapula.

In addition to the sound and the development of irritation as the shoulder blade is swung, the patients complain of pain, particularly on shoulder girdle action, because soft tissue irritation leads to an aching type of shoulder neck discomfort that pervades the region.

TREATMENT. When the condition has been accurately defined the most satisfactory treatment is resection of the bony abnormality. In most instances removal of the corner of the scapula that includes the hooklike formation is a simple and effective remedy.

Technique. The patient is placed on his face with the arm hanging over the side of the table so that the vertebral border of the scapula is prominent. The arm is prepared, however, so that adequate manipulation can be carried out. A longitudinal incision just medial to the medial border of the scapula and curving above and below the spine for a distance of two inches is made (Fig. 7–16). Muscle layers are split in the direction of their fibers, and blunt dissection exposes the medial border of the scapula. Deep protractors are needed to retract the soft tissues because the bone lies deeper than is usually appreciated. Depending upon the size and the length of the spur, a piece of scapula roughly triangular in shape, one inch by three-quarters of an inch in size, is excised. The bone edges are smoothed and bleeding is carefully controlled by a local coagulant such as Surgicel to prevent recurrence of the spur. As soon as the wound is satisfactorily healed, active movement is started and continued.

SEVERE SAGGING SHOULDER

An extreme form of scapulothoracic disorder may develop from either of the preceding problems or after frank rupture of the suspensory (coracoclavicular) ligament. In some instances irritation from the scraping of the scapula across the posterior chest becomes so troublesome that the patient continues to pull the arm and shoulder more and

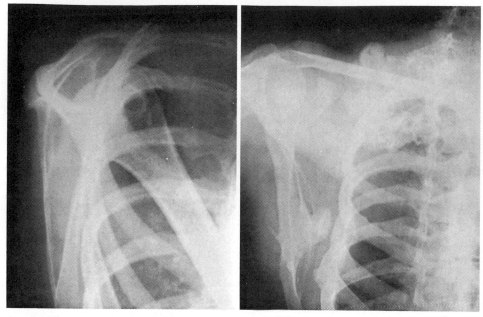

Figure 7–15 Scapular spurs producing snapping scapulae. *A*, Spur of upper corner of scapula. *B*, Large spur near inferior angle.

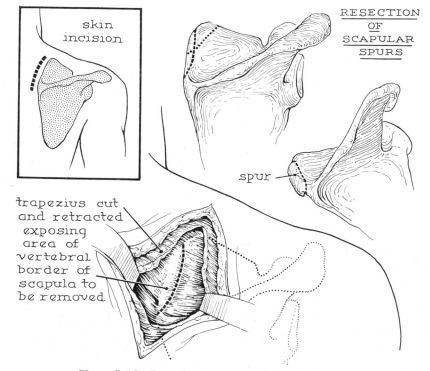

Figure 7–16 Operative treatment for snapping scapula.

more away from the irritating site. In this way he develops a habit or spasm in which he twists and pulls the shoulder and neck apart, as it were. This is continued to such a degree that the muscles become lax and weak and the excursion of the scapula on the chest is grossly increased. A point is reached at which the affected side sags and drops to the front in abnormal fashion. The whole girdle then sags, not just the head of the humerus in the glenoid cavity. On examination the shoulder may be grasped, and shifting of the scapula back and forth on the chest will reproduce the most unpleasant element of the discomfort. Middle-aged, thin, poorly muscled, somewhat introspective women seem to be the ones who most often develop this disorder. Because of a relatively minor focus of soft tissue irritation in the region of the vertebral border of the scapula, they consistently tense and shrug themselves into a state of extreme discomfort.

Several years may be necessary to develop the severe form of the discomfort as the muscle atony increases and the sag becomes greater. At this point radiating pain to the arm and hand may develop from compression of the neurovascular bundle anteriorly. A very similar situation develops much more rapidly if the suspensory ligaments have been ruptured or excised. Cutting of the conoid or trapezoid ligaments, such as may develop from too radical excision of the lateral one third of the scapula, will allow the shoulder girdle to sag forward, producing constant shoulder drop and, later, neurovascular symptoms (Figs. 7–17, 7–18 and 7–19).

Treatment. Muscle education and exercise designed to improve the tone of the suspensory muscles should be tried most conscientiously, along with the simple measures outlined previously for injection of trigger points. In some instances the disorder will progress to the point that only surgical treatment offers significant assistance. The principle of operative treatment is to remove any obvious irritation at the scapulothoracic junction and to resuspend the scapula so that the extreme muscle atony of the suspensory muscles is counteracted. This is done by inserting fascial slings which extend from the posterior spinous process of the cervical spine to the scapula so that it is suspended in proper relation to the chest again. At first this would seem to be a somewhat major procedure for the amount of discomfort, but it is a most satisfactory operation when the proper indications are present. It should be stressed that minor degrees of the atonic type of the disorder should not be treated surgically; however, when patients have had constant distress for a period of three or four years and present the evidence of obvious scapular sag, the

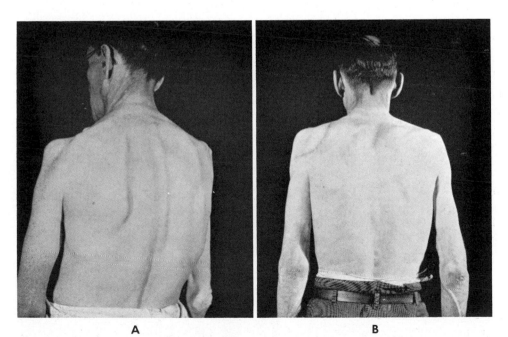

A   **B**

Figure 7–17 Severe sagging shoulder following too extensive resection of outer end of the clavicle, including conoid and trapezoid ligaments. *A*, Before operation. *B*, After fascial suspension.

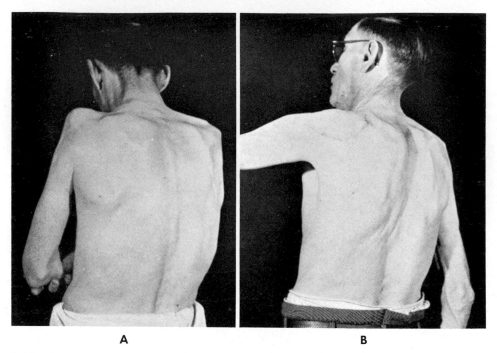

A   **B**

Figure 7–18 *A,* Preoperatively, function requires the support of the opposite arm. *B,* Independent movement is possible after surgery.

insertion of the fascial supports can initiate a dramatic improvement.

SURGICAL TECHNIQUE. The operation is extremely effective for the sagging scapula that develops following excision of the outer end of the clavicle when this has included the suspensory mechanism. The patient is placed in the prone position on the operating table with the arm hanging at the side over the table. The whole upper extremity is prepared, including the posterior scapular and lower cervical regions. The incision is made parallel to the spine, curving gently downward and extending

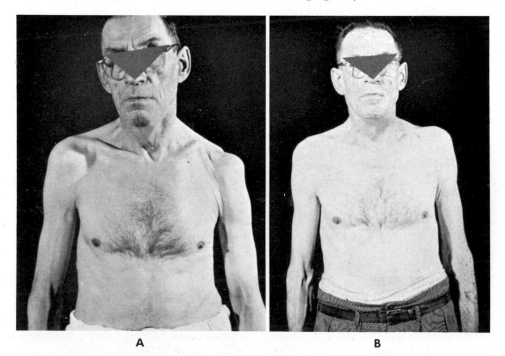

A   **B**

Figure 7–19 Appearance from the front before and after fascial suspension.

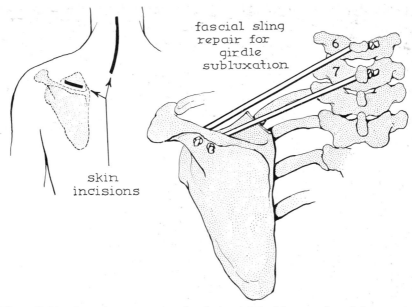

Figure 7–20   Operative exposure and technique of fascial suspension of the scapula.

from near the scapular notch to below the root of the spine; the medial edge is exposed (Fig. 7–20). The first step of the operation is exposure of the root of the spine of the scapula and excision of any osteophytes or hook formation that may be encountered. The next step is exposure of the posterior spinous processes of the lower two cervical vertebrae. This is accomplished through a midline incision over the tips of spines of C.6 and C.7. A hole is drilled through each of these spines, with care being taken not to split the spines since they are sometimes poorly developed; usually a three-sixteenths inch drill is the maximum which can be accommodated. Two strong fascial slings are then made from fascia removed from the thigh and are anchored through the drill holes in the spinous processes and carried subcutaneously to the first incision close to the notch of the spine. The whole upper extremity is then lifted, elevating the shoulder girdle as far as possible, and the fascial slings are fastened securely. In this way the tension on the slings holds the scapula up and back. The wounds are closed in the usual fashion. A pelvic forearm plaster is applied, keeping the arm in the fascial suspended position. This is fashioned from a broad band of plaster around the iliac crests, which are well padded, with the plaster encircling the body and resting on the crests. The operative side is elevated and held in this position

by a plaster ledge around the forearm and fastened to the body band (Fig. 7–21). The plaster remains in place for six weeks.

This form of fixation is preferable in patients in whom there has been excision of the clavicle. In some instances, when the sagging is not quite so extreme, a body

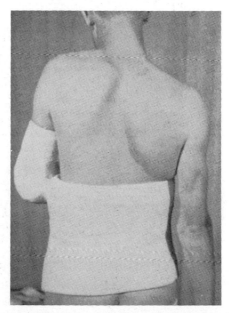

Figure 7–21   Type of plaster applied postoperatively to hold the scapula suspended in new position.

swathe with a stockinette shirt which is held firmly in place will be sufficient to hold the shoulder in the corrected position. Following the removal of the fixation at the end of six weeks, exercises for the arm and shoulder are initiated, but vigorous exercise for the shoulder girdle is discouraged.

NERVE LESIONS PRODUCING SHOULDER-NECK PAIN

There is a group of neural disorders in this region which may come into clinical focus by the production of shoulder-neck pain. These include trapezius strain, serratus anterior paralysis, scapular dystrophies and suprascapular neurodynia. They are described completely in the chapter on nerve disturbances.

The two common lesions to be particularly kept in mind are trapezius and serratus anterior paralysis. Since these may have an insidious onset, they may go unrecognized for some time. Either lesion may be present as a chronic shoulder-neck complaint, with an aching quality similar to the other entities described previously.

TRAPEZIUS PARALYSIS

The trapezius is a most important muscle in the shoulder girdle. When it is paralyzed by injury to the accessory nerve, serious deformity and disability result. The nerve is frequently damaged in operations on the neck such as biopsies, in wounds of the neck or from pressure or traction trauma (Fig. 7–22).

Mechanism of Injury. The trapezius is supplied largely by the accessory nerve; the contributions from C.3 and C.4 are not prominent. The nerve follows a vulnerable course through the upper portion of the posterior triangle in the neck, entering into the sternomastoid muscle and crossing the apex to reach the trapezius muscle an inch above the clavicle. In the posterior triangle the neck lies just beneath the deep fascia and is the highest structure crossing this triangle. At this point, it is intimately related to cervical lymph glands and is covered only by skin and fascia, making it particularly susceptible to injury.

Signs and Symptoms. Paralysis of the trapezius results in abnormal shoulder contour, particularly as seen from the back. The shoulder slope is replaced by a sharp right-angled appearance. The shoulder drops and the scapula tilts, with the inferior angle riding closer to the midline. Loss of power in the trapezius produces winging of the scapula of a rotatory nature because stability is decreased. Weakness in elevating the shoulder against resistance then develops because of loss of the rotatory stabilization. This is in contrast to serratus paralysis, in which the direct anteroposterior clamping effect is lost, and the winging in this instance is more from front to back. The trapezius aids extension of the neck against pressure in conjunction with the muscle of the opposite side. Loss of trapezius power can be insidious, and sometimes the only complaint may be a persistent shoulder-neck ache or a dragging sensation when wearing an overcoat or other heavy garment. Examination demonstrates weakness of shoulder abduction and circumduction. Sometimes the contour alteration is not easily recognized because of superficial soft tissue padding, but the lack of rotatory fixation of the scapula should be apparent.

Treatment. The accessory nerve is large enough to be repaired surgically and when

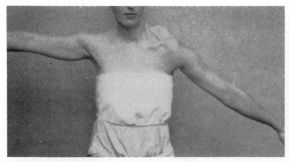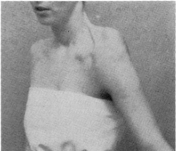

Figure 7–22 Patient with trapezius and levator paralysis following cervical gland biopsy. Note extensive deformity, with altered neck contour and winging at scapula.

there is persistence of paralysis, clinically and electrically, the nerve should be repaired as quickly as may be feasible. Electrical stimulation is applied to the muscle, and exercises for the accessory muscles such as the levator scapulae, serratus, deltoid and rhomboids are initiated. In irreparable lesions, fascial suspension can be carried out. In some instances the two procedures can be combined in the same operation, with the fascial suspension being carried out and after this the accessory nerve being explored and repaired.

TECHNIQUE. Exposure of the accessory nerve is obtained by an incision extending across the upper portion of the posterior triangle. The lateral border of the sterno-mastoid is identified and retracted medially. The accessory nerve is identified coming out from under the posterior margin about the center of this muscle. It is the highest structure in the triangle and lies superficially just beneath the fascia and surrounded by lymph vessels. A small nerve, the lesser occipital, curves up and over from below and is intimately associated. The nerve leaves the triangle laterally under the anterior border of the trapezius about 1½ inches above the clavicle. Extra length for suture of the accessory nerve is gained by mobilizing it and bending the neck toward the side of the lesion.

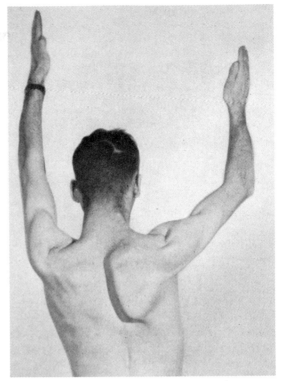

Figure 7–23 Injury of long thoracic nerve producing paralysis of serratus anterior.

PARALYSIS OF THE SERRATUS ANTERIOR MUSCLE, INJURY OF THE LONG THORACIC NERVE

The long thoracic nerve is the highest branch of the brachial plexus. It may be involved in the extensive plexus injuries or may be injured directly from pressure or traction trauma (Fig. 7–23).

Mechanism of Injury. The long thoracic nerve follows a tortuous course, arising from roots C.5, C.6 and C.7. After it has been formed it appears at the scalenus medius and descends behind the brachial plexus to cross the axilla close to the chest wall. Thence it descends on the outer surface of the serratus anterior muscle.

In the upper portion of its course, the nerve may be exposed to pressure such as in carrying heavy loads on the shoulder. Similarly, some athletic activities involving violent use of the shoulder girdle as a unit, like discus or javelin throwing, may result in traction injuries to the nerve. In the lower portion of its course, dissections on the axilla, as for example in carrying out the operation of

radical mastectomy, may injure the nerve, or it can be involved in the pathological process. Because the nerve lies close to the chest wall, undue pressure may inadvertently be applied in this region in very thin people, such as in frail elderly women encased in body plasters who are not turned frequently enough and have continued pressure on one side for a considerable length of time.

Signs and Symptoms. Injury to the long thoracic nerve produces paralysis of the serratus anterior muscle. This results in flaring or winging of the scapula when abduction of the arm is attempted, particularly against resistance. The serratus anterior contributes significantly to the stability of the scapula and, along with the trapezius, clamps it to the chest wall, providing a firm base for the hoisting mechanism of the shoulder and arm. When this stability is lost, the scapula stands out from the chest in an anteroposterior direction and the vertebral body projects backward.

Treatment. Persistent paralysis of the serratus anterior leaves a weak extremity; this is particularly disabling in a workman. The muscle is difficult to treat by electrical stimulation because of its position. Usually, however, it may be reached by applying an electrode to the chest in front of the posterior axillary fold. In some instances the use of a sling or a brace which holds the scapula to the chest wall is effective in controlling the winging action.

SURGICAL THERAPY. Patients who do not recover in a reasonable time should be treated surgically. If damage is suspected in the supraclavicular portion of the nerve, this is exposed through the same incision as is indicated for plexus exploration. The nerve is identified behind the plexus, piercing the scalenus medius. In the distal portion of its course it is exposed by an incision across the anterior fold of the axilla to the chest wall. In either position the nerve is exposed and the pathology dealt with as indicated.

IRREPARABLE LESIONS OF THE LONG THORACIC NERVE. Sometimes the nerve fails to recover. This can be offset somewhat by exercises designed to increase the power of the upper trapezius, rhomboids and levator scapular muscles. When this is not sufficient, several operations have been advised. The principle of these procedures is to anchor the flaring medial border of the scapula to the chest wall. This restores the clamping action and stabilizes the scapula in abduction. There is some limitation of movement, but this is not significant.

Surgical Techniques. In the Whitman technique, fascial strips are used to anchor the vertebral border to the posterior spines of T.4, T.5, T.6 and T.7. In the Dixon technique, a strip of fascia is used to anchor the inferior angle to adjacent musculature.

The most effective procedure, however, is that devised by Lowman. The principle of this method is to insert a strip of fascia at the distal portion of the medial border, carry it across the midline subcutaneously and attach it to the medial border of the opposite scapula. This restores the clamping action and stabilizes the scapula. Postoperatively the arm is carried in a sling, with the scapula fixed to the chest wall until fixation has become solid, usually at the end of three to four weeks.

REFERENCES

Brooker, A. E., et al.: Cervical spondylosis. A clinical study with comparative radiology. Brain *88*:925–936, 1965.

Claessens, H., et al.: Rehabilitation in shoulder lesions. J. Belg. Rheum. Med. Phys. *20*:69–72, 1965.

Copeman, W. S. C., and Ackerman, W. L.: Fibrositis of back. Quart. J. Med. *13*:50, 1944.

Dixon, F. D.: Fascial transplants in paralytic and other conditions. J. Bone Joint Surg. *405*:19, 1937.

Fierro, D., et al.: On the significance of calcifications and limited ossifications of the posterior cervical ligament. Minerva Radiol. *11*:157–165, 1966.

Hunt, J. C., et al.: A convalescent cervical collar. Amer. J. Orthop. 7:109, 1965.

Moyson, F., et al.: Acute pseudotorticollis: A little known disease. Acta Paediat. Belg. *20*:259–270, 1966.

Rose, D. L., et al.: The painful shoulder. The scapulocostal syndrome in shoulder pain. J. Kansas Med. Soc. *67*:112–114, 1966.

Saha, N. C.: Painful shoulder in patients with chronic bronchitis and emphysema. Amer. Rev. Resp. Dis. *94*:455–456, 1966.

Schein, A. J.: Back and neck pain and associated nerve root irritation in the New York City Fire Department. Clin. Orthop. *59*:119–124, 1968.

Whitman, A.: Congenital elevation of the scapula and paralysis of serratus magnus muscle. Operation. J.A.M.A. *99*:1332, 1932.

Chapter VIII

LESIONS PRODUCING SHOULDER PAIN PREDOMINANTLY

Pain in the shoulder arises more often from disease of the glenohumeral or shoulder joint proper than from any other structure. The cardinal symptoms are clearly localized pain and soreness. Patients point this out in typical fashion by grasping the shoulder point firmly with the opposite hand. They have a clear conception of the zone of their discomfort; vague ache in the neck or sharp, radiating pain to the forearm is not a part of the picture. They learn early that it is the movement of "the arm in the socket" that causes them most distress. Neck action or body position affect it little or not at all. All acute derangements of the shoulder come to attention in this fashion. In long standing lesions the area of deltoid insertion is often implicated. After the shoulder pain has been present for some time, added discomfort may be experienced in the scapular zone, or it may extend to the elbow. Questioning shows that such extension is secondary and that the dominant and initial discomfort originates in the shoulder.

There is a long list of causes of this type of pain, including degenerative tendinitis, calcified tendinitis, cuff ruptures and bicipital lesions as the common entities. It will be noted that the terms "subacromial bursitis" and "frozen shoulder" are usually avoided in such lists. As our knowledge of shoulder pathology increases, it is apparent that these are insufficiently descriptive names that are often inaccurately applied to many syndromes of varied etiology. Both these conditions do occur, but they are a result of other lesions, rather than a primary disease entity.

DEGENERATIVE TENDINITIS
(Subacromial bursitis, subdeltoid bursitis, supraspinatus tendinitis, etc.)

For many years the commonest ailment involving the shoulder has been labeled "bursitis," but as a clearer understanding of the pathological processes has developed, it has become apparent that a degeneration of the rotator cuff or a tendinitis is the common foundation of shoulder disorders. In some degree, accompanied by acute or repeated minor trauma, this lesion accounts for nearly all persistent shoulder disability. The degenerative process involves the musculotendinous cuff and the bicipital apparatus. At times either the cuff or the bicipital apparatus may be the most prominently involved, and frequently both are. Since these are intimate glenohumeral structures, it is logical that disorders affecting them are reflected by predominantly localized shoulder pain.

In the adaptive adjustments of mammals the upright position has greatly increased the stress and strain on the cervicobrachial and the lumbosacral zones. In the upper body region the object has been to free the arm and provide motion to the hand. Shoulder elements have contributed significantly to this development, but inevitably certain parts, the rotator cuff for example, have been exposed to greatly increased mechanical stress (Fig. 1–3). We work either by standing or sitting with a task in front of us, using the shoulder to bring the hand into the arc of function. This has not only changed the configuration of the forelimb, but has also exposed some parts to greater stress. Development has enabled man to use his arms in the overhead position also, so that in addition to normal adaptative strain, greatly increased occupational stress can also develop. Disturbances in the cuff come to light initially as irritation of the overlying subacromial bursa, but the bursal reaction is a result rather than a primary cause.

SIGNS AND SYMPTOMS

Degenerative tendinitis is characterized by pain in the shoulder which the patient localizes accurately and indicates by placing the hand firmly over the point of the shoulder (Fig. 8–1). Shortly, a catching discomfort on certain movement is appreciated, chiefly when lifting the arm. Gradual limitation of movement, particularly rotation, follows. Everyday tasks initiate pain which increases to a persistent gnawing ache. No significant episode, accident or acute incident is associated as a rule. Little by little, on certain movements, general soreness develops and is accompanied by occasional sharp twinges. A little later, movements which cause the twinge are avoided and aching pain at night becomes bothersome. These patients have difficulty finding a comfortable position for sleeping. They attempt to obtain relief by holding the shoulder, but no position is comfortable. Later, pain may appear to come from a point lower down in the arm, in the region of the deltoid insertion. It is usually at the stage when sleep is disturbed and the back trousers pocket cannot be reached or the hair cannot be combed that the patient seeks relief. This is a disease of middle age; housewives, painters, carpenters, bricklayers

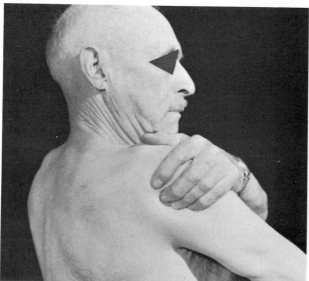 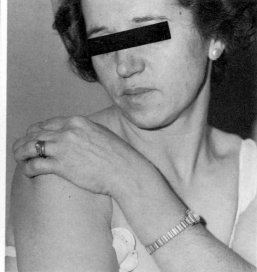

Figure 8–1 "Shoulder grasp" of patients with localized shoulder disorders, in this case degenerative tendinitis.

and hard swinging golfers are most commonly afflicted.

Examination demonstrates a typical painful catch as the arm is lifted and rotated, bringing the head of the humerus under the acromial arch (Fig. 8–1). There is some limitation of movement, but the shoulder is not frozen. Active movement is done hesitantly. Often crepitus can be felt, and occasionally the patient has noted something slipping or a soft grinding element as the arm is lifted. Active movement to 70 or 80 degrees is possible. External and internal rotation are limited slightly. Study from the back shows some atrophy of supra- and infraspinatus and deltoid. Atrophy is never so severe at this stage as when the lesion has progressed to the typical frozen shoulder or when there has been a rupture of the cuff.

Examination of the upper aspect will reveal tenderness directly over the upper end of the humerus (Fig. 8–2). The zone of maximum tenderness is over the cuff—not over the acromion, and not over the biceps tendon. The region is sore, but there is not the exquisite tenderness encountered in the typical tendinitis with calcification. The patient is certain of the general area of soreness but sometimes has to hunt for the really tender points. Often he grasps the shoulder and feels for it, progressing from the tip down toward the deltoid insertion. This region may be implicated and may be a little tender on palpation. Flexion of the forearm against resistance does not produce significant pain, although a little generalized discomfort may ensue. There is no complaint of pain along the front of the shoulder or down the medial aspect of the arm. Palpation along the long head of the biceps does

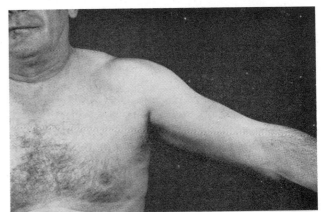

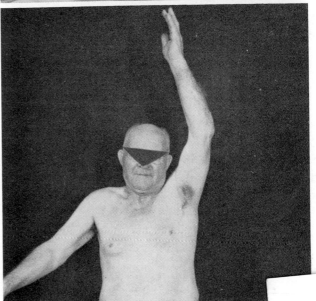

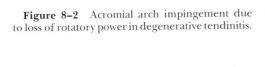

Figure 8–2 Acromial arch impingement due to loss of rotatory power in degenerative tendinitis.

not cause significant discomfort. When the pain has been noticeable for some weeks, other areas are implicated, the posterior aspect of the shoulder and root of the neck, for example, or pain may extend to the elbow. Questioning shows such discomfort is transient and less severe than the persistent and primary shoulder ache.

At this point the picture is clear, but the longer the lesion is neglected, the hazier the picture becomes. The patient learns to avoid the painful arc, so that the range is gradually decreased and the atrophy is increased. The process may continue in this way until a typical frozen shoulder develops if proper treatment is not instituted (Fig. 8–3).

X-RAY EXAMINATION

X-rays are not very helpful, but they should be taken and examined carefully. No abnormality may be apparent on cursory examination, but systematic search often shows minute changes. Subcortical cysts, flattening and eburnation of the greater tuberosity, sharpening of the tuberosity, small detached spicules or a roughened facet may be seen (Fig. 8–4). If the disturbance is sufficiently severe to warrant contrast studies, the arthrogram demonstrates an intact capsule with no subacromial leak. The inferior joint fold is still lax and redundant and has not been obliterated, nor has the capsule shrunk as in adhesive capsuli-

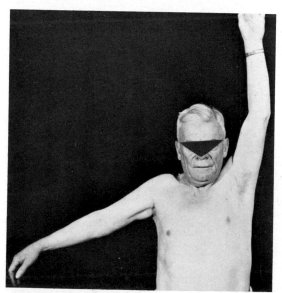

Figure 8–3 A later stage of degenerative tendinitis. Freezing has started. Note tendency to hump the right shoulder, which is not seen in the patient in Figure 8–2.

tis. The upper edge is sometimes a little ragged when compared with a normal cuff and it may extend further out on the greater tuberosity, suggesting some laxity or stretching of the cuff in this area (Fig. 8–5). If there is a leak into the bursa, a tear is present in addition to the tendon degeneration. If the shadow has a rectangular box-like configuration, the adhesive capsulitis stage has developed.

COURSE AND PROGRESS

The progress of the patient depends upon the severity of the lesion, situational factors and, often, the patient's occupation. If adequate treatment is applied and movement is retained in spite of some pain, the disabling adhesive or freezing stage is avoided. In less stoical and more apprehensive patients, the tendinitis stage may quickly blend with a pernicious adhesive capsulitis, and freezing of the joint occurs. Many of these patients may recall some traumatic episode, but it has seldom been severe. If significant injury is added, the degenerated fibers give way easily, tearing the cuff. Rarely, the discomfort from the degenerative process is not prominent and persistent, and extensive questioning is necessary to bring the patient to admit that shoulder ache has been present for some time. This form of tendinitis develops over a period of weeks and does not assume the fulminating characteristics of tendinitis with calcification.

ETIOLOGY AND PATHOLOGY

General Description of the Process

Degenerative tendinitis is a reaction to mechanical stress and strain plus a process of degeneration. It has been labeled tendinitis for want of a more accurately descriptive term. The impression of infection should not be conveyed because the process is a mechanical, degenerative, nonbacterial one. All our joints have a weak spot: in the knee it is the menisci and the undersurface of the patella; in the hip it is the head of the femur and its vascular supply; in the shoulder the weak spot is the musculotendinous cuff and biceps tendon. Just as we recognize small changes starting in these vulnerable areas and progressing to wide damage, a similar but slightly different process can be seen in

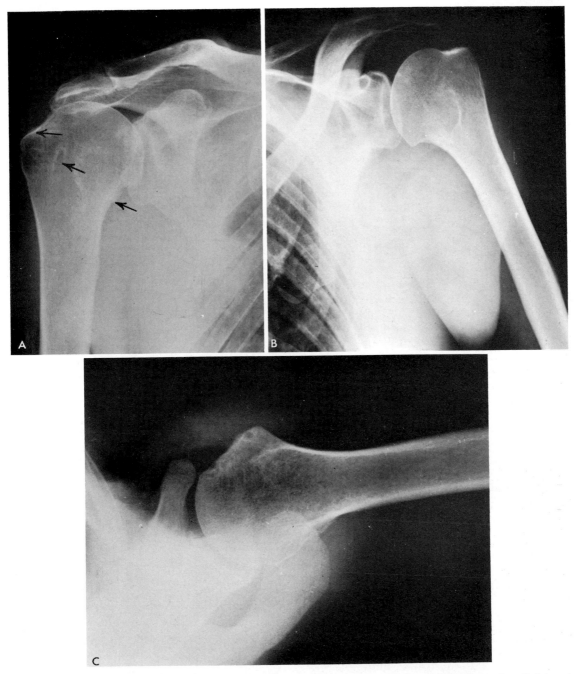

Figure 8–4 X-ray changes in degenerative tendinitis. *A*, Roughening, eburnation and cyst formation. *B*, Sclerosis and eburnation at cuff insertion. *C*, Erosion, roughening and cyst formation of greater tuberosity.

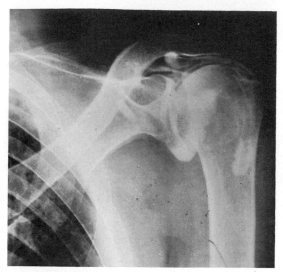

Figure 8–5 Arthrogram in a patient with degenerative tendinitis. The cuff is not torn, but the space between the head of the humerus and the undersurface of the capsule is increased, suggesting laxity and thinning of the cuff.

the shoulder. The development of a wear and tear or degenerative arthritis in the knee and hip is common and well recognized. Degeneration in the shoulder begins in the intimate soft parts, and the severe bone changes encountered in the hip and the knee do not develop. The rotator cuff bears the brunt of the wear and tear, leading to premature aging. The anatomical position, allowing exposure to mechanical stress, rather than any deficiency in its intrinsic structure, favors this aging process.

Extensive studies of this wear and tear damage of capsular structures have been done by Grant, Meyer, DePalma, Wilson and Duff, and Keys. Wear increases with age until, according to Codman, a histologically normal tendon in old people is rare. The underlying degenerative process is the early change, but in many instances the cuff gives way, resulting in tears and defects. Tendinitis is interpreted as the early and less serious lesion.

We look for torn cartilages in coal miners and in soccer players and we can expect cuff disturbances in painters, in carpenters and in housewives who do much ironing. Lumping, fraying and cracking of the cuff near its insertion occurs, which upsets the closely adjusted relation to the overhanging coracoacromial arch. Gradually the patient becomes conscious of this as a painful catch or a clicking sensation when the arm is lifted. From this simple beginning widespread changes

develop in bursa, capsule, bone and cartilage. They progress from a small focus, just as they may in the knee and hip, increasing to extensive joint damage.

Changes in the Tendon

The primary change is in tendon, which then disturbs structures above and below; the bursa is irritated and cartilage is roughened and eroded. Normally the tendon is a stout ribbon composed of bundles of collagen fibers. Between the bundles are narrow spaces that contain a few blood vessels and are sparsely lined with fibroblasts. The fibers spread a little as they are anchored into the tuberosity, so that the thinnest, most compact portion lies a short distance away from the bone attachment. Degeneration starts in the collagen fiber and in the ground substance between the fibers. The first area involved is the juxtainsertional belt, the part a little medial to the insertion zone. Grossly this appears as a slight thickening or roughening on the surface—an oval, somewhat granular area (Fig. 8–6). When such a region

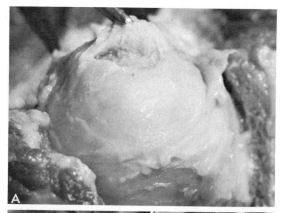

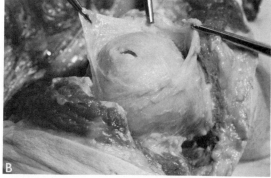

Figure 8–6 *A,* Early degeneration of cuff with roughening and separation of superficial fibers. *B,* Later stage with cracking of the cuff.

is examined under the microscope, changes are apparent in fiber and ground substance. The fibers become straight, loose and thin, changing from the normal, compact, wavy, symmetrical composition; the margins are less well defined, and staining qualities are altered (Fig. 8–7). Changes in the ground substance appear in the form of mucoid swelling which later leads to a characteristic fibrinoid change. Oval areas lose their collagen fiber composition with the fibrinoid change and later are replaced by fibrous tissue. As more devitalization, fibrinoid and fibrotic changes occur, the tensile strength of tendon is decreased and more direct strain is focused on the insertion fibers and adjacent cortex.

Studies by Mosely and his associates have made a fundamental contribution to the elucidation of the vascular supply of the rotator cuff, which is supplied by three principal sets of vessels.

Osseous Arteries. A group of vessels from the bicipital groove branch of the anterior circumflex enters the greater tuberosity and penetrates to the tendinous attachments.

Muscular Branches. From supra- and subscapular arteries, a profound network extends into the tendinous zone, through the musculotendinous junction.

Tendinous Vessels. In addition to anastomoses of the muscular and osseous branches, the supraspinatus zone receives a branch from the arcuate artery, which runs beneath the bursa and extends to the supraspinatus tendon to anastomose with these vessels.

The suggestion has been made that a critical zone exists at the point of anastomosis, but practical experience suggests that this zone cannot be extensive. It is common experience at operation for removal of calcium deposits or cuff repair to encounter insistent oozing from the conjoint tendon if it is pricked with a needle or resected for suture; the area is anything but an avascular or ischemic zone. These observations support the modern theory of calcifinolaxis, that calcium is precipitated on living collagen, but not necessarily in an area of ischemia. Similarly, as one studies cuff ruptures it becomes evident that they do not all occur in any one place, nor do they have a similar configuration. The variation in size, shape and position does not indicate that any initial separation has a fixed source.

Synovium atrophies and disappears at the point of reflection from tuberosity on the capsule. Changes similar to those in the cuff appear in the sheath and the long head of the biceps tendon. The sheath becomes thickened and adherent, and zones of fragmentation and hyaline degeneration appear. The

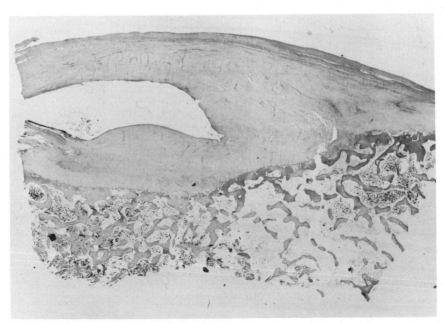

Figure 8–7 Microscopic appearance of cuff insertion zone showing early signs of degeneration. Three definite changes are apparent: (1) separation of layer of deep fibers; (2) loosening of anchoring zone; and (3) beginning of changes in cancellous bone.

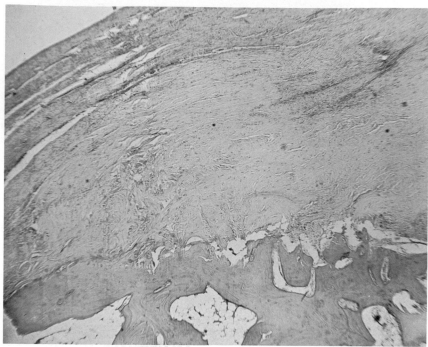

Figure 8–8 Early microscopic changes in degenerative tendinitis. Separation and fibrillation of collagen fibers, changes in ground substances between the fibers, cracking of cartilage plate and disruption of normal cancellous architecture are apparent from above downward.

tendon is roughened, tensile strength is decreased and areas of fibrinoid degeneration develop, to be followed by fibrosis. The weakened area may give way as these changes progress.

The cuff is anchored by rows of perpendicularly placed cells that infiltrate the osseocartilaginous junction. Beneath these roots is a thin line of compact bone roofing the cancellous upper end of humerus. In the aging process, cells of the anchoring zone show degenerative changes too; they become loose and vacuolated and the compact cortical line is disrupted (Fig. 8–8). Some areas of cortex become eburnated and hardened, and small portions may be avulsed. Beneath the cortical layer, small cystic cavities develop in the cancellous zone from the coalescence of several trabeculae. As the tendon weakens further, it becomes stretched as a hat does when blocked or a rubber tube in blistering so that it may be creased or folded and caught as the head of the humerus swings under the coraco-acromial arch. What happens to a cuff once this stage is reached depends on the activities, age and occupation of the patient. In younger people calcification may occur in the disturbed area; in laborers who handle heavy work a fall may produce a

massive rupture. In older, more sedentary patients the wearing, fraying and cracking continues in varying degrees.

Bursa

The bursa during this process loses its filamentous proportions. The thin, pinkish envelope develops thick walls with redundant folds. Thick, cord-like adhesions appear firmly anchored to the floor and are most obvious at the musculotendinous junction, away from the tuberosity. When movement is decreased, the bursa shrinks and the walls tend to fall together, becoming adherent. On microscopic examination the normal, smooth, synovial surface is deficient, with patchy areas being replaced by fibrous tissue. Zones of hyaline degeneration in the walls and villous folds are present. The extent of the fibrosis varies; in some patients only a few normal areas remain, and the walls become thick, stiff and adherent (Fig. 8–9).

Cartilage and Bone

The smooth surface of cartilage immediately beneath tendon also reflects the

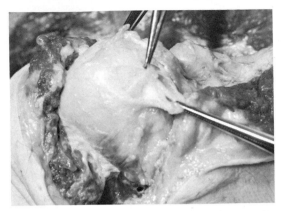

Figure 8–9 Thick adherent bursa of degenerative tendinitis.

triangular-shaped area, with the base at the edge and the apex pointing into the joint (Fig. 8–10). Bare cortical bone lies under the tendon, then at the rim. Cortex becomes eburnated and, as tendon fibers pull out, it is roughened and heaped up. All these changes—the fraying and thickening of tendon, heaping up of bone, roughening of cartilage, gluing of bursa—take place in the critical subacromial zone and will then tend to obstruct the swing of the tuberosity beneath the coraco-acromial arch. As movement continues, the wearing process grinds on. Subcortical trabeculae atrophy, and small cystic areas develop and are filled with fibrofatty substance.

changes of the degenerative wear and tear process. The sheen is lost first as it becomes scratched, blister formation develops and superficial flakes are dislodged. As the eroding pressure from the roughened tendon continues, cartilage disappears over a

TREATMENT

Degenerative tendinitis is a chronic process which can usually be treated quite successfully by conservative measures. The

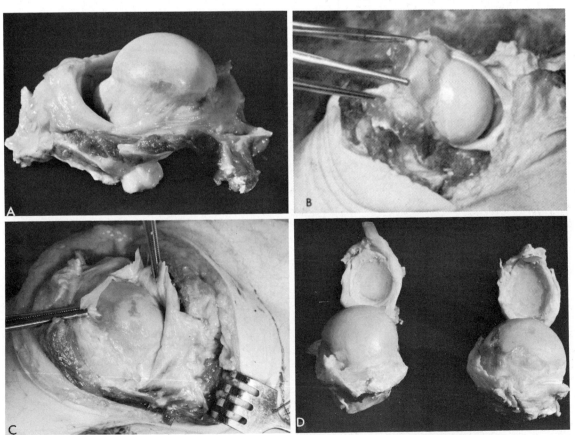

Figure 8–10 Joint changes at various stages of degenerative tendinitis. *A*, Normal head and capsule at age 50. *B*, Cracking and fraying of cuff, erosion of cartilage. *C*, More advanced changes in tendon and bone. *D*, Advanced changes in head and glenoid compared with normal.

principles are to relieve the pain, preserve joint movement and help the patient plan how to avoid obviously irritating activities. These patients have had shoulder pain for some time and often fear they have some serious disease such as a malignant lesion or crippling arthritis. It helps considerably to explain the nature of this disturbance; patients are most grateful for having their fears allayed.

Injection Therapy

The quickest and most effective relief is obtained from injections of anesthetic agents into the subacromial bursa. One or several injections at intervals of one to two weeks are necessary. The author prefers 2 per cent Novocain, or a similar local anesthetic, with 5 to 12 cc injected as an office procedure; 1 cc of a steroid may be added. After receiving the injection, the patient moves the arm through as full a range as possible, assisted by the doctor if necessary. The relief of pain is always sufficient to increase the range. The probable duration of the maximum pain relief is explained, so that the patients will not be disconcerted by the return of some discomfort. Increased movement is encouraged within reasonable discomfort limits, and the patient is instructed in exercises and proper sleeping posture.

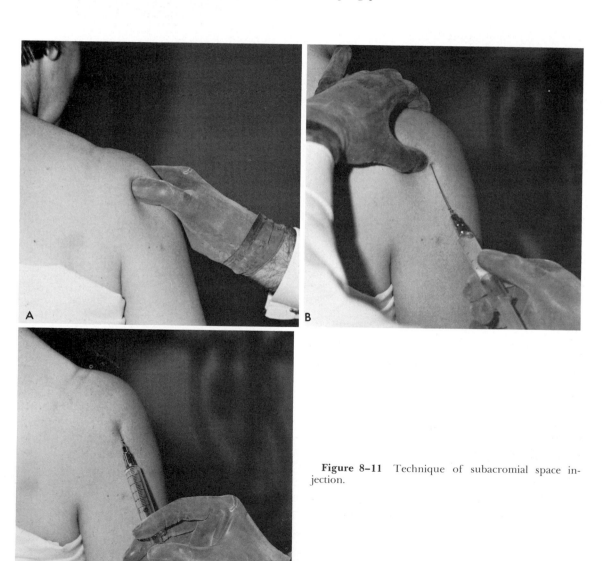

Figure 8–11 Technique of subacromial space injection.

Table position for shoulder surgery.

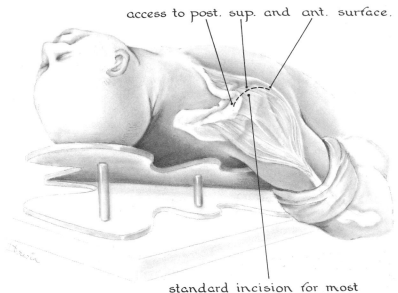

access to post. sup. and ant. surface.

standard incision for most
shoulder reconstruction.

Figure 8–11A   Table position for shoulder surgery.

Since the principle of injection therapy is to decrease subacromial reaction, the injection is made into the subacromial bursa, not into the joint. It is much easier to do this from a posterior aspect; otherwise, it is difficult to be certain the injected material is placed subacromially so that it will bathe the irritated zones.

A point just below and medial to the angle of the acromion is selected and a 21-gauge 1½ inch needle is used. It is insinuated under the acromion on top of the humerus until it comes to rest in the subacromial space, where it is discharged (Fig. 8–11). If the head of the humerus is hit with the needle, the needle is angled upward slightly to parallel the undersurface of the acromion. Injections into the deltoid insertion are ineffective and sometimes made in error because this is the point of pain as a result of the fiber conversions. The disease is not located here, but lies under the acromion. Similarly, injections from the front into capsule substance are ineffective because the solution fails to reach the zone of maximum irritation with certainty.

Local block of the suprascapular nerve has been recommended, but the author's experience has been that a more direct approach to the main problem by subacromial injection is much more effective.

Systemic Medication

Drug therapy, accompanying subacromial injections and physiotherapy, is extremely useful when the suitable drugs can be tolerated by the patient. Some form of steroid or phenylbutazone, or a combination of these, is the most effective. Phenylbutazone, preferably buffered, is given in sufficient quantity to produce an effective blood level. Such a routine usually includes 2 tablets three times a day for two days, then 1 tablet three times a day for three days, followed by 1 tablet twice daily for an additional period of approximately two weeks. The maintenance dose of 1 tablet twice daily may be continued for three to six weeks, depending upon the response. Beyond this point, the blood state must be checked and the drug discontinued if there is any suggestion of leukopenia or anemia. Many other side effects and allergic reactions must also be guarded against. The drug should be avoided in patients with hypertension, anemia, cardiovascular problems, gastric ulcer or kidney disease. It is usually quite feasible to use the drug carefully.

Steroid preparations are similarly effective, particularly when there is extensive freezing or adhesive capsulitis. If cortisone is used, a useful dosage schedule is 25 mg three times a day for three to five days, then 25 mg once a day for nine or ten days. Proper precautions in the administration of this drug are also essential. Swelling of the feet and ankles is an indication for discontinuation of phenylbutazone or the steroid.

Sedation and Physiotherapy

Some light sedation is used for a short while at night in support of injection therapy. A preparation containing acetylsalicylic acid, codeine and phenacetin is best; however, this is usually not necessary when cortisone or phenylbutazone is being used. Injection or cortisone therapy should be accompanied by a program of active exercises. The amount of physiotherapy needed depends on the extent of movement restriction. When this is so great that the patient can go no further in abduction than a right angle, or less, and there is limitation of rotation, supervision of the program by a physiotherapist is recommended. When this help is not available, the physician can outline a program of home exercises, such as is set forth here. Prolonged physiotherapy is not necessary, and the application of heat alone is useless. It is an increase in range of motion and strengthening of the muscles that is most beneficial. Exercises must not be so rough that pain is increased or the patient will not cooperate and will lose ground and freezing may occur. If too much pain is initiated, exercises should be decreased and kept within the pain toleration range and then gradually increased as toleration grows. Injection, systemic therapy and sedation are all means of decreasing the pain on movement so that a gentle active process of manipulation can be carried on. Forceful manipulation is not recommended.

If the disturbance has progressed to a point bordering on the frozen shoulder syndrome, treatment other than that outlined previously is necessary. Rugged manipulation, however, will tear the capsule rather than the adhesion, thereby aggravating the whole process.

Home Routine of Shoulder Exercises

Shrugging Shoulders. Start with a circular motion upward, downward, forward and backward.

Wall Creeping. Holding the arm out at full length, let the hand creep up the wall as high as possible. Start with the body facing the wall a little to the front rather than directly sideways. As range and strength increase, turn the body so the motion is more one of abduction.

Arm Swinging. Start in the forward position and gently swing the arms in rotation, then graduate to the vertical position, swnging the arm forward and backward and then sideways.

Arm Rotation. Swing forearms across abdomen, starting with the arm steady at the side. As the range increases, reach behind the back and behind the neck.

Recumbent Swinging. When pain is prominent, initiate the circumduction motion with the patient lying supine. In this position, abduction is possible to a greater range and girdle movement is discarded.

More Advanced Exercises. Circle arms at right angles in abduction. Swing the arms above the head and clasp the hands. Swing the arms at shoulder height.

Exercises should be started gradually, with each exercise being performed six times twice a day, and slowly increased to a dozen times.

Operative Treatment

Eighty to 90 per cent of patients with degenerative tendinitis recover with conservative treatment. If in spite of adequate treatment pain and limitation of movement persist, interfering with productive activity, surgical therapy should be considered. The most satisfactory procedure is exploration of the joint and debridement of the degenerated tendon area. The underlying disease is a degenerative process in the tendon which results in mechanical obstruction of shoulder movement. Little can be done about the degenerative process, but the mechanics of the glenohumeral joint can be improved. This is accomplished by altering the overhanging coracoacromial arch so that less obstruction faces the greater tuberosity as it swings in abduction. The operation should not be applied carelessly for all shoulder disabilities but used only when the diagnosis is clear and conservative treatment has failed. Indications will be clear for the small percentage of patients who require this procedure. Chronicity and economy are controlling factors; it seems unreasonable to expose patients to months of pain and limitation of movement, favoring the onset of a frozen shoulder, when there is an operative procedure of benefit.

Recently the author has discarded total excision of the acromion in favor of acromioclavicular arthroplasty. Several reasons have dictated this course. Acromionectomy, although effective in improving coracoacromial relations by decreasing overhanging obstruction, is usually too extensive a procedure. All the acromion seldom needs to be removed, since it is usually the medial portion that causes obstruction rather than the whole or the lateral segment. An anteromedial quarter inch can be removed to increase arch height and to serve as an arthroplasty of the acromioclavicular joint. More often, excision of the outer half inch of the clavicle is done to produce the acromioclavicular arthroplasty. This increases the space beneath the arch quite adequately.

Repair of the deltoid after total acromionectomy is sometimes difficult and may be unsatisfactory. Acromioclavicular joint irritation is an extremely common concomitant lesion in these conditions, and obtaining the additional swinging space for the head of the humerus in this fashion also removes possible irritation at the acromioclavicular joint. When rotation of the humerus is lost due to capsular irritation, the patient cannot swing the humerus under the arch nearly so well and he tends to supplement this defect by replacing glenohumeral motion with acromioclavicular action at a much earlier stage of the abduction swing. Such substitution wears the acromioclavicular joint, and irritation develops in this area as a secondary painful symptom. Arthroplasty of the acromioclavicular joint has been a very successful development in the technique of operative treatment for degenerative tendinitis and adhesive capsulitis and in repair of massive cuff defects.

Incision. The utility shoulder incision is made, which is a cut 3 inches in length extending distally from the anterior aspect of the acromioclavicular joint along the direction of the deltoid fibers (Fig. 8–11A). Once the problem within the joint has been identified and the operative management decided, the incision may be extended posteriorly over the clavicle to complete the arthroplasty, or distally to deal with disease located more inferoanteriorly (Fig. 8–12).

Exposure. Fibers of the deltoid are separated and the joint inspected (Fig. 8–13). Acromioclavicular arthroplasty is nearly always required, unless very minimal cuff irritation and bursal reaction are encoun-

tered. The incision is extended posteriorly over the joint for 1 to 1½ inches. The acromioclavicular superior capsule is incised and reflected medially beneath the outer half inch of the clavicle, and this is cut with the reciprocating saw. The piece of clavicle is pulled out, usually leaving a strong posterior capsule intact as a stabilizing guard (Fig. 8–14). The coracoacromial ligament is cut and the bursa and cuff debrided (Figs. 8–15 and 8–16).

When the major irritation embracing cuff margin and cortex of humerus lies more laterally, acromioclavicular arthroplasty is accomplished by removing the anteromedial ¼ to ⅜ inch of the acromion. This has a similar result as far as the joint is concerned and does not jeopardize deltoid attachment nearly so much as total excision of the acromion. This maneuver is frequently used in repairing cuff tears which lie well lateral on the head of the humerus.

The clavicle or acromion should be cut cleanly with the saw and not rongeured away or split with a bone cutting forceps. Coagulant material such as Surgicel or Gelfoam is packed around the cut surface to prevent future spur formation (Figs. 8–17 and 8–18).

Closure is effected with a synthetic suture such as Mersilene; catgut and silk are to be avoided because of frequent granuloma formation. The deltoid fibers are repaired with a light continuous suture, a few subcutaneous stitches are inserted and the skin is sewn, preferably with an intracuticular running synthetic suture.

Postoperative Routine. The arm is suspended for 24 hours at the side and then placed in springs and slings. If there is any tendency to freezing, suspension is continued at night and the limb is placed in the swinging apparatus in the daytime (Fig. 8–19). The patient is allowed up in 48 hours with the arm in a sling. If the patient is reluctant to move the shoulder, a cantilever brace is applied when he is up (Fig. 8–20).

Active motion at a right angle is started in the swinging suspension at once and continued in the brace or in the sling. Systemic medication is started at 48 hours (phenylbutazone) and continued for four to six weeks.

The patient is discharged when the postoperative reaction has subsided and the limb is comfortable. This often is five to seven days, but may take longer if the patient is reluctant to use the limb. Sutures are re-

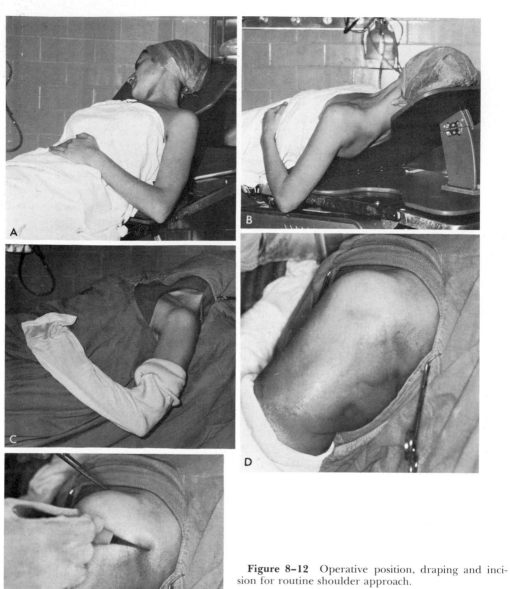

Figure 8–12 Operative position, draping and incision for routine shoulder approach.

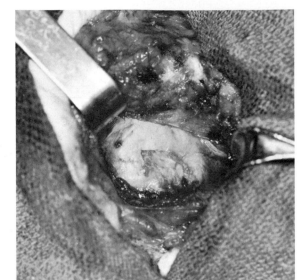

Figure 8–13 Separation of deltoid fibers for exploratory view.

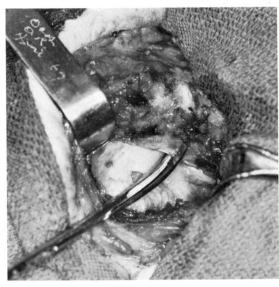

Figure 8–14 Extension of the deep parts of the incision proximally by sectioning the coracoacromial ligament.

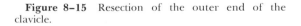

Figure 8–15 Resection of the outer end of the clavicle.

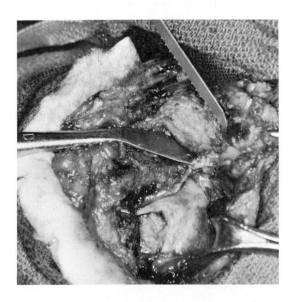

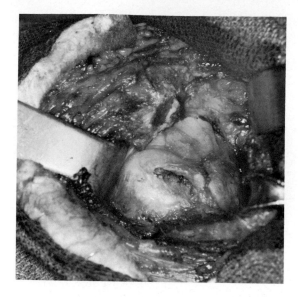

Figure 8–16 Debridement of roughened area of humeral head.

Figure 8–17 Mobilization of bursa to cover uneven zone.

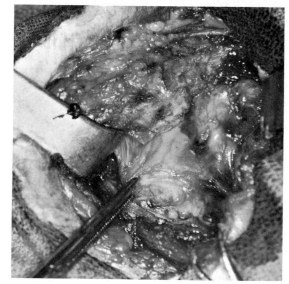

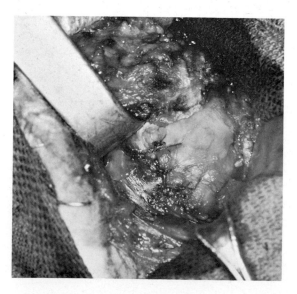

Figure 8–18 Bursa sutured into place.

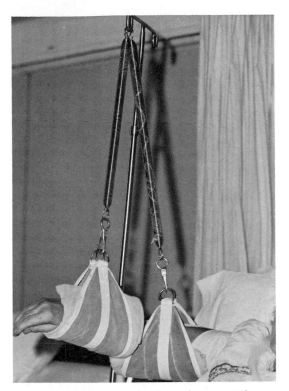

Figure 8–19   Postoperative spring suspension.

moved at three weeks, and supervised for a further six weeks and are varied according to the patient's progress and limb control. The goal should be free motion, well above a right angle, with marked decrease in pain.

TENDINITIS WITH CALCIFICATION

The most painful affliction of the shoulder is acute tendinitis with calcification. It is a common condition usually encountered in younger, more active patients than those with degenerative tendinitis. The deposits occur in the rotator cuff, right in tendon substance. They are most often related to the supraspinatus area but may occur in relation to infraspinatus, subscapularis and teres minor also. Deposits may be present for years without causing trouble, but an acute disturbance may develop suddenly.

SIGNS AND SYMPTOMS OF TENDINITIS WITH CALCIFICATION

Patients seeking attention for this disorder come when the pain is acute and present a typical picture. They often wear an anxious

expression and come into the office holding the afflicted extremity like a Ming vase with the uninvolved arm. They have had sleepless nights and seek prompt relief. Pain is the dominating complaint, and they localize it quickly and accurately to the shoulder. Any movement of the arm is distressing, and they cannot use it to dress or undress. A sudden jar precipitates paroxysms of discomfort. There is limitation of movement in all directions because of pain and muscle spasms. If the patient can tolerate the movement, it is possible to demonstrate that the typical impingement arc from 70 to 100 degrees of abduction evokes maximum discomfort. The course of the disorder may be fulminatingly acute over a period of 48 hours, or more commonly a little less acute over a period of five to seven days. The pain starts as a slight catch or stab on lifting actions and is followed shortly by a persistent ache on all movements. In acute cases this quickly reaches a climax where any movement is most distressing. The shoulder is swollen and warm (Fig. 8–21). The patient pinpoints an exquisitely tender area on the upper aspect. When the process is subacute, some pain is referred to the insertion zone of the deltoid. No gross changes are apparent in this zone, but the muscle feels a little tense. Patients may complain of a lump at this point, but examination invariably shows only a

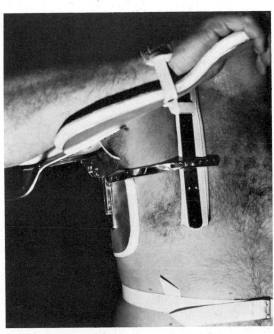

Figure 8–20   The cantilever brace.

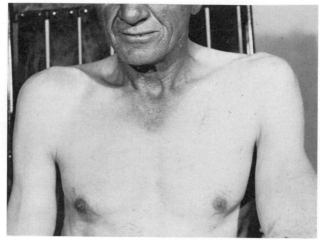

Figure 8–21 Acute tendinitis with calcification. Note swollen right shoulder.

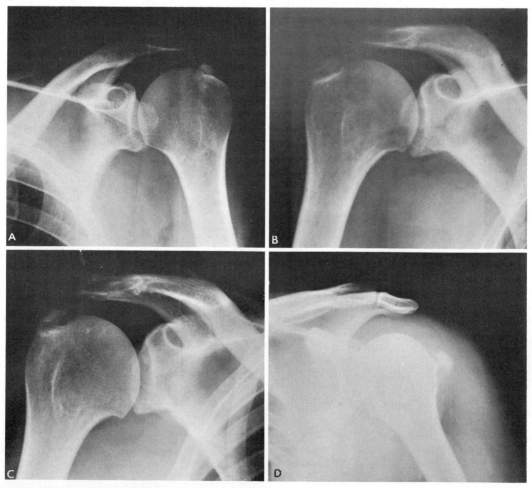

Figure 8–22 Appearance of calcium deposits. *A* and *B*, Typical small deposits. *C*, Deposit and acromioclavicular arthritis. *D*, Deposit in infraspinatus insertion.

little tenderness and possibly a little prominence of the deltoid fibers as a result of the increased tension and spasm.

These patients are very uncomfortable and demand some relief quickly. Their period of disability varies with the efficacy of the therapy and the extent of the local disease process. Symptoms can occasionally be made to subside with no treatment at all other than keeping the shoulder immobilized at the side. Such examples are rare, however, and this management is apt to be followed by limitation of movement or complete freezing of the shoulder. Peculiarly enough, recurrence is uncommon if the deposit disappears. Once the acute symp-

toms have started, the episode usually follows through its full distressing course.

Clinical progress is not significantly altered by the appearance or position of the calcified deposit. The common location is on the supero-anterior aspect. The size of the deposit bears little relationship to the severity of the symptoms. As seen in x-rays the deposits may vary from a stringy, crescentic formation to a sharply defined, billowy cloud (Fig. 8–22). The consistency of the deposit is related to the therapeutic result, since cloudy, diffuse deposits are easily aspirated, or tend to absorb quickly, whereas small, granular concretions are resistant. Night pain is an accompaniment of all shoulder

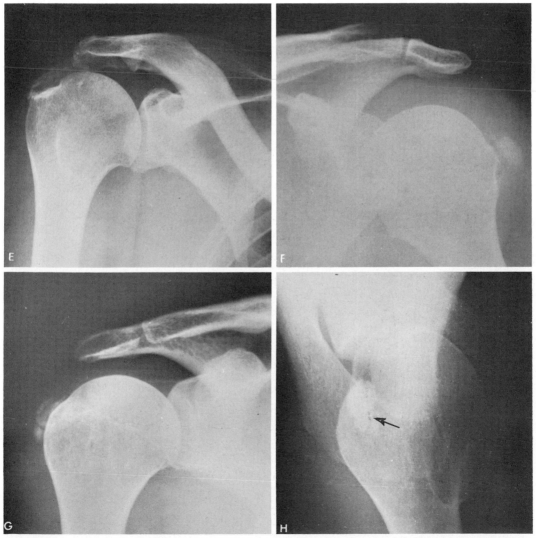

Figure 8–22 *(Continued.)* Variations in calcium deposits. *E*, Linear "inspissated" type, difficult to locate at operation. *F*, Large deposit situated posteriorly. *G*, Multiple deposits anteriorly. *H*, Deposit in a more superior than usual locatiion.

disorders and is very prominent in calcified tendinitis. It begins as a vague aching discomfort that makes it difficult for the patient to lie on the involved side. No position is comfortable and sedation is needed for relief. The patient may be awakened by the acute pain, due to pressure or irritation of the inflamed area in the tendon. During sleep there is a release of muscle spasms, allowing rotation; sudden movement or elevation brings the tender area into contact with the overhanging obstructing coracoacromial arch, producing a sharp twinge of pain.

ETIOLOGY AND PATHOLOGY

Periarticular calcification is found more often in the shoulder than in any other joint in the body. It occurs in a relatively young age group, 25 to 50, so that it differs from degenerative tendinitis. The concretions are granules of calcium phosphate that develop right in tendon substance. They are not part of a generalized calcification process such as may develop in hyperparathyroidism; no profound metabolic upset occurs, and the reaction is independent of increased calcium in the blood. The precipitating factor appears to be local change in the tendon substance. Usually only one shoulder is involved acutely at a time, but both shoulders may be affected. The deposits vary in consistency from a watery paste to powdery granules; no bony elements are encountered. Strangely enough, deposits often rupture into the bursa but rarely go the opposite way into the

joint. The supraspinatus insertion is the zone most often disturbed, but deposits are found also in infraspinatus, subscapularis and teres minor muscles.

The appearance at operation is characteristic. When deltoid fibers are retracted, a distended subacromial bursa is encountered and the surroundings are grossly injected, almost to the extent seen in an inflammatory process. Tissues are moist and edematous, contributing to the swelling of the shoulder. A small incision is used in exploring these lesions; the humerus is rotated, bringing into view the deposit on the floor of the bursa as a rounded, boil-like elevation. The peak has a yellowish white center, like a pimple about to break open. The surrounding tissues are reddened, edematous and injected. Cutting into the deposit will permit 1 or 2 cc of whitish paste to escape as if under pressure (Fig. 8–23). Beneath and around this fluid center there is a zone of dry, granular powder, which gradually fades into tendon substance. The deposits lie close to the tendon edge and may burrow into the cortex of the bone, but rarely enter the joint. The granules are firmly embedded and need to be dug out with a curette after the more liquid part has been evacuated.

Microscopically a small portion of the tendon has disappeared completely and is replaced by amorphous granules. These have been described by Codman as having a concentric, striated formation, somewhat comparable to pigment gallstones. The deposit is sharply demarcated from tendon. At one

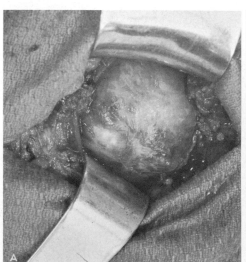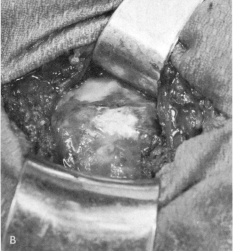

Figure 8–23 Appearance of deposits at operation. *A,* Small inspissated deposit. *B,* Large, almost liquefied deposit.

point there is apparently normal tendon and, at the next, it is gone completely. There is no zone of gradual change. In many patients there is little inflammatory reaction except in the region of the bursa. There is a possibility that acute changes such as vascular dilatation, granulation tissue formation and cellular infiltration come from the bursal layer and develop only when the bursa has been involved.

Why these deposits occur and what provokes their eruption has long been a puzzle. They start in tendon substance toward, but not quite at the edge of, the common capsule cuff. At this point, over an area of 1/2 to 3/4 inch, the cuff has a homogenous collagenous structure, with blending and interlacing of fibers from all the muscles. It is relatively avascular and composed of tightly packed collagen fibers. To this zone are transmitted forces from many directions. In addition to rotatory and torsional stress, there is the constant function of stabilization by the capsule in holding the head of the humerus and the glenoid in contact. The cuff capsule remains efficient and strong for all acts under most circumstances. However, it is easy to visualize the development of areas of relative weakness from constant torsion strain or unbalanced forces focused continually on one zone. Presumably, abnormal aging of collagen fibers initiates the calcification mechanism.

The aging process in collagen has been studied as it occurs in the skin of patients with scleroderma. The fibers become hypertrophied first, showing evidence of swelling and edema. Later they become atrophied, spaces appear between them, and the nuclei are decreased. Atrophy progresses as a result of deficient blood supply. The collagen alters in degenerated fibers, with the process starting in a few fibers and gradually involving a wider area. In devitalized tissue faulty oxygenation occurs, reducing carbon dioxide formation and shifting the pH to the alkaline side. Precipitation of calcium in the more devitalized fibers is then favored. Chemical examination of the deposits shows that calcium carbonate and phosphate are the main constituents. The calcium formation occurs over periods of weeks or months; only after it is well established do signs and symptoms develop. Routine x-ray examinations have revealed a great many deposits that have not produced any symptoms; they may disappear without ever coming into clinical focus.

Change in the deposit varies considerably: it may remain the same size or regress without symptoms; it may continue to enlarge and rupture into the subacromial bursa, producing the acute picture; it may be asymptomatic for a long time and suddenly produce acute pain. When this occurs, something new has happened to the deposit. From the pathological standpoint, delineation of the activating mechanism is largely conjectural. It has been suggested that swelling or increase in size of the deposit occurs as the result of a liquefaction process or a vascular hyperemia that enlarges the zone and so irritates the overlying bursa. Possibly continued movement after a little swelling has occurred repeatedly squeezes or pinches the granular mass, favoring liquefaction. Such a process sets off the whole chain of clinical events, resulting in acute pain, mechanical obstruction and reactive muscle spasm. The liquefaction process with edema and increased blood flow favors softening and erosion of the floor of the bursa, and the deposit ruptures into the subacromial bursa. This process is accompanied by exquisite pain, but sometimes when it has occurred, calcium is absorbed and symptoms subside.

If the bursa is examined during the acute stage, the lining is red and injected. Microscopically there is vasodilatation, cellular infiltration and accumulation of granules in the synovial lining cells. Possibly the calcium acts as a chemical irritant of the bursa, calling forth a greatly increased vascular response, which speeds absorption. The deposit breaks its way into the bursal floor as a small pinkish white nodule. There are a yellowish white apex and a button-like surrounding zone of dilated vessels. The synovium is irritated and injected. When the deposit is curetted, a small pit is left in the tendon, which becomes filled in later with fibrous tissue. The site rarely gives rise to future trouble. Once the calcium has been absorbed, recurrences are unlikely. Rupture of the cuff in this zone is rarely encountered.

TREATMENT OF CALCIFIED TENDINITIS

Acute Cases

Injection Therapy. The quickest and most satisfactory procedure is infiltration of the subacromial area and aspiration of the deposit. Not all patients respond to this method, but an attempt should be made. When the deposit is a fluffy, cloud-like mass,

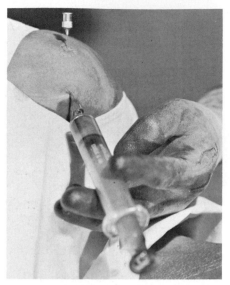

Figure 8–24 Two-needle irrigation technique for removing semifluid calcified deposit.

satisfactory results usually follow aspiration. If it is a small granular inspissated deposit, aspiration is not so successful. The technique of local infiltration has been outlined previously. Two needles are used following local infiltration (Fig. 8–24). Number 22 gauge intramuscular needles are adequate. One needle is inserted from the side and the other from the front toward the calcified deposit. Frequently the deposit can be withdrawn from the bursa through one needle as Novocain or saline is inserted through the other. When the deposit is localized and granular, it should be broken up as much as possible with the point of the needle to set it free into the bursa so that it may be aspirated. As in degenerative tendinitis, injection of hydrocortone may be beneficial.

Medication. Most of these patients require sedation for the relief of pain and this should be provided. A course of phenylbutazone or cortisone should be given if there are no contraindications.

Immobilization. During the very acute stage, the arm should be supported in a sling or on a light abduction splint, if this can be tolerated. However, even during this period, gentle active movement should be encouraged.

Exercise Program. Once the acute stage has subsided, exercises must be carried out faithfully. As a rule, these patients develop a good range of movement quickly and freezing does not become a problem unless the patient has an unusually low pain threshold.

SUPINE EXERCISES. In the early stages keep the arm at rest or supported in a sling when not exercising.

1. Flex elbow and touch shoulder.
2. Hands over chest, lift elbows off bed.
3. With arms across chest gradually lift elbows from the side.

STANDING EXERCISES. These can be started three to four days after supine program, when pain is less acute. Perform once an hour at first, and then every two hours.

1. Lift arm forward.
2. Touch opposite shoulder.
3. Reach to back of neck.
4. Reach to back of waist.
5. Start at shoulder level and crawl upward.
6. In stooping position start pendulum circles.

LATER EXERCISES. After pain has decreased considerably, stronger muscle contraction is started.

1. With hands behind head, extend elbows and increase range.

X-ray Treatment. Conflicting reports on the effectiveness of radiation therapy are present in the literature. All reports stress the need of early application if satisfactory results are to be obtained. It is also apparent that only well qualified radiotherapists should be entrusted with this procedure. The rationale is not clear, but it is assumed that x-radiation increases local vasodilatation, and the active hyperemia speeds solution and absorption of the calcium deposit. This may be the initial response in the early case, but repeated radiation favors fibrosis, which is most harmful. It must be emphasized that x-radiation is detrimental if the lesion has progressed to the point at which there is any suggestion of freezing of the shoulder. A short course of only two to three treatments, or possibly a single treatment, should be used but abandoned if there is no immediate improvement. Roentgen therapy should be accompanied by proper physiotherapy to achieve satisfactory results. Gradual decrease in pain may ensue, but movement must be retained and the muscles strengthened. Chronic cases do not respond well to x-ray treatment, and complete freezing of the shoulder may result from persistent use of this method.

Operative Treatment of Calcified Tendinitis. The majority of these patients do well on the conservative regime which has been outlined, but there are some who do not respond or in whom the pain is of such fulminating severity that it cannot be tolerated. When extremely acute symptoms develop and are not quickly relieved by conservative measures, patients should not be subjected to a prolonged course of pain and discomfort. The intense pain keeps the shoulder at the side, favoring capsular contraction, adhesion formation and gluing of the inferior capsular folds. Surgical excision of the deposit is the method of choice in those who do not respond quickly and should not be delayed until a frozen shoulder has developed. The operation is not extensive and results in immediate and dramatic relief. The period of disability is shortened considerably. Occasionally, young women will ask that conservative treatment be continued in spite of fulminating pain so that they may avoid even a minute scar on a glamorous shoulder, but this should not be the determining consideration.

TECHNIQUE OF EXCISION OF CALCIFIED DEPOSITS. General anesthesia is preferable, but the operation can be done under a local. When the latter is used, the surgeon must be certain of the site of the deposit and thoroughly familiar with the anatomy of bursa and cuff. This is a vascular region and one may be confused easily by bleeding, which adds to the difficulties if the operation is being done under a local anesthetic; light general anesthesia is preferable. A small longitudinal incision 1½ to 2 inches long is made in the direction of the deltoid fibers, starting just anterior to the acromioclavicular joint and extending distally (Fig. 8–25). Skin towels are applied. Hemostasis is obtained, preferably by using the electric coagulator. The deltoid fibers are separated and the incision is deepened until the bursa is reached. Small ribbon retractors are inserted. A moist filamentous sac is encountered. Bursal and subbursal structures are reddened and injected. The assistant rotates the head of the humerus and the deposit comes into view as a small pimple-like elevation (Fig. 8–26). It has a yellowish white center and is surrounded by a tense, angry-appearing zone. Several deposits may be present, but only one appears acutely irritated. The bursa may contain white milk-like material or be quite clear. When the projecting nubbin is incised, toothpaste-like substance escapes under tension. This is sucked out, leaving an irregular cavity. Around this small hole is a granular or powdery ring of calcium, extending into the tendon substance. A small

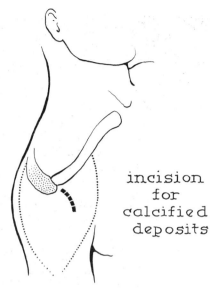

Figure 8–25 Incision for exposure of calcified deposits. A short superoanterior cut is used which may be elongated to the usual utility-incision length.

curette is necessary to remove this part. The deposit does not involve the whole thickness of tendon substance and it is rarely necessary to penetrate into the joint in removing the deposit. Only the deposit should be excised, and the tendon should not be disturbed sufficiently to produce a significant defect. Sometimes a single suture is needed to pull the fibers together after removal of the deposit.

The deposit is usually apparent at once on incision of the bursa. When search is necessary, the best guide for orientation is the bicipital groove. When the elbow is at the side with the palm upward, the groove is felt at the inside border of the incision. This may be verified by palpation as the upper end of the humerus is rotated. The humerus is gently rotated through as complete a range as possible to restore movement. In this process adhesions may be felt to give way. The cuff is inspected carefully for any extra deposits after the initial one has been removed.

LOCATING HARD-TO-FIND DEPOSITS. A deposit may be difficult to locate after opening the bursa, even when its position can be gauged by identifiable landmarks and it is quite visible in the x-ray. Often this is due to a layer of cuff substance over the deposit. Under these circumstances a 20-gauge 1½ inch hypodermic needle is used as a "seeker" (Fig. 8–27). The suspected zone is needled and, when the deposit is located, a gritty

Fig. 8–26

Fig. 8–27

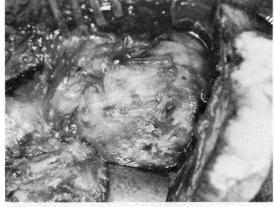

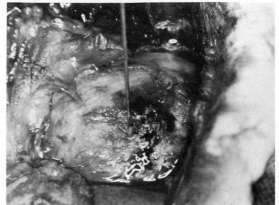

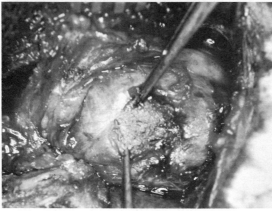

Figure 8–26 Exposure for calcified deposits.
Figure 8–27 Identification of deposit by needling suspected area.
Figure 8–28 Deposit is identified and evacuated.

Fig. 8–28

sensation will be felt as the needle is pressed into the cuff. Some granules will adhere to the point of the needle as it is withdrawn; these can be identified with careful scrutiny. The extent of the deposit, can then be outlined (Fig. 8–28). X-rays should always be done shortly before surgery to be sure the deposit has not been absorbed since the previous examination.

Postoperative x-rays frequently show a small amount of calcium remaining, but this is not significant and rarely causes further symptoms. After operation the arm is kept in traction for 24 to 48 hours; movement is initiated as soon as local pain will allow. Physiotherapy is started and continued until a full range of movement is present. In early cases and those without significant freezing, little help is needed; In longstanding, more chronic problems, considerable supervised physiotherapy is required. Systemic medication may need to be continued for four to six weeks or until a good range of motion has returned.

RUPTURES OF THE ROTATOR CUFF

Deficiencies in cuff substance, full thickness in nature, are much more common than has previously been suspected. They can occur in all adult age groups and may or may not have resulted from a remembered traumatic episode. They are commonest in middle-aged workmen, but athletes, housewives, nurses and professional men may also rip the rotator cuff. The classic picture is of a middle-aged workman with no previous shoulder trouble who stumbles, taking weight on the outstretched arm for protection, or slips, landing on his elbow. Once the patient gets to the upright position, his shoulder is sore and he notices difficulty in lifting the arm. Pain, weakness, and restriction of motion persist. A nurse lifting a patient, a skier tumbling on a slope, a housewife reaching for and lifting the laundry may all suffer a full thickness cuff tear.

A few signs or symptoms may be present

immediately after a fall, but persistence of some discomfort, slight weakness and, particularly, failure to improve extensively over a period of six weeks with competent conservative treatment are strongly suggestive of a cuff tear rather than a simple "supraspinatus sprain."

SIGNS AND SYMPTOMS

History. There may be a good history of injury like a tumble or a slip or backward fall, a fall from a height with the arm striking an outrigging projection, or a projectile tumble on the point of the shoulder. Incidents like this quickly bring the lesion to mind. However, the damaging episode may not be nearly so dramatic. A simple act of reaching at a difficult angle or continually repeated much less strenuous acts can tear the cuff. Predisposing occupational activities can also contribute. All workmen consistently engaged in above shoulder level activities may fray and wear the rotator cuff so that a relatively trivial strain can then rip it. Extensive stress on the shoulder, as, for example, by the hard-throwing shortstop, can also tear the cuff. Elderly individuals are particularly susceptible, and falls which could easily have precipitated the syndrome may not be remembered.

Pain. As the result of a fall or a similar incident the patient often experiences a sharp twinge of pain related to the shoulder region. Subsequently less acute aching discomfort appears which the patient can clearly localize to the joint area. Twinges of pain result from attempting to get the arm above the shoulder, causing the patient to let it drop limply to the side. The pain continues on effort and increases as weakness develops. The shoulder hurts at night, and it becomes difficult for the patient to lie on the involved side. In later stages pain extends to the deltoid insertion and, at a still later period, if motion is restricted, discomfort in the shoulder-neck angle develops as the patient, in an effort to compensate for his weakness, puts extra stress on the suspensory muscles.

If the examiner passively moves the head of the humerus under the acromion, the patient frequently has a sharp twinge of pain. This sequence of weak, painless motion, followed by a painful arc on passive motion, and then decreased pain as the arm is swung above the shoulder level, is referred to as a typical painful arc, or arc of impingement syndrome (Fig. 8–29).

Stiffness. Restriction of motion develops some weeks after the fall and reaches a point at which it is difficult to raise the arm to a right angle, either in abduction or flexion. Inability to get the hand behind the back, to fasten a dress or reach into a hip pocket, is clear evidence of rotatory restriction (Fig. 8–30).

Weakness. The cardinal sign of cuff ruptures is persistent weakness. The patient may

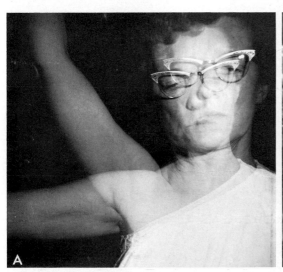
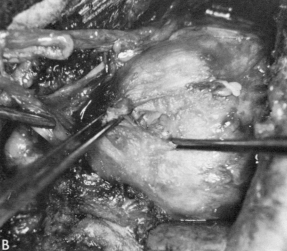

Figure 8–29 *A*, Double exposure showing impingement point causing lag in abduction in a case of cuff tear. *B*, The lesion as it appeared at operation.

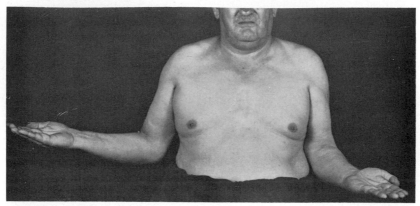

Figure 8–30 Stiffness leading to restriction of rotation.

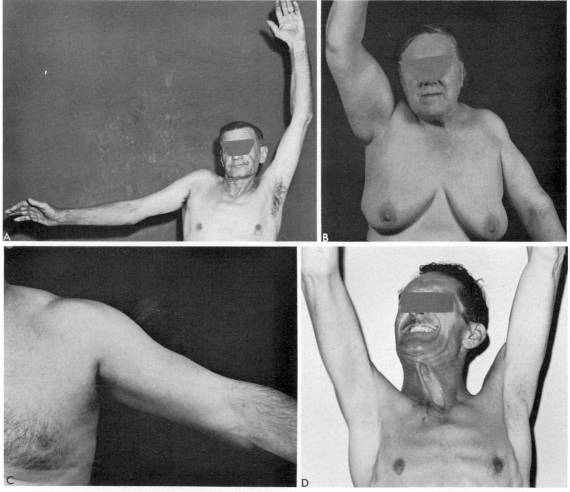

Figure 8–31 Weakness in abduction in full thickness cuff tear. *A*, Typical weakness in extensive tear. *B*, Cuff tears occur in women also. Gross weakness in a massive tear. *C*, Moderate weakness with considerable motion masking a full thickness tear. *D*, Full thickness tear in which extensive motion is possible if unresisted.

be conscious of this in his work, but often the examiner must demonstrate it and sometimes it is easily overlooked. The patient may be able to lift the arm into full abduction or beyond when he has a full thickness cuff tear. However, if this action is resisted a little, sometimes by as little as the pressure of one finger, even a strapping patient may be unable to abduct or flex the shoulder well (Fig. 8–31).

The old fashioned concept of the hunching girdle rhythm as the tell-tale mark of cuff rupture has been discarded. Without resistance, no decrease in range may be apparent, but it behooves the examiner to always assess motion against resistance. The presence of consistent weakness helps to differentiate a tear from a simple chronic tendinitis.

Muscle Atrophy. Some decrease in bulk of supra- or infraspinatus can often be seen, but this is not always apparent. In the later stages, four to six months after the tear has occurred, it can nearly always be identified. The deltoid shows some slight flattening also, but the loss of substance is much more apparent as related to the spinati (Fig. 8–32).

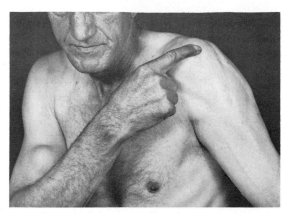

Figure 8–33 Point of tenderness in cuff rupture.

Tenderness. The torn cuff is always sensitive. The area chiefly to be palpated is the upper end of the humerus, holding the elbow in slight extension to uncover more of the cuff substance in front of the overhanging coraco-acromial arch. One needs to press firmly to penetrate pressure through the deltoid to reach cuff substance. In thin people a defect can sometimes be made out with firm pressure. Rotating the head of the humerus and palpating at the same time is also helpful. Some sensitivity of acromio-clavicular joint in longstanding cases is usually present, too, because of the substitution of motion at this joint for the loss of rotation (Figs. 8–33 and 8–34).

In early cases only a few weeks old, soreness in the supra- and infraspinous fossa is found in addition to tenderness over the end of the humerus (Fig. 8–35). When the tear involves the anterior quadrant, the bicipital sulcus may be implicated, in which case the maximum soreness is in this area. A less common rupture implicates the subscapularis, and tenderness can quite precisely be localized to the antero-inferior aspect. Localization of soreness more distally and inferiorly at the front is characteristic of this lesion.

"Crepitus and Clicking." A subjective clicking sensation is often experienced by the patient, principally on abduction or rotation. On examination it is possible to detect a coarse crepitus over the supero-anterior aspect that is accentuated by passive swinging of the head of the humerus. Crepitus is not always diagnostic of a cuff tear, because chronic bursitis and tendinitis can also evoke this sign; however, the crepitus is of a softer nature, not so painful and less likely to be a persistent point at which the maximum

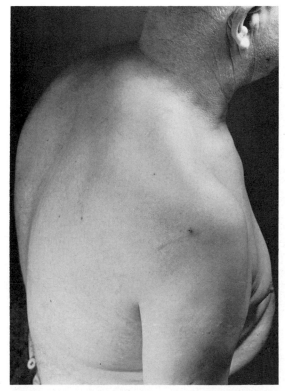

Figure 8–32 Atrophy of supraspinatus can often be identified when the tear is some months old.

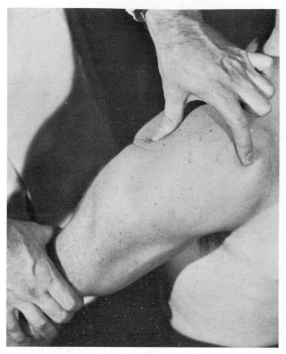

Figure 8–34 Examination of zone of most frequent cuff tears is facilitated by shoving the head of the humerus forward with the thumb and palpating with the index finger, with the subject's arm extended.

clicking is appreciated. In cuff tears, if the split is impinging, it is more apt to evoke a louder and coarser crepitus.

SPECIAL INVESTIGATION

Local Anesthetic Insertion. When the subacromial tissues are anesthetized, the patient may overcome overhanging arch "obstruction" as a result of obliteration of the pain. Ability to abduct, flex or even circumduct after local instillation, however, is not a sign of an intact cuff; it is the persistence of weakness that is significant, and this can usually be shown in spite of the local injection. Since it has been apparent so often that the patient retains the power of abduction and even circumduction in the presence of the tear, the local anesthetic test no longer can be regarded as a reliable guide to diagnosis.

Electrical Examination of the Muscles. In some instances the use of electrical stimulation of the muscle is helpful. When there is an intact but degenerated cuff, stimulation of supra- and infraspinatus produces a good response of abduction. However, if there is a full thickness tear, the stimulation of the muscle substance produces a poor response because of the defect, and the patient experiences considerably greater pain.

Arthrography. Contrast studies have become by far the most reliable means of identifying full thickness cuff defects. No other method of assessment, either clinical or radiological, begins to have the accuracy of this examination. The author has had the opportunity of assessing many cuff tears but still finds that the arthrogram is more consistently accurate than clinical appraisal.

Contrast studies should be carried out at the first suspicion that a cuff tear may be present. In some instances this will be after conservative treatment for what appears as a supraspinatus sprain has failed to cure the patient over a period of six weeks. In other

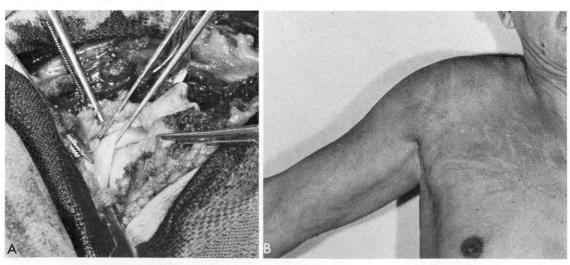

Figure 8–35 Anterior quadrant tear; pain and weakness on abduction.

instances the signs and symptoms shortly after an injury may be sufficiently suggestive to prompt immediate use of the arthrogram.

The author has found repeatedly that it is most difficult to distinguish between a sprain and a tear. Clinically they may be almost identical, but the failure of consistent improvement following treatment for a sprain points to the need for contrast studies, which will settle the issue (Fig. 8–36).

ETIOLOGY AND PATHOLOGY

Preliminary wear and tear were formerly regarded as essential to the development of this lesion. Observations now show that this

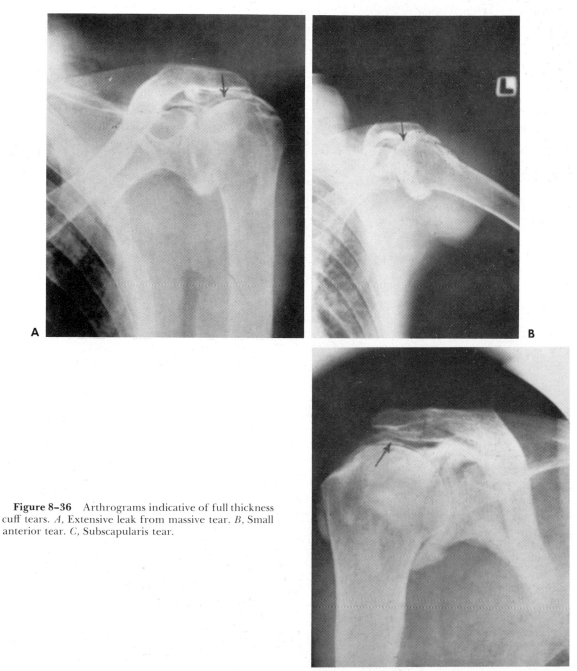

Figure 8–36 Arthrograms indicative of full thickness cuff tears. *A*, Extensive leak from massive tear. *B*, Small anterior tear. *C*, Subscapularis tear.

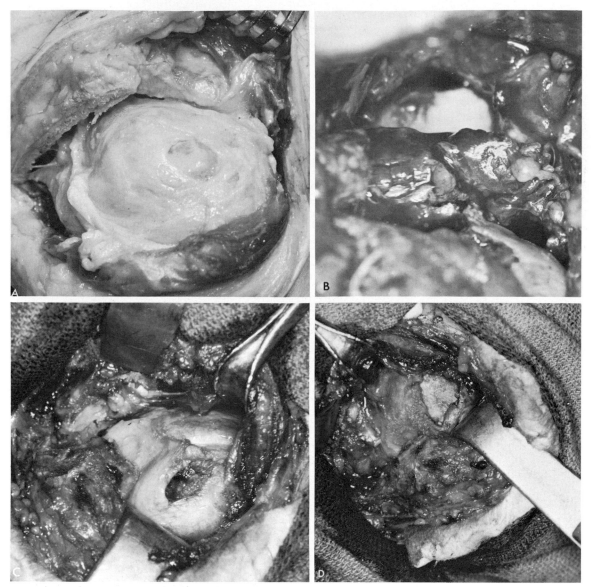

Figure 8–37 Pathology of cuff tears. *A,* "Erosion" type tear. *B,* Small tear. Note sharp edges in contrast to *A. C,* Recent complete rupture. Note sharp edges of defect. *D,* Marginal evulsion from bone.

is not so. Some antecedent fraying of the cuff may be anticipated in the 40 to 50 age group, but ruptures also occur in younger patients in whom there has not been time for such changes to develop. Some cuff tears are really better considered as erosions resulting from a gradual thinning of cuff, which then gives way following some further insult, or gradually just wears through. Others, however, are sharp splits of cuff substance that appear as linear cracks, like a split in a piece of fiberglass. In some other instances the

insertion of the tendons has been wrenched from its attachment to bone (Fig. 8–37).

The primary wearing force is the constant rotatory shift of the head of the humerus in the capsule (Fig. 8–38). The coupling of a myriad of forces can be postulated, so that the position and extent of the rupture are subject to many influences. The universal mobility of the joint, in addition to the constant wearing process, allows a widespread acceptance of a passive stress, also contributed to by the long lever of the humerus, which

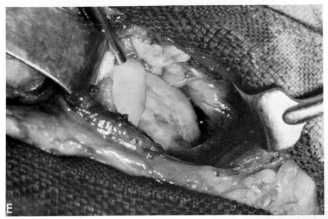
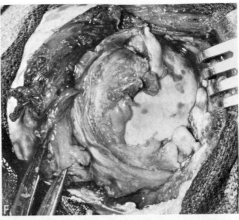
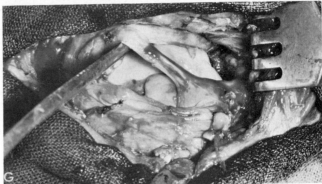

Figure 8–37 *Continued. E,* Massive tear (recent) with retraction. *F,* Massive tear with retraction. *G,* Erosional tear at later stage.

acts as an avulsing force on capsular attachments, as well as stretching cuff substance in between its points of anchorage.

For some time it was postulated that the blood supply played a part in the origin of cuff tears, but this aspect could only be applied to the erosion type of lesion and plays no part in other configurations. At the time of surgical repair of a torn cuff, one is impressed by the amount of vascularity rather than the degree of ischemia.

Recent investigation with contrast and video studies has thrown new light on the hydraulics of joint lubrication. In the case of the shoulder it would appear that there are some significant observations relative to the way the joint is lubricated. The motion studies show quite clearly that, as the arm is abducted and rotated, the major amount of contrast media collects in the inferior aspect of the cuff, as would the synovial fluid (Fig. 8–39). In contrast, in this active abduction and external rotation there is a minimal amount of lubricating material remaining in the superior portion of the joint, so that during this phase of motion it would appear that less lubricating material is available to protect the structures at the top of the joint. This distribution of lubricant may favor the wearing process and would be a further explanation for the localization of wear and tear changes in this zone.

In Figure 8–40 it will be seen that, as the arm is brought to the side, much less of the lubricant and contrast media is in the inferior aspect of the joint and more is over the upper

blow on top of shoulder

STATIC FUNCTION OF CUFF

pull of weight being carried plus pull of gravity

force of falling

Figure 8–38 Forces acting on the upper end of the humerus and cuff area that favor rupture.

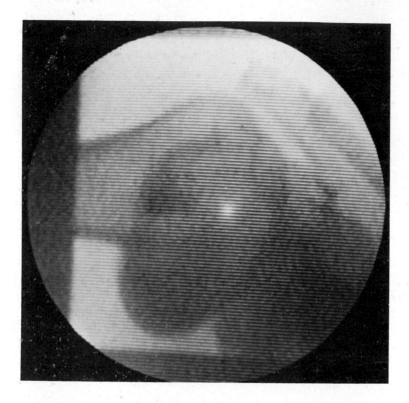

Figure 8–39 Arthrogram showing flow of dye and lubricant to the inferior aspect of the joint as the shoulder is abducted in the act of throwing. Note that a minimal amount of dye remains over the superior and critical contact aspect of the cuff and the head of the humerus with the coracoacromial arch.

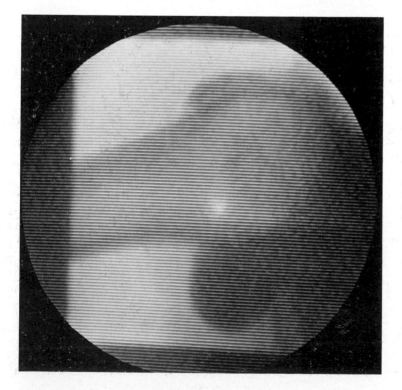

Figure 8–40 Flow of dye is free through the joint on adduction, with much less dye in the anterior aspect and much more dye over the upper end of the humerus.

aspect of the humerus. It would appear that it is in this phase of shoulder motion that the major lubrication of the superior aspect takes place, but during the critical abduction external rotation phase there is minimal protection from the lubricant.

Many different types of tears are recognized, but most of these injuries can be considered under the heads of massive avulsions, rim tears, concealed tears, anterior or bicipital tears, and subscapular tears (Fig. 8–41).

Massive Avulsion

Massive avulsion is seen, as a rule, only in those shoulders in which the cuff has already been worn and devitalized. When such a case is exposed at operation, as soon as the deltoid is retracted the surgeon sees the cartilage on the upper end of the humerus (Fig. 8–42); the layers of bursa and cuff have disintegrated. As the incision is enlarged, the cartilage of the humerus comes more clearly into view and the remnants of the cuff are identified as a few bulbous tags, like a fringe around a bald head. The defect is the size of a 25 to 50 cent piece (Fig. 8–42, D and E). There may be very little tendon substance left. The head is riding higher than normal, and the assistant needs to apply traction at the elbow so that the cuff fringes may be "fished out" from under the acromion. Depending on the age of the lesion, there are changes in articular cartilage consisting of a roughening and minute blister formation, extending inward from the periphery. The junction belt of the cartilage and tuberosity is roughened, and cartilage disappears over an oval or triangular area, extending inward. Cortex or rough cancellous bone appears in the bottom of the pitted zone. Microscopic examination shows a degenerated tendon with fragmentation of fibers, areas of fibrinoid reaction, separation, and splitting of layers with fibrous infiltration.

Rim or Partial Tears

The commonest configuration of tear is a crack at the rim. This is a partial tear which starts in the insertion zone as a linear rent and later enlarges into a triangular defect in somewhat the way a piece of cellophane tears (Fig. 8–43). In the early stages a crack or linear separation only is seen, but continued activity and repeated trauma from abducting and flexing the shoulder and tensing the rotator cuff make the defect larger. The edges are thin; the margins are not normal healthy tendon and tear easily

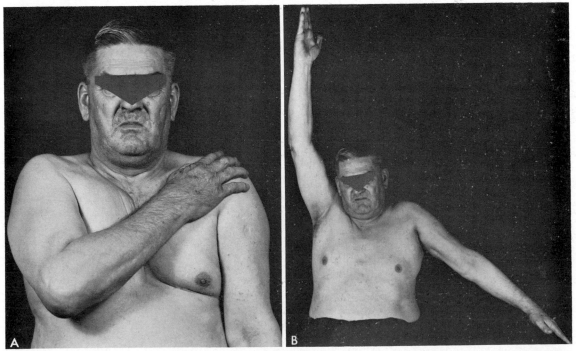

Figure 8–41   Clinical picture of massive cuff evulsion in a middle-aged workman: shoulder joint pain with marked weakness, girdle-type shoulder action.

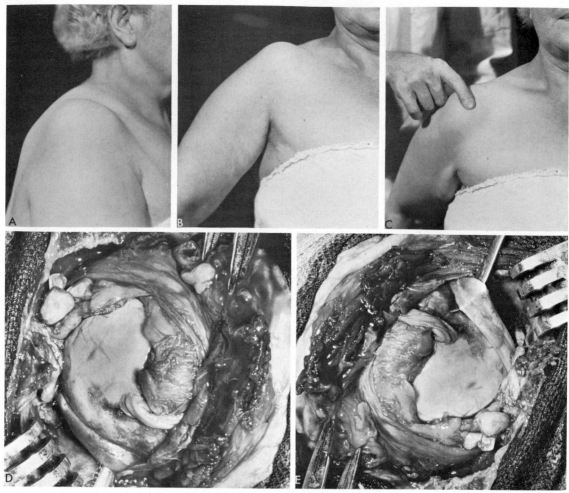

Figure 8–42 A massive tear with displacement of long head of the biceps. *A*, Point of maximum tenderness supero-anteriorly. *B*, Attempted abduction merely jumps the head of the humerus up in the socket when the depressor effect of the cuff or long head of the biceps is lost. *C*, Obvious atrophy. *D*, Appearance at operation. *E*, The biceps tendon is dislocated medially. The bare head of humerus sticks up with a fringe of cuff about it. The cartilage is eroded at the bicipital groove.

when sutures are inserted. When the tear has been present for some months, changes appear in cartilage and the bone beneath. Blistering and roughening of the smooth cartilage occurs over a triangular area, corresponding to the defect. Many massive avulsions begin in this fashion; the partial tear is ripped by further, more severe trauma, and the cuff disintegrates over a large area. Microscopic sections show fibrinoid degeneration in the tissue at the edge of the defect, gradually disappearing over a radius of ¼ to ½ inch from the edge.

Concealed Tears

The musculotendinous cuff is a thick, laminated thong with its layers anchored in sequence as it arches over the head of the

humerus (Fig. 8–44). This laminated construction allows deep fibers to be torn while superficial layers may remain intact. Such avulsion of the deep fibers constitutes the so-called concealed tear. It is a more common lesion than has previously been appreciated, and in the past many shoulders have been explored and closed without the entity being recognized. Normally when capsule is exposed at operation, it is smooth and glistening. Any roughening, thickening or granular erosion is suggestive of degenerative or traumatic change beneath. Deep fibers give way in step-like fashion much as one pulls out drawers from the bottom in a chest of drawers. A small, oval "hump" appears, covered by the intact top layers. When it is incised, the deep part appears cracked and separated into layers (Fig. 8–44).

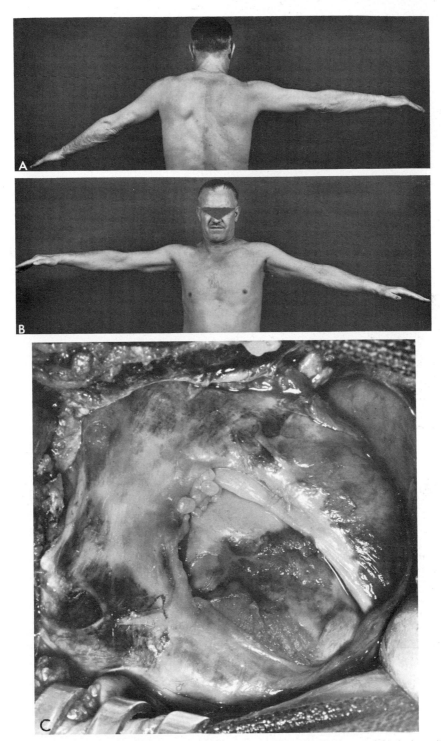

Figure 8–43 A rim rupture of the cuff. *A* and *B*, Obvious weakness on abduction. *C*, The lesion of this patient as it appeared at operation. There is an oval defect in the cuff through which a small triangular area of articular cartilage can be seen fading into a roughened pitted cortical zone.

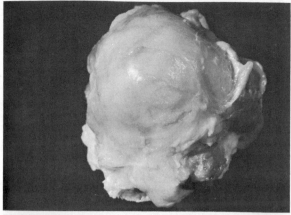

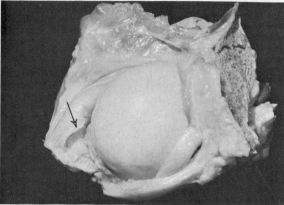

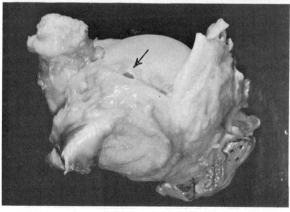

Figure 8–44 Appearance of concealed tears. The cuff apparently is intact, judging by the appearance of the surface. Incision of swollen zone shows splitting of the deep fibers and a concealed tear.

Cartilage under the cracked zone is rough and eroded. The separation and detachment of the deep fibers disturbs the normal, smooth contour, forming a hump or ridge which impinges on the overhanging coracoacromial arch. As arm motion continues, the superficial layers are compressed and eventually damaged also. Microscopically, whole layers of fibers have degenerated, with fibrosis infiltrating between the layers. Some zones show sharply avulsed fibers that are similar to the posttraumatic changes in a fresh tear of the cuff.

Anterior or Bicipital Tears

Tears of the musculotendinous cuff related to the biceps tendon are not common and are quite distinctive. They result in signs and symptoms implicating the bicipital apparatus in addition to indications of rotator cuff rupture. Their position and extent frequently present special problems in reconstruction. These tears lie anteriorly over the long head of the biceps and are usually oblong or rectangular in shape. The anterior zone of the capsule covering the head of the humerus and the biceps is less well protected by the coraco-acromial arch than the lateral and posterior parts (Sec Fig. 8–45). Backward falls particularly put major stress on this part of the capsule. The biceps acts as a deterrent to upward displacement of the humerus and assumes some of the protecting function in such falls.

When sufficient force is applied so that the cuff gives way anteriorly, the defect is enlarged by the strong and quite direct pull of the infraspinatus. This is a more powerful traction than that exerted by the supraspinatus and a defect may result, uncovering a large part of the anterior zone of the head. This region of cuff performs a further special function which places added strain on it.

Just above the bicipital groove, the capsule blends with the intertubercular fibers, forming the transverse humeral ligament and contributing to maintenance of the tendon in the groove. Rotatory strain in particular stretches this zone; abduction and external rotation may rupture the retaining fibers as the tendon is "sprung" from its trough. Less severe strain merely weakens this area, allowing increased play of the long tendon. A vicious cycle results, so that a small defect is stretched by both biceps and the usual cuff tension. Sometimes a double defect results, with the cuff giving way from the tuberosity on both sides of the tendon. Cuff laxity at this point seriously interferes with biceps function, and the tendon may slip medially over the lesser tuberosity off the head (Figs. 8–42 and 8–46).

Microscopically the cuff changes are similar to those described in the other types of

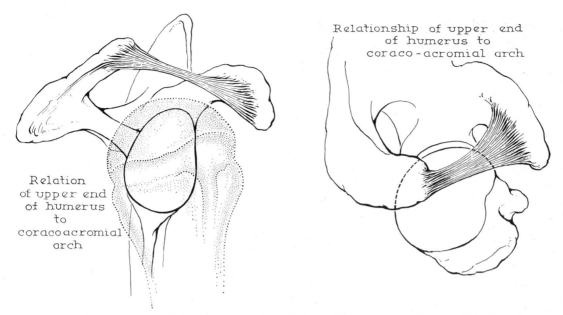

Figure 8–45 Superior aspect of the humerus and its relation to the coracoacromial arch. Note that a large part of the upper end of the humerus is unprotected.

tear but, in addition, the biceps tendon shows degeneration, shredding and fragmentation of the fibers in the zone under the defect.

TREATMENT OF RUPTURES OF THE ROTATOR CUFF

General Considerations

The best treatment for a torn tendon anywhere in the body is, first, restoration of its continuity and then careful re-education of its action complex. These are the principles applied in tears of the rotator cuff also. Most of the confusion and many of the unsatisfactory results in treating these cases result from inaccurate diagnosis. If the cuff is not torn through its substance completely, recovery will follow good conservative treatment. If there is a definite defect completely through the cuff, such as may be demonstrated in the arthrogram, operative repair is the method of choice. Once these general principles are clear, it is possible to consider the various factors and situations which may modify this general plan.

Cuff tears occur most frequently in middle or later life because the wear and tear degeneration of constant use has weakened the tendon. Workmen, particularly those in the vulnerable age group, are susceptible to cuff ruptures. A considerable number of ruptures

are encountered in patients over the age of 60, so that the general condition of the patient, the extent and type of tear, the occupation, the age of the lesion and the operative and postoperative facilities available must be

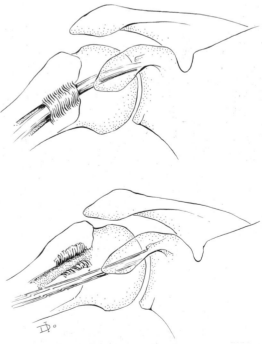

Figure 8–46 Diagram of mechanism of bicipital dislocation and rupture of the intertubercular ligament.

taken into consideration. Common sense application and interpretation of these factors is all that is necessary.

Type of Lesion. Most complete ruptures, that is, involving the whole thickness of the tendon, should be repaired when circumstances permit. Arthrography is of the greatest help in demonstrating the complete defect. If it is massive, the indications are clear; however, controversy may arise over therapy of the small defect. One has only to see a few of these lesions at operation to realize how easily small tears become big ones. The tension exerted by the rotators snubbing the head in the glenoid is a constant "pulling apart" traction no matter where the defect starts. If shoulder level activity is not required, the therapy may take a different course.

Age of the Lesion. The earlier the operation is carried out, the easier it is to do a snug repair of the defect; there is no comparison of the ease with which the gap may be closed at six weeks as opposed to six months. This is true no matter what the configuration of the tear may be or where the defect is located. Delay allows the gap to increase. Of equal importance is the state of the tissues; in long-standing ruptures, tissue of the edge of the defect is of poor quality, it holds sutures poorly, and needles tear through it easily. For a distance of $1/4$ to $1/2$ inch there may be no good anchorage for the repair stitches. Constant tension retracts the edges, and the rotator muscles shorten and become glued down in their retracted position; mobilization to close the defect is immeasurably more difficult the longer the lesion is left unrepaired. This does not mean that no attempt should be made even at six or eight months, because much can still be accomplished, but it is more difficult. The passage of time alone should not be the prime consideration. It is very rare that some improvement cannot be obtained by operation, but superior results are possible in earlier treatment.

Age of the Patient. Since this is usually a disturbance of middle and later life, and is a major operation, reasonable considerations must be given to the age and the general condition of the patient. Chest and prostatic complications occur easily. Some form of immobilization, either traction or abduction splint, is essential postoperatively. This hampers chest movement somewhat, and the prone position favors urinary stasis and prostatic obstruction and also invites phelbo-

thrombosis and embolism. These are all preventable by reasonable postoperative care but are deterrents in poor risk patients such as those with chest or cardiac weaknesses. In assessing the age of the patient, it is the physiological rather than the chronological figure that should be considered. Some at 65 are a physiological 55, others at 58 are closer to 70, so that common sense must be used in gauging age and operability. In all doubtful instances, the opinion of a well qualified internist is of inestimable value in settling the issue.

Occupation of the Patient. Cuff tears are encountered most frequently in workmen such as carpenters, painters, bricklayers, paperhangers, machinists, laundrymen or construction workers. Activity at the shoulder level or in the above shoulder range is often vital to the occupation. Every effort and the best treatment possible should be made available to restore this function. The results of operative repair are superior, residual disability is less and time loss is decreased. The office worker, salesman or clerk, on the other hand, may be able to carry on relatively satisfactorily with residual weakness and considerable limitation of movement.

Persistent pain, however, is an indication for surgical treatment. Even in those instances in which extensive motion is not restored by repair, a significant decrease in the pain may almost always be counted upon. Many patients reach a stage at which the persistent discomfort, particularly at night, is most bothersome. It is characteristic of these lesions that, if any improvement is effected by reconstruction, the pain is almost entirely obliterated.

Facilities Available. Attention should be given also to the facilities available for treating these patients. Proper operative repair is a major procedure requiring first class operating room facilities and at least one assistant; more are necessary if fascia is to be used and an extensive defect to be repaired. Despite the described approach, strong retraction is needed for proper exposure. The facilities for postoperative care are of equal importance. Precise procedure is needed at operation, but the most perfect repair may end dismally if the postoperative program is not conscientiously supervised. This applies to the immediate as well as the late postoperative period. Once the immediate reaction has subsided, these patients are best handled at a center where a fully planned curriculum of physiotherapy and occupational therapy may be carried out.

Conservative Treatment

In those patients in whom the diagnosis of rupture of the cuff has been made but, for some of the various reasons outlined previously, operation is not advised, considerable help can be given by a conservative program. The arm may be held in a cantilever splint for three weeks, if the lesion is encountered early (Fig. 8–47). Supervised physiotherapy is essential. These patients develop reflex dystrophy easily. Contractures in elbow, wrist and fingers can be much more disabling than the shoulder disease and must be prevented. This immobilization of the shoulder should be continued for a period of three weeks, but immediate and free movement of the elbow, wrist and fingers is started. Sometimes this needs to be supplemented by electrical stimulation of the muscles. At the end of three weeks active motion is started

and the arm may be lowered gradually. The shoulder muscles are strengthened as the splint is lowered by degrees and then discarded, usually at the end of six weeks.

Some therapists prefer to avoid any period of immobilization because of the danger of forearm and hand contractures. Under these circumstances, active movement is encouraged from the beginning, with pain relieved at intervals by local anesthetic injection, similar to the course followed in degenerative tendinitis. Success in this regime depends on strengthening the accessory muscles, trapezius, biceps and triceps, to replace the snubbing action of the cuff. Not too much should be expected of this routine, particularly if the long head of the biceps is ruptured or displaced.

Techniques of Cuff Repair

Anesthesia. The use of general anesthesia is preferred by the author (Fig. 8–48). Electrocoagulation is used for hemostasis.

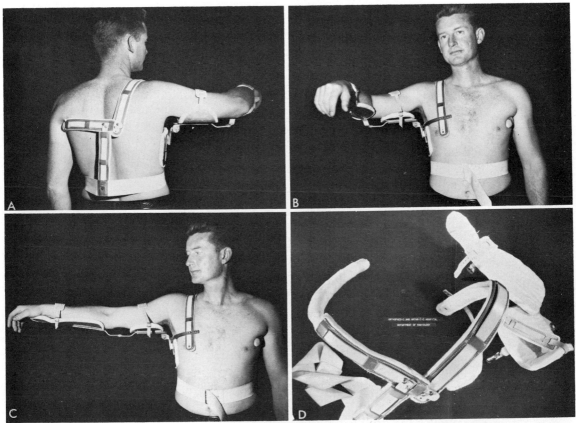

Figure 8–47 Cantilever brace useful in conservative treatment and postoperative program for cuff tears. *A,* From the back. *B,* From the front. *C,* Shoulder rotation and elbow action. *D,* Brace for a right shoulder as it appears when not in use.

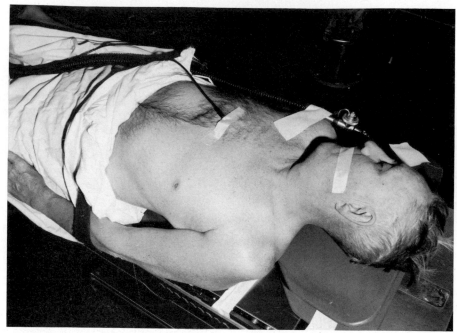

Figure 8–48 The surgeon should have full access to the shoulder-neck region when operating on this area. It is desirable for the anesthetist to intubate and prepare the patient so that the head and shoulders are left quite free. Note the tube going to the machine at the foot of the patient.

Careful preoperative investigation for concomitant disability is essential in these patients since many come to surgery after the age of 40. As the joint may be open for some time at operation and considerable traction and pressure on the tissues may be necessary, the author has felt it best to use prophylactic antibiotics. Such a routine may be governed and altered by many considerations, but precise precautions must be observed in all open joint surgery.

Position for Operation. The sitting shoulder position is a significant help in these operations. The patient should be elevated about 45 degrees and so placed on the table that the arm hangs free at the side after it has been draped (Fig. 8–49). The shoulder should rise above the back of the rest so that there is access to the postclavicular and supraspinous fossae. The arm is prepared and draped with stockinette and allowed to hang free at the side; this is essential to allow the traction and manipulation that assist significantly in exposure and repair.

Incision and Exposure. The most useful

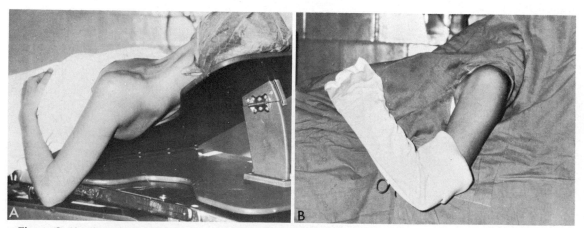

Figure 8–49 Operating position for shoulder surgery. The arm is draped free, so that access to the top, back and front of the shoulder is provided.

approach for cuff repair is an incision that allows exploration and assessment of the disease first and may then be easily enlarged as necessary to permit repair of the type of full thickness defect which is encountered. The complete skin cut is made, but the deeper exposure is not made until it has been decided whether it is needed laterally over the tuberosity, inferiorly over the subscapularis or posteriorly into the supra- and infraspinous fossae (Fig. 8–50).

A supero-anterior utility incision is used, starting from 1 inch behind the acromioclavicular joint, extending distally for 3 inches, centered over the acromioclavicular joint and extending forward in the direction of the deltoid fibers. The upper anterior portion of this is deepened, and the deltoid fibers are separated by blunt dissection and retracted. The coraco-acromial ligament comes into view superiorly and the roof of the subdeltoid bursa appears just beyond this. The bursa is incised and retracted, but this is done in such a way as to preserve it if it is not extensively thickened and constituting a subacromial obstruction. A special curved humeral head retractor is helpful at this point, but ordinary right angle retractors can be used to separate the deltoid fibers enough to rotate the head of the humerus for complete inspection of the joint.

Exposure is completed on the basis of whether a massive tear, a lateral tear, a rim

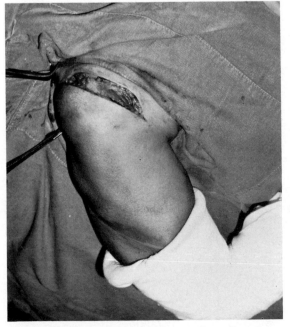

Figure 8–50 Incision and exposure for cuff surgery.

rent, a bicipital or a subscapular lesion has been encountered.

Small Complete Cuff Tears. The simplest tear to repair is the small slit or rim rent. It is encountered in two locations principally, the junction of the supraspinatus and subscapularis or anterolaterally in the supraspinatus.

In either location the exposure, as outlined previously, is the same. Following the exploratory process, the coraco-acromial ligament is resected, cutting it at its acromial attachment and retracting it medially (Fig. 8–51). A small artery of the thoraco-acromial axis is almost always encountered in cutting this ligament and must be electrically coagulated because it will continue to bleed. Sufficient exposure now is available to allow mobilization of the cuff. The assistant pulls on the arm, and the dissecting finger probes into the supra- and infraspinous fossae, loosening the cuff. These acts of traction and digital freeing usually are sufficient to let torn edges fall together, and repair may be accomplished with a few interrupted Mersilene mattress sutures. If possible, the bursa is then repaired and the wound is closed in layers.

Massive Tears. Repair of massive ruptures requires extensive exposure and special techniques. The position, incision and preliminary inspection are the same as described previously. When a massive defect is identified, the first step is a complete manipulation of the shoulder to release adhesions, particularly those resulting from infraglenoid contractures. It is an error to attempt to repair such tears without first carrying out this maneuver. Often the humerus is riding at a higher than normal level, squeezed to this point by the infraglenoid adhesions and the unresisted upward thrust of the head of the humerus, which occurs when the patient attempts to abduct it (Fig. 8–52).

When the capsule has been completely loosened, it is not uncommon to find that the cuff defect has decreased by as much as one third. This allows insertion of the finger beneath the acromion and over the head to further free cuff substance.

Exposure is continued by resecting the coraco-acromial ligament and then performing an acromioclavicular arthroplasty. This last step makes feasible mobilization of the supra- and infraspinatus muscles well down to their origins in the fossae. It also makes possible a further 15 to 20 degrees of

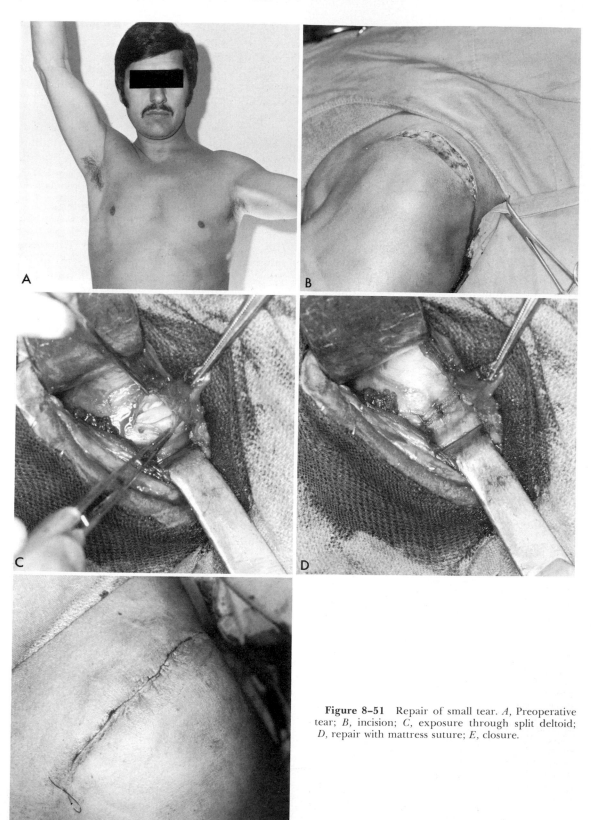

Figure 8–51 Repair of small tear. *A*, Preoperative tear; *B*, incision; *C*, exposure through split deltoid; *D*, repair with mattress suture; *E*, closure.

abduction without rotation or acromio-clavicular impingement. In all massive cuff repairs some decrease in rotation may be expected, so that this maneuver is extremely helpful and adds significantly to the range of pain-free motion subsequently obtained.

Some tears of considerable size are sufficiently obliterated by these manipulations that they may be approximated edge to edge (Fig. 8–52). In others, it is necessary to shorten the insertion by modifying the attachment into the upper end of the humerus. This is accomplished by cutting a face in the head of the humerus, appropriately angled to allow the cuff to be pulled over it and secured in place. The segment of humeral head removed will have some articular cartilage on it and often is shaped like an orange segment. The placing of this cut can only be determined by pulling the cuff over the head with the arm slightly abducted, marking with an osteotome the point of

desired attachment and then making the cut appropriately (Fig. 8–53).

The edges of the tear are freshened and fastened to the humerus with fascia through small drill holes. Some surgeons prefer to use a small staple at this point, but a form of firm bone fixation is necessary to retain a strong repair. In making this cut, one face will serve for cuff adhesion and the other allows anchorage of the stitches. The incision is then closed in the routine fashion. When it is possible, the bursa is repaired over the zone of cuff attachment in the same way one closes the peritoneum in the abdomen.

Lateral Tears. When examination through the exploratory segment of the incision indicates that the defect is extensive, but quite laterally placed, a slightly different routine is followed (Fig. 8–54).

An acromioclavicular arthroplasty is done, but the medial 5/16 to 3/8 inch of the acromion is resected, including usually a little of the

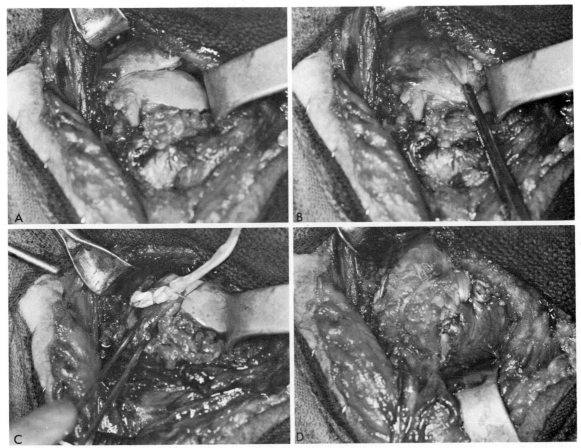

Figure 8–52 Steps in obliterating an extensive defect using fascia. *A,* Extensive gap prior to mobilization. *B,* The cuff is then mobilized by dissection into the spinous fossae and loosened from its attachment to the spine by digital dissection. *C,* Suturing of rotator cuff in position with fascia fixed to Gallie needle. *D,* Appearance following obliteration of gap.

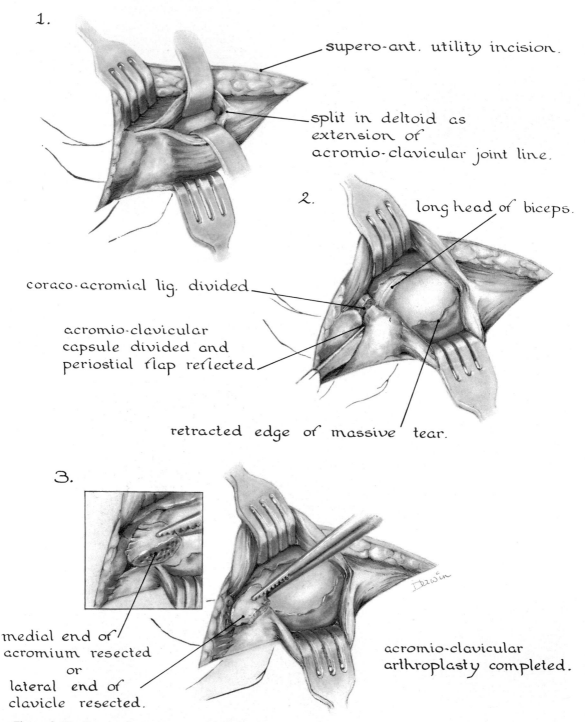

1.

supero-ant. utility incision.

split in deltoid as extension of acromio-clavicular joint line.

2.

long head of biceps.

coraco-acromial lig. divided

acromio-clavicular capsule divided and periostial flap reflected

retracted edge of massive tear.

3.

medial end of acromium resected or lateral end of clavicle resected.

acromio-clavicular arthroplasty completed.

Figure 8–53 Repair of massive tear with the cuff insertion shortened by resecting the head of the humerus and suturing the cuff into the defect.

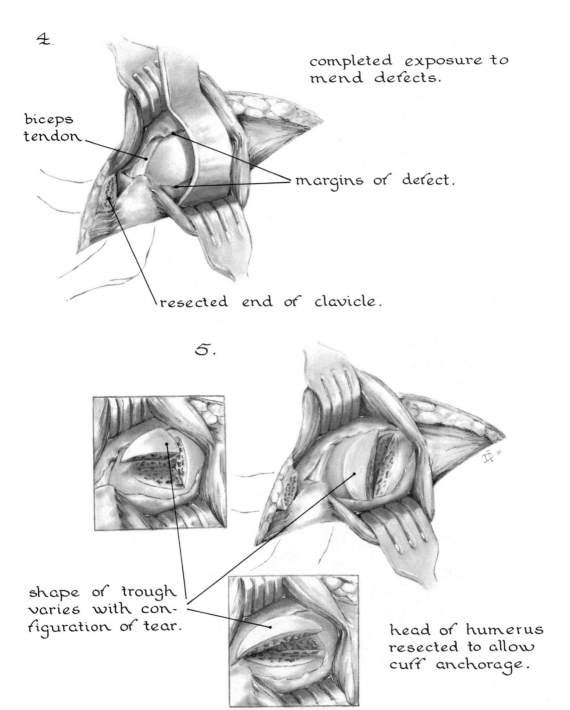

4.

completed exposure to mend defects.

biceps tendon

margins of defect.

resected end of clavicle.

5.

shape of trough varies with configuration of tear.

head of humerus resected to allow cuff anchorage.

Figure 8–53 *Continued.*

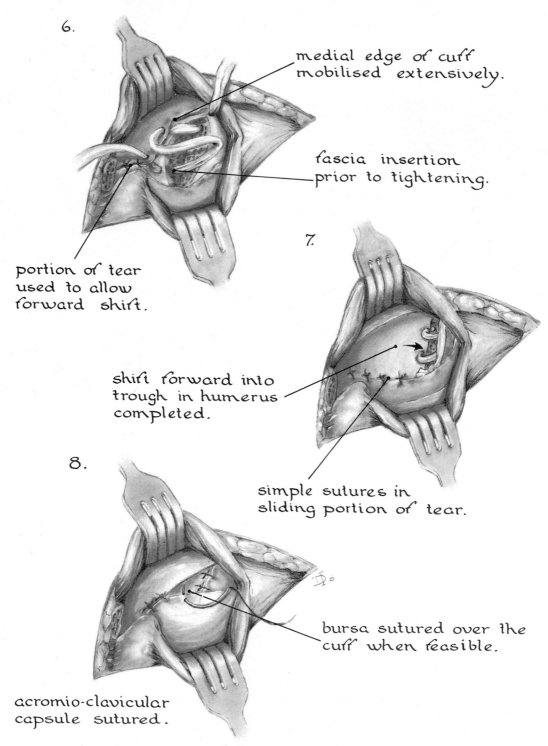

6.

medial edge of cuff
mobilised extensively.

fascia insertion
prior to tightening.

portion of tear
used to allow
forward shift.

7.

shift forward into
trough in humerus
completed.

simple sutures in
sliding portion of tear.

8.

bursa sutured over the
cuff when feasible.

acromio-clavicular
capsule sutured.

Figure 8–53 *Continued.*

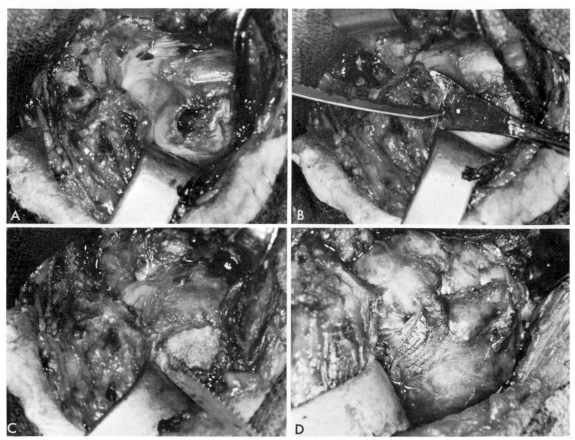

Figure 8–54 Repair of a laterally placed tear is facilitated by a "lateral" acromioclavicular arthroplasty. *A,* Cuff tear with the edge of the acromion almost digging into it. *B,* Anteromedial portion of acromion is resected. *C,* A surface is prepared on the humerus. *D,* Cuff has been sutured to the edge of the prepared surface with fascia.

anterior point of the acromion. In this way better access is provided to the lateral side of the head of the humerus, and this makes the freeing of the cuff in this region much easier. Exposure of a superior site for humeral head troughing is available and the cuff can be transfixed with greater facility. An arthroplasty is effected by removing the medial acromion just as well as by removing the lateral end of the clavicle, but the clavicle is left intact if the acromion is removed.

Total resection of the acromion is avoided because of the difficulty of fixing the origin of the deltoid securely. In some instances it is quite feasible, but often experience has been that the deltoid pulls off the attachment, leaving an unsatisfactory repair. For this reason a partial acromionectomy, which will contribute all the advantages of an acromioclavicular arthroplasty, appears much better.

Bicipital Tears. A further, quite different configuration of tear is not uncommonly encountered in the form of a split, extending along the course of the biceps toward and sometimes implicating the bicipital groove. It frequently happens that the intertubercular fibers are damaged in a tear such as this, allowing the long head of the humerus to dislocate medially. Often this leads to a most unstable shoulder, with extensive impairment of use.

When this lesion is encountered, the exposure involves extension of the deltoid separation a little further distally. The coracoacromial ligament is resected, and the acromioclavicular arthroplasty is carried out in the usual fashion. The defect is repaired with fascia, using a lacing stitch made with two needles. The fascia is inserted at the top of the defect and laced toward the intertubercular sulcus. The long head of the biceps is replaced in its groove, and the fascia is anchored through two drill holes in the upper end of the humerus on either side of

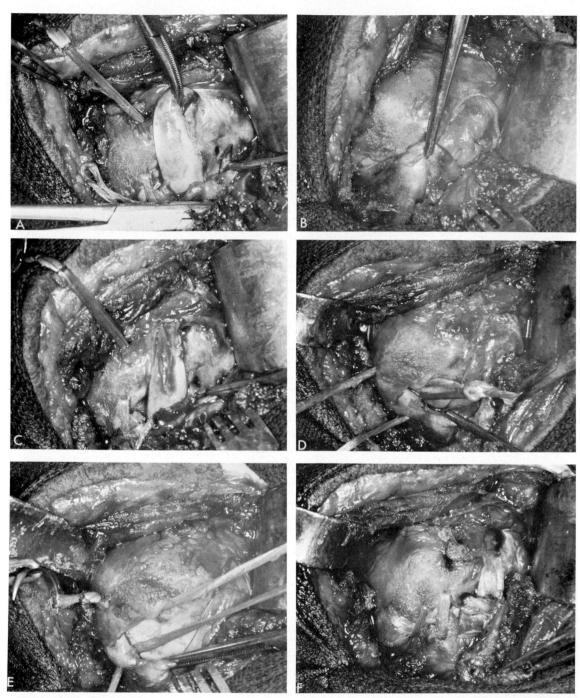

Figure 8–55 Repair of anterior or "bicipital" tear with complete dislocation of the biceps from the groove. Defect is obliterated and intertubercular fibers are reconstructed. *A*, Biceps is replaced in the groove from its dislocated position. *B*, Gap is obliterated by mobilization of cuff. *C*, The fascial suture laces edges together and then is anchored in bone on either side of the groove (*D*) and (*E*). *F*, Completion of the repair with new intertubercular ligament formed, tendon replaced and gap obliterated.

the intertubercular sulcus so that as the fascia is tied, it forms a new roof of intertubercular fibers. The tendon can be firmly held in its proper position by this maneuver. Closure is effected in the usual fashion (Fig. 8–55).

Subscapular Tears. Powerful rotatory stress can split the subscapularis or avulse it from its moorings. The lesion is usually seen in young athletes or the younger age group. Some suggestion of the location of these tears is obtained in the examination and contrast studies. The tenderness is antero-inferior, with the plane often extending toward the chest; in an arthrogram, the dye leaks medially instead of superiorly (Fig. 8–56).

When this tear is encountered, the incision is extended slightly distal; resection of the coraco-acromial ligament and acromio-clavicular arthroplasty are not required. As a rule, replacement of the tendon is not difficult, although reaching it is somewhat awk-

ward. In some instances a tear such as this is best approached by the inferior axillary incision, which is used for repair of recurrent dislocation in women.

When exploratory incision superiorly indicates this type of tear, a further cut is made in the inferior axillary fold, extending across the roof of the axilla. The deep fascia is incised, and the principle is to retract the anterior wall of the axilla, consisting of pectoralis major and deltoid superiorly. When this has been done, dissection continues along the coracobrachialis and biceps on their lateral side, exposing the subscapularis. As a rule, the rupture occurs toward the medial aspect of this area, with the tendon being avulsed from the margin of the glenoid tuberosity. The tendon of subscapularis is mobilized in both directions and, with some internal rotation, is usually possible to bridge this gap adequately. The repair is carried out with interrupted mattress sutures, but

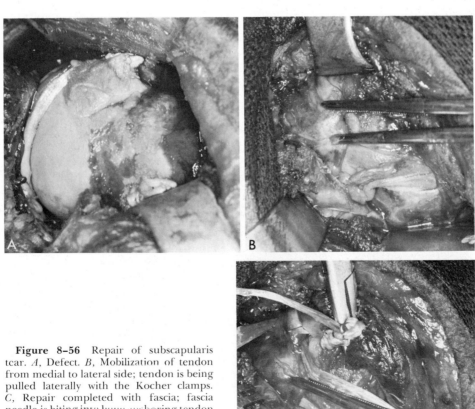

Figure 8–56 Repair of subscapularis tear. *A,* Defect. *B,* Mobilization of tendon from medial to lateral side; tendon is being pulled laterally with the Kocher clamps. *C,* Repair completed with fascia; fascia needle is biting into bone anchoring tendon with the fascia.

in longstanding defects, it should be laced with fascia.

PREPARATION OF FASCIA. The use of fascia lata has been extremely helpful in the author's hands. In the repair of cuff defects it affords an autogenous suture material that has a degree of resiliency after fixation, which is beneficial as applied to many of the tears. In addition, it forms a scaffolding of "living" suture, which is particularly helpful in large, massive tears. The lacing technique offers a method of obliterating defects effectively when there is considerable decrease in cuff substance.

A small transverse incision 2 inches long is made and centered over the tensor fascia, roughly a hand's breadth above the patella. The incision is carried down to the fascia, and the fat is separated from the tensor fascia, which can be easily palpated. A strip about 5/16 inch in width is cut with a scalpel and dissected free and then removed with a fascia stripper.

The stripper removes a piece of fascia approximately 9 to 10 inches in length and this is fixed to a fascia needle. The needle is a stout one with an appropriately large eye. The fascia is sewn on with two separate binding stitches. When it is desired to use a side-to-side lacing stitch, needles are sewn on each end. When a single stitch suture is required, an anchoring knot may be placed on one end and a needle on the other.

Concealed or Partial Thickness Tears. Symptoms from many of these tears subside with conservative treatment. Persistent trouble develops as a result of continued "overhanging arch impingement." Incision and exposure are carried out as described previously for the repair of small tears. Identification of the torn area is accomplished purely by palpation and observation. Nearly always it is a heaped-up zone, 1/2 to 3/4 inch in diameter and lying near the lateral edge of the humerus. Impingement on the coracoacromial arch by abduction and rotation of the head can be demonstrated. The principle is to resect this elevated area, carrying the incision down to the cortex of the humerus. A wedge-shaped segment about 3/4 inch is removed, and the detached fibers are dissected; the edges are smoothed so that they may be tacked into place along the edge of the defect. In placing the defect in this fashion, the repaired edges lie without obstructing the overhanging arch. It is usually possible to carry out the repair with interrupted mattress sutures, although a small strip of fascia occasionally is required as suture.

Postoperative Management. Because of the variation in size, shape and age of the cuff defects, and the different techniques required for repair, it has seemed advisable to establish a grading system so that a systematic postopeative routine can be established. Only in this way is it possible for physiotherapists and others to pace the patients intelligently. Three grades, based on severity, are recognized; nearly all tears fall clearly into one of these categories.

GRADE I. Small and partial tears, which have been repaired without the use of fascia, usually with mattress sutures only and without acromioclavicular arthroplasty, constitute this group. After operation the shoulder is placed in suspension at a right angle for 24 to 48 hours, depending on the patient's tolerance, and active motion is then instituted immediately. The patients are allowed up as soon as they feel comfortable with the arm supported in a sling.

GRADE II. Tears of moderate size are included in this group, which will have required an acromioclavicular arthroplasty and fascial repair; however, the repair will usually have been accomplished without resection of the humeral head or advancement of the insertion. Such patients are placed in sling traction for 24 to 48 hours and then suspended in swinging traction for 7 to 10 days (Fig. 8–57). They are given bathroom privileges at once and are allowed up with the arm supported at right angles or in a cantilever brace. When they can move the shoulder comfortably in the springs and slings, they continue entirely in a brace, which is removed at night. As soon as the patient can raise the arm in flexion and abduction, against gravity, the brace is lowered; it is continually lowered until it is resting at the side and is then discarded.

GRADE III. Massive tears and most other extensive defects are included under this heading. The repair needs longer protection for healing, and the muscular weakness and imbalance are always more extensive. This means that more skillful physiotherapy and supervision are essential. The cardinal principle in recovering shoulder function is to concentrate on the act of flexion and not on abduction (Fig. 8–57). Care must be taken not to allow the shoulder to set in extension in the early postoperative period. If the arm is allowed to drift posteriorly, even although it is kept in a right angle splint, it is extremely

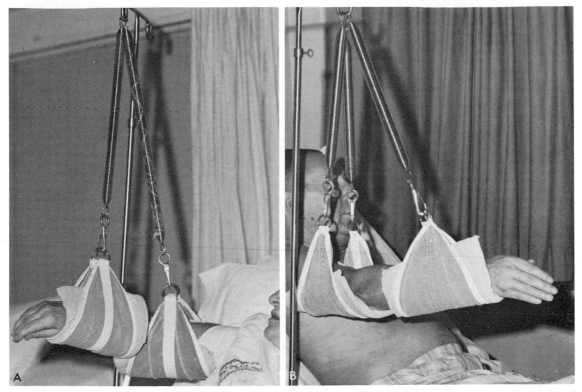

Figure 8–57 "Springs and slings." Postoperative suspension of shoulders with full thickness tears of grades 2 and 3.

difficult to get it forward again to a point where it may be brought up to the mouth, which is the essential act.

The cantilever splint has been designed to maintain a position that keeps tension from the suture line but allows a forward and backward swing at this level, preventing capsular freezing. The weight of the injured arm is taken on the opposite axilla, not on the iliac crest of the same side. The fulcrum for the suspension of the injured shoulder is at the glenohumeral joint, not on the chest wall as is usually the case in other abduction braces.

The arc of swinging movement in the pivot carries well forward to the front of the body, and there is a lock on the pivot joint to prevent excursion backward too far into extension.

The arm may be lowered to the side by degrees and still swing in this lower locked position. The bar over the shoulder on the side of the injury is placed medial to the acromioclavicular joint to avoid pressure on the usual operative incision (Fig. 8–58). A cantilever bar extends under the opposite axilla and is padded to avoid irritation from pressure, but the patient is then able to wear it

continually, with the weight of the injured arm supported by the uninjured one.

The splint has been put together in sections so that is can be quite simply taken apart and adjusted to various sizes of limb and chest. It also may be assembled for either right or left side from the same set of parts.

Grade III tears remain in a splint for at least three weeks, lowering or removal depending upon the progress (Fig. 8–59). The patient is taught to gradually assume the weight of gravity in the splint, starting about two weeks postoperatively; in more extensive defects this interval may be somewhat longer. As he gradually is able to assume the weight, and the rhythm of lifting into flexion is obtained, the arm is lowered in the brace. This is continued until, at about six weeks, he usually has enough power to lift the arm from the side against gravity to the level of a right angle. When this point has been reached, the brace is discarded.

A program of concentrating on active and assisted active motion is continued for a further six weeks, but with much less supervision. Patients report once or twice a week at this stage to check their home exercise

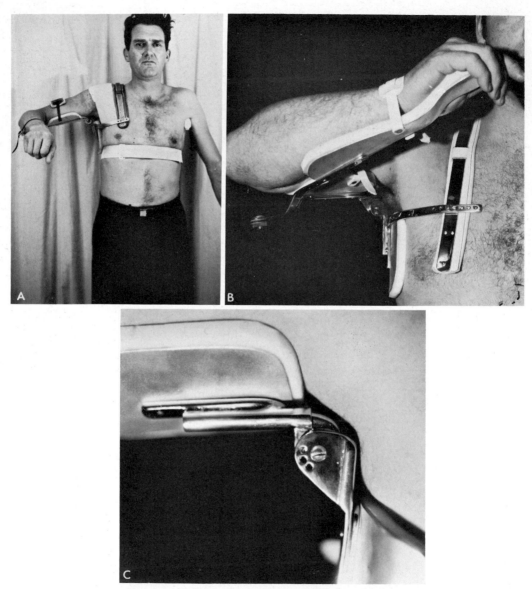

Figure 8–58 Cantilever splint. *A*, Weight of arm is taken on uninjured side. The shoulder strap rests medially to the incision so as to avoid pressure on the operative area. *B*, A swivel joint allows motion at a right angle, preventing stress on the suture line. *C*, Brace may be progressively lowered and swivel action retained.

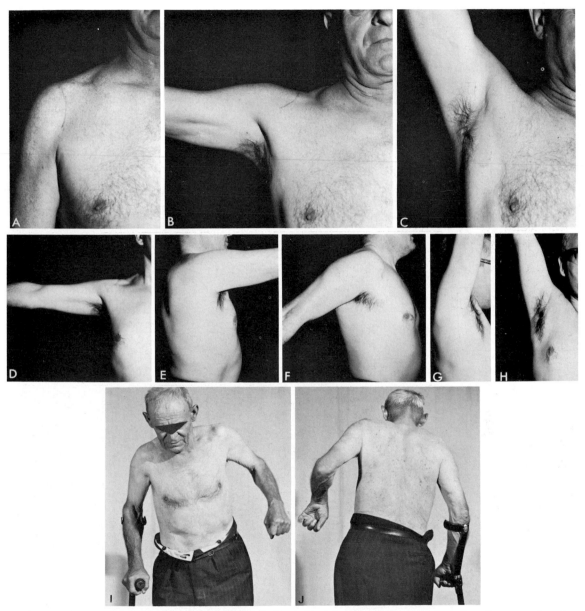

Figure 8–59 Results of cuff injuries. *A, B* and *C,* Healed incision and full range of motion, three months after operation for a full thickness tear. *D, E, F, G* and *H,* Result of repair of massive tear with fascia, four months after operation. *I* and *J,* Result eight months after conservative treatment only of a full thickness tear proved by arthrography.

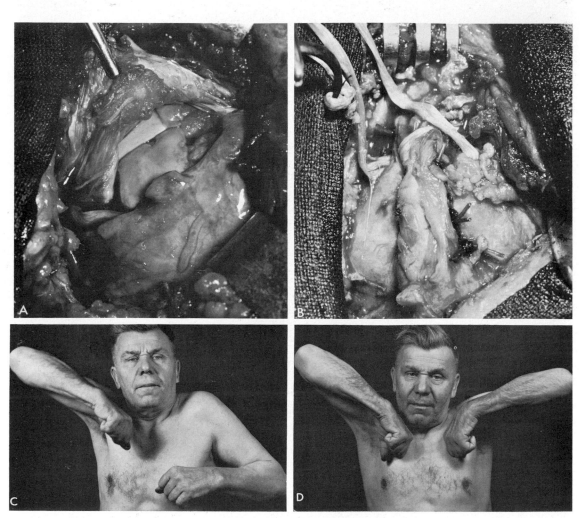

Figure 8–60 Anterior bicipital tear repaired by fascia before and after operation. *A*, lesion. *B*, Repair techniques. *C*, Range of power preoperatively. *D*, Result four months postoperatively.

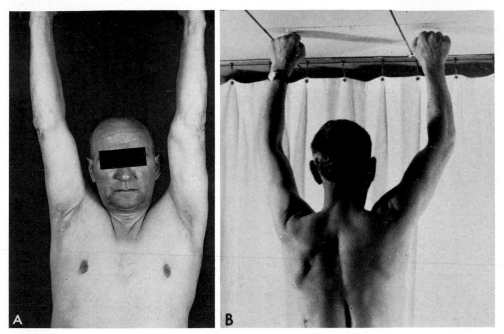

Figure 8–61 Postoperative results of bilateral cuff repairs. *A,* One shoulder two months and one, eight months after operation. *B,* One shoulder three months and the other, one year after operation.

progress. Laborers with these extensive lesions usually cannot resume work for 10 to 12 weeks postoperatively. For patients in less strenuous occupations the period of inactivity is considerably less.

Postoperative Program Beyond Acute Phase. The immediate postoperative plan is outlined in the previous discussion. All patients reach a point at which the operative reaction has subsided: the wound has healed, the pain has gone, and constant rigid support or traction is no longer needed. The time at which such a stage will be reached will depend on the site and extent of the cuff defect, the security of the repair, and the general pain tolerance of the patient. In massive avulsions it is usually six weeks or more; in rim or concealed tears three weeks; in anterior or bicipital tears, about four weeks (Figs. 8–60, 8–61, 8–62 and 8–63). At this point a program of planned exercises and instruction should be started. This is the phase that leads to successful rehabilitation of the patient, and its importance cannot be overestimated. In dealing with workmen in particular, a rehabilitation center has much to offer; if possible the program should be carried out at such a center.

The muscle developing routine embraces three principal components: specific exercises for the shoulder and accessory shoulder muscles, remedial gymnastics as group exercises, and occupational therapy designed to develop creative and purposeful function.

SPECIFIC EXERCISE PROGRAM FOR PATIENTS WITH CUFF LESIONS. The plan is to start with assisted active movement of each group of muscles and progress gradually. As the range is increased, resistance is added. This may be started with attention to individual muscles such as triceps, biceps, and rotators, but later should be directed to movement patterns rather than individual muscle actions. For example, shoulder flexion should be encouraged by substituting biceps and pectoral contraction for deltoid and rotator contribution, and so on. In many patients the greatest barrier to good recovery is the initial fear and reluctance to move, which may have become so fixed that it is translated into physical inability to move. In these circumstances relearning and education of the movement pattern may be aided by electrical stimulation of the muscles coupled with painstaking instruction by the physiotherapist. Once the idea of the pattern has been relearned, further use is easy and the program proceeds well. Progress varies from patient to patient and the individual lesion, but the change from assisted movement, to active and then to resisted movement is made as quickly as is reasonable. These exer-

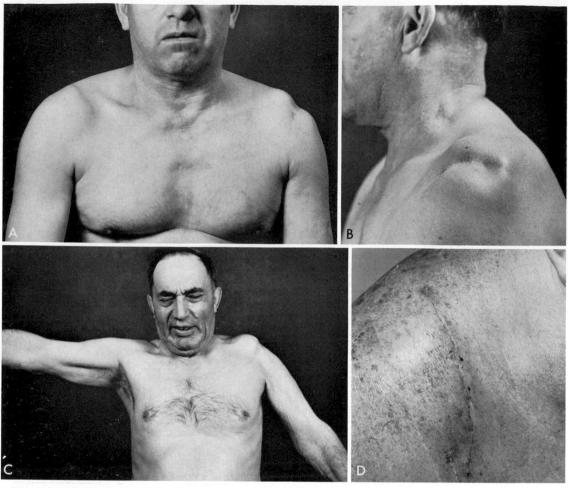

Figure 8–62 Result of cuff repairs. *A*, Repair using old method of complete acromionectomy. *B* and *C*, Note poor purchase for the deltoid which mars the result. *D*, Present incision as it usually heals.

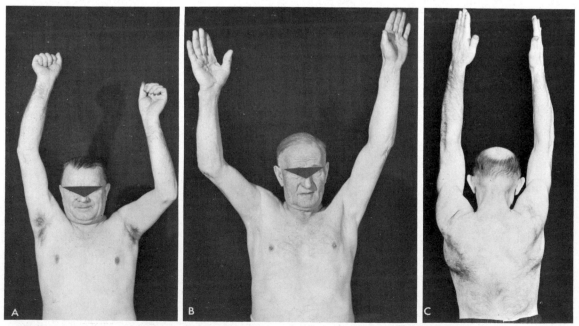

Figure 8–63 Results of repair. *A*, Three months; *B*, four months; and *C*, five months postoperatively in patients in a slightly older age group.

cises are presented in Table 8–1. An attempt has been made to recognize at least two types of clinical level in each group.

One principle in all exercise routines for the shoulder should be emphasized: the

Table 8–1 REHABILITATION PROGRAM AFTER CUFF REPAIR

GROUP I	Still using splint, but gradually discarding it		
Class	Physiotherapy	Group Exercises	Occupational Therapy
Class I Some pain and considerable weakness	Pendulum exercises, standing and prone	Smooth board movements, supine and rotatory	Wall work, assisted by weighted sling
Class II Less pain and a little more power	Wall climbing	Rotation exercises, seated	Bench work with elbows supported on bench or at various levels
GROUP II	Splint support still needed, plus encouragement in coordination and control		
Class I Some pain and weakness plus poor control and coordination	Spring elevation with normal hand supporting	Cradle motion	Sanding, two-handed, standing; sawing, two-handed
Class II Less pain but still with weakness and some stiffness	Double spring rotation	Stick exercises	Sanding, one-handed; planing
GROUP III	Much less pain, some weakness, splint discarded, various degrees of stiffness		
Class I Active exercises with some assistance	Pulley exercises, two-handed	Spring rotation	Shuffleboard; basketry
Class II Active	Standing before mirror to improve control	Swinging bean-bag	Quoits; horseshoes; gardening
Class III Active, sustained	Pulley and routine active	Swinging and lifting, progressing to overhead activity	Basketry; weaving; wall work
Class IV Active, resisted	Manual resistance and weight lifting	Indian club swinging and lifting	Painting; shoulder wheel; hoisting; climbing

movement that is most easily learned and restored is forward flexion, and this should be the starting exercise. It has a simple pendulum quality that is easily accomplished. If one starts by attempting to do the much more complicated abduction motion, the program may stall. Once something simple has been learned, the patient is ready for the next step because he has regained some confidence in his capabilities. In the plans outlined the flexion action at various levels, to the shoulder and then above the shoulder, is mastered first. Should abduction never be recovered, the patient can always manage simply by turning his body so that the hand enters what was previously the abduction zone. This simple plan has a further beneficial reaction; it teaches a movement pattern again. Often much of the persistent disability results from loss or forgetting by the higher centers of the brain of the technique of putting isolated actions together as a pattern. The above may be learned easily and, once started, the pitch and pattern are retained.

POWER BUILDING EXERCISES

1. Weights are added to the pendulum regime.

2. Weights are added to flexion and abduction regime.

Active Exercises
1. Flexion exercises.
2. Abduction exercises.
3. Rotation exercises.
4. Combination movements.

Assisted Maneuvers
1. Stretching of abduction contracture.
2. Stretching gentle external rotation.
3. Stretching flexion contracture with hands behind head.

DISORDERS OF THE BICIPITAL APPARATUS

The long head of the biceps tendon is intimately related to the shoulder joint and is affected by all movements of the humerus on the scapula. In addition, it serves its own function of anchoring a powerful muscle. As a result of its position and intrinsic function, it contributes significantly to shoulder action. Disorders and disease arising from this mechanism have long been overlooked. Pioneer work in this field has been done by Meyers in demonstrating bicipital pathology, and further contributions have been made by

Moseley, Gilcrest, Lippman and Bechtol. Disturbances of the bicipital apparatus are common and disabling, and their recognition and separation from other entities marks an advance in our understanding of shoulder disorders.

There are many sources of damage to the bicipital mechanism. It is exposed to friction in everyday exertion; it is subject to greatly increased stress and strain in heavy laboring activities, particularly overhead work. In its role of stabilizing the head of the humerus at the front, it bears the brunt in injuries such as backward falls when the extended arm is used involuntarily for protection (Fig. 8–64). Bicipital lesions as a group have some characteristic signs and symptoms which separate them from other shoulder lesions, and further differentiation is possible into several common syndromes.

GENERAL SIGNS AND SYMPTOMS OF BICIPITAL INVOLVEMENT

Some episode of trauma is common in the patient's history. This may be minor, such as an unaccustomed repetitive motion, or may be a major injury. Apparently inconsequential details are often significant in determining the cause. A history of continued and unaccustomed use of a screwdriver, a sudden lift in the overhead position with the arm externally rotated as in lifting a car hood, a sharp pain in holding a weight at arm's length, or an unexpected backward fall with the arm extended posteriorly to take the weight are significant examples. These patients complain of pain that is clearly localized to the shoulder and becomes identified with movements of the arm. It is not related to the neck or the girdle as a whole, nor are the forearm and the head implicated.

When the initial episode is clearly defined, a snapping sensation is often mentioned or a feeling of something giving way in the shoulder. Sometimes this snap becomes repetitive and later can be felt and heard in shoulder action. It is sharply painful and is followed by a persistent more general ache. Later in the process weakness and limitation of movement become apparent. Some pain may radiate from the shoulder a short distance along the inside of the upper arm and is related to the course of the long head of the biceps. Still later, as pain and weakness continue, the patient often adopts a characteristic attitude, with the arm held close to the side and supported by the good hand; he has probably learned that the forearm and hand can be used with the arm in this posi-

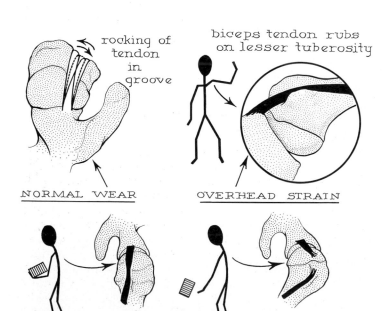

NORMAL WEAR — rocking of tendon in groove

OVERHEAD STRAIN — biceps tendon rubs on lesser tuberosity

EXTENSION INJURY — man dropping heavy object suddenly, rips tendon where frayed

Figure 8–64 Mechanics of bicipital ruptures.

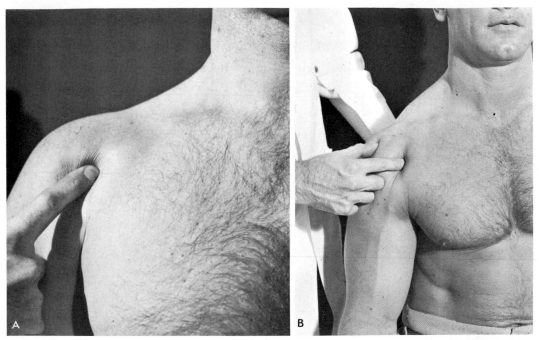

Figure 8–65 *A,* The bicipital point. *B,* The bicipital point (index finger) is compared with the tender point in cuff tears (thumb).

tion, because the painful tendon is splinted in the groove by keeping the arm at the side. All rotatory movements are carefully avoided.

Examination discloses certain findings which are characteristic of these lesions. The tenderness in the shoulder is definitely related to the bicipital apparatus (Fig. 8–65). This may be supero-anteriorly over the intra-articular tendon (Fig. 8–66), anteriorly over the groove and transverse ligament, or antero-inferiorly along the biceps tendon (Fig. 8–65). Such a tender zone differs sharply from that usually found in rotator cuff lesions or calcified tendinitis (Fig. 8–65*B*). Tests for the biceps function of supination and flexion are most helpful in identifying these lesions. Zergason's test of flexing the elbow and supinating the wrist against resistance may elicit pain referred to the antero-medial aspect of the shoulder. Often it is on the release of tension that a maximum response is obtained. A negative response to this test does not rule out a bicipital disturbance, however. In some lesions gross laxity of the tendon can be demonstrated, and it may be moved from side to side when the arm is abducted and internally rotated. The tendon is slack in this position and abnormal laxity is easily demonstrated (see Fig. 8–71). In all cases of suspected bicipital damage, special x-rays of the upper end of the hu-

merus should be made to outline the bicipital groove (Fig. 8–67). There are specific abnormalities of the groove which are suggestive of bicipital disturbances and which will be discussed under the individual lesions. Once the general syndrome has been appreciated, further investigation identifies several common types.

BICIPITAL LESIONS

Bicipital Tendinitis and Tenosynovitis

The long head of the biceps follows a tortuous and hemmed-in course from its origin in the muscle belly to the supraglenoid tubercle. It is not unreasonable to expect reaction to trauma and strain to develop just as may occur in tendons and tendon sheaths elsewhere in the body. The type of trauma which usually produces tenosynovitis (for example, in the wrist) is one heavy blow or repeated blows resulting in constrictive adhesions. This is not the mechanism commonly encountered in the case of the long tendon of the biceps (Fig. 8–68). The bicipital area is not nearly so vulnerable to direct trauma as the more distal regions of the extremity, so that tendinitis and tenosynovi-

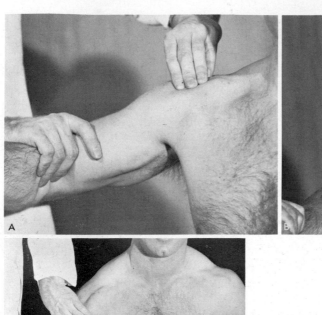
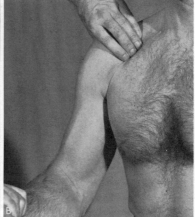
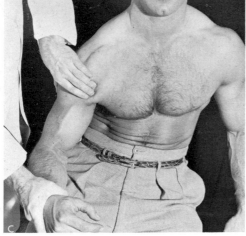

Figure 8–66   Points of tenderness in bicipital involvement. *A,* Over intra-articular part of tendon. *B,* Over groove and transverse ligament. *C,* Anteroinferiorly along the bicipital tendon.

tis may develop gradually without definite acute episodes of injury.

Signs and Symptoms of Bicipital Tendinitis and Tenosynovitis.   Following an activity such as the first game of badminton or tennis of the season, or a jerking strain in lifting with the outstretched arms, discomfort is noted in the shoulder (Figs. 8–65 and 8–66). An indefinite ache is present first and is not plainly related to motions that use the biceps tendon. More acute pain develops, and the patient avoids lifting acts, keeping the arm at the side with the elbow flexed since this is the position of maximum comfort.

Examination shows tenderness at the top and front related to the tendon course across the upper end of the humerus. It follows into the bicipital groove and along the tendon into the arm. Deep palpation at the medial border of the deltoid delineates tenderness on pressure along the tendon as the arm is rotated externally and internally. Flexion of the elbow and supination of the hand against resistance (Zergason's sign) may produce pain referred to the front and inner aspects of the shoulder (Fig. 8–69). In all shoulder lesions in which involvement of the biceps mechanism is suspected, special x-rays that show the groove in profile should be done. In a tendinitis or tenosynovitis, bony abnormalities are not usual, but any abnormal contour of the groove may set the stage for development of the disability. If the groove is too flat or shallow, the tendon may slip out; if it is too deep, it may be roughened and squeezed; and if there is spur formation, it will become frayed.

Treatment of Bicipital Tendinitis and Tenosynovitis.   This is the mildest of the bicipital syndromes and responds quickly to conservative treatment.

LOCAL ANESTHETIC INFILTRATION.   Using a 2 per cent solution of Novocain, infiltrate the groove and adjacent area of the capsule.

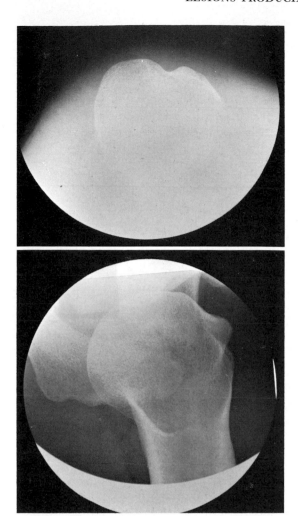

Figure 8–67 X-rays showing the bicipital groove.

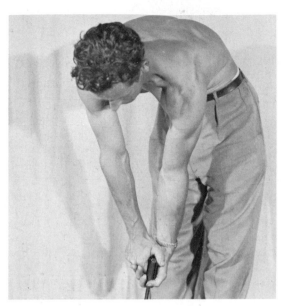

Figure 8–68 One common mechanism producing bicipital irritation. Strong supination as in using a screwdriver or lifting and externally rotating the forearm in the extended position.

PERSISTENT SIGNS AND SYMPTOMS. If the signs and symptoms continue or increase, the lesion is more than a simple tenosynovitis or traumatic tendinitis, and one of the severer grades of bicipital disturbance should be suspected, such as rupture of the inter-

Sometimes several injections at five- to seven-day intervals are needed. The first injection, if inserted properly, produces prompt relief.

IMMOBILIZATION. During the acute stage, which is usually a matter of days only, the arm should be carried in a sling. The patient is encouraged in gentle movement to prevent freezing of the rest of the shoulder structures.

MEDICATION. Acute discomfort requires appropriate light sedation such as an aspirin-codeine combination to allow gentle movement. A course of an anti-inflammatory drug like phenylbutazone also helps.

ACTIVE EXERCISES. Following subsidence of the acute discomfort, active movement is encouraged. If there is any reluctance, the patient must be placed under the care of a competent physiotherapist at once. Mobilization must be persisted with to prevent extensive freezing of the glenohumeral joint.

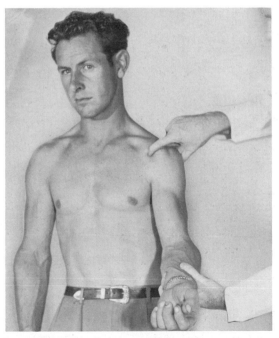

Figure 8–69 Testing for biceps action. Flexion and supination of the forearm against resistance.

tubercular fibers or partial rupture of the tendon.

Rupture of the Intertubercular Fibers or Transverse Humeral Ligament

The long head of the biceps tendon is held in the intertubercular groove by a fascial roof which is strengthened at the top to form a transverse ligament, stretching between the greater and lesser tuberosities (Fig. 8–70). These are stout fibers that blend smoothly with the cuff capsule. They perform an important function in retaining the long head in position, contributing to the fulcrum function of the groove as the tendon changes course across the head of the humerus. These fibers may be ruptured by certain forcible movements when the tendon is placed under strong tension. The maneuver which places most strain on these fibers is abduction and external rotation. In this motion the tendency is for the long head to shift medially over the head of the humerus as the humerus is rotated externally (see Fig. 8–70). In this motion the tendon would slip out of the groove if the intertubercular fibers did not curb it. When abduction is added, the strain is increased and any sudden external rotation of the humerus with the biceps flexed under tension will "spring" the intertubercular fibers (Fig. 8–46).

A similar result may occur when groove or tendon develops abnormally. The long head and the groove have a reciprocal relationship so that alterations in the groove are frequently associated with variations in the tendon. A broad, shallow groove may be associated with a thick, fat tendon, favoring insecure fixation in the tunnel and placing extra strain on the intertubercular fibers. Similarly a deep, narrow groove favors secure fixation, but an element of constriction is added, which may irritate the tendon.

Signs and Symptoms. These patients present the general signs suggestive of damage to the bicipital apparatus, but there are further findings which distinguish this particular lesion. A history of injury is common and has usually been a twisting and lifting strain of the arm. The mechanism is an external rotation strain placed on the long head when it is taut. A typical example is the patient bending under the front of a car hood and lifting it with his abducted externally rotated arm. A sudden catch is felt in the shoulder as the weight is increased. The twisting and rotation strain is added to an already tensed, flexed, supinated elbow and hand. With the arm in such a position the biceps is shortened, producing maximum bulk along the groove so that it may be easily "sprung," sliding medially as the head of the humerus continues external rotation. Frequently there is a snapping sensation which can be felt by the patient; sometimes similar snapping is heard by the examiner later. This is due to the swinging back and forth of the tendon when it has been freed from the groove. The patient subsequently

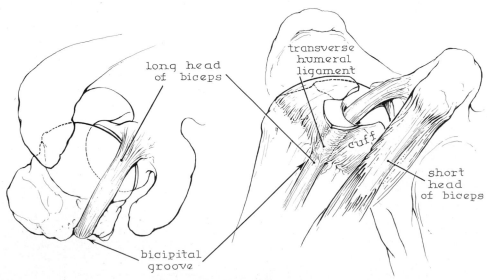

Figure 8–70 The bicipital apparatus.

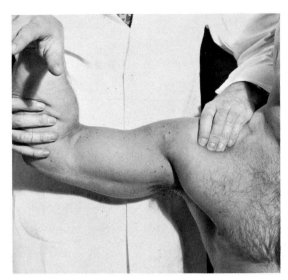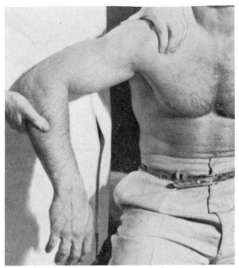

Figure 8–71 Demonstrating slipping of the long head of the biceps from the groove. The tendon may be felt to jump under the fingers as the head of the humerus is rotated.

notices something jumping in the shoulder as he flexes his elbow and rotates his arm.

Examination shows tenderness along the tendon, but a point of acute and maximum tenderness exists over the tip of the bicipital groove. An important test in demonstrating a slipping tendon is to have the patient abduct and internally rotate the arm with the elbow flexed (Fig. 8–71). With the arm in this position the examiner palpates the tendon with one hand, rotating the arm with the other. In this maneuver the tendon can often be felt slipping back and forth, free of its moorings. It can be restored to the groove and held in position by externally rotating and then extending the arm in supination. X-rays of the upper end of the humerus, outlining the tuberosities in profile, may show a shallow groove. The disturbance can occur, however, when no abnormalities of the groove are apparent.

Treatment. Various degrees of this lesion are encountered, all the way from a mild strain to complete rupture, and the treatment varies accordingly.

STRAIN OF INTERTUBERCULAR FIBERS. The intertubercular area is infiltrated with a local anesthetic and the patient is instructed to avoid flexion and external rotation strains for ten days to two weeks. Immobilization of the arm in a sling for seven to ten days is necessary. The lesion is most commonly encountered in the younger age group so that any danger of immobilization producing

stiffening is minimal but must always be kept in mind. Active movement is encouraged as soon as the acute discomfort subsides.

FRANK RUPTURE OF INTERTUBERCULAR FIBERS. A flopping tendon, uncomfortable snapping sensation and localized shoulder pain become quite disabling, so that operative treatment is the method of choice in this stage. The principles of the procedure are to expose and explore the intertubercular area and deal with the tendon according to the extent of damage that is encountered. In some instances it is best to transfer the loose long head medially to the coracoid process. When there is obvious discrepancy in tendon and groove size or the tendon is worn or frayed extensively, transfer of the tendon to the coracoid is done. However, with less extensive tendon damage it may be feasible to replace it and to reconstruct the torn intertubercular fibers with fascia. There are occasions when rupture of the intertubercular fibers is a part of an anterior tear in the rotator cuff, in which case the cuff is repaired and the intertubercular fibers are restored at that time.

Technique of Transfer of Long Head of Biceps. The patient is placed in the sitting shoulder position as illustrated in Figure 8–72. The supero-anterior incision is used to approach the bicipital region, but the anterior limb is made a little long and the posterior limb is shorter. The incision extends from the tip of the acromion distally for 4 inches, just

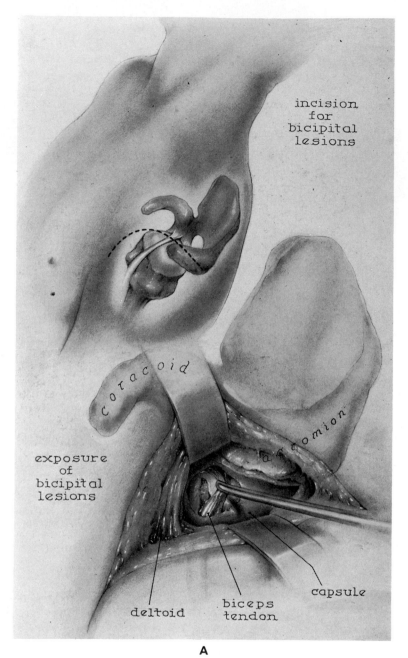

incision
for
bicipital
lesions

coracoid

acromion

exposure
of
bicipital
lesions

deltoid

biceps
tendon

capsule

A

Figure 8–72 Operative technique for transfer of the long head of the biceps to the coracoid process. *A*, Incision and exposure of the long head.

medial to the bicipital groove. The deltoid fibers are split longitudinally, exposing the sulcus. The tendon will be found loose in the groove or out of the groove completely, lying on the medial side of the head. The retaining intertubercular fibers are torn; sometimes only remnants of these fibers are left. The tendon of the long head of the biceps may be frayed or it may be thicker than normal, appearing too bulky for a shallow groove. The long head is identified and pulled up into the wound. This elevates the capsule like a tent and it is possible to follow along the tendon and cut it close to the glenoid rim (Fig. 8–72). The severed tendon is then retracted to be transferred to the attachment of the short head.

The coracoid process is exposed by blunt dissection, retracting the medial edge of the incision. A long curved Kelly is used to make

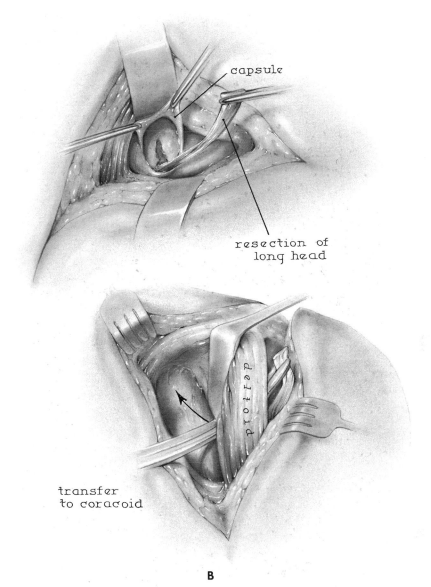

B

Figure 8–72 *(Continued.)* *B,* Tendon transferred medially beneath the coracoid.

Illustration continued.

a tunnel underneath the medial portion of the deltoid, and the long tendon is pulled underneath to the coracoid. A hole is drilled in the coracoid process. The tendon of the long head is split and tied to the coracoid, half being pulled through the prepared hole. It is fixed under slight tension; usually there is barely enough tendon to tie so that the traction exerted in tying the knot imposes the right amount of tension. Any small tear in the capsule can be repaired with interrupted mattress sutures.

Postoperative Regime. The arm is placed in a sling and an adhesive or Elastoplast dressing applied, keeping the elbow flexed. This dressing is left in place for two weeks, and the patient carries the arm in a sling for an additional two weeks. Gentle active flexion of the elbow is started at the end of two weeks, and movements are increased gradually after the fixation is removed.

Ruptures of the Biceps Tendon

Ruptures of the long head of the biceps tendon are much more common than has

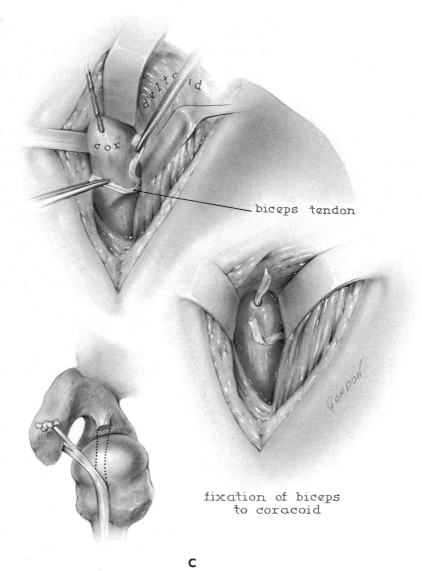

fixation of biceps
to coracoid

C

Figure 8–72 *(Continued)* C, The tendon is split in two and tied through a drill hole in the coracoid process under tension.

been appreciated. They occur following moderately severe trauma in the younger age group, but result more often and from less obvious injuries in an older group. Ruptures are most commonly encountered in workmen, and sometimes the history of injury is sufficiently characteristic to indicate the diagnosis. The general findings suggestive of involvement of the bicipital apparatus are present, but the symptoms can be more disabling than bicipital tendinitis or rupture of the intertubercular fibers.

Signs and symptoms. A typical candidate for rupture is a middle-aged workman who lifts a heavy load in front of him with his hands supinated and his elbows extended. If a sudden jerking element is unexpectedly

added to his burden he almost lets go what he is holding or the weight slips. A sharp stab of pain is experienced as the sudden, increased strain is applied to his arms in this extended position. Often there is a sensation of weakness and sometimes a snapping sound in the shoulder. The arm may "give way" completely and the workman be unable to continue because of weakness and pain. Shortly an unusual swelling or lump is noticed on the front of the arm, and just below the shoulder the arm seems thinner than usual; examination at this point demonstrates weakness in the biceps and pain referred to the forearm when the elbow is flexed and supinated against resistance (Fig. 8–73). There is limitation of shoulder rotation and

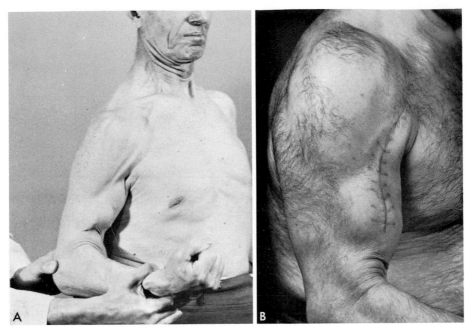

Figure 8–73 Ruptures of the long head of the biceps. *A*, Note distal position of muscle belly of the long head and distress on contraction. The short head is intact. *B*, An ineffective repair for rupture of long head of biceps. The tendon was fixed to the bicipital groove instead of being transplanted to the coracoid. Lack of power in the biceps is apparent and the accessory function of the long head in abduction and flexion of the shoulder is lost when the long head is fixed to the humerus.

abduction. Pressure over the bicipital groove is painful and the tenderness extends down the arm along the groove. Palpation of the belly of the biceps shows it to be relaxed and moving ineffectively on flexion. It usually comes to rest just below the middle of the arm, producing a typical abnormal contour; this abnormality is not always obvious, however. Electrical stimulation of the biceps produces pain referred to the shoulder and demonstrates the decreased power.

X-ray Examination. X-ray examination may show very little disturbance of the bicipital groove, but the head of the humerus is often riding higher than normal in the glenoid socket.

Etiology and Pathology. The biceps is a powerful muscle, but the long head is subject to constant wear and tear from movement of the head of the humerus in addition to the role it plays in flexing and supinating the forearm. The long head is fixed to the glenoid and the intra-articular portion is relatively inert, so the humerus glides back and forth on the tendon more than the tendon shifts on the humerus. Because of its long course and intimate relationship to the head, it is affected by nearly all shoulder motion, whether or not the muscle belly is contracting actively. The tendon is a stout strap of tissue which helps to stabilize the

head, improving its relation and approximation to the glenoid fossa. When its own intrinsic function of anchoring the powerful contractile mechanism is added to the stabilizing function and to exposure to the irritation of routine movement, it is amazing that it is not more often and more extensively involved in pathological processes.

In its course through the joint from the supraglenoid tubercle, the tendon is lax and mobile; its first point of anchorage is as it turns into the tunnel around the corner of the lesser tuberosity (Fig. 8–64). At this point the intertubercular fibers and adjacent area of articular capsule blend, completing the retaining mechanism. Constant pressure can be exerted on different facets of this fulcrum. In some positions the strain and relationship are such as to place maximum force on the intertubercular fibers as has been described previously; more commonly, constant pressure is exerted by the tendon inferiorly on the articular cartilage of the humeral head just above the bicipital sulcus. Constant use or irritating occupations, such as those involving much overhead activity, reaching, holding or lifting, irritate the canal exit. The smooth cartilage becomes worn and roughened (Fig. 8–74). The tendon frays a little, and a vicious cycle is established. The wearing and erosion of the floor is in-

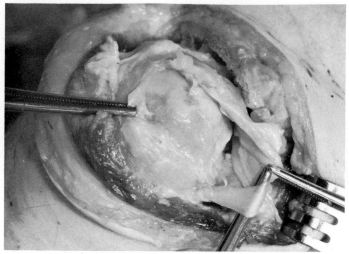

Figure 8–74 Erosion of cartilage on the head of the humerus beneath the biceps tendon. Tendon has shifted medially as a result of weakening of the transverse humeral ligament.

creased by the fraying, and the roughening of the floor breaks more tendon fibers (Fig. 8–75). The tendon weakens and becomes a little lax. Greater play and laxity favor erosion, until bare cortical bone is exposed. Sudden extra strain cuts the remaining fibers as they are pulled across the sharp surface, and the tendon ruptures.

When the joint is examined at operation, it presents a typical picture. The floor of the upper end of the bicipital groove is roughened and adjacent articular cartilage has a bubble-like or pebble-like appearance and fans out over the head of the humerus in a spray or fountain-like fashion. The width of the pebbled area corresponds to the sway of the lax tendon. The tendon may have been worn through completely, in which case the bared cortical zones have become smoothed over. The capsule roofing the

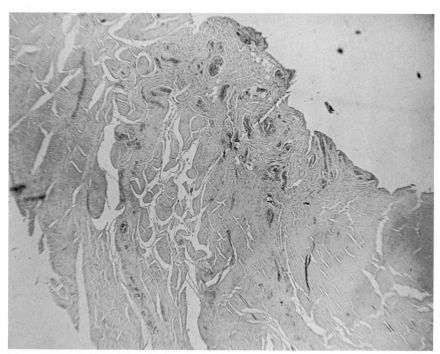

Figure 8–75 A microscopic section of the biceps tendon showing extensive degenerative changes. The collagen fibers are loose and poorly stained. Patchy areas of mucoid and fibrinoid change are apparent. Surface fibers are frayed and the zone is avascular.

tunnel or former path of the long head is thinned, lax and of abnormal consistency.

The foundation of the disturbance is the wear and tear of degeneration, and when sudden increased stress is added, several changes result. The frayed tendon gives way suddenly or gradually. If it happens quickly, the syndrome of rupture is apparent and unmistakable. If it happens gradually, the tendon may become fixed in the groove and stretch apart gradually. The gradual process produces weakness and general shoulder soreness rather than acute symptoms. The process may grind on without a dramatic episode until, at some point, pain caused by the mechanical derangement limits movement and the typical frozen shoulder or adhesive capsulitis results. This is a common ailment and one which contributes significantly to the frozen shoulder syndrome. A degree of tendinitis plus the bicipital lesion is often encountered.

The most important predisposing cause of bicipital disturbance is trauma, but abnormalities in the groove and tendon due to developmental and structural changes contribute also. Monumental work by Bechtol and his associates has shown that variations in the contour of the superior bony margin of the bicipital sulcus are important. In the development of the animal scale, the bicipital groove is gradually deepened as the prehensile and climbing upper extremity is evolved. The supra sulcus tubercle is a property of man's upper extremity stabilization, and variations in individuals can reasonably be expected. Abnormalities in tendon groove relationship have previously been alluded to (see Chapter I). The reason that more symptoms are not apparent from bicipital changes is that the damage to the articular cartilage and the head of the humerus occurs at a point well away from the glenoid fossa and in an area not frequently closely applied to the socket. The shoulder is a non-weight-bearing joint, so that articular damage is not so disturbing as in the hip, where weight transmission results in more complete disintegration of the joint. Rupture of the tendon is rarely encountered inside the joint or in the region of the muscle belly; it occurs in the region of the intertubercular fulcrum because this is the area exposed to maximum stress. The rupture sometimes occurs just above the sulcus and the tendon becomes fixed by natural processes to the groove. The rupture in such cases has been a gradual tearing and weakening separation. In more acute ruptures the proximal tendon may retract into the joint, producing an internal derangement of the joint.

Treatment. The acute episode is usually a disabling one, the persistent weakness, limitation of movement and shoulder pain, particularly in workmen, often being incapacitating and requiring immediate treatment. For those who need to use the arm to earn a living, operative treatment has proved best. The principles are exploration of the biceps and transfixion of the long head to the coracoid under suitable tension. Two methods have been advocated: fixation of the tendon in the groove, and transfer to the coracoid process; the author has found the latter procedure to be the more satisfactory. When the long head is fixed to the groove, insecure anchorage is often obtained or the tendon is not fixed under proper physiological tension. A further important consideration is that the biceps function of contributing some flexion to the shoulder is completely lost if the tendon is fixed to the humerus. Only when it is shifted to the coracoid and again crosses the glenohumeral joint will some influence of this tendon be retained in flexion of the shoulder.

TECHNIQUE OF BICEPS TENDON TRANSFER. The operation should be done as soon as the rupture has been identified because of changes which may occur in the torn tendon. The distal segment recoils to the upper portion of the arm and lies in a curled-up mass which becomes encysted, and the fibers subsequently degenerate (Fig. 8–76). Operation is best carried out within six weeks, if possible, so that there will be sufficient strong tendon without degeneration for the most satisfactory type of transfer. The proximal portion of the tendon retracts into the joint and sometimes constitutes a source of internal derangement because it lies loose. At the time of transplantation of the ruptured portion, the bicipital groove should be explored and, if feasible, the proximal segment should be excised.

Surgical Technique. A longitudinal incision extending from just above the coracoid process along the bicipital groove to the midpoint of the arm is carried out. As this incision is deepened, palpation in the distal portion will identify the coiled-up biceps tendon. Care is taken in dissecting the tendon free from the encysting fibrotic reaction. The proximal portion of the belly of the biceps

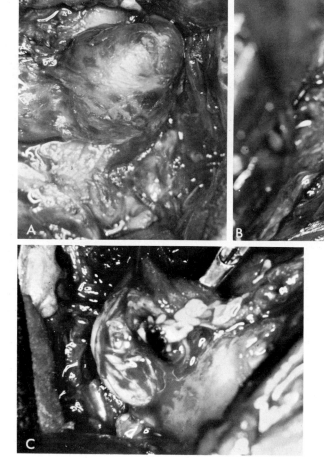

Figure 8–76 Rupture of the long head of the biceps. *A,* The tendon recoils distally and becomes encysted. *B,* The "cyst" is incised, revealing the coiled-up tendon. *C,* The tendon may be dissected out of the cyst and straightened for transplantation to the coracoid. The longer the tendon remains in the encysted state, the more difficult it is to effect this.

is carefully mobilized because the fibrosis extends downward for some distance. Care is taken to avoid injury to the nerve supply of the biceps from the musculocutaneous nerve, which reaches it along the lateral bicipital groove.

Mobilization allows the tendon to be stretched and, as a rule, with the elbow flexed enough length is obtained to pull the tendon under the deltoid to be attached to the coracoid. The tendon is split and a small hole is drilled in the coracoid through which one of the split segments is threaded and tied to the other.

In mobilizing the tendon distally, care must also be taken to avoid injury to the circumflex nerve reaching the deltoid from the medial aspect on the undersurface.

Postoperative Care. Postoperatively the arm is placed in a sling. Shoulder motion is initiated early, but active use of the tendon is delayed for three weeks until the wound is healed and the anchoring sutures are solidly fixed.

Technique of Repair in Late Cases. Transplantation of the head to the coracoid is difficult when the lesion is of many months' standing. The process of fibrosis and encystment, which envelops the retracted distal segment of the tendon, usually makes it difficult to find sufficient substance to carry out the transfer. If it is wished to persevere with this maneuver, the tendon can be elongated by a piece of fascia lata removed from the thigh and laced into the musculotendinous junction. In this way prolongation of the tendon can be obtained, and it is then feasible to reach the coracoid process for fixation in the same fashion. Such a repair is not nearly so strong as when there is enough length of biceps tendon, but it does provide a degree of improvement in strength and also improves the appearance (Fig. 8–77).

Ruptures of Biceps Tendon and Rotator Cuff Plus Nerve Damage

Attention is called to a serious injury belonging to this group of tendon cuff disturbances which has not been emphasized heretofore. It involves rupture of the biceps tendon, often extensive damage to the rotator cuff and, in addition, a varying degree of brachial plexus paralysis. This syndrome is almost invariably encountered in an elderly patient. The history of injury is characteristic and frequently is the clue to the damaging process. The patient slips and, in losing balance, falls backward, so that the weight of the body is taken on the outstretched arm, which has been placed backward. This will have forced the head of the humerus forward and upward, so that it escapes the protection of the overhanging coraco-acromial arch (see Fig. 3–19). The maximum stress is then taken on the long head of the biceps, the shoulder capsule and the anteromedial soft tissues. Sometimes the shoulder subluxes or partially dislocates. Invariably there is extensive ecchymosis over the anteromedial aspect of the shoulder

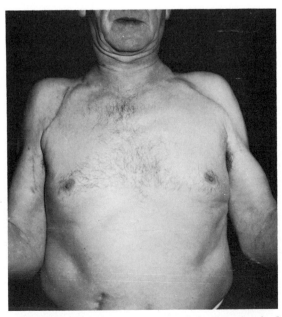

Figure 8–77 Bilateral rupture of the long head of the biceps. The right side has been repaired, with improvement in contour and power.

and adjacent chest areas, indicating extensive soft tissue disruption. Examination shows damage to the rotator cuff, weakness or rupture of the biceps and variable nerve damage. Paralysis of the deltoid and partial median or musculocutaneous lesions are often encountered.

Treatment. The combination of tendon damage and paralysis not only produces a serious disability, but the interaction decreases the effectiveness of treatment of all components. The nerve damage is a stretching or bruising, a lesion in continuity, which recovers with adequate conservative treatment that includes electrical stimulation and muscle education. The cuff and tendon damage remain disabling, and operative treatment is directed toward these.

Acute Stage. Any dislocation or subluxation is reduced, and the arm is immobilized in a light shoulder spica. Care must be taken to be sure that the dislocation remains reduced because the tendon and capsule damage leave a very lax joint, and it is possible to have subluxation or dislocation occur within the plaster. The importance of this complication in all dislocations cannot be too strongly emphasized because the nerve damage may be increased. It is also important to look for nerve damage beforehand, rather than have to assume later that it happened beneath the plaster. The upper half of the plaster is cut at the end of two weeks and physiotherapy, including electrical stimulation and assisted active exercise is started. Sometimes the age and activity of the patient are such that this conservative program is all that should be carried out. The plaster is removed at the end of six weeks and physiotherapy is continued.

Later Stages. When the circumstances and age of the patient are such that use of the arm is needed for carrying on an occupation, reconstruction of the capsule and tendon damage is carried out.

Technique. The shoulder is approached through the supero-anterior incision, and the capsule tendon region is exposed. As a rule the cuff is more extensively damaged than the biceps tendon. Attention is focused on restoring this as well as possible. Depending on the extent of rupture, it may be repaired by mobilization and the insertion of mattress sutures, or it may be necessary to use fascia, as outlined previously (see repair of ruptured cuff). Repairing the cuff and transplanting the biceps tendon is an extensive procedure and may tax the patient's general condition at one operation. The operator must be guided by the individual's reaction at the time. In repairing the cuff, if the biceps tendon is still intact but loose, the intertubercular fibers can be reconstructed so that the tendon is retained in its groove (see Fig. 8–60). This is an important step since the stability afforded by the tendon improves the abductor power markedly. When there has been frank rupture of the tendon in addition to the cuff damage, transplantation to the coracoid is recommended.

Postoperative Regimen. Sometimes it is preferable to have these patients in a light abduction plaster for two to three weeks because of the extensive soft tissue damage and shoulder laxity. The upper half of the plaster is removed soon after operation, and particular attention is paid to the elbow and hand movements, so that reflex dystrophy does not develop, particularly in the older age group. A light shoulder spica with the arm bivalved or a cantilever splint is applied for three weeks. Hand and forearm movement is started early, the shoulder being lowered gradually until active shoulder movement can be started.

ACROMIOCLAVICULAR ARTHRITIS

Pain localized to the shoulder sometimes arises from arthritis in the acromioclavicular joint; this is accompanied by a characteristic group of findings. Unless careful examination is done, acromioclavicular arthritis can be overlooked and cuff disturbances diagnosed in error.

SIGNS AND SYMPTOMS

The joint normally shows considerable variation in contour, but the two sides are usually the same. The joint line has varying degrees of obliquity and often there is a large, bulbous end of the clavicle (Fig. 8–78). Injury and degeneration are the common causes of acromioclavicular disruption. There is aching pain in the general shoulder area which the patients do not, as a rule, recognize as coming from the top, but rather implicates the general shoulder region. The patient is uncomfortable when sleeping on the sore side. Sharp pain is noted after the arm is

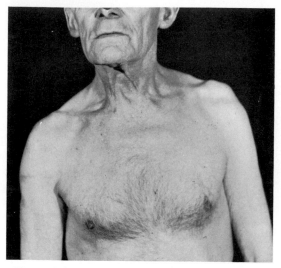

Figure 8–78 Marked distortion of the outer end of the clavicle in acromioclavicular arthritis.

raised to a right angle. Activities below the shoulder level do not cause discomfort, but once the arm is elevated above the right angle, the pain is acute. The arc or zone in which this pain is felt contrasts sharply with that caused by cuff lesions like degenerative tendinitis, in which the pain occurs at a lower level just as the tuberosity is swinging under the arch.

Examination of the superior aspect of the shoulder elicits tenderness over the joint line; often there is some irregularity of the end of the clavicle. Sometimes crepitus can be felt as the arm is abducted above a right angle. Occasionally a jumping sensation is experienced as a result of the slipping of the lateral end of the clavicle. A characteristic sign is the production of pain by passive flexing of the arm across the chest at a right angle. This maneuver rubs the acromion and clavicle together as the acromion follows a crescentic course along the lateral end of the clavicle. Crepitus is also often apparent as this is carried out and is accompanied by pain. There may be considerable joint destruction without significant alteration in the skin contour. Some joints appear subluxed or dislocated when actually there is a little enlargement of the end of the clavicle only, without articular damage. Acute pain is reproduced by pressure over the clavicle with one hand and elevation of the acromion by pushing up on the elbow with the other, thereby causing the joint surfaces to rub together (Fig. 8–79).

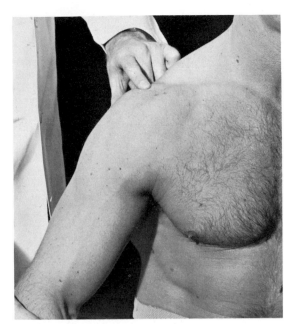

Figure 8–79 Tender point in acromioclavicular arthritis.

ETIOLOGY AND PATHOLOGY

The commonest cause of acromioclavicular discomfort is posttraumatic arthritis. As a part of the overhanging coraco-acromial arch, the joint is exposed to trauma from above and from below. This region of the shoulder is used in carrying, holding, levering, and so forth, so that it is commonly susceptible to occupational stress. Blows on the shoulder tend to be taken in this general region, too, so that the joint is actually in a somewhat vulnerable area. Significant symptoms do not appear until roughening and narrowing of the joint are moderately well established. In elevating the arm, motion at this joint does not occur until the scapula starts to rotate with the humerus and the clavicle fixed; this occurs at about 85 to 90 degrees (see Figs. 3–5 and 3–6). For this reason, abnormalities of the joint cause maximum pain in the arc above a right angle, which helps to distinguish them from other shoulder disorders. Anatomically there is broad variation in the size of the contiguous facets, the angle of the joint and the site of articulation. Structural abnormalities, which may show up on routine x-rays, are not significant unless accompanied by signs and symptoms (Fig. 8–80).

A somewhat similar clinical picture results from the congenital deformity of coraco-clavicular bar (see Chapter I). In these circumstances there is a bar of bone extending from the clavicle down to the coracoid process; somewhere along the bar there is an articulation at a point between the clavicle and the coracoid process. The strut acts as an obstruction to rotation of the clavicle during shoulder girdle circumduction, and discomfort arises in the later zones of abduction (see Congenital Anomalies of the Scapula, Chapter I).

TREATMENT

The principle of treatment is to avoid irritation of the acromioclavicular joint. When overhead work and similar activities can be decreased, considerable relief is obtained. For those people, who wish to carry on without being hampered in movement or by pain, acromioclavicular arthroplasty is the most satisfactory solution. This operation was popularized by F. B. Gurd and provides effective relief. It is not an extensive procedure, and the period of incapacity is short. Obliteration of the acromioclavicular joint by arthrodesis is not recommended because it hampers the movement of circumduction. During the phase of circumduction, movement occurs at the acromioclavicular joint; if the acromion has been fixed to the clavicle, the circumduction range may be decreased by 15 to 20 degrees.

Technique of Acromioclavicular Arthroplasty

The patient is given a general anesthetic and placed in the sitting shoulder position. A supero-anterior incision 3 inches long is made just medial to the acromioclavicular joint. The acromioclavicular capsule is incised and an osseoperiosteal flap is raised from the lateral ¾ inch of the clavicle and reflected medially. This flap is preserved for closure after the joint has been resected.

At this point the possibility of associated capsular contracture should be assessed. A frequent development with acromioclavicular arthritis is some degree of adhesive capsulitis. When this is present, gentle manipulation of the humerus in the glenoid is carried out, with pressure maintained on the head as passive rotation is done. By maintaining pressure in the head and doing the rotation with care, it is possible to gently free adhesions and avoid rupture of the cuff. When the adhesions are extensive or this

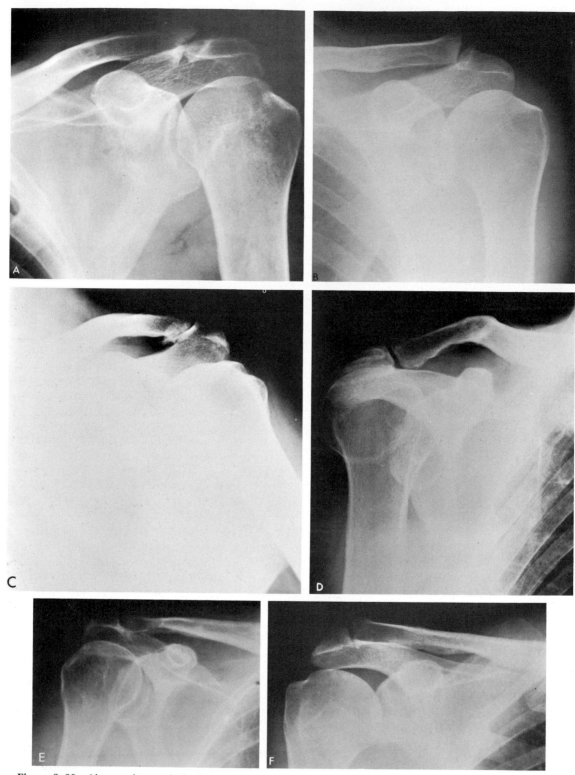

Figure 8–80 Abnormal acromioclavicular joints. *A*, Subluxation with arthritis. *B*, Posttraumatic arthritis. *C*, Osteoarthritis. *D*, Normal joint lines. *E* and *F*, Marked spur formations.

maneuver is carried out in blind fashion, the cuff may be ruptured, adding considerably to the impairment.

A general anesthetic is preferable, although the operation can be done under local anesthesia (Figs. 8–48 and 8–49). The acromioclavicular joint and the outer half inch of clavicle are exposed. The outer 1/2 to 3/4 inch of the clavicle is denuded and freed by subperiosteal dissection. This piece of clavicle is excised cleanly. The principle is to put the acromioclavicular joint out of action and yet leave the clavicle stable. Stability is most important, and care is exercised to remove not more than the outer 1/2 to 3/4 inch so that the suspensory, coranoid and trapezoid ligaments are preserved. If the suspensory ligaments are cut, major disability results from shoulder laxity and instability. Coagulant gauze is packed along the outer end of the clavicle to diminish osteophyte formation (Fig. 8–81).

After the outer half inch of the clavicle has been cut free, it is pulled out of the capsule, usually preserving the posterior fibers which serve as a stabilizing factor and do not contribute obstruction to the overhanging swing of the head of the humerus.

Postoperative Regimen. The arm is suspended for 24 hours and then supported in a sling for seven to ten days. Active motion is started immediately. Frequently there is a degree of adhesive capsulitis; in these cases longer supervision is required. If the freezing has been extensive, the patient should be immobilized in a cantilever splint for a week or two to be certain that capsular adhesions do not recur. The patient with this problem can usually be treated as for a Grade I cuff tear; he will require systemic medication such as phenylbutazone along with physiotherapeutic supervision for six to eight weeks.

Treatment of Coracoclavicular Joint

This anomaly may be noted as an incidental finding on routine chest examination and may be present without causing significant disturbance. As a rule when symptoms develop, considerable sclerosis of the articulation is apparent. The treatment of choice is excision of the bar of bone, including the joint (see Chapter I).

Technique. The coracoclavicular articulation is approached through a linear incision parallel to and just distal to the middle third of the clavicle. By blunt dissection the coracoid process is exposed and the obstructing bar traced to the clavicle. The bar is exposed and an appropriate portion excised, care being taken again to preserve the suspensory ligaments. The site of excision is packed with Surgicel to minimize spur formation.

Postoperatively the arm is supported in a sling until the wound is healed. Physiotherapy consisting mainly of assisted active glenohumeral motion is started and continued for seven to ten days with care being taken to avoid irritating the excision site.

ARTHRITIS OF THE GLENOHUMERAL JOINT

The shoulder joint is less frequently afflicted by the common forms of arthritis than are many other joints; however, it is susceptible to posttraumatic, osteo, rheumatoid and tuberculous arthritis. Acute infectious arthritis and metabolic arthritis are much less common. Arthritis of the shoulder produces pain that is well localized to the shoulder point and is aggravated by shoulder movement; tenderness is localized to the joint zone. These findings separate the arthritides from disturbances of the neck because of the lack of relation to neck movements, and from conditions causing radiating pain because of the distribution of the discomfort.

POSTTRAUMATIC ARTHRITIS

Serious injury to the head of the humerus or glenoid is the commonest cause of arthritis in the shoulder. It develops following fractures of the head or anatomical neck of the humerus or fractures of the glenoid. Injuries producing distortion of the head of the humerus are the commonest source (Fig. 8–1).

Signs and Symptoms

In contrast to knee and hip, it takes some little time for arthritis changes to reach clinical proportions after injury to the shoulder. There may be considerable distortion of the head, malunion following fractures, for instance, with no incapacitating symptoms developing for some time. This is because of the configuration of the joint

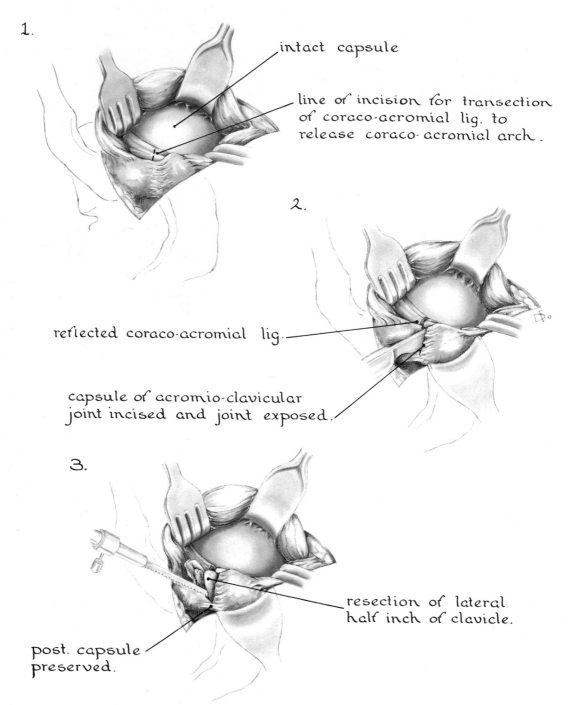

1.

intact capsule

line of incision for transection
of coraco-acromial lig. to
release coraco-acromial arch.

2.

reflected coraco-acromial lig.

capsule of acromio-clavicular
joint incised and joint exposed.

3.

resection of lateral
half inch of clavicle.

post. capsule
preserved.

Figure 8–81   Operative technique for acromioclavicular arthroplasty.

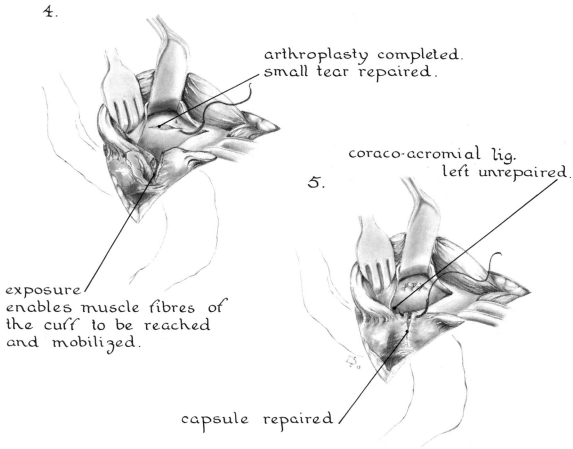

4.

arthroplasty completed.
small tear repaired.

coraco-acromial lig.
left unrepaired.

5.

exposure
enables muscle fibres of
the cuff to be reached
and mobilized.

capsule repaired

Figure 8–81 *Continued.*

surfaces, which are not nearly so intimately applied to each other as is the case of the hip and knee. The laxity of the joint is also a buffer, and since it is not a weight-bearing articulation, constant stress is not present as an irritant. Frequently the patient has learned to avoid the several movements which may initiate the pain, and the natural laxity of the joint accommodates motion sufficiently to prevent acute distress. Considerable limitation of movement may be made up for by increased mobility at the accessory joints of the shoulder. This maneuver, accompanied by adaptation of the soft parts, allows the patient to perform many activities without distress. Obvious deformity of the head can be made out on palpation, rotating the head beneath the palpating hand.

Etiology and Pathology

Fractures and malunion result in incongruous articulating areas, and the articular cartilage becomes scratched and eroded, eventually disappearing in places. The changes occur most frequently in the head of the humerus, and the glenoid fossa, as a rule, does not reflect damage to the same extent. This is because the whole head of the humerus is not in contact with the glenoid and may not be constantly exposed to the irregular, roughened regions.

Treatment

The principle of treatment is to avoid the painful zone of movement. If this can be done simply by limiting the activities of the patient, sufficient relief may be produced. Most of the time patients demand more than this, so that either arthroplasty or arthrodesis should be carried out.

Technique of Arthrodesis. Arthrodesis of the shoulder in cases of posttraumatic arthritis is not nearly so difficult as, for example, in the case of neurotrophic disease. There are several effective methods, and the selection depends upon the surgeon's preference. An intra-articular procedure can be done. The joint is exposed from the front or from above, the head of the humerus is denuded of cartilage, and the glenoid fossa is similarly treated. Heavy wood screws may be used as an additional support, being placed on either side of the graft and drilled through the head of the humerus into the glenoid. The position of maximum function is 60 degrees abduction, 10 to 15 degrees flexion and some internal rotation.

POSTERIOR ARTHRODESIS. The technique of arthrodesis preferred by the author and popularized by Dr. Joseph Davis is fusion from the posterior aspect, utilizing the acromion as the bone graft.

The patient is placed either in the sitting shoulder position or lying on the opposite side. The aim is to have the shoulder clearly exposed from back, top and front, and the arm draped free at the side for proper positioning.

A curvilinear incision is made from the base of the scapular spine, along it, and reaching over the acromion anteriorly. The principle is to osteotomize the acromion and use it as a graft inserted in key fashion into the top of the humerus across the glenoid. Cutting the acromion provides an excellent exposure and free access to all aspects of the joint.

The cortical surfaces of the glenoid and the head of humerus are removed and suitably approximated. A trough of sufficient width, approximately 5/16 inch wide, is cut into the glenoid from the top and continued across the joint into the humeral head for a distance of 1½ inches. The detached piece of acromion is then fitted into this slot, locking the glenoid and humerus together in the desired position. In some instances, as emphasized by Davis, the soft tissue is left attached to the acromial graft so that a pedicle graft is utilized.

In carrying out shoulder fusion it is extremely helpful to have prepared beforehand the abduction plaster for immobilization after the operation; then it can be slipped onto the patient without difficulty when the operation is finished. If this procedure is followed, it is a considerable help also to be certain that the proper degree of abduction and forward flexion is attained; this facilitates the completion of the procedure.

OSTEOARTHRITIS OF THE SHOULDER

As in all other joints, this type of arthritis develops from two sources: progressive wear and tear or the aging process of degeneration, and posttraumatic reaction. The underlying changes are similar in both, but because of the extreme mobility and lack of weight bearing, symptoms do not appear so quickly or so severely as they do in hip and knee. The degenerative or true osteoarthritic process arises from progressive disturbance initiated by primary soft tissue injury. Wearing, tearing and fraying of the cuff and biceps tendon scrape and roughen articular cartilage, interfering with movement (Fig. 8–82).

Signs and Symptoms

Osteoarthritis of the shoulder produces persistent localized shoulder pain which is aggravated by movement of the arm. It is not related to cervical movement, nor do significant radiating symptoms develop. There is gradual limitation of motion, increasing pain at night, a grating sensation, atrophy of the muscles and eventual limitation of all movements. On examination tenderness is present diffusely over the joint. Passive movement demonstrates altered articular contours and crepitus. X-rays usually show gross change in the articular surfaces, often with subchondral cystic formation, cartilage erosion and tear-drop osteophytes on the inferior surfaces.

Etiology and Pathology

The degenerative type arises from the progressive disturbance initiated by soft tissue injury. As indicated under injuries of cuff and biceps tendon, damage to these soft tissues alters the normal function and introduces obstacles to movement. The frayed or ruptured cuff favors roughening of the smooth cartilage and gradual erosion. Abnormalities in the biceps fixation result in unaccustomed pressure on the humeral head, with blistering and pebbling of the adjacent articular surface. Because of the extensive mobility, the patient is able to avoid rubbing roughened surfaces together, so that the course of this disease is toward soft tissue fixation and freezing rather than extensive lipping and spur formation (Fig. 8–83).

Treatment

The management of these cases depends a great deal on the occupation, the age and the activities of the patient. In older patients

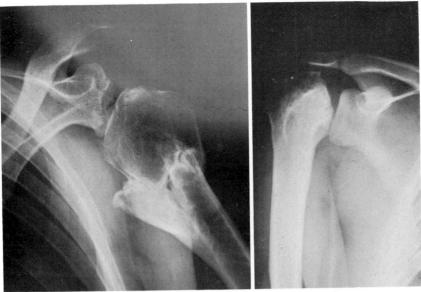

Figure 8–82 Examples of posttraumatic arthritis of the shoulder due to fractures through the head and neck of the humerus, and posttraumatic glenohumeral arthritis.

who lead a sedentary existence a conservative program only is indicated. Pain is avoided by limiting movement and activity, and a light sedative relieves any acute discomfort. Some movement is encouraged to prevent freezing, but this should be kept within the limits of the pain threshold. Such movement is desirable also to prevent secondary vascu-

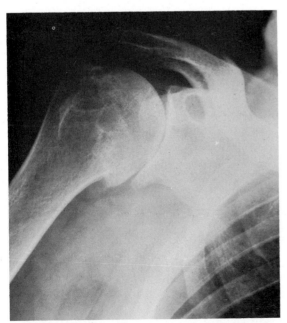

Figure 8–83 Degenerative arthritis of the shoulder, decreased joint space, lipping of humerus and glenoid and avascular-appearing head.

lar and reflex dystrophy changes in the hand and fingers.

In younger, more active people and those who must use the extremity in earning a livelihood, operative treatment may be indicated. Osteoarthritic changes are so often accompanied by extensive soft tissue damage that arthrodesis may be desirable to provide stability as well as to decrease the pain. The shoulder is fixed at 55 to 60 degrees abduction and 15 to 20 degrees flexion; this provides a painless stable base for the action of forearm and hand and is quite satisfactory, particularly for laborers.

Technique of Arthrodesis. As a rule, an intra-articular arthrodesis is done; the principles are excision of the cartilaginous surfaces and adequate transfixion supported by bone grafts. There are many good methods embodying these principles. (See also following arthroplasty technique.)

WATSON-JONES TECHNIQUE. This is an excellent method of arthrodesis (Fig. 8–84A). It involves preparing a bony flap of the outer portion of the acromion and the clavicle, which are partially fractured so that they may be bent down and fitted into a transverse trough, fish-mouthwise, in the head of the humerus. Up to this point it is an extra-articular procedure and may be supplemented by preparation of the humerus and glenoid cavity in the usual fashion.

PUTTI PROCEDURE. This differs from the

Watson-Jones procedure in that the flap from the spine and the acromion is fashioned by splitting the portion of the spine longitudinally and sliding this separate posterior piece into a trough for the upper end of the humerus.

GILL TECHNIQUE. This technique is similar to the preceding procedures, but the acromion is prepared by roughening top and bottom surfaces. The joint surfaces are denuded of cartilage and the upper aspect of the humerus is split to receive the tongue-like process of the acromion (Fig. 8–84*B*).

BRITTAIN PROCEDURE. This is an extra-articular scapulohumeral arthrodesis by an ingenious technique. It embodies the application of a massive graft from the tibia which is fixed in a hole in the humerus and in a slot in the lateral border of the scapula. The procedure is done with the patient prone and the affected arm hanging over the edge of the operating table. An incision is made over the posterior axillary area in an L-shaped fashion. A hole is drilled in the medial aspect of the humerus and an arrow-shaped graft is fashioned from the tibia. The graft is inserted in the slot in the scapula and wedged into the hole in the humerus (Fig. 8–84*C*).

Posterior Arthrodesis. In many conditions for which arthrodesis of the shoulder is required the author has found it desirable to carry out the procedure from the posterior aspect. Significant advantages are apparent. Dr. Joseph Davis introduced a technique for posterior arthrodesis using a pedicle graft of acromion and inserting it posteriorly into the glenoid and head of the humerus. The author has used a similar technique but has not used the pedicle graft.

TECHNIQUE. The patient is placed on the operating table lying partly on his face and with the diseased side upward. The entire upper extremity is prepared along with an area extending to the midline posteriorly. The shoulder is approached through a transverse incision curved slightly forward but made along the upper border of the spine of the scapula and extending from the root of the spine to beyond the acromion laterally; this incision is deepened. The muscular attachments are then retracted from the acromion and the adjacent spine of the scapula for a distance of 1½ inches medially. The spine is osteotomized at this point, and the acromion and this part of the spine are then used as a graft to be inserted later.

A trough is then cut through the head of the humerus and into the glenoid which is now most adequately exposed with the removal of the acromion. Soft tissues are removed and the trough is deepened to a sufficient length to receive the graft formed by the acromion. The trough is cut about 5/16 of an inch wide and should be about 2 inches in length. If there are extensive irregularities the surfaces of the glenoid and the head of the humerus may be shaved and approximated to the proper angle in creating the trough for the graft.

The head of the humerus and the glenoid should be placed in proper apposition 60 degrees abduction, 30 degrees forward flexion and neutral rotation prior to inserting the graft. Once the tough has been cut the graft is then fashioned to proper size and tacked into the trough, locking the head of the humerus to the glenoid. The outer ½ inch of the clavicle is excised. The soft tissues are then closed firmly and the arm is placed in a previously prepared spica at the desired angle of arthrodesis.

Postoperative Management. In all these procedures the shoulder is immobilized in a plaster spica at the desired angle, and fixation is maintained for 12 to 16 weeks. Since these are long procedures, it is preferable to have the plaster prepared beforehand or to use prepared plaster patterns which can be applied quickly at the time of completion of the operation (Figs. 8–85 and 8–86).

Arthroplasty of the Shoulder. In post-traumatic and osteoarthritis, when capsule and muscles have not deteriorated and the patient is anxious to preserve movement, arthroplasty may be used. It is not recommended if there has been extensive damage to the rotator cuff because merely improving the articular surface will not provide the power and control needed for good active movement. It is a major operation to be done only if the general condition of the patient warrants. Fullest cooperation and stubborn persistence on the part of the patient are essential in the postoperative regimen. Reconstruction of the shoulder is more difficult than the hip because of the vital part played by the rotator cuff and the shoulder muscles. Care is necessary to preserve the cuff or to repair it if necessary to prevent mediocre results. In the hip, on the other hand, preservation of the intimate joint structures is not so essential and important muscles are so disposed at a distance that they do not interfere

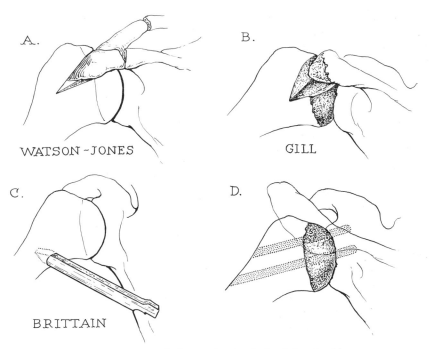

A. WATSON-JONES

B. GILL

C. BRITTAIN

D.

Figure 8–84   Techniques of arthrodesis of the shoulder.

or may be easily reconstructed. Shoulder muscles should be innervated and functioning satisfactorily before operation.

Prime indications for arthroplasty include comminuted fractures of the head of the humerus, posttraumatic arthritis, osteoarthritis and rheumatoid arthritis. Fractures of the head often leave an incongruous surface, impairing cuff function. For this reason the author advises arthrography in these cases before an arthroplasty. In this way any extensive cuff damage is revealed, and reconstruction can be planned accordingly. It may be necessary to repair the cuff first before correcting the joint deformity.

TECHNIQUE.   Pioneer work in this field has been done by Dr. C. S. Neer. He is responsible for the development of successful operative techniques and a standard stem prosthesis. The principle of shoulder arthroplasty is to renovate joint surfaces in such a way that capsule and cuff structures are

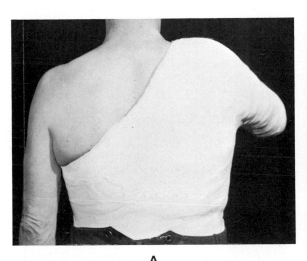

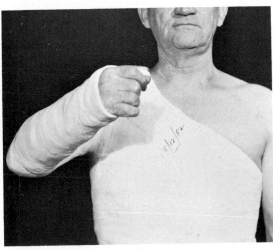

A

B

Figure 8–85   *A,* Postoperative result of posterior method of fusion. *B,* Proper fixation following arthrodesis of humerus of shoulder.

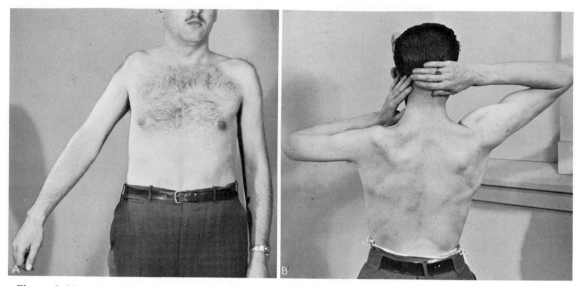

Figure 8–86 *A,* In adults, fusion angle may be lowered somewhat, leaving a useful extremity with the patient able to reach his pocket and posteriorly more easily. *B,* Range of motion possible when arthrodesis is carried out at the standard angle. Children usually show much greater powers of adaptation, and the preferred position remains approximately 60 degrees abduction.

preserved with as little disturbance as possible. It is essential to convert these to as workable a state as possible and to carry out repair meticulously.

Neer Technique. A 5-inch incision is made over the deltopectoral interval, starting at the clavicle and curving outward sufficiently to avoid crossing the axillary skinfold. The deltopectoral interval is identified, and the cephalic vein ligated and removed. The anterior 2 inches of the deltoid are detached from the clavicle and retracted laterally; sufficient tissue is left on the clavicle to facilitate repair of this muscle. The coracoid may be divided for better exposure, but this is usually not necessary.

The subscapularis tendon is secured with a stay suture and detached from the lesser tuberosity. The anterior half of the glenohumeral joint is exposed by blunt dissection with great care to avoid injury to the axillary nerve, which lies against the capsule inferiorly. The anterior half of the capsule along with the glenohumeral ligaments is then divided. The long head of the biceps is detached from the superior glenoid and this tendon is withdrawn from the bicipital groove. The arm is then externally rotated, delivering the humeral head forward into full view. The portion of the head normally covered by articular cartilage is removed with a broad osteotome. Marginal excrescences, when present, are first removed to identify this level; otherwise, osteophytes inferiorly

tend to mislead the operator into excessive removal of the neck.

The medullary canal is identified with a long instrument (such as a Nicola gouge). A prosthesis is selected which permits seating to within 1½ inches by hand. Reaming or gouging of the medullary canal is rarely necessary. The articular surface is placed in 20 degrees retroversion and the prosthesis is protected from erosion with a saline sponge as it is driven into the medullary canal. Just prior to final seating, prominences may be trimmed from the neck for more accurate contact. The joint is then irrigated and the arm is internally rotated, causing the replacement to virtually disappear from view as it points backward toward the scapula. In osteoarthritis, although glenoid osteophytes are often seen radiologically, they have with one exception been left undisturbed. When the lesion is of long standing, no attempt is made to repair the capsule. The subscapularis is accurately sutured to the lesser tuberosity with chromic catgut. The biceps tendon is anchored in the bicipital groove and the excess tendon removed. The deltoid is reattached to the clavicle, and the fascia is closed with interrupted sutures.

Postoperative Care. A sling and swathe are applied in the operating room, except in posterior fracture dislocations, in which case the arm is immediately suspended in abduction and slight external rotation. Mobilization varies according to the specific problem.

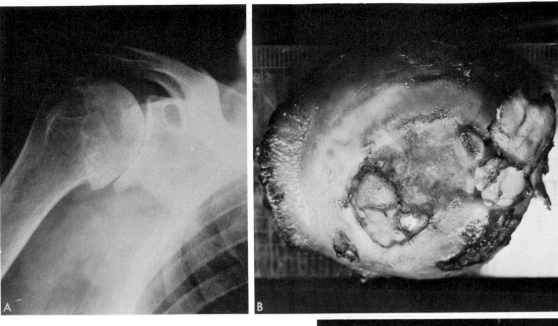

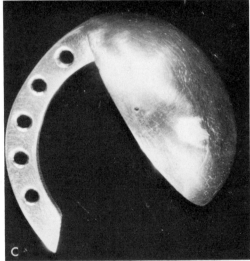

Figure 8–87 Arthroplasty of the shoulder. *A*, Osteoarthritis well established. *B*, Articular changes in resected head. *C*, Cortical fixation type prosthesis. Perforated arch penetrates cortex and is fixed in this position.

Pendulum exercises are started, as a rule, after 48 hours, but abduction and external rotation are postponed until after the third week when the attachment of the subscapularis tendon is felt to be adequate to allow a full exercise program. After the fifth day the arm is permitted freedom during the daytime, but a sling and swathe are used at night for three weeks. Wall climbing and forward elevation with the pulley are started after the first three weeks. A full program of limbering and, later, strengthening exercises is followed progressively after the third week.

(*Comment:* The author has used the Neer prosthesis but has not found it necessary to remove the long head of the biceps and has preferred to repair the cuff carefully afterward.)

Bateman Technique. A sitting shoulder posture is used and a utility incision extending over the shoulder just medial to the acromioclavicular joint is made. The incision is 5 inches long, starting 1 inch behind the clavicle, going over the lateral end and extending distally along the line of the fibers of the deltoid muscle. The deltoid fibers are retracted and joint surfaces are inspected to plan reconstruction. Further exposure is necessary and, as a rule, this is best obtained by doing an acromioclavicular arthroplasty in routine fashion. The coraco-acromial ligament is resected. An incision is made in the anterior portion of the capsule medial to the subscapularis insertion and bicipital groove. This is extended distally far enough to allow the articular surface to be brought into view. As the humerus is externally rotated and abducted through this incision, the long head of the biceps remains in its groove and is retracted superiorly.

The arthroplasty is started by carrying out the reconstruction of the humeral head first. Gross irregularities are removed with the reciprocating saw or the power grinder. The head is resected at a point which is gauged by placing the prosthesis beside the head, with the stem along the shaft of the humerus. Care is taken to stop the cut of the humeral head before it reaches the tuberosity and cuff insertions. Removal of the head allows free access to the glenoid.

The glenoid is then debrided but, as a rule, not much modeling is required. The surface can be smoothed with the power burr.

When a stem prosthesis is used, a cut is made in the cancellous layer in the shape of the triangular stem to allow a start and it is then pounded firmly into place. As a rule the stem proceeds through the cancellous layers without further resection; this also allows a firm grip by the bone on the stem. The capsule is then carefully sewn and the wound is closed in layers.

Various models of prosthesis can be used. The author has constructed a prosthesis with a shorter stem and also designed one that transfixes the cortex (Fig. 8–88) rather than being inserted into the medullary canal. The latter is much easier to insert and appears most useful in arthroplasty for arthritis.

Fractures with extensive shattering of the head can be better handled with the stem type of prosthesis. The approach, capsular repair and postoperative management are the same regardless of the precise configuration of the prosthesis that is used.

Postoperative Routine. The arm is placed in suspension at a right angle for 48 hours and then the cantilever brace is applied. Across the chest, right-angled movement is initiated at once, but abduction, flexion and rotation are not started for three weeks, by which time the capsule and wound are usually healed. A program of gradual lowering of the brace, along with active and assisted active motion is started; the brace is usually discarded at six to eight weeks. In-hospital patients are kept in springs and slings until they are well enough to be ambulatory and

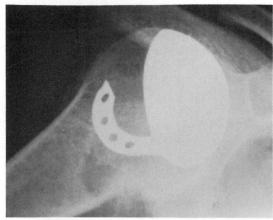
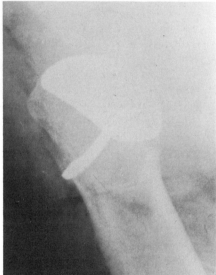

Figure 8–88 Radiographic appearance of prosthesis after insertion in a case of osteoarthritis.

use the brace when up and about (Fig. 8–89). For the first five days they sleep with the arm in suspension and, after that, lower it onto pillows at the side. A program of constant encouragement and conscientious therapy is essential to obtain a good result following all these procedures. The continuing effect of gravity in pulling the arm to the side poses a constant threat of infra-articular adhesion formation, and this would significantly limit the amount of motion that could be obtained.

RHEUMATOID ARTHRITIS OF SHOULDER

The shoulder is not commonly involved in atrophic or rheumatoid arthritis; this is al-

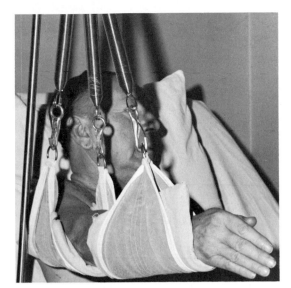

Figure 8–89 Slings and springs fixation for postoperative treatment in prosthetic arthroplasty.

most always a late complication after many other joints have been afflicted. The history and development are straightforward, with pain, tenderness and limitation of movement developing. There is obvious involvement of other joints; eventually gross limi-

tation of shoulder movement and atrophy of the muscles occur (Fig. 8–91).

Treatment

Systemic Therapy. See the treatment for rheumatoid arthritis outlined in Chapter XV.

TREATMENT OF THE JOINT. During the acute phase the joint should be splinted in the position of function, 50 to 60 degrees abduction, with slight flexion and in the midposition of rotation. The joint must not be allowed to become stiff at the side or fixed in internal rotation. A light plaster bivalved splint may be used, but the cantilever base is much better.

Reconstruction or arthroplasty is unsatisfactory unless it can be done at a very early stage after subsidence of the acute phase, provided the acute phase has been short. Shoulder movement is so dependent on muscle function that, as a rule, the motors are very poor after a prolonged period of immobilization. Replacement arthroplasty has not been extensively applied for these reasons also, but may prove to be of some

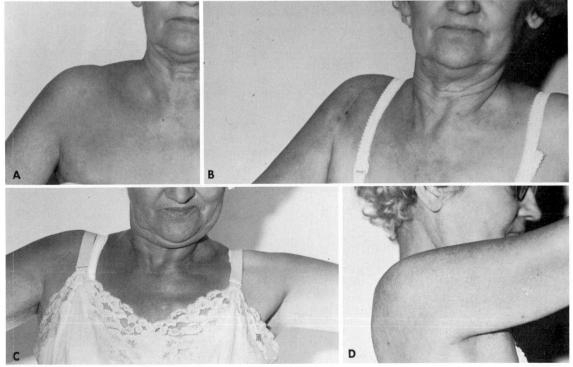

Figure 8–90 Postoperative result of arthroplasty. *A,* Two weeks after operation. *B,* Healed incision (three weeks). *C,* Six weeks. *D,* Twelve weeks.

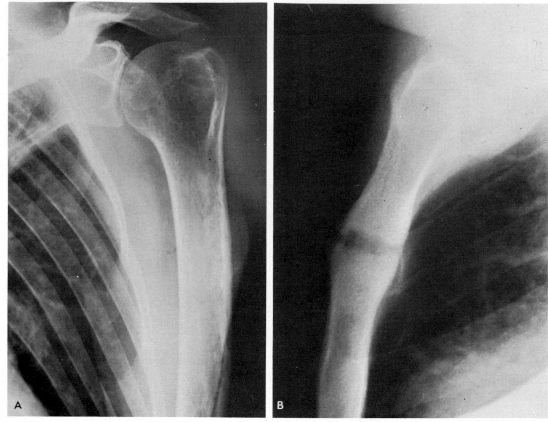

Figure 8–91 Rheumatoid arthritis of the shoulder. *A*, Note extensive atrophy and scalloping of internal cortex line and atrophy of the shoulder girdle. *B*, Associated change in the sternum.

use when there is more effective control of the acute stage.

TUBERCULOSIS OF THE SHOULDER (Caries Sicca)

This entity is now extremely rare. Tuberculosis does occur in the shoulder but is not common. Probably less than 1 per cent of cases of bone and joint tuberculosis involve the shoulder.

Cardinal Signs and Symptoms

Two distinct types are recognized. The most commonly encountered is the caries sicca type, which occurs in adults. It is ushered in by discomfort that gradually increases until any movement is painful. Pain is localized to the shoulder without involvement of the neck or significant peripheral radiation; it is quickly followed by limitation of movement in all directions, and this

continues until the joint is almost completely fixed. Extensive atrophy of the muscle occurs, and the only movement possible is a girdle type of action. The x-rays are characteristic, showing decalcification of the humerus and the scapula, narrowing of the joint space, cystic formation in the humerus and absence of new bone formation (Fig. 8–92). The insidious progress of the changes is characteristic.

Pathology

The disease starts as a focus in the margin of the head of the humerus, producing cystic formation and erosion at the point of attachment of the capsule. This results in a characteristic punched-out appearance on x-rays. The process is not a suppurative one, which accounts for the term sicca, indicating a low-grade subacute, shriveling process. In children the disease follows a more acute and devastating course, with the development of swelling, pain, fever and synovial thickening.

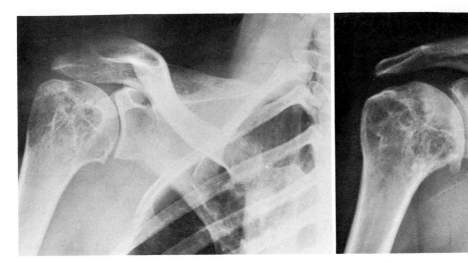

Figure 8–92 Tuberculosis of the shoulder.

There is extensive decalcification and the joint space is obliterated, but less cystic formation is seen than in the adult form.

Differential Diagnosis

Giant Cell Tumor. The cystic appearance which is sometimes encountered in caries sicca can be confused with giant cell tumor. The involvement of the glenoid, obliteration of the joint space and extreme atrophy clearly differentiate the two lesions.

Infectious Arthritis. Staphylococcal arthritis or other pyogenic foci in the shoulder are rare and run a much more acute course in contrast to the extensive bone atrophy which is characteristic of tuberculosis. There is sclerosis and production of new bone in the pyogenic process. Usually little difficulty is encountered in distinguishing between these states.

Fibrocystic Disease. The cystic formation of fibrocystic disease may be confused with tuberculosis, but it is localized to the humerus without involvement of the joint or glenoid and there are no systemic signs or symptoms.

Osteogenic Sarcoma. Occasionally osteogenic sarcoma, particularly in the early stages, may resemble the acute tuberculous process in children. The x-ray picture quickly differentiates the two; invasion of soft tissue by the neoplasm is characteristic.

Osteoarthritis. Longstanding wear and tear arthritis that involves the humerus and glenoid presents a picture very similar to caries sicca. The extensive atrophy, the fixation of the joint and the progressive course in tuberculosis separate it from osteoarthritis.

Treatment

General Treatment. Tuberculosis of the shoulder is secondary to a focus elsewhere, so that systematic investigation of chest, kidney, and so forth, should be carried out. The general condition of the patient must be bolstered as in all tuberculous processes. Chemotherapy now plays an important part in the management of all tuberculosis. In early cases it alone may effectively control the lesion, but in most instances it is used in conjunction with other accepted routines. A variety of agents are available, and new, more effective ones continue to appear. Streptomycin is of proved value when it is tolerated. It is administered, 1 gram a day, concomitantly with P.A.S. A course may be given over one to three months, depending on the severity of the lesion and the patient's tolerance.

Local Treatment

CHILDREN. The joint is immobilized in a position of function, which in a child is about 80 degrees of abduction and 20 degrees of flexion. The reason the arm may be placed so high is that young people show greater adaptation and are able to bring the arm to their side from this position, whereas adults find it difficult from such an angle. After the acute process has subsided, arthrodesis should be done. In this instance an extra-articular method, such as that of Brittain, is preferable.

ADULTS. Since the disease follows a less

virulent and more subacute course in adults, arthrodesis can be performed at an earlier stage. The choice of the type of arthrodesis depends on the extent of joint involvement and the amount of bone destruction. The position desired is 60 degrees abduction and 15 degrees flexion. Adults do not accommodate themselves to a greater degree of abduction than this and are unable to get the arm to the side because of limitation of scapular rotation. In this less virulent adult type, intra-articular arthrodesis may be done, but some prefer adhering to an extra-articular approach.

Arthrodesis in Tuberculosis. The shoulder is approached through a lateral longitudinal incision of 2 inches, which exposes the acromion, the upper end of the humerus and the distal aspect of the shaft. The joint is opened and debrided. The upper end of the humerus and glenoid are denuded of cartilage and desquamated debris. They are fashioned so raw cancellous surfaces are accurately applied in the desired position. A heavy Kirchner or threaded wire is inserted from the lateral aspect, fixing the joint surfaces in satisfactory position. Above and below this wire two holes are drilled and fashioned with chisels to receive grafts. Two cortical grafts are removed from the tibia, the ends are pointed and they are inserted into prepared holes (Fig. 8–84, *D*). Extra fixation by a large screw inserted between the grafts may be desired, but if possible this should be avoided in tuberculous joints. The acromion is cut at the junction of the spine; the undersurfaces are rawed and laid over the denuded humerus. Cancellous bone is packed around the articular surface. The arm is immobilized in a body spica in the desired position. It is most helpful in these cases to have the spica prepared beforehand or to use a prepared pattern; either reduces the operating time and insures consolidation of the position obtained at operation. Immobilization is continued until the shoulder is solid when checked by x-ray examination — usually four to six months. Concurrent systemic treatment is continued.

ACUTE INFECTIOUS ARTHRITIS OF THE SHOULDER

The shoulder is not often involved by acute arthritis, but it can occur. The widespread and effective use of antibiotics has controlled infection following compound fractures and osteomyelitis of the upper end of the humerus, which were the usual sources of articular involvement. Contamination after penetrating wounds and compound fractures remain the common causes. Metastatic involvement is rare.

Signs and Symptoms

The diagnosis is usually obvious, with exquisite pain localized unequivocally to the shoulder area. The pain persists on any action and there is increasing limitation of movement because of muscle spasm and acute soreness. On examination the whole shoulder contour is distorted by a generalized enlargement. Tenderness is present all over, but the supero-anterior aspect is the most sensitive. The muscles are stiffly contracted, and the shoulder and arm are held close to the side. The signs and symptoms of an acute systemic process, fever, leukocytosis, and raised sedimentation rate, are present too. The x-rays show a narrowing of joint space and osteoporosis of humerus and glenoid.

Treatment

Aspiration. The joint should be aspirated and as much exudate as possible removed. Penicillin or an appropriate antibiotic, depending on the susceptiblity of the causative organism, is placed in the joint. Repeated aspiration and antibiotic injection may be necessary. Systemic antibiotic therapy is also given. The shoulder is immobilized in a sling or light abduction plaster with the upper half removed. Immobilization is continued until the acute process has subsided, and then active movement is started.

Drainage. It is rare that the process is so rapid and fulminating that it is not controlled by repeated aspiration and antibiotic injection. When this does happen, the joint must be drained. An incision is made over the supero-anterior and posterior aspects. Through and through Penrose drains are inserted, the drains being removed as soon as the discharge has stopped.

GOUT OF THE SHOULDER

The shoulder may be involved in a metabolic arthritis, but this is not common. Deposits of uric acid crystals occur at the articu-

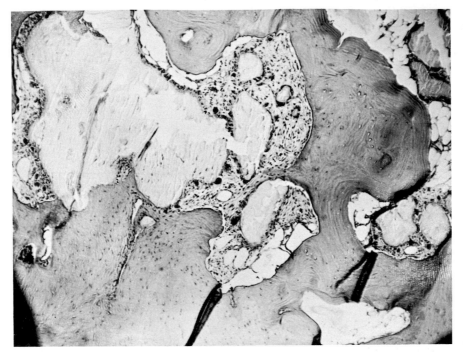

Figure 8-93   Gout of the shoulder.

lar margins in the region of the cuff insertion and may simulate calcific deposits. This produces a localized, small cystic or eroded area in the region of the greater tuberosity (Fig. 8-93).

Signs and Symptoms

The signs and symptoms of systemic metabolic disorder are present and diagnosis is made on the basis of these findings rather than on the local joint disturbance. Acute pain of rapid onset without significant antecedent trauma is the usual history. Pain is localized to the shoulder without neck or peripheral radiation; it is sore to lie on and to move. At this stage the shoulder lesion closely resembles acute tendinitis with calcification. A diagnostic dose of colchicum and laboratory tests which indicate a high uric acid level settle the issue.

Treatment

Colchicum tablets, 0.5 mg ($^{1}/_{120}$ gr), three to four times a day are given for two or three days, depending upon the response. In recurrent severe attacks the drug may be needed more often. Chronic and refractive cases may respond to ACTH and phenylbutazone.

TYPHOID ARTHRITIS

This is a rare condition today, but the shoulder may be involved in severe typhoid, along with the spine. The systemic picture overshadows articular complications and therapy is so directed. The joint is rested in the position of function. The lesion is seen more often as a chronic or longstanding disturbance and may give rise to diagnostic speculation when the shoulder is investigated for other conditions. The past history is usually sufficient to make one suspect the true nature of the disturbance.

NEOPLASMS OF THE SHOULDER

Tumors of the shoulder are mentioned at this point only to stress the fact that they may give rise to persistent shoulder pain. It is a continuing gnawing discomfort localized to the shoulder, unrelieved by rest and unrelated to activity. The pain may be most obvious at night and has a progressive character; frequently it keeps the patient awake because of a throbbing sensation. The whole subject of tumors is considered in detail in Chapter XVII.

REFERRED PAIN

One tends to forget that lesions apart from the locomotor system may be reflected in the shoulder area. Pain interpreted in the shoulder without radiation to the neck or the arm may arise from lesions some distance away. Some of the disturbances which produce such pain are common and serious. Myocardial infarction or tumors of the lung may first become apparent through pain in the shoulder. Any pathological process which irritates the undersurface of the diaphragm may refer pain to the upper aspect of the shoulder, so that perforated ulcer, biliary disease, subphrenic abscess or splenic abnormalities may produce localized shoulder pain.

FROZEN SHOULDER (Adhesive capsulitis, periarthritis, painful contracted shoulder)

This condition has been left to the last for discussion under the head of shoulder pain because it results from any of the foregoing states and must be considered as an end stage rather than a primary condition. It is a collective term, denoting a painful stiffening of the shoulder which has progressed to the point where all normal free action is lost and the arm is elevated with a typical girdle hunching action (Fig. 8–94). For too long this term has served as a convenient "catchall" for shoulder disorders, and it is apparent that efficient treatment of the condition depends on early recognition of the primary disorder. Older patients are most susceptible, and any relatively mild disturbance from a simple bruise to supraspinatus tendinitis to bicipital lesions may end as a frozen shoulder. The periarticular tissues become tight and stiff and the joint gradually freezes. If the primary cause is treated properly, frozen shoulder can be prevented.

SIGNS AND SYMPTOMS

This condition is easily diagnosed, but the underlying cause is sometimes more obscure. The typical patient is 50 or over and complains of pain clearly localized to the shoulder. This has usually been present for some weeks and has become increasingly troublesome at night. The pain is aggravated by arm movement, and relief is obtained by gradually decreasing the use of the extremity. A painful stiffening sets in and progresses until the normal free swing of the arm and shoulder is lost completely. The patient attempts to overcome hampered shoulder action by using accessory muscles, so that later on pain is prominent over the posterior aspect of the shoulder and in the neck-shoulder region because of the increased strain on accessory muscles such as the trapezius.

Examination at this stage shows the humerus glued in the glenoid, all movement being lost; any remaining action is accomplished by shift of the whole girdle on the chest. Rotation and abduction are markedly affected. Depending upon the length of establishment of the freezing process, there is atrophy of all muscles about the shoulder. The top of the humerus at front and at the side is tender on palpation. Often it is difficult to localize the point of maximum tenderness because the whole region is sore.

X-ray examination shows no startling change beyond some osteoporosis of the glenoid and the head of humerus. The humerus appears to be riding at a little higher level in the glenoid than normal. An arthrogram shows a typical picture (Fig. 8–95). There is loss of the normal redundant folds at the inferior aspect of the joint, and the articular shadow has a square box-like appearance because of the contracted capsule.

PATHOLOGY

In the severest form of this disorder, profound changes occur in the intimate joint lining. The synovial layer alterations have been the basis for the term "adhesive capsulitis." In a relatively early and acute case, at operation the synovium is stuck to articular cartilage and needs to be pulled from the surface, giving way in the same fashion adhesive tape does from any smooth surface. Normal intra-articular space is almost completely obliterated, and the joint cavity is filled with the juicy redundant injected lining. The normal lax, pleat-like folding at the inferior aspect is lost as the synovial surfaces become glued together. The capsule is thickened and contracted, which also limits movement. The muscle layers, tense and spastic from pain stimulation, remain con-

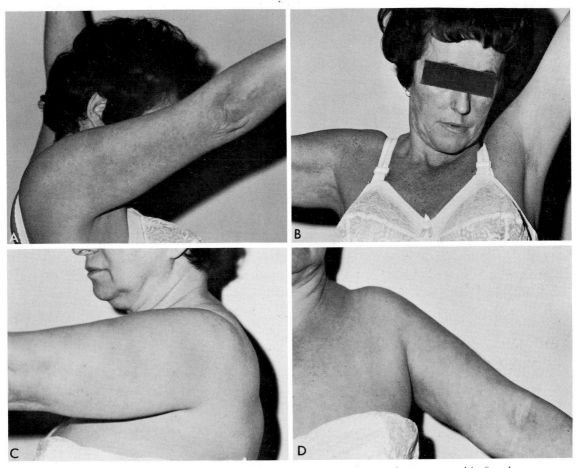

Figure 8–94 Frozen shoulders. Adhesive capsulitis is more commonly encountered in females.

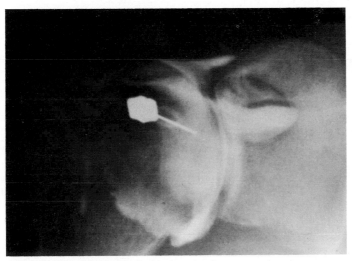

Figure 8–95 Arthrogram of a frozen shoulder. Note small amount of dye that can be injected, and shrunken inferior recess.

tracted and later atrophy. As the joint structures contract layer by layer, the freezing process becomes complete. In later stages the adhesions become thick and fixed, tying capsule to bone. The joint cavity is dry and small and the head of the humerus is drawn up close to the glenoid.

The changes are not indolent, passive degeneration and are not the result of lack of movement only. The appearance of degenerative tendinitis differs profoundly from this lesion, and joints, the seat of the paralytic disorder, never appear like this even though movement may have been absent for a long time. There is some independent active change setting off the profound synovial condition, capsule and muscle response probably being secondary to lining irritation. Some antecedent episode can normally be found, but a percentage may be regarded as an idiopathic adhesive capsulitis. This is the term which should be reserved for the condition since it most accurately depicts the pathological picture. Periarthritis is much too general and would include a multitude of lesions.

In the late stages more profound changes are found in the capsular and extracapsular structures. The rotator cuff is thick and inelastic, the biceps tendon frequently is glued to its groove, and the normal synovial lining sleeve protection is completely obliterated. The subacromial bursa is thin, dry and brittle. Tough adhesions traverse the subacromial space at the margins of the bursa. They are firmly implanted in the cuff, usually at the musculotendinous junction. These adhesions are so strong and firmly attached that they may pull pieces out of the cuff on rugged manipulation just as one pulls up soil on the roots of a plant. Accessory ligaments become thickened, gluing joint structures together; for example, at operation of these shoulders the coracohumeral ligament appears as a tight checkrein, tautly stretched from the coracoid and holding the humerus in internal rotation.

TREATMENT

Prevention is the best therapy for this condition. If any painful shoulder condition is given early attention, the freezing process can largely be prevented.

Treatment of Primary Lesion. So many of these cases follow acromioclavicular arthritis, tendinitis, muscle tears, fractures and bicipital lesions that the primary condition governs the treatment routine, which has been outlined previously. A recent survey shows that acromioclavicular irritation is an extremely common accompanying lesion. In some instances this is unquestionably the primary disturbance and, since it deters active abduction, capsular contracture then is favored. An important corollary is that in a capsulitis from any source, the loss of rotation means much greater acromioclavicular use because failure to swing the humeral head brings this joint into action at a much earlier phase in the circumduction swing than would ordinarily be the case.

Idiopathic Frozen Shoulder. There is a percentage of patients in whom the primary cause is obscure or the process appears simply as progressive, painful limitation of movement without implication of any one structure significantly. Females age 40 to 50 are the commonest sufferers; men in some age groups are afflicted also, but less frequently. This has been labeled idiopathic periarthritis or true adhesive capsulitis. It would appear that acromioclavicular joint, rotator cuff or bicipital degenerative changes provide the impetus, but a more fulminating than normal sequence in synovial reaction occurs, resulting in the more intense adhesive process.

The principles of treatment are to relieve pain, restore movement and improve muscle power.

Pain Relief

This is necessary only in the early stages. Light sedation is sufficient; salicylates and codeine compounds are effective. Cortisone and phenylbutazone also relieve the pain.

Cortisone or Steroid Routine in Frozen Shoulder. Cortisone has proved an effective aid in treating these conditions. It is not used routinely but if, after a week of proper physiotherapy, no improvement is apparent, it may be started. Dosage varies from patient to patient, but one routine is administration of

100 mg for 2 days, followed by
75 mg for 3 days, followed by
50 mg for 5 days, followed by
25 mg daily for 2 weeks.

The benefit derived is the relief from pain

rather than any permanent effect on joint structures.

Physiotherapy

Good physiotherapy is the basis of treatment of this condition. Once reasonable relief from pain has been obtained, a competent physiotherapist should take over and direct a program of gradually increasing active movement and gentle passive assistance. Rugged manipulation is to be avoided; the best results are from gentle help at the end of the active range, and gradual increase in this. The good physiotherapist has a sense of "pace," so that the patient does not go beyond the pain threshold to stir up more muscle spasm and favor more reactive freezing. The postoperative spring exercises outlined for cuff repairs are particularly good for frozen shoulder.

Surgical Treatment

Most patients respond to physiotherapy, regaining sufficient painless motion so that they are not hampered. Some show very little change, despite adequate sedation, cortisone and physiotherapy. This group needs something more radical because the adhesions have become too strong, the capsular contractions too rigid and the muscles too firmly fixed. In the past the vogue was to manipulate the shoulder of such patients under anesthesia and, depending on the enthusiasm of the operator, various results have been reported. Undoubtedly some patients are helped, but it is felt that these are the ones who would do well under a conscientious conservative routine anyway.

The author recommends a more direct approach in refractive patients, particularly in those who are not elderly and in whom there is no contraindication to a minor surgical procedure. All these patients should be treated conservatively first, but in those who do not improve in a reasonable time, say four to six months, surgical manipulation is desirable. It is much more effective to carry out manipulation with cuff structures under direct vision than as a blind procedure. When it is done in this fashion, undesirable complications are avoided and a better freeing of contractures is obtained. In addition, accessory helpful procedures such as acromioclavicular arthroplasty can be done at the same time. It is possible to tear the shoulder capsule very easily in a blind manipulation, and the author has done this even under direct vision. However, when it is done with the joint exposed, any damage can be repaired. A further consideration is that at the time of surgical manipulation, it is possible to depress the head of the humerus gently so that the tear, if it occurs, does not as a rule implicate the important part of the rotator cuff that tends to be confined to the inferior aspect. In this zone, the tear is not nearly so serious.

So many of these cases are complicated by acromioclavicular irritation, either as a primary or a secondary reaction, that it appears extremely worthwhile to do an acromioclavicular arthroplasty at the same time. In this way greater leeway of abduction, some 15 to 20 degrees, is possible; this is important, particularly if there is any residual decrease in rotation.

Technique of Surgical Manipulation of Shoulder. Light general anesthesia is given and the patient is placed in the usual sitting shoulder position. An incision 4 inches in length is made, extending from the posterior aspect of the acromioclavicular joint, and constituting the usual utility incision. The deltoid fibers are separated, and the coracoacromial ligament is resected. At this point the joint is inspected by retracting the fibers of the deltoid, and the operator gently maneuvers the upper end of the humerus. The elbow is grasped with the right hand and the other hand depresses the head of the humerus as it is gradually abducted and externally rotated. At a point of about 80 degrees, considerable resistance is encountered and capsular adhesions can be heard to give as the abduction rotation force is gently continued. In elderly patients and in those in whom the contracture is of long standing, rotatory freeing is done first of all, aided by a periosteal elevator and digital dissection; adhesions are removed from around the cuff prior to the abduction type of rotation. By carrying out the manipulation under direct vision it is possible to minimize the extent of cuff rupture, although it will sometimes still occur.

POSTOPERATIVE TREATMENT. These patients are placed in springs and slings, and early active motion is instituted, along with continued systemic therapy, including adequate sedation and anti-inflammatory medication.

Principles of Exercise Therapy in Frozen Shoulder. The frozen shoulder is one of the more difficult problems the physiatrist and physiotherapist are called upon to treat. In the ensuing discussion it is assumed that obvious causes of the lesion have had adequate and appropriate treatment, as outlined previously, so that it is the idiopathic or neglected adhesive capsulitis lesion which is being treated. Remembering that it is a contracting pincer-like freezing process which intimately binds humerus and glenoid together, the effort is toward loosening constricting adhesions and improving muscle power to retain the increased movement obtained from the process of release. Because of the constricting nature, it is gentle, persistent stretching of the adhesions that is needed. This may best be initiated by active movement which allows a paced stretching within pain limits. When this has reached a maximum, assistance is provided through gentle passive stretching. The joint surfaces are not seriously altered, muscles are intact,

and the nerve supply is working, so that once range is regained it can be retained.

Something more is needed than mere instruction to develop the active exercise routine to an efficient plane. The effort must be made to a maximum in each movement to obtain stretching. This is a slow process and may be ineffective despite a skilled physiotherapists' supervision. In this connection a colleague, Dr. J. Berkley, has introduced the term "encouraged exercises" and applied it to a plan of repetitive movement that uses rhythm and assisting forces by means of springs. The exercises are familiar ones, but a little thought and planning bring into play assisting forces, such as gravity, pull of the normal limb, and a stretched spring as a set of two opposite springs. The principle is to encourage a rhythmic movement like the pendulum swing of the clock. At first, gravity is used. Other aids are added as progress indicates. The "encouragement" factor is sound psychological aid to these patients; it becomes a visible assisting force, an attainable

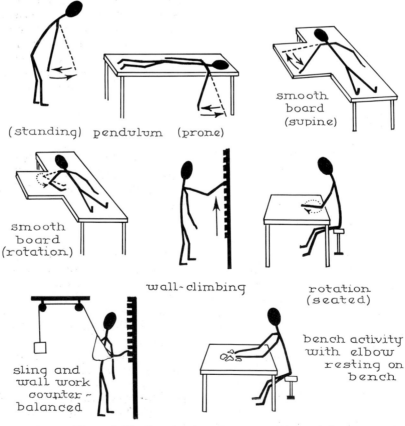

(standing) pendulum (prone)

smooth board (supine)

smooth board (rotation)

wall-climbing

rotation (seated)

sling and wall work counter-balanced

bench activity with elbow resting on bench

Figure 8–96 Exercises in early postoperative period.

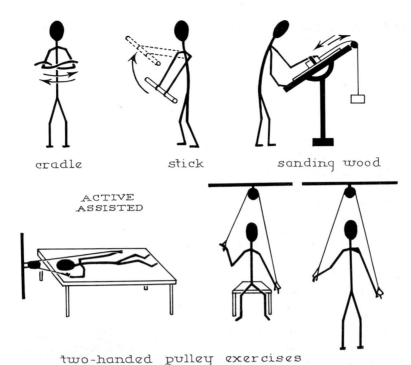

cradle   stick   sanding wood

ACTIVE
ASSISTED

two-handed pulley exercises

Figure 8–97 Exercises for patients with shoulder weakness and some pain and limited motion. (Courtesy Dr. J. Berkely.)

work goal for their efforts. Some of these patients may be described as "exercise resistant" as a result of apprehension, indolence, hypersensitivity or frank neurosis. In this group particularly, the encouraged exercise method is helpful (Figs. 8–96, 8–97 and 8–98).

STERNOCLAVICULAR ARTHRITIS

Disease of the sternoclavicular joint is not common, but occasionally significant changes are encountered. Posttraumatic arthritis following fracture or dislocation is the commonest abnormality. Occasionally the joint is involved in a rheumatoid or osteoarthritic process (Fig. 8–99). Patients complain of pain and tenderness in the sternoclavicular area. Often they have noticed a slight swelling which has increased gradually. Maximum discomfort occurs during the midrange of abduction or flexion. The clavicle elevates, rotates and slides backward and forward at this point, so that acts such as pushing or shoving at shoulder level are particularly painful (Fig. 3–5).

TREATMENT

Surgical treatment is required only occasionally, chiefly for posttraumatic arthritis.

When symptoms are sufficiently severe, the medial end may be excised. Occasionally excision of exostoses and smoothing of joint margins is sufficient. When rupture of the intra-articular ligament has occurred, producing symptoms similar to an internal derangement, excision is advised (see Chapters XI and XIII).

TREATMENT SUMMARY FOR CONDITIONS WITH PREDOMINATING SHOULDER PAIN

Degenerative Tendinitis

1. Inject subacromial area with a mixture of local anesthetic and steroid.
2. Administer systemic anti-inflammatory drugs.
3. Relieve night pain by light sedatives and hypnotics.
4. Illustrate a routine of exercises that may be done at home.
5. In chronic recurrent cases do arthrogram, looking for cuff tears. Resect acromion.
6. This is a common chronic ailment, and patients are at once relieved if they can be assured no serious disease is present.

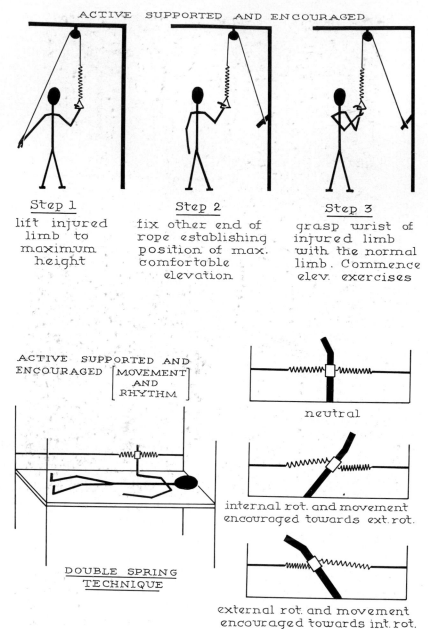

ACTIVE SUPPORTED AND ENCOURAGED

Step 1
lift injured
limb to
maximum
height

Step 2
fix other end of
rope establishing
position of max.
comfortable
elevation

Step 3
grasp wrist of
injured limb
with the normal
limb. Commence
elev. exercises

ACTIVE SUPPORTED AND
ENCOURAGED [MOVEMENT
AND
RHYTHM]

neutral

internal rot. and movement
encouraged towards ext. rot.

DOUBLE SPRING
TECHNIQUE

external rot. and movement
encouraged towards int. rot.

Figure 8-98 Use of springs is particularly helpful in therapy of stiff shoulders. (Courtesy Dr. J. Berkely.)

Tendinitis with Calcification

1. This is an acutely painful process, requiring urgent attention.

2. Aspirate the deposit, if possible.

3. Relieve the pain.

4. Limit movement in acute stage.

5. Ammonium chloride in 7½ gr capsules may be used as a supplementary drug but is not always effective.

6. If x-ray therapy is used, avoid repeated application.

7. All remedies should be accompanied by exercises when acute symptoms have subsided.

8. Surgical excision is the method of choice in refractive or chronic lesions.

Ruptures of Rotator Cuff

1. Suspect cuff tears in workmen with history of injury that is followed by persistent shoulder weakness.

2. If in doubt, do an arthrogram.

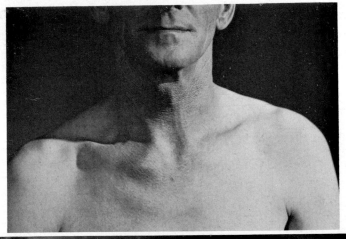

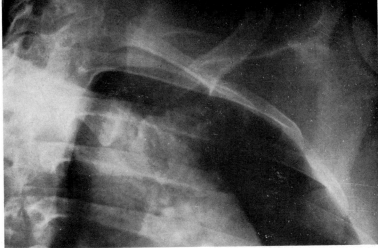

Figure 8-99 Osteoarthritis of right sternoclavicular joints. Note enlarged end of clavicle and joint dislocation in the x-ray.

3. Treat partial tears conservatively.

4. Operate on complete tears and those without improvement after six weeks.

5. Repair the cuff as early as possible.

6. Resect acromion and do a snug repair.

7. Use traction rather than plaster fixation postoperatively.

8. Follow up with conscientious physiotherapy.

9. Do not operate on elderly sedentary patients.

10. Do not permit haphazard physiotherapy regime.

Bicipital Lesions

1. Consider these lesions in patients with pain and tenderness at the front of the joint.

2. Recognize three grades: tendinitis, rupture of intertubercular fibers, and complete rupture of the tendon.

3. Treat tendinitis conservatively.

4. Transfer the long head to the coracoid process in slipping and ruptured forms.

5. Remember combination injuries of tendon, cuff and nerves are not uncommon.

Acromioclavicular Arthritis

1. Think of this lesion in patients who complain of pain in abduction above the right angle.

2. Resect the outer ¾ inch of acromion in those with persistent symptoms.

Glenohumeral Arthritis

1. Posttraumatic and osteoarthritis

a. Do arthrodesis in workmen with persistent pain.

b. Evaluate possibility of arthroplasty in more sedentary patients.

2. Rheumatoid arthritis

Treatment of primary disease and arthroplasty predominate.

3. Metabolic arthritis

Treatment of primary disease and arthroplasty predominate.

4. Tuberculosis
   a. General measures.
   b. Chemotherapy.
   c. Arthrodesis.
5. Acute infectious arthritis
   a. Chemotherapy.
   b. Aspiration.

Frozen Shoulder

1. Remember this is a result and rarely a primary entity.
2. Treat the underlying cause.
3. Administer cortisone.
4. Use concentrated, supervised, conscientious physiotherapy.

REFERENCES

Bateman, J. E.: The diagnosis and treatment of ruptures of the rotator cuff. Surg. Clin. N. Amer. *43*:1523–1530, 1963.

Bateman, J. E.: Gallie technique for repair of recurrent dislocation of the shoulder. Surg. Clin. N. Amer. *43*:1655–1662, 1963.

Bosworth, D. M.: Calcium deposits in the shoulder and subacromial bursitis. A survey of 12,122 shoulders. J.A.M.A. *106*:2477, 1941.

Brickner, W. M.: Prevalent fallacies concerning subacromial bursitis. Its pathogenesis and rational operative treatment. Amer. J. Med. Sci. *149*:351, 1915.

Caldwell, G. A., and Unkauf, B. M.: Results of treatment of subacromial brusitis in three hundred and forty cases. Ann. Surg. *132*:432–442, 1950.

Claessens, H., et al.: Incidence, treatment and outcome of ruptures of the cuff of the short rotator muscles of the shoulder. Acta Orthop. Belg. *32*:407–422, 1966.

Codman, E. A.: The Shoulder. Rupture of the Supraspinatus Tendon and Other Lesions in or about the Subacromial Bursa. Privately printed, Boston, 1934.

Codman, E. A.: Ruptures of the supraspinatous – 1834 to 1934. J. Bone Joint Surg. *19*:643, 1937.

Compere, E. L.: The painful shoulder. J.A.M.A. *189*:845–846, 1964.

Crenshaw, A. H., et al.: Surgical treatment of bicipital tenosynovitis. J. Bone Joint Surg. *48A*:1496–1502, 1966.

Debeyre, J., et al.: Repair of ruptures of the rotator cuff of the shoulder. J. Bone Joint Surg. (Brit.) *47B*:32–35, 1965.

Debeyre, J., et al.: Surgical treatment of ruptures of the rotator cuff of the shoulder Technics, results, surgical indications. Acta Orthop. Belg. *32*:391–406, 1966.

Duncan, G. A.: Surgical treatment of calcific subacromial tendinitis. Virginia Med. Monthly *95*:11–14, 1968.

Durbin, F. C.: Frozen Shoulder. Nurs. Times *62*:743–745, 1966.

Garrett, T. R., et al.: Portable shoulder exerciser. Phys Ther. *46*:50–51, 1966.

Goldie, I.: Calcified deposits in the shoulder joint produced by calciphylaxis and their inhibition by triamcinolone. An experimental model. Bull. Soc. Int. Chir. *24*:51–56, 1965.

Haguenauer, J. P., et al.: Scapulo-humeral periarthritis of the "frozen shoulder" type following cervical lymph node involvement. Rheumatologie *18*:231–235, 1966.

Hitchcock, H. H., and Bechtol, C. O.: Painful shoulder. Observations on the role of the tendon of the long head of the biceps brachii in its causation. J. Bone Joint Surg. *30A*:263–273, 1948.

Hodgkinson, R.: Surgery for the painful shoulder. Med. J. Aust. *2*:318–319, 1966.

Joyce, J. J., et al.: Surgical exposure of the shoulder. J. Bone Joint Surg. *49A*:547–554, 1967.

Leriche, R., and Jung, A.: Les calcifications sous-deltoidiennes de l'épaule. Rev. O'Orthop. *20*:289, 1933.

Lippman, R. K.: Bicipital tenosynovitis. N.Y. State J. Med. *44*:2235–2240, 1944.

Lundberg, B. J.: The frozen shoulder. Clinical and radiographical observations. The effect of manipulation under general anaesthesia. Structure and glycosaminoglycan content of the joint capsule. Local bone metabolism. Acta Orthop. Scand. Suppl. 119, 1969.

McKenna, D. E.: Tendinitis of the shoulder. Med. Times, *68*:295, 1940.

McLaughlin, H. L.: Mascular and tendinous defects at the shoulder and their repair. Lectures on reconstruction surgery of the extremities, American Academy of Orthopedic Surgeons. Ann Arbor, J. W. Edwards, 1944, pp. 343–358.

McLaughlin, H. L.: The selection of calcium deposits for operation; the technique and results of operation. Surg. Clin. N. Amer. *43*:1501–1504, 1963.

McLaughlin, H. L.: Repair of major cuff ruptures. Surg. Clin. N. Amer. *43*:1535–1540, 1963.

Moseley, H. F.: Shoulder Lesions. 2nd ed. New York, Paul B. Hoeber, Inc., 1953.

Moseley, H. F.: The results of nonoperative and operative treatment of calcified deposits. Surg. Clin. N. Amer. *43*:1505–1506, 1963.

Moseley, H. F.: The natural history and clinical syndromes produced by calcified deposits in the rotator cuff. Surg. Clin. N. Amer. *43*:1489–1493, 1963.

Parsons, J. L., et al.: DMSO, an adjutant to physical therapy in the chronic frozen shoulder. Ann. N.Y. Acad. Sci. *141*:569–571, 1967.

Pizio, Z., et al.: Posterior dislocation of the shoulder joint. Wiad. Lek. *21*:985–987, 1968.

Quigley, T. B., and Renold, A. E.: Acute calcific tendinitis and "frozen shoulder": Their treatment with ACTH. New Eng. J. Med. *246*:1012–1014, 1952.

Quigley, T. G.: The nonoperative treatment of symptomatic calcareous deposits in the shoulder. Surg. Clin. N. Amer. *43*:1495–1499, 1963.

Rose, D. L.: Diagnosis and management of bursitis. Texas Med. *64*:63–65, 1968.

Schaer, H.: Tendinitis und pseudobursitis calcarea-nicht; bursitis subdeltoidea calcarea. Zbl. Chir. *66*:1126, 1939.

Seze, S. de, et al.: Rupture of the tendinous cuff of the rotator muscles of the shoulder. Anatomical, radiological, and clinical study. Sem. Hop. Paris *41*:2375–2384, 1965.

Welfing, J., et al.: Calcifications of the shoulder. 11. The disease of multiple tendinous calcifications. Rev. Rhum. *32*:325–334, 1965.

Worcester, J. N.: Osteoarthritis of the acromioclavicular joint. Clin. Orthop. *58*:69–73, 1968.

Chapter IX

LESIONS PRODUCING SHOULDER PLUS RADIATING PAIN

Shoulder pain with distal radiation frequently represents a problem requiring careful assessment. Because it is the fulcrum of the extremity, many clinical states are reflected initially in the shoulder region, but shortly the discomfort experienced implicates the arm, forearm, hand or whole limb. Patients often have difficulty in localizing this type of pain and describe it as up and down the arm or whole arm pain (Fig. 9–1).

Since the shoulder serves as the universal joint of the limb, its action may appear as the irritant when actually it just happens to be the most frequently used motion in a wholly painful limb. Neck action also is involved in many shoulder motions, either as a stabilizing element or accompanying movement, and this may be the precipitating irritant rather than the glenohumeral action.

The source of shoulder and radiating pain may lie centrally in the spinal cord or distally in the axilla (Fig. 9–2). An extensive group of lesions belong in this category, including disorders of the cervical nerve roots, supraclavicular neurovascular disturbances like cervical ribs and the scalene lesions, sub-clavicular abnormalities and the broad group of clavipectoral compression syndromes.

CHARACTERISTICS OF NEURAL VERSUS VASCULAR PAIN

Disturbances at different levels in this region implicate different pain-producing elements. Thus, a pattern of pain resulting from a purely neural irritation can be recognized, a further one resulting from vascular involvement is encountered and, finally, states evincing a combination of these mechanisms occur.

The extensive network of nerves in this region provides many sites for pathological irritation—spinal cord, intervertebral foramen, brachial plexus, trunks above clavicle, plexus cords behind and below the clavicle.

Regardless of the site, certain basic qualities of the pain characteristic of neural irritation can be recognized. Headache and shoulder-neck ache may usher in a disorder, but shortly the pain is consistently extended below the insertion of the deltoid, reaching

293

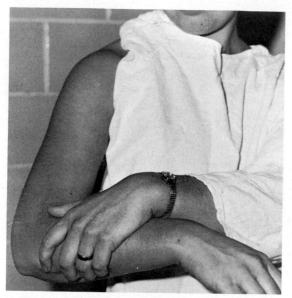

Figure 9–1 Typical designation of pain distribution in the group of patients with shoulder and radiating pain.

are common accompaniments. When this discomfort has been present for any length of time, the effect is to leave a constant imprint in the form of hypesthesia or other altered sensation.

The great vessels of the limb also course through this region and may be implicated by lesions which compress them or exert unusual traction, or by a combination of these forces setting up vascular symptoms. A type of radiating pain quite different as to pattern and quality then results. Vascular pain has a less well defined distribution and frequently involves the whole forearm, all the hand or all the fingers. A sensation of fullness or bursting thickness may be experienced. Some pins and needles or a sleepy feeling is frequent, but it often is evanescent, disappearing completely and leaving no sensory imprint or aftermath. Sudden and simple changes in position alter this type of pain quickly and completely. Discoloration may occur, but usually only in long established and severe disturbances. The pain from vascular irritation may be due to direct constriction or traction on a main vessel.

elbow, forearm and fingers. One rough way of quickly assessing a presenting pattern is to ascertain its consistent extension below the elbow. In by far the majority of instances such radiation means the source of the disorder is other than the glenohumeral mechanism.

Neural pain has a sharp tingling element, a sudden darting or lancinating quality, often of very sudden onset. In its extension to the periphery it will keep on involving one specific area, being more constantly at one side of the hand or the other or in one group of fingers. It is intermittent, often disappearing quite completely until evoked again by the irritating disease mechanism. Paresthesia, tingling and numbness or a burning element

A further chronic but less well defined discomfort develops as a secondary change and results from interference with the metabolic processes; abnormal metabolites then act as an irritant in the area of supply. Ligation of a main artery alone does not cause pain, but if an irritating solution is injected it immediately causes discomfort as a result of constriction in the zone of peripheral distribution. Subsequently a more vague discomfort in the area then develops owing to the interference with nutrition and the resulting ischemia. Persistence of the phase of constriction keeps up the pain; ultimately con-

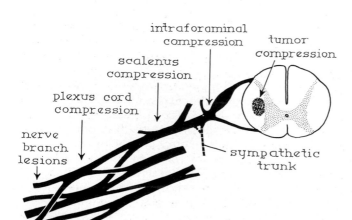

Figure 9–2 Sites of pathology evoking neural type radiating pain.

siderable dulling of all sensation ensues. These, however, are late changes following severe vascular obstruction.

CERVICAL ROOT SYNDROMES

TUMORS OF THE SPINAL CORD

Although tumors of the cervical cord are not common, they should be kept in mind because of their seriousness and the dramatically successful surgical treatment that is possible. The signs and symptoms are usually clear-cut, but it is important to be aware of these in investigating shoulder and radiating pain. When profound motor and sensory changes are encountered in addition to persistent pain without a history of injury, the possibility of a space-taking lesion should be kept in mind. In all other diseases of this group, neurological findings are not nearly so definite as they are in a cord tumor. The pain starts in a gradual fashion but continues in the shoulder and neck and is followed later by sharper radiating discomfort to the periphery of the extremity. Characteristically the patient complains of difficulty in finding a comfortable position, and pain may persist at night with a boring, aching quality.

Pathology, signs and symptoms and treatment have all been covered in detail in Chapter XVI, Neurological and Dystrophic Lesions.

INTERVERTEBRAL DISC LESIONS

Nerve root compression resulting from intervertebral disc abnormalities evokes an aching type of shoulder pain, followed shortly by extension of a characteristic neural discomfort to the hand and fingers (Fig. 9–3). The recognition and proper treatment of this disturbance have helped to clarify this broad class of shoulder and radiating pain considerably. All necks are subject to some wear and tear change, with some signs of intervertebral pathology occurring as early as age 35 in many people. In the cervical spine the root normally occupies one third of the foramen, so that considerable adjustment from encroachment by an extruded nucleus is possible. In addition to frank extrusion of the nucleus, narrowing of the intervertebral foramen as a result of spondylosis implicates nerve roots also. In this fashion one may distinguish an acute episode

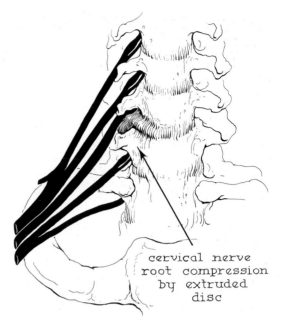

cervical nerve root compression by extruded disc

Figure 9–3 Nerve root pressure due to disc herniation.

or trauma caused by posttraumatic extrusion of a nucleus through the annulus from a so-called "hard" disc, which is a compression developing gradually from a combination of disc degeneration and osteophyte formation; in still more chronic states, cord compression may be added.

Etiology and Pathology

Foraminal compression of the nerve root is often a combination of slow disc extrusion along with growth of encroaching osteophytes. The deterioration of the intervertebral discs involves annulus, nucleus and the cartilaginous plates (Fig. 9–4). In the annulus a cracking or fissure formation occurs as a result of trauma or the aging process, favoring some displacement of nuclear material from its usual confines. The tendency is for the cracks in the annulus to occur on either side, rather than in the midline, because of the bolstering strength of the anterior and posterior longitudinal ligaments, particularly in the midline. The effect of this tendency to lateral weakness is that the bulging is then closer to the foramen and the nerve roots. When the forces of vertical compression are added to this wandering of the nucleus, further extrusion occurs (Fig. 9–5).

The changes in the nucleus are toward a shrinking and dehydration, with loss of

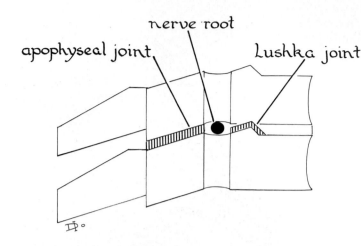

Figure 9–4 Circumferential articular relations of the nerve root.

elasticity and resilience; some deterioration in its shock absorbing and supporting characteristics then results, so that it does not act so effectively as it ages. However, a wide margin of elasticity is retained and is sufficient to last as long as is necessary if changes in the annulus and cartilaginous plate did not further favor a diminution of the nuclear contribution. The third element in this mechanism, the cartilaginous plates, exhibits progressive deformation also. Cracking of the plate in the center portion of the disc may occur, but much greater changes occur around the edge. At the lateral edges of the vertebral bodies, from C.2 to T.1, a series of accessory joints, the joints of Luschka, have been identified. Much of the recent interest in this area has been aroused by the pioneering work of Compere. The joints of Luschka

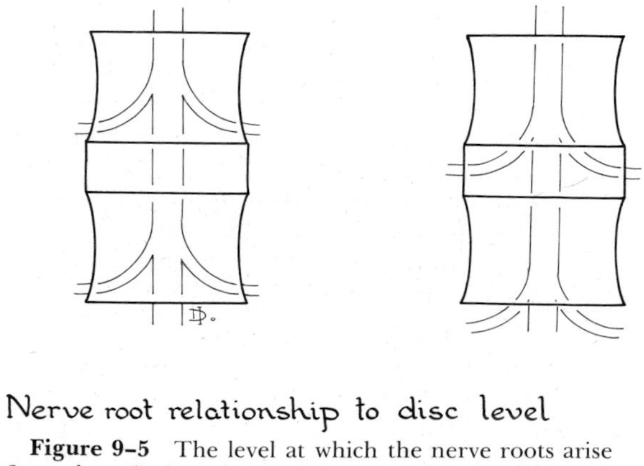

lie anteromedial to the nerve root and posteromedial to the vertebral artery and veins (Fig. 9–6). They consist of small spur-like lips on the upper surface and constitute a type of accessory joint. These small islands are covered with cartilage, and a capsule with synovial tissue has been identified, making it appear that these represent a true arthrodial mechanism.

The significance of these zones is that they appear considerably more susceptible than the rest of the cartilaginous plate to wear and tear change because of their position and shape. They really constitute an accessory ball bearing type of mechanism which is principally concerned with controlling the gliding action of one vertebral body corner on the other (Fig. 9–7).

The action of flexion and extension in the cervical spine is not one of pure bending, but rather consists to a considerable degree of a gliding or sliding motion, with one cartilaginous plate really rolling to a controlled degree on the other. These lock at the corners and constitute a significant block or guard of this gliding element. In order to carry out this function, they require this corner type of seating but this also brings them into contact with the intervertebral foramen, so that if there is any reaction related to these joints, it may encroach upon the foramen, initiating spur formation (Fig. 9–8).

Signs and Symptoms of Root Syndrome due to Disc Lesions

Acute Herniated Cervical Disc. Pain is the cardinal symptom, usually coming on after some definite injury. This may be a vertebral compression type of injury, such

Nerve root relationship to disc level

Figure 9–5 The level at which the nerve roots arise from the spinal cord is slightly above the annulus in the cervical area as compared to a lower level in the lumbar region.

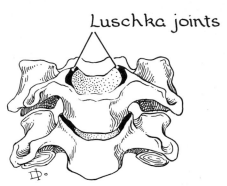

Luschka joints

Figure 9-6 Joints of Luschka.

as a fall or diving accident or one of severe voluntary muscular contracture, as in lifting a heavy object. The pain starts in the shoulder but quickly extends to the upper arm, then to the forearm and fingers. It usually involves only one nerve root, so that the involvement in the hand corresponds to the individual nerve root distribution. The common distribution is to the thumb and index finger from the sixth root, middle fingers from the seventh root and the fourth and fifth fingers from the eighth root. A great deal of variation in the peripheral distribution is encountered, and although the pain characteristics are quite definite, the anatomical distribution may be confusing. Shortly there is associated a feeling of numbness and tingling in the zone of the pain distribution. This often is brought on by positioning the neck or moving the neck so that the patient automatically spares the spine, and there is considerable restriction of neck motion.

Signs of Motor Involvement. These follow very shortly after the acute pain. This is interpreted initially as difficulty in carrying out certain complete acts, such as lifting and holding a cup or attempting to get the arm out at the side. After a while the patient then more clearly localizes his weakness to the thumb, the index finger, the little finger or all of the hand, depending upon the nerve root which is involved. Alteration in the biceps and triceps jerk frequently occurs in this acute lesion. Electromyographic investigation will usually identify a zone of denervation as well as alteration in the nerve conduction times.

Chronic Extrusion or Hard Disc. The common development is a gradual onset of discomfort, starting with some pain in the neck, then extending to the shoulder and eventually implicating the forearm and hand.

The course may be punctuated by more acute exacerbations, but most often it follows a gradually progressive and persistent development. The definite history of injury or significant antecedent trauma is not usually obtained. On examination there is some restriction of neck motion, particularly in forward bending, and a complaint of pain in attempting to extend the neck. Movement to the side of the pain increases the root compression and reproduces the radiating symptoms. Decrease of the discomfort is apparent when tilting the head away. Tenderness related to the midportion of the neck posteriorly, both in the midline and at either side, is common. Pressure on the posterior spinous processes sometimes initiates the radiating discomfort. Pain and tenderness sometimes implicate the front of the neck, with sensitivity involving the scalenus anticus particularly; in many instances pressure here initiates the radiating discomfort.

Extension of pain to involve the chest is a frequent complaint, as is also some headache and suboccipital pain. Signs of weakness and atrophy gradually develop in lesions implicating the space between C.5 and C.6, and

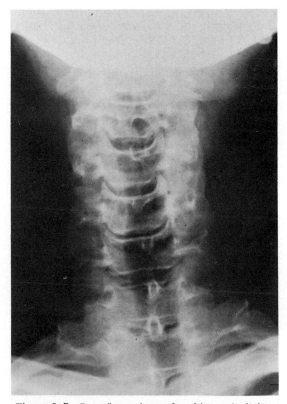

Figure 9-7 Spur formation at Luschka, articulation.

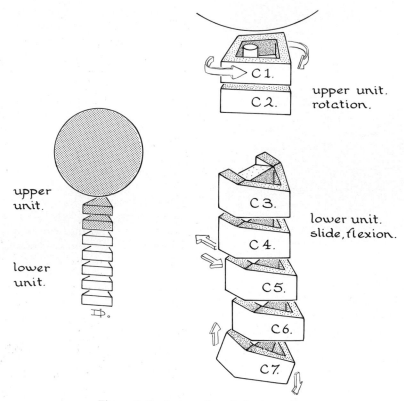

upper unit.

lower unit.

C 1.

C 2. upper unit. rotation.

C 3.

C 4. lower unit. slide, flexion.

C 5.

C 6.

C 7.

Figure 9–8 Action of cervical spine units.

the biceps and deltoid are involved; in lesions implicating the space between C.6 and C.7, the triceps is weak. Involvement of the small muscles of the hand suggests implication of the eighth cervical root. The pattern of cutaneous disturbance follows the individual nerve roots, weakness of the hands and clumsiness in certain motions being a frequent complaint. Sensory change is difficult to outline; alteration in appreciation of light touch and pinprick, involving the base of the thumb and lateral border of the forearm, usually results from involvement of the sixth root, C.7; the thumb and index finger, and sometimes the middle finger, are implicated. In C.8 compression it is the medial border of the palm, the fifth and, occasionally, the fourth finger which are involved (Figs. 9–9 and 9–10).

Electromyographic Change. Electromyographic examination is extremely useful in diagnosing these lesions (Fig. 9–11). In addition to implication of the muscles in the forearm and hand, which results from pressure on the anterior root, in many instances it is possible to detect some involvement of the segmental muscles in the paraspinal area,

which would be allied to the posterior root. If an electromyographic examination of the erector spinae shows definite evidence of some denervation, such as fibrillation action potentials, it is highly suggestive of nerve root involvement. This test is of particular significance in differentiating the lesion from a carpal tunnel syndrome. When there is compression of the median nerve at the wrist in the carpal tunnel, precise involvement of the thumb, index and middle fingers occurs with a quite constant sensory pattern. In addition, there will be alteration in the nerve conduction times at this level, but no alteration in the nerve conduction times at the elbow or elsewhere. There would be no evidence of denervation in the paraspinal muscles unless the nerve root had been implicated.

Cervical Myelopathy. Extension of the compressive forces may implicate the spinal cord in addition to foraminal compression of a nerve root. In some instances this can be so extensive that it appears as a space-taking lesion such as a cord tumor. Cord involvement almost always develops only in those patients in whom the symptoms have been present for some time and is suggestive

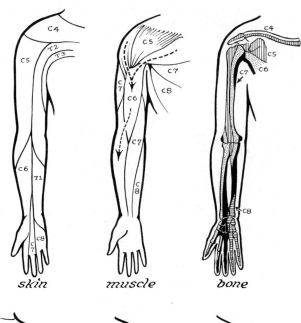

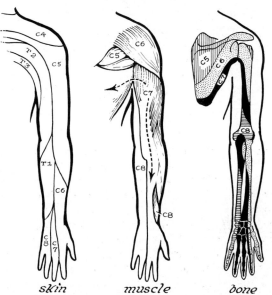

Figure 9-9 Comparison of segmental innervation of superficial and deep structures.

of root compression. The cardinal indication of cord involvement is the development of changes involving the lower limbs. This may be a slight degree of spasticity, or some frank weakness in one limb or the other. Commonly both sides are involved to an equal degree. The usual picture is spastic weakness, and this may progress to a frank Brown-Séquard syndrome of dissociated anesthesia. In cord involvement the signs in the upper limb always are more severe, with weakness, atrophy and electromyographic changes being prominent. The reflexes will be absent in the corresponding root area, but in the lower limb, they will probably be increased as a result of the spasticity. A positive Babinski reflex is also frequently obtained (Fig. 9-12).

Radiological Findings

Plain films of the cervical spine in young people will show interbody and foraminal changes in all but the very acute extruded disc. In these cases there is usually a significant history of antecedent trauma in addition to the radiating pain and signs of nerve root involvement. Under these circumstances contrast studies are mandatory to identify the level of the lesion (Fig. 9-13). Cervical

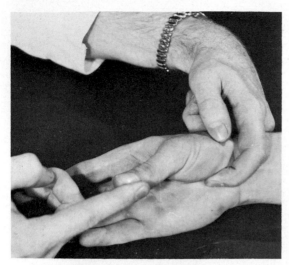

Figure 9–10 Testing for thenar weakness.

myelography is extremely helpful in demarcating the level, with its greatest assistance occurring in the acute extrusion and in those cases in which there is some cord involvement. In the average chronic case the level of involvement is indicated by the interbody changes and these will be quite clear in the x-rays, so that myelography is not always required (Fig. 9–14).

In those instances of cord involvement the changes can be so extensive that there is a complete block with a positive Queckenstedt test. The total protein in the spinal fluid will also be increased. In some instances, if a complete block is present, the contrast studies do not distinguish between a tumor, an extruded disc or a spondylotic lesion (Fig. 9–12).

A further method of investigation is discography, which may be done under a local anesthetic. For the details of this and the methods of conservative and operative treatment of disc lesions, see Chapter XVI, Neurological and Dystrophic Lesions.

CERVICAL NEUROVASCULAR SYNDROMES

CERVICAL RIB AND ABNORMALITIES OF THE FIRST RIB

As the evolutionary scale is ascended from reptiles to man the cervical spine gradually loses its outrigging rib elements. This has enabled man to have a movable neck and has paved the way for specialization of the upper extremity. Abnormalities in this zone are to be expected, just as they occur in the transitional area related to the lower limb, the lumbosacral region. In addition to developmental abnormalities, similar symptoms result from derangement of normal elements, so that consideration must be given to: (1) extra or abnormal first ribs, (2) disturbances of normally placed first ribs, and (3) abnormally positioned first ribs.

Abnormal development of the costal element on the seventh cervical vertebra is found in roughly six patients per 1000. In half the patients the condition is bilateral. When there is a unilateral rib, a supernumery costal tubercle frequently exists on the opposite side. Most cervical ribs are found incidentally during routine x-ray examination for other conditions (Fig. 9–15).

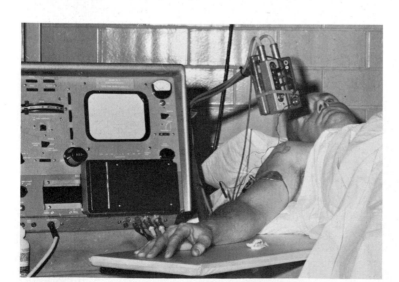

Figure 9–11 Electromyographic examination.

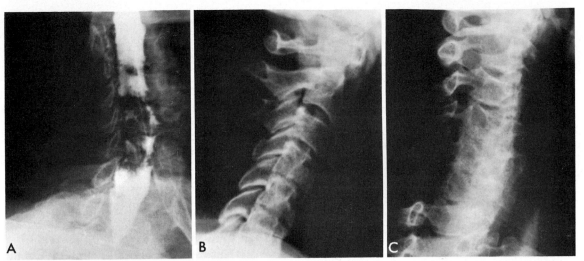

Figure 9–12 Appearance of myelogram in a case of extensive spondylosis producing myelopathy suggestive of a cord tumor (*A*). *B*, Posterior laminectomy to decompress the cords. *C*, Anterior interbody fusion for stability.

Cardinal Signs and Symptoms

Pain is the cardinal symptom and is frequently initiated as aching in the shoulder, but quickly extends to the inner border of the forearm, the hand and the fingers; a tingling, numbness and a pins-and-needles sensation develop and are aggravated by sudden, jerking movements of shoulder and neck. Such activities as lifting, reaching, sweeping, craning and cleaning bring on the pain. It is the lifting motion of the arms to the front, side or above the head that causes vascular constriction by the first rib. Patients learn that keeping the arm by the side and supporting it alleviates the discomfort. In

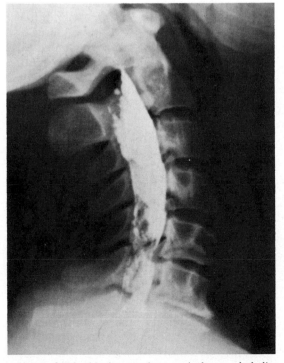

Figure 9–13 Myelogram in a typical extruded disc defect.

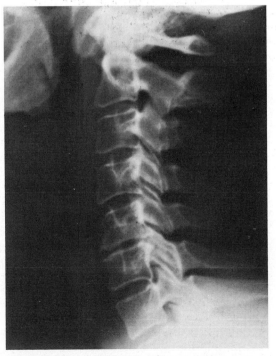

Figure 9–14 Typical interbody narrowing and posterior marginal spur formation producing cervical root syndrome.

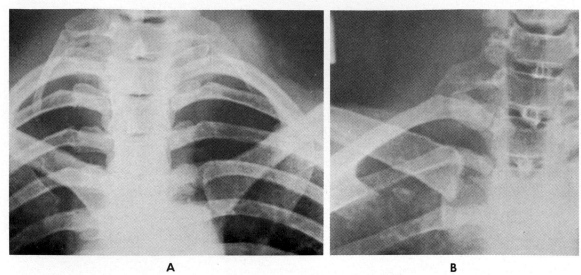

A   **B**

Figure 9–15 Cervical ribs. *A,* Typical complete rib on both sides. *B,* Elongated process only where a complete osseofibrous bar is indicated by the small calcified point below the clavicle, indicating the tip of the extra rib.

longstanding cases, more severe symptoms develop; the whole hand has a bursting tense feeling and it is discolored, clammy and cold. The weakness of the hand, particularly on gripping, becomes apparent and, much later, typical intrinsic muscle atrophy develops. Sometimes signs and symptoms develop very rapidly and it is possible for a patient to retire one night quite free of discomfort apart from some vague shoulder ache and awake the following morning with intense pain in the hands and fingers. Chest movement, particularly inspiration, intensifies the symptoms. Palpation of the neck will often demonstrate the rib.

Examination in the early stages shows very few changes in shoulder, arm or hand. The most significant finding is the reproduction of the radiating symptoms by compression of the vascular bundle above the clavicle. Adson has called attention to a most useful test: the patient lifts his chin and tilts it to the affected side; this is done with the patient sitting upright, arms resting on knees. At the same time the radial pulse or blood pressure is checked. Obliteration or significant weakening of the pulse is indicative of subclavian vascular compression due to rib abnormality or scalenus anticus constriction. X-ray examination demonstrates the rib abnormality and, with the above reaction, is diagnostic of this disturbance. Any abnormal calcification above the first rib should arouse suspicion of a cervical rib. Identification of a cervical element versus a first dorsal transverse process is aided by the observation that

the cervical rib points downward, while the first thoracic is frankly transverse.

Late in these cases signs of nerve trunk compression appear in the form of motor and sensory changes in the hand. It is the inferior trunk of the plexus which springs from C.8 and C.7 nerve roots that is most often stretched or compressed. This results in weakness or paralysis of the muscles supplied by the ulnar nerve, interossei, hypothenar group, flexor carpi ulnaris and flexor digitorum profundus to the fourth and fifth fingers. More extensive muscle involvement is rarely encountered, which serves to differentiate the lesion from progressive muscular atrophy, in which a wider group of intrinsic muscles, both thenar and hypothenar are involved. Sensory changes, consisting of hypesthesia and, rarely, anesthesia, also follow the ulnar distribution. Vascular changes, including cyanosis, sweating and fullness of superficial veins, occur later also. Trophic changes, minute ulceration, may occur. The diagnosis rests on the x-ray demonstration of the cervical bony anomaly and the radiating signs and symptoms. Other neurovascular syndromes resemble it closely, but with these findings, the diagnosis is clear-cut.

Etiology and Pathology

Cervical rib has been an interesting anatomical and embryological study for a long time. Eminent authorities have differed on some aspects of the precise mechanism of

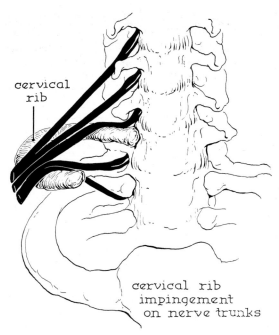

cervical
rib

cervical rib
impingement
on nerve trunks

Figure 9–16 Cervical rib relation to brachial plexus.

production but the general principles have been well accepted. Wood, Jones and Todd, in particular, have made extensive studies. The origin of this anomaly has been traced to the reptilian class, in which lower forms such as snakes have ribs on all vertebrae. Ribless regions gradually appear as the scale is ascended to lizard forms, where elements of limbs appear. The more complicated the limb replica becomes, the more complete do the ribless zones become to allow freedom of movement of the limb. In the early embryo, segments and nerves to segments are well defined. The neural element is dominant, but there is segmental bone and rib develop-

ment (Fig. 9–16). This arrangement of symmetrical nerve and bone contribution persists in snakes, but as limb buds appear there must be a coalescence of elements in the limb bud zone to innervate and support an appendage. The dominant neural element streams into the limb bud, blocking or discouraging corresponding intersegmental bony elements such as ribs.

The limb bud grows at right angles to the vertebral column as a derivative of several body segments, funneling and drawing nerve roots of several segments into it. These roots form a plexus at the base of the limb, preventing costal development (Fig. 9–17). In the cervical region, the brachial plexus is formed and the ribless vertebral zone follows. Lower in the body the lumbosacral plexus similarly favors a ribless lumbar region. If the limb bud fails to develop exactly at the proper segmental level, variations in the elements extending into it may be expected. When it takes off at a segment higher than normal, the main plexus contribution starts from C.4 and consequently less comes from T.1. It is argued that in such circumstances the minute T.1 strand offers less than normal resistance to development of the costal element and a cervical rib appears. This is a so-called prefixed plexus. A postfixed plexus is composed of major contributions, starting at C.6 and extending to C.2. It is not settled whether such a construction occurs and prevents growth of a normal first rib. Presumably, however, nature does recognize neural development as more important than rib and it becomes the controlling force. One remnant of nerve pressure can still be seen in the cervical region in man in the form of the groove on the upper surface of the first rib.

Figure 9–17 Development of cervical rib from conflict of body and neural segments.

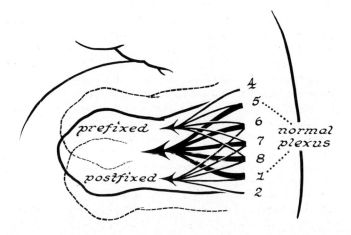

prefixed

postfixed

4
5
6
7
8
1
2

normal
plexus

This is interpreted as arising from pressure of the lower trunk of the plexus against the rib in the nerve conflict described. The depth of this groove increases as the extent of contribution to the brachial plexus from T.1 increases, which supports this theory of primitive nerve dominance. The signs and symptoms arise from pressure on the neurovascular bundle in the neck. The abnormal bone is an obstruction or elevation projecting laterally, lifting up the lower trunk and subclavian vessels.

Treatment of Cervical Rib

Many cervical ribs are found that have caused no symptoms, and no treatment is needed. Many of these having trouble with a demonstrable abnormality need no more than advice and an explanation. Those with persistent signs and symptoms require surgical treatment.

Conservative Treatment

EXPLANATION AND REASSURANCE. Many of these patients become alarmed when told they have an extra bone in the neck, and unlimited disability is imagined. A simple explanation and reassurance that it is a controllable, well understood disturbance helps considerably.

EXERCISE AND POSTURAL INSTRUCTION. Significant signs and symptoms usually do not develop until past middle life and may be initiated by general debility, a recent illness or a postural habit that has favored atony of the suspensory muscles. It may be a transient systemic disturbance that brings the signs and symptoms into focus, and once this has been controlled, the cervical rib manifestations subside. Unless signs and symptoms persist and increase, proper postural instruction and exercises should be tried. Development of the muscles that pull the shoulder back is helpful, since this will decrease the forward drop of the arm.

Surgical Treatment.
Persistent pain, increasing signs of nerve pressure and sympathetic irritation after a conservative trial has proved unsuccessful are indications for operative removal of the obstruction.

TECHNIQUE. A collar incision across the posterior triangle from the sternoclavicular joint is made (Fig. 9–18). Dissection is continued deeply through the platysma, exposing the sternomastoid muscle. The attachment of this muscle may need to be divided or it can be retracted medially, exposing the omohyoid muscle. Transverse cervical and suprascapular arteries appear in the field at this point and usually need to be ligated and divided. There is now exposed the scalenus anterior with the phrenic nerve on its surface. The subclavian artery will then be apparent, compressed by the scalenus against the cervical rib and brachial plexus. The phrenic nerve is retracted and the scalenus anticus is dissected free from the pleura with special care, particularly at the inner border. The muscle is cut obliquely and the fibers retract, decompressing the artery. Sometimes the artery needs to be gently dissected free from the lower roots of the plexus. Frequently, the muscle is thick and bulky and it must be divided carefully, sometimes excising a centimeter or two from the lower attachment.

When there is a large well formed cervical rib, it compresses the lower trunk of the plexus, compelling it to ride up over the top before continuing laterally. The rib is removed by separating the trunk of the plexus, holding the lower trunk down and the middle trunk upward. Adson has suggested reflecting a flap of muscle between the brachial plexus and the subclavian artery to minimize adhesions and scarring. Suture of the omohyoid tendon is done if this has been divided. Postoperatively the patient is allowed up the day after the operation and is discharged as soon as the wound is healed.

DISTURBANCES OF A NORMAL FIRST RIB

Belonging to the group of neurovascular disturbances are several abnormalities of the first rib which are uncommon but will be encountered in clinical practice. Included in these are fractures or an abnormal configuration or position of the rib. These are in contrast to a group of disorders in which the disturbance, although related to the first rib, really results from alteration in the space between the clavicle and the first rib.

The sudden onset of pain in the shoulder, with radiating symptoms, following strenuous unaccustomed activity may sometimes be traced to a fracture of the first rib. It has been suggested that there are predisposing sources, such as the groove for the neurovascular bundle and the point of the scalene muscle attachment to the rib. Strong muscle tow with the scalenus attached posteriorly

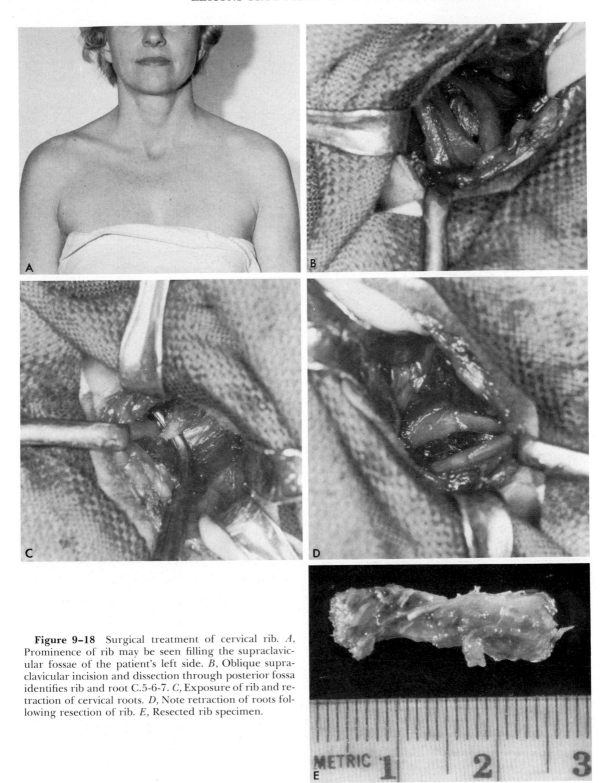

Figure 9-18 Surgical treatment of cervical rib. *A,* Prominence of rib may be seen filling the supraclavicular fossae of the patient's left side. *B,* Oblique supraclavicular incision and dissection through posterior fossa identifies rib and root C.5-6-7. *C,* Exposure of rib and retraction of cervical roots. *D,* Note retraction of roots following resection of rib. *E,* Resected rib specimen.

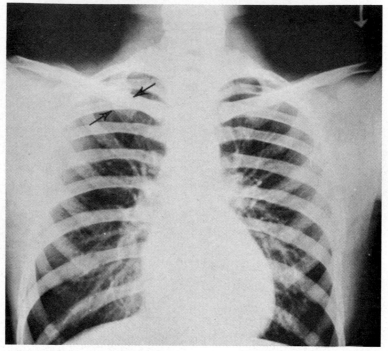

Figure 9–19 Fracture of first rib.

and the subclavius anteriorly may produce sufficient torsion stress reflected to the groove in the bone that it fractures. X-ray examination may initially appear negative, but close scrutiny will show a faint line which later becomes much more apparent as healing progresses and callous formation develops much like that seen in a stress fracture in the foot (Fig. 9–19).

Treatment

No specific therapy is required other than limitation of activity until symptoms have subsided. Sometimes wearing a sling for a period of three weeks diminishes the discomfort.

ABNORMAL POSITION OF THE FIRST RIB

A normally developed first rib may be altered in position so that it interferes with the neurovascular bundle. Frequently improper posture or associated congenital deformities of the cervical spine usher in this disturbance (Fig. 9–20).

The normal axis of the first rib is down and forward. When this plane is altered so that the anterior end is tipped up, the rib becomes more horizontal and abnormal stress on the neurovascular bundle develops as it goes over the top of the horizontal rib. Cervical scoliosis contributes to such a disturbance, as does a congenital hemivertebra. The rib on the convex side of the curve would be higher, with resultant traction on the neurovascular bundle. Shoulder and radiating symptoms develop but may not be apparent until middle life because of early body adaptation. Sometimes symptoms from this disturbance follow a debilitating illness or injury, especially in women. Conservative

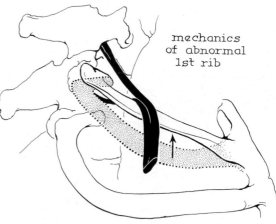

mechanics of abnormal 1st rib

Figure 9–20 Abnormal angle of normal first rib causing pressure on nerve trunks.

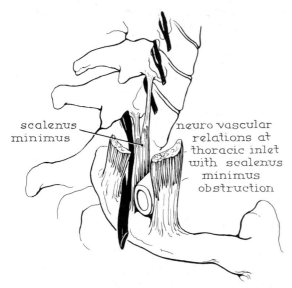

Figure 9–21 Attachments of the scalene group.

treatment is usually sufficient, but occasionally resection of the first rib or scalenotomy is necessary.

SCALENE SYNDROMES

Many anatomical studies have established the variations in the contour, size, incidence and attachment of the scalene muscles (Fig. 9–21). A short hypertrophic muscle can compress subclavian vessels and the lower nerve trunk, resulting in significant symptoms almost identical with those of a cervical

rib. There has been a tendency to lump many disorders under this heading, which accounts for some of the unsatisfactory results of scalenotomy. However, careful attention to the symptomatology of this disturbance identifies a precise syndrome which can be materially helped by scalenotomy.

Treatment

Conservative Treatment. In many patients proper postural training, exercises and avoidance of irritating positions will produce sufficient relief. The extensor position of neck and shoulder aggravates the radiating symptoms, so that resting with a pillow under the head, lifting up the involved shoulder, produces relief (Fig. 9–22). Injection of the scalenus with a local anesthetic relieves acute symptoms, and repeated careful injection reduces further discomfort.

Operative Treatment. Persistent symptoms are relieved by scalenotomy. A 2 inch transverse incision is made over the clavicle about one finger's breadth and an inch from the sternal end (Fig. 9–23). The platysma and deep fascia are divided, and supraclavicular nerves which may be encountered are retracted. The external jugular vein may course across this incision; if it appears to complicate the exposure, it is resected. However, it may often be retracted medially. Dissection at this point brings into view the posterior border of the sternocleidomastoid muscle.

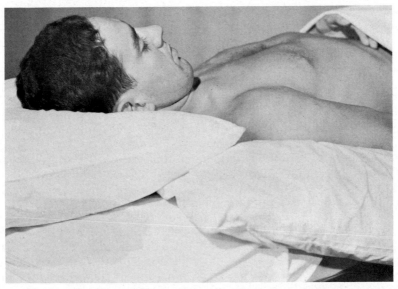

Figure 9–22 Pillow position to relieve scalene tension.

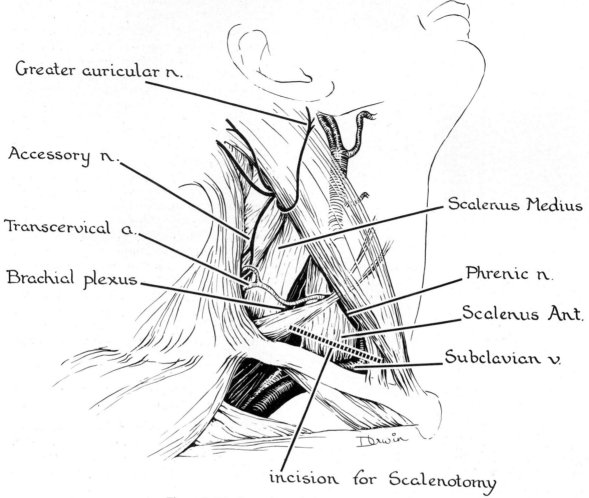

Greater auricular n.

Accessory n.

Transcervical a.

Brachial plexus

Scalenus Medius

Phrenic n.

Scalenus Ant.

Subclavian v.

incision for Scalenotomy

Figure 9–23 Operative technique for scalenotomy.

This is elevated gently and retracted medially, bringing into view the subjacent scalenus anticus. On the anterior surface of this muscle the phrenic nerve crosses in a diagonal fashion. Immediately lateral to the scalenus anticus digital palpation will identify the upper roots C.5 and C.6 of the brachial plexus. Frequently the transcervical vessels course across this field just lateral to the border of the scalenus anticus and they may need to be clamped and resected; if not controlled they may bleed quite vigorously. Retraction of the vessels occurs rapidly and it may be difficult to find them, considerably complicating the exposure. For this reason, if encountered they should be clamped and tied meticulously as one advances deeper into the incision.

The author believes it is extremely important to identify the C.5 and C.6 roots and retract these prior to cutting the scalenus anticus. Considerable variation in the normal anatomy of the scalenus anticus may be encountered; it may be thicker, shorter, much broader or thinner than normal. The significance of the variations is that they often implicate the brachial plexus and the root C.5 and C.6 may run directly through the scalenus substance. This means that if the nerves are not identified initially and retracted, they could easily be cut as the scalenus anticus is severed.

Once the plexus has been carefully identified and retracted, a curved hemostat or a Luer forceps is inserted posteriorly and medially, and the scalenus anticus is gradually elevated so that it may be cut under direct vision. This will help to prevent damage to adjacent structures, particularly the jugular vein or carotid artery.

THORACIC INLET OR CLAVIPECTORAL COMPRESSION SYNDROMES

In addition to the well recognized and clearly described disturbances from cervical ribs and tight scalene muscles, it is apparent that there is a large group of similar but, as a rule, less severe disorders not explained by these two entities. They arise from abnormalities along the course of the nerves and vessels as they pass from thorax to arm and have been variously described as inlet or outlet syndromes. Actually, cervical, rib and scalene disturbances form a part of this group, but the terms inlet and outlet are used to describe those cases which are not adequately explained by such abnormalities. In the past they have probably been called scalene disturbances, and many of the unsatisfactory results that have occurred from scalenotomy may possibly be explained by the recognition of this different etiology.

One thinks of the outlet as the inferior margin of the opening, as, for example, of the pelvis, but these disturbances really have to do with the upper margin or limit of the arm segment much more than with the exit from the thorax. Symptoms come about as a result of brachial activities rather than thoracic function so that the term inlet syndrome would appear to be more appropriate. A more accurate description still is clavipectoral compression syndromes.

The cases under consideration do not fit well into the previous classifications since they are not the result of disc pathology or cervical, rib or scalene disturbances even though they have a somewhat similar symptomatology. Certain distinguishing characteristics of the group can be recognized. The patients have a little shoulder pain, but forearm, hand and finger discomfort is much more prominent; it is vague and indefinitely localized, rarely severe and frequently bilateral. No history of injury or sudden onset is obtained, as a rule. Middle-aged and older persons are affected mostly, and women are involved more often than men; they seek attention after the disability has been noted for some time. There are no clear-cut neurological signs, and disturbances rarely progress to such severity. The subjective discomfort, however, is very real; remissions occur often, to be followed by the return of the same symptoms with similar or increased intensity. Studies of these disorders have been carried out in depth by Wright, Eden, Leday, Kelford, Todd and others and have brought these abnormalities into clearer focus. They result from disturbance of the axillary or brachial inlet area and implicate the neurovascular bundle. A multitude of names have been used, some of which are appropriate to a degree, but none embraces the group as a whole. Outlet syndrome, inlet syndrome, nocturnal dysesthesias, costoclavicular disturbances, pectoralis minor lesions, postural disturbances, posterior triangle lesions, sleep palsy, awakening numbness and sleep tetany are terms that have been variously used. Out of this large assortment several distinct groups are recognized: (1) costoclavicular disturbances; (2) postural syndrome group; (3) hyperabduction syndrome; and (4) sleep dysesthesias. Since the maximum disturbance arises along the course of the neurovascular bundle as it passes under the clavicle and the pectoral muscles, the author has referred to these disorders as a whole as the clavipectoral compression syndromes (Fig. 9–24).

ETIOLOGY AND PATHOLOGY OF THE GROUP AS A WHOLE

The vascular bundle follows a tortuous course from the mediastinum to the arm. Halfway through, it becomes associated with the major nerve trunks, and it is from this

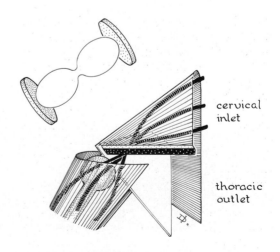

cervical inlet

thoracic outlet

Constricting effect of clavicle. Hourglass configuration.

Figure 9–24 Constricting role of clavicle on the neurovascular bundle.

point on that the neurovascular bundle may be disturbed. Of necessity there must be a mobile segment in the root of this bundle to allow for the activities of the arm. The function of the upper extremity, having progressed to extensive mobility and prehension, demands much more freedom than was necessary in former plantigrade or weight-bearing duty. This mobile area occurs in a zone from under the clavicle to below the pectoralis minor border. Above and below this segment the bundle is anchored so that movement of the arm does not transmit movement to the vessels. The scalenus anterior lies above this area and does not take part in this zone so that it is not a factor in the present group. The channel that the neurovascular bundle follows is roofed by the clavicle, the clavipectoral fascia and, finally, the pectoralis minor (Fig. 9–25). This zone lies opposite the shoulder joint so that both nerve and vessels crossing are irritated more by movement here than either above or below (Fig. 9–26).

The interval between clavicle and pectoralis minor is bridged by the costocoracoid membrane, which is a remnant of the precoracoid (Fig. 1–5). This membrane may be thickened at the lower edge or rolled into a taut string at its margin as it arches onto the chest. Cadaver studies have shown considerable variation in this structure. It may be a thin filamentous layer or a snug band which hampers and constricts the vascular bundle when the arm is abducted and rotated (Fig. 9–27).

Confusion exists as to the role of the clavicle. Ordinarily it would appear that ample room remains for the exit of the vessels underneath, and this is increased on abduction of the arm because the clavicle rolls upward, allowing the curved medial portion to lift and providing more room over the vessels (Fig. 9–25). It is conceivable that on extension, direct backward traction of the shoulder without rotation or abduction of the arm, the space occupied by the subclavian vein is decreased. Further along the course it can be demonstrated that the bundle is embarrassed by abduction and external rotation in the region of the head of the humerus and beneath the pectoralis minor. At the extreme of abduction and rotation, the vessels are hooked around the coracoid process and the pectoralis minor (Fig. 9–26, *A*). When there is a strong costocoracoid ligament this structure compresses the vessels first, at a higher level (Fig. 9–27).

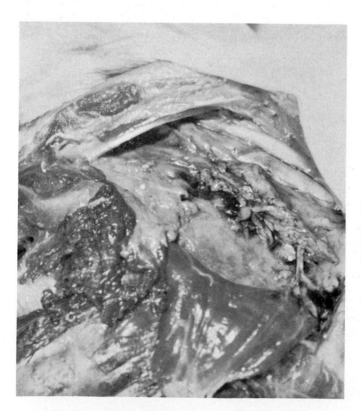

Figure 9–25 Dissection of clavipectoral area of left shoulder showing relation of subclavicular structures to the neurovascular bundle. The subclavius muscle is at the top below the clavicle and arches over the nerves and vessels. It has a stout sharply defined tendinous lower border. The pectoralis minor has been reflected in the lower part of the field.

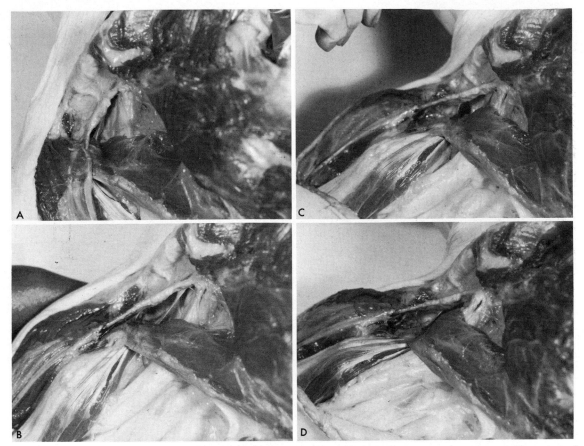

Figure 9–26 Relation of the pectoralis minor and the neurovascular bundle on arm movement. *A*, Dissection of pectoral region shows the pectoralis minor relaxed and slack when the arm is at the side. *B*, As abduction is started the pectoralis minor tenses and the neurovascular bundle becomes tensed. *C*, Increased tension is apparent as the arm reaches 70 degrees. *D*, At a right angle, with the elbow extended, the pectoralis minor is taut and wraps around the neurovascular bundle.

COSTOCLAVICULAR DISTURBANCES

The cleft behind the clavicle may be encroached upon by distortion of the clavicle and this may occur either as an acute process or as a complication some time after a fracture of the clavicle.

Pathology of Subclavicular Lesions

Acute Injury. Tremendous force is needed to break the clavicle in the area which is directly above the nerves and vessels. In this region the clavicle has its strongest construction, being tubular in section so that it serves as a rugged overlying protection to the important elements beneath it. Fractures of the medial third or sometimes at the junction of the inner middle thirds result from an overpowering application of force, such as heavy weights falling on the shoulder. The

vessels and nerves may be injured as the clavicle is shattered. In some instances a crushing injury creates sharp segments which lacerate the structures after the clavicle has largely dissipated the force of the impact. In other instances the force of the impact continues and acts as a dragging traction mechanism, further traumatizing the subjacent structures. In this fashion the great vessels may be torn or lacerated as they are pulled over the first rib, which then acts as a fulcrum in this injury process. In the acute phase, the clinical picture is a dramatic one, with extensive swelling above the clavicle and formation of a large hematoma in the axilla and anterior chest region. Arterial rupture may be apparent from the very extensive swelling and the compromise of the blood supply to the rest of the extremity. Sometimes it is the vein which is involved, and this leads to considerable, but much less, swelling

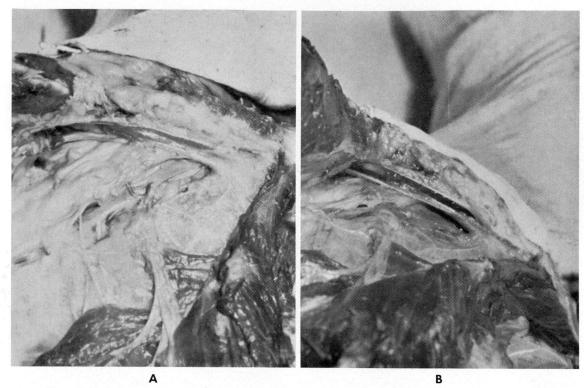

Figure 9–27 Reaction of costocoracoid membrane to the neurovascular bundle. *A,* The fascia is prolonged around the bundle from subclavicular structures. *B,* The costocoracoid ligament is intimately related above.

than when the artery is punctured; the gradual formation of a large hematoma indicates the source.

In some instances an arteriovenous aneurysm will develop from a puncture wound of the artery and vein. Few symptoms may be apparent in the initial stage, but within a matter of days radiating discomfort develops as a result of the compression of the nerve elements. Intractible pain of the radiating variety with altered sensation in the hand, as well as the local changes, is characteristic of this stage. An anterior venous aneurysm at this site can quickly erode the nerves; once it has been identified, it constitutes a surgical emergency.

In the chronic process exuberant callus developing at the seat of what usually has been a comminuted fracture gradually implicates the subjacent structures (Fig. 9–28). In these instances radiating symptoms are a gradual development, with symptoms of the vascular compression appearing first and disturbances of the neural elements developing afterward. Peripheral pain, intermittent whole hand numbness, frequent color change and, eventually, intermittent swelling are encountered.

Treatment

Acute Injuries. Immediate exposure of the subclavicular structures with sufficient extension of the incision to enable mobilization of the neural and vascular trunks above and below the clavicle is essential. The fracture fragments are retracted and the vascular lesion identified. In most instances it is possible to repair the arterial damage. A bayonet type of incision is employed; this begins above the medial end of the clavicle, extends in the transverse fashion along the clavicle to its midpoint and then distally for about 6 inches below the clavicle.

Chronic Problems. Chronic subclavicular compression is a much less formidable lesion to control. Surgical measures are required and involve exposure and resection of the zone of exuberant callus. In some instances it is necessary to completely transect the clavicle and remove a portion for adequate decompression. This has a beneficial effect on the neurovascular bundle in that it decompresses both the nerves and the vessels. Recently, resection of the first rib has been suggested in cases such as this. This could be done through a posterior axillary approach, with

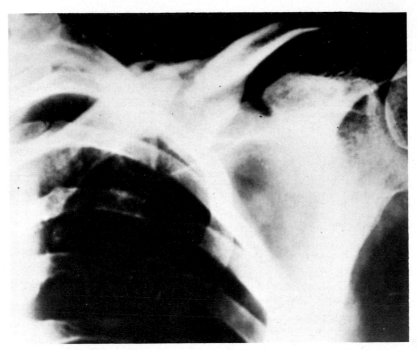

Figure 9–28 Costoclavicular pressure behind clavicle caused by callus.

removal of the segment of the rib, which would increase the space in the cleft between the clavicle and first rib.

POSTURAL LESIONS

Altered relative position of the shoulder girdle to the neurovascular bundle, or vice versa, is a common element in all these disorders. However, a group may be separated in which there is a relatively static process, or one which comes on gradually as a more general development without specific, separate, irritating incidents. They are labeled "postural" because of the alteration of the normal girdle relationship to the rest of the body. This group of patients is to be separated from those who experience discomfort from a specific action but have no structural abnormality.

Clinical Picture

Thin, middle-aged or elderly women are most frequently affected. They complain of bilateral numbness and tingling in the fingers and a vague aching shoulder neck discomfort. Symmetrical sagging of both shoulders is apparent and is the result of muscle atony and the aging process. Paralytic disorders develop this same sensation. Loss of the suspensory muscle tone, as in complete paralysis of trapezius and levator scapulae, allows the shoulder girdle to drop, embarrassing the neurovascular bundle (Fig. 9–29). Relative, or nonstructural, decompensation is seen in patients after a serious illness in which debilitation and general poor body development favor an extremely slouched posture. Those who have changed their work to a more strenuous activity with altered postural requirements may have similar

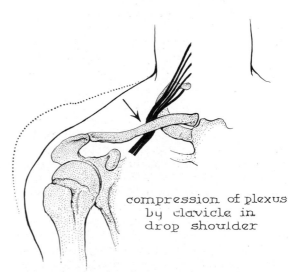

compression of plexus
by clavicle in
drop shoulder

Figure 9–29 Compression behind the clavicle.

transient symptoms. Motor and sensory signs rarely develop, but the subjective paresthesias are very real. A common error is to blame the symptoms on the normal bone changes in the cervical spine. The vascular symptoms of a feeling of fullness in the fingers, fingertip tingling, and involvement of the whole hand usually are distinguishing features.

Treatment

Local. Any obvious predisposing disorder is eradicated. Drop shoulder, paralytic lesions, and so forth, are treated. In permanent paralysis, suspensory operative procedures (see Chapters VII and XIV) are necessary. Sling support for both arms for four to six weeks is advised in the acute or convalescent postural group. Physiotherapy aided by electrical stimulation is started, with attention to developing suspensory muscles. Proper working and sleeping postures are outlined.

Systemic. Often a general body building program is needed. Nutrition is improved by proper diet and food supplements. Assistance of a skilled internist in correcting and regulating any associated cardiac, thoracic or renal abnormalities is indicated. This group of patients may be confused with those with the acroparesthesias discussed later.

HYPERABDUCTION SYNDROMES

The neurovascular bundle may be compressed in the zone distal to the clavicle as it passes beneath the costocoracoid membrane and pectoralis minor. I.S. Wright has called particular attention to the contribution of the pectoralis minor in this mechanism, and it appears as a significant factor in this broad group with shoulder and radiating symptoms.

Clinical Picture

This syndrome is seen most frequently in young male adults of short, thick-set, stocky stature. It is a more acute condition than the preceding disorders. Shoulder discomfort is related chiefly to the front and in the region of the coracoid process. Numbness and tingling in the fingers, a feeling of the hand going asleep, and a sense of fullness are the chief complaints. These symptoms may be noticed on awakening, but the greatest discomfort

occurs during working hours. Investigation frequently shows that the patient is working with his arms in the overhead or above-shoulder position, or his duties require much lifting and tension in the shoulder flexed position. Abduction usually is a most irritating maneuver, and the patient will note relief from keeping the arm at the side.

Tenderness over the coracoid is a frequent finding. The cardinal sign is reproduction of the discomfort by pressure over the pectoralis minor just below the coracoid. At this point deep pressure compresses the neurovascular bundle against the chest, reproducing the radiating signs (Fig. 9–30). Definite motor, sensory or reflex changes are lacking. The hand may be a little swollen at times and all fingers will be involved. Frequently the patient himself has observed the position that initiates the discomfort. As a rule, the radial pulse is obliterated on abduction or manipulation of the arm much more easily than on the uninvolved side. Wright has pointed out that in 80 to 90 per cent of normals, the radial pulse is obliterated on hyperabduction, but in this group are some in whom it is produced much more easily and with less extensive change in posture. Not many patients normally retain this posture for any length of time.

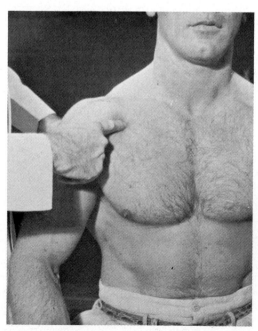

Figure 9–30 Testing for subcoracoid compression of the neurovascular bundle.

Treatment

1. Remove the occupational strain or postural habit initiating the discomfort. Sometimes patients work out a satisfactory routine themselves once the disturbance is explained.

2. In longstanding problems, tension on the pectoralis minor may become sufficiently severe to warrant cutting the muscle close to the coracoid. When conservative measures fail and the symptoms are definitely related to hyperabduction, this is a satisfactory procedure.

Operative Technique. The arm, axilla and shoulder area are suitably prepared. The patient is placed in the supine position. The neurovascular bundle is approached through a linear incision 6 inches long, just below the coracoid and centered over the pectoralis minor insertion (Figs. 9–31, 9–32). The pectoralis major is split in the direction of its fibers. Beneath this muscle, the pectoralis minor can be identified at its attachment to the coracoid process. The muscle is cut close to the insertion, between a pair of inserted clamps. It is retracted medially, exposing the neurovascular bundle. By gentle dissection the bundle is freed of any adhesions. The pectoralis minor is allowed to retract as it will. Sometimes a thick costocoracoid ligament is encountered and this is cut also.

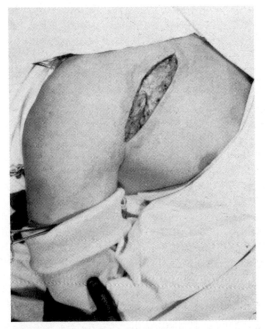

Figure 9–31 Incision for exposure and cutting the pectoralis minor.

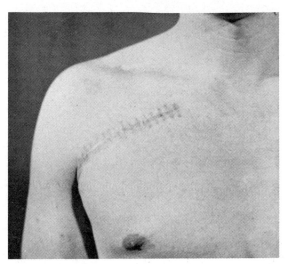

Figure 9–32 Healed incision, postoperatively.

Any obvious adhesions involving the neurovascular bundle are excised.

SLEEP DYSESTHESIAS OR NOCTURNAL ARM DISTURBANCES

The final group of patients manifesting radiating discomfort due to neurovascular compression are those whose symptoms are associated with sleep or recumbency. This is a common disturbance and many descriptive terms are applied, such as nocturnal dysesthesia (Wartenberg), sleep tetany, waking numbness, nocturnal palsy and morning numbness. The experience of awakening with the arm and hand asleep is common to all. For example, the neurovascular bundle may be compressed by lying on the side with the arm under the body. Resting with the arm in the abducted and externally rotated position may stretch the nerves and vessels, leading to the typical tingling discomfort in hand and fingers. This may assume pathological proportions if the irritation is prolonged. One of the most interesting clinical experiments ever reported is that of T.W. Wood, who produced the signs and symptoms of this group by sleeping with the arm in the abducted position (Fig. 9–33). Numbness, tingling, paresis and even trophic changes appear to be dramatically relieved by the assumption of a normal posture.

Clinical Picture

These patients are usually between 40 and 60 years of age and complain of some mild

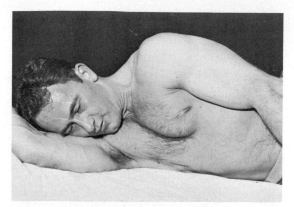

Figure 9–33 Sleep compression of the neurovascular bundle. Note venous distension of the forearm and arm after 3 minutes in this position.

shoulder ache, but the dominant discomfort is in hand and fingers. It is noted chiefly on awakening in the morning or after resting for a period. It often wakes the patients at night and they get up and walk around the room, flicking the hand and arm to restore feeling and circulation. The discomfort goes quickly, since almost any movement brings relief. They may return to bed and go through the same performance again. Often they learn to sleep with the arm hanging over the side of the bed or in some other unusual position. A common cause is some change in the normal sleeping habits because of a different bed, new surroundings or having to lie in the same position to avoid irritating some sore part of the body. It is not a serious disorder and almost never progresses far enough to produce motor, sensory or trophic disturbances. Paresthesias involve the whole hand, but the medial border more prominently. This has been ascribed to traction on the inferior cord of the plexus, which produces discomfort in the ulnar nerve distribution.

Treatment

Avoiding the irritating position relieves the discomfort. Patients often are a little credulous when this is suggested as a remedy. Some study and effort are needed to break sleep habits at times since the provoking attitude varies widely. A short or too small bed is a common cause since it forces the patient to sleep in a cramped position or to keep the arm at an unusual angle. It may be necessary to keep the arm at the side by tying the wrist to the side of the bed. Sedation is to be avoided because deep sleep aggravates the condition.

RAYNAUD'S DISEASE, ACROPARESTHESIAS, THROMBOANGIITIS OBLITERANS

Mention is made of these disorders because they may be confused with some of the preceding conditions. They differ profoundly in that there is no mention of shoulder discomfort, no relation to arm or shoulder movement, and body posture has no effect. The peripheral symptoms, however, are very similar, accounting for the confusion. Raynaud's disease is manifested by profound peripheral vasomotor upset. Blanching of the fingertips occurs in spasm, followed by painful reddening or cyanotic suffusion of the same zone. Exposure to cold precipitates these attacks, both hands usually being involved. Acroparesthesia is a much milder disorder encountered chiefly in women about the menopausal age. Painful reddening of the fingers is the common finding and is sometimes, but not always, related to exposure to cold. Alleviation of symptoms has been reported following proper hormonal therapy. Acrosclerosis or acroscleroderma is a condition with similar finger and hand discomfort distinguished by skin disturbances such as excess corneal layers and thickening. Thromboangiitis obliterans involves the upper extremity, producing finger discomfort also. The altered radial pulsation, progressive nature of the disease, usual relationship to smoking, phlebitic episodes and trophic ulceration are distinctive.

REFLEX DYSTROPHY OF THE UPPER EXTREMITY (SHOULDER-HAND SYNDROMES)

The shoulder is linked with the hand in a symptom complex presenting the features of a reflex sympathetic disturbance. This is a picture of neurovascular upset which develops as a result of sympathetic stimulation. In the majority of cases it is secondary to some other factor, but the reflex dystrophy phenomena becomes so predominant that common usage has labeled it a cause when it is really a result (Fig. 9–34).

We are familiar with reflex sympathetic dystrophy in the lower extremity such as that established by Sudeck's classic descrip-

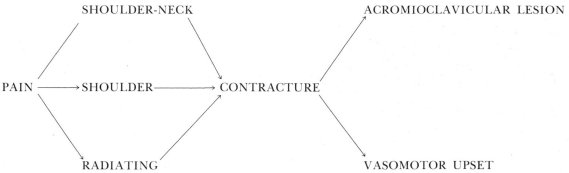

PRIMARY   *SECONDARY*   *TERTIARY*

Figure 9–34 Stages in the development of reflex dystrophy.

tion of posttraumatic osteoporosis. It is reasonable to anticipate that a similar disturbance may occur in the upper extremity. Recent observations show clearly that, in addition to injury, other disorders occur of a purely medical nature, resulting in a dystrophy involving shoulder and hand. The underlying construction of the upper extremity is such that reflex sympathetic disturbances will draw together the shoulder and hand if there is involvement of either as a primary episode. The swollen hand following a Colles' fracture in the elderly female is a classic example; the shoulder movement is unconsciously limited when the peripheral grasping end is thrown out of kilter. The stimulus for use of the whole extremity is no longer active so that parts at a distance are affected. Similarly, by the same mechanism, a shoulder bruised by a fall on a slippery kitchen floor may result in a painful swollen hand.

The shoulder-hand syndrome is a clinical complex which can arise following heart disease, hemiplegia, herpes zoster, thoracic disease, thrombophlebitis and trauma. In addition, there is a group of cases in which no clear incident or primary factor may be found. These patients have the typical dystrophic hand with profound shoulder involvement and constitute the so-called idiopathic group; however, they are a minority. Budeck, Steinbrocker and De Takats have done outstanding studies of this whole group of disorders. In many cases, when primary etiology is not apprent, more careful search will show trauma as the cause.

SIGNS AND SYMPTOMS

Pains begin in the shoulder area, but shortly shift to the periphery and are accompanied by limitation of movement, swelling and a dusky hue to the skin (Figs. 9–35, 9–36 and 9–37). The hand is warm at first but later becomes cold and sweating is increased. The pain is diffuse and does not conform to isolated nerve patterns. The part is sensitive to pressure or manipulation, and the sensitivity increases to a point at which the patient wears an anxious expression and is fearful of the slightest movement. The complex obviously involves the shoulder, but the most painful aspect develops in the hand. The elderly patient with a fracture of any kind that must be immobilized in a plaster or sling may develop the whole complex, which becomes far more difficult to treat than the initial injury. Since not all cases of stiff shoulder develop the severe vasomotor upset in the hand, the controlling causes are not quite clear.

There is limitation of shoulder movement in all directions, the pain is a dull, burning ache rather than a lancinating, sharp discomfort of nerve root irritation. The hand is uniformly swollen, painful and tender. The important aspect of diagnosis is determination of the source of the primary disturbances rather than being satisfied with recognizing the secondary syndrome. The presenting reflex dystrophy often masks the underlying disturbance; danger lies in treating this syndrome and not recognizing it as a result rather than a primary cause. For instance,

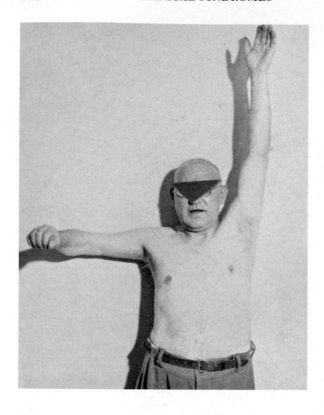

Figure 9-35 Shoulder-hand syndrome. Note limitation of shoulder motion and the swollen right hand.

a heart problem may be neglected while the hand and shoulder are treated. The common causes of this syndrome are found in: (1) the shoulder, (2) trauma to any part of the upper extremity, (3) the heart, (4) the chest, (5) the neck, and (6) the nervous system.

ETIOLOGY AND PATHOLOGY

Sympathetic stimulation is presumed to be the cause of this disorder. Clinical observation and response to therapy rather than a definite physiological demonstration are the basis for this conclusion. Similar disorders elsewhere in the body, like Sudeck's atrophy, are explained on the same grounds. It is a profound neurovascular upset, but the various trigger mechanisms setting it off are not all clearly understood. One form of sympathetic upset which has a proved neural association is the symptom complex known as causalgia. It is featured by burning pain, swollen hand, glassy skin and a trigger-like response to certain stimuli. An overirritated sympathetic reaction is the suggested cause of this condition, and possibly somewhat similar mechanisms operate in the shoulder-hand complex. A course of afferent stimuli is set up which calls forth both a peripheral and central response which, in turn, develops

hyperreactive or hypersensitive properties, and a vicious cycle is established. A study of this mechanism involves analysis of both the central and peripheral contributions.

Central Mechanism. In the spinal cord a network of connecting neurons is present in the gray matter. It extends up and down the cord, connecting many segments, and is described as the "internuncial pool" (see Fig. 3-23). Trauma to the upper extremity produces painful sensation or afferent impulses that are recorded in this area. Such impulses may connect with sympathetic or anterior horn motor neurons and be reflected as neurovascular signs and symptoms. Pain is set up in the usual fashion by irritation of afferent receptors in the injured area. Normally this subsides, but if a state of hyperexcitability or hyperacceptability in this central connecting network occurs, there will be a continued or persistent source of irritative impulses bombarding neurovascular connections. Why this imbalance should persist has many conjectural explanations. It has been postulated that persistent pain impulses are due to scar and fibrosis about the injured area, producing the hyperexcitable internuncial pool. If this reflex is interrupted at any point, the cyclic persistent chain of symptoms is broken. Apparently the

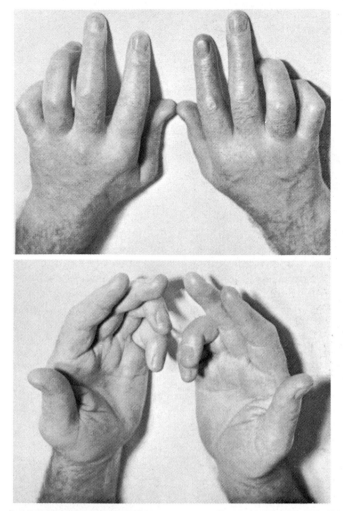

Figure 9-36 Shoulder hand syndrome. Note swollen tense fingers with shiny tips.

result of this persistent pain irritation is the production of a preliminary sympathetic paralysis, which would account for the vasodilatation seen clinically, which, in turn, is followed by a sympathetic overactivity, resulting in vasoconstriction. The late changes in the disorder are caused by vasoconstriction. The osteoporosis is due to the hyperemia which occurs in the early stages.

Peripheral Changes. The peripheral changes are a little more clearly defined because sweating, congestion, blushing and

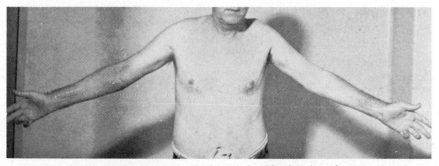

Figure 9-37 Example of bilateral shoulder-hand syndrome.

swelling are mediated by sympathetic fibers. In the main nerve trunks lies the vasoconstrictor control from which fibers are distributed to the periphery. The arterioles are principally supplied, and there is a greater concentration of these in the hand than in the shoulder, which explains the profound involvement of the hand in a sympathetic upset. Normally a restraining constrictor tone is maintained, and when this is cut or released, vasodilatation occurs. Sympathetic irritation also increases sweating because the sweat glands have sympathetic supply. A local axon reflex is at work as well because local pain stimuli produce vasodilatation which may persist as long as the pain lasts. The reaction in the shoulder follows the appreciation of pain. Possibly in an effort to avoid any stimuli, the joint is kept still, and secondary changes develop in synovium and capsule. Movement at the shoulder then initiates further pain, which falls on a system already hyperactive to such stimuli so that the whole process is reinforced.

Shoulder Disorders Initiating Reflex Dystrophies. This syndrome can develop in almost any of the shoulder disorders that have been discussed. The onset of pain sufficiently severe to cause the patient to immobilize the shoulder, and hence, the extremity, can be followed by sympathetic upset. Quickly the peripheral pain may dominate the situation and the shoulder becomes of secondary importance.

What produces the sympathetic disturbance in one patient and not in the other is not clear. Thus, tendinitis, calcific tendinitis, cuff rupture, bicipital lesions, cervical discs, cervical arthritis, scalenus disturbances, cervical rib, and so forth, can all be followed by this sympathetic upset. In general, the shoulder conditions which result in reflex dystrophy occur in the older age group. Reflex dystrophy is not seen in the disorders of industry and occupation unless some other factor, such as indiscriminate immobilization, has been added.

Trauma. In the older age group almost any injury to the upper extremity may be followed by limitation of shoulder movement and a painful swollen hand. A Colles' fracture or sprained wrist may be followed by a profound sympathetic upset. Carrying the arm in a sling for two weeks in treatment of a sprained wrist may be enough to set off a full-blown reflex dystrophy. The mechanism in this instance is that of synovial and capsular contraction at the inferior aspect of the joint

as the beginning of the freezing process. This restricts shoulder movement, and when an attempt is made to break down this process, the pain occurs which the patient instinctively interprets as an indication to keep the arm tight at the side, so that the whole process starts over. We are all familiar with such a shoulder lesion arising from a slight sprain in older people. The late changes of soft tissue contracture are similar to those resulting from immobilization, but in this instance the immobilization was produced by the pain. The ulnar supply to the forearm is chiefly involved and possibly this is due to greater susceptibility of the inferior cord, along with the vessels, to irritation (Fig. 9–38).

Cardiac Etiology. It has long been known that this syndrome can develop after myocardial infarction. A stiff painful shoulder is noted three to four weeks after a cardiovascular accident, to be followed later by changes in the hand. Sometimes after subsidence of the acute symptoms, atypical ulnar, nerve-like flexion contracture of the hand remains. All the structures, periarticular as well as soft parts, are involved and may become fixed.

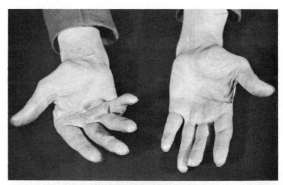
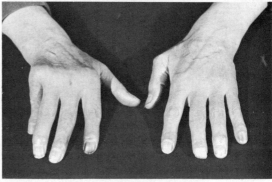

Figure 9–38 Late changes in shoulder-hand syndrome; contracture of the fingers is almost like Dupuytren's contracture.

Myocardial damage can be reflected in the internuncial or spinal cord connecting network through superior, middle and inferior cardiac nerves. Impulses passing along these nerves to the pool radiate to sympathetic synapses, initiating the characteristic vasomotor changes. The cardiac infarction may heal, but it is presumed that the internuncial pool continues to reflect afferent impulses that perpetuate the sympathetic stimulation. It is more probable that the sympathetic upset, once initiated, is difficult to correct and that under some as yet not understood circumstances it may be a self-perpetuating process. Added to this chain is the damage from immobilization and disuse, which augments the whole process. The hand signs frequently appear on both sides in the postmyocardial group, but the left predominates. This is, as would be expected, the result of the central location of the primary disorder. Cardiac infarction is not needed to produce the syndrome since other heart abnormalities such as persistent angina and auricular fibrillation have been recorded as being followed by the typical reflex disturbances.

Cerebral Lesions. The paralyzed extremity of the hemiplegic often presents the typical picture of sympathetic dystrophy. The cerebrovascular accident interferes with autonomic control, in addition to disrupting motor function. The paralytic extremity is fertile ground for the development of reflex abnormalities from the process of immobilization. It does not seem necessary to postulate a separate cerebral mechanism. Disuse atrophy and capsular contraction are common unless specific steps are taken early to prevent them.

Miscellaneous Disorders. Many other conditions have been reported as causing the shoulder-hand syndrome. Herpes zoster affecting the neck-shoulder zone is frequently followed by the sympathetic changes. Once the primary disorder comes under control, the sympathetic disturbances subside as a rule.

TREATMENT OF SHOULDER-HAND SYNDROME

Treatment of the Underlying Condition. It should be emphasized that this is a symptom complex arising from a great many completely unrelated disorders. All these conditions must have appropriate treatment first, and if this does not improve the sympathetic dystrophic disturbance, attention is paid to the local condition. If the syndrome is recognized, it may be possible to treat the primary and the complicating condition at the same time.

Treatment of Sympathetic Upset. Interruption of the sympathetic supply by stellate ganglion injection has been the most effective therapy. The stellate ganglion may be injected with a local anesthetic, thereby changing the sympathetic imbalance. It must be done with great care under the best of conditions. It is a safe procedure in skilled hands, but serious complications can develop. Performing it in the hospital or in the hospital outpatient department is preferable, since oxygen and resuscitation facilities are available if needed. Depending upon the response, it may be repeated at three- to seven-day intervals.

TECHNIQUE OF STELLATE BLOCK. Most techniques of stellate block are based upon the anatomic relationship of the stellate ganglion to cervical prevertebral fascia. The ganglion lies behind the tough prevertebral fascia in front of the transverse process at the level of C.7 and T.1. The fascia is penetrated above the ganglion zone and the local anesthetic allowed to run down, diffusing over the sympathetic trunk and the ganglia. The fascia prevents a superficial leak of the solution. Caldwell and associates have presented a most careful study on the "short-needle" technique, which is safer, quicker and more effective than those previously described. The simplest approach is that of Patzer. With the patient lying down, the chin is tilted up and away from the sore side. The thumb of one hand displaces the transverse process of C.6. This is felt by noting the prominent C.7 spine posteriorly and the cricoid cartilage lower border anteriorly. The needle is inserted just behind the thumb and angled medially until the transverse process is felt. It is then slid over the anterior aspect a little, ending medial to the scalenus anticus muscle. Before injection of the solution, the needle is observed for cerebrospinal fluid regurgitation. One cubic centimeter of 2 per cent Novocain is inserted slowly; after a short pause to observe any response, a further 4 cc is inserted. A good block produces ptosis, enophthalmos, myosis, and ipsilateral anhydrosis in addition to pain relief and increased warmth of the extremity.

Complications may occur such as pneumothorax, hemothorax, subarachnoid injection and reaction to the anesthetic agent. It is well for the procedure to be done in a hospital where oxygen and resuscitation are immediately available; only those completely familiar with the technique should use it. Intravenous administration of Pentothal or other barbiturates counteracts anesthetic reaction. Despite this formidable list of possible accidents, they are infrequent and should not constitute a contraindication if reasonable precautions are taken. There are other techniques, for which the reader is referred to the listed references.

Specific Physiotherapy in Shoulder-Hand Syndrome. Since both shoulder and hand are involved, this is a painful condition and exercise therapy must be initiated gradually, with care to avoid the brusque approach. More tact is needed to deal with these patients because they are older and a little less pliable, and other disorders often complicate the picture. Cooperation is essential in all exercise programs, and a special effort is needed in this disorder. The usual program is to give the stellate blocks at weekly intervals. It is in the period shortly after the block when pain is most effectively relieved that exercise should be started. Once there has been some relief of pain, much of the limiting spasm disappears and the patient volunteers a sense of freedom.

HAND EXERCISES. Opening and closing the hand as a whole is started. This is repeated until a rhythm is developed, and the same routine is carried out with the opposite hand, which reinforces the movement pattern. This movement is done 10 to 15 times, depending upon the patient's response and tolerance. A short rest period is allowed, followed by a similar effort. When the fist is opened, the fingers are fanned. In clenching the fist the thumb is brought alternately inside and outside of the fingers. Attention is paid then to strengthening the finger action, to individual finger action and to increasing wrist movement. If finger movement is particularly sluggish, or if the stellate block effects have worn off, hydrotherapy may help. An ordinary basin of warm water or a whirlpool bath seems to ease the pain and spasm, and the buoyancy favors movement. Some gentle passive assistance can be added, but movements must be kept within the pain threshold. One suggested routine is five minutes of exercise every hour, then ten minutes every two hours, then 15 minutes four times a day.

SHOULDER EXERCISES. The nature of the underlying lesion governs the amount and the extent of the shoulder exercise. In most patients it is preferable to start in the supine position. The elbow is flexed and the arm is lifted forward. This exercise is repeated until rhythmic movement is possible. With the confidence gained on flexion, abduction then is attempted, repeated and carried to the pain limit. Keeping the elbow flexed aids this movement. Rotation is then started with the forearm at a right angle and the hand resting on the bed. External rotation is attempted and gradually increased over a week, when some improvement should be noted and some confidence restored. The shoulder routine is alternated with the hand routine and done for the same periods.

Supine, pendulum or standing exercises are started next. These also are not so extensive as in other shoulder routines because of the pain and the usual general condition. Flexion with elbows flexed is started, then abduction with elbows flexed is added. Rotation is started with the arm at the side. Later, with elbow extended, flexion and abduction are initiated. Gradually these fundamental movements are put together in composite acts, such a touching the back of the neck, reaching the hand behind into the back pocket, and crawling up the back to the shoulder blade. When pain is controlled, gentle passive stretching is added in acts such as placing both hands behind the head and pushing elbows backward. Heavy resistance and powerful pulley exercises are not used in these conditions. Over a period of three to four weeks stellate blocks are continued along with the exercise instruction. After six weeks the patient is encouraged to carry on the routine without assistance, but supervision for a longer period is necessary in refractive cases.

PHYSIOTHERAPY. Supervised physiotherapy is most important and should be combined with the other techniques. There is little use in paying attention to the vascular disturbance alone, unless the supporting muscle function keeps pace with it.

SURGERY. In intractable cases, when there is no serious primary disease or primary disturbances do not contraindicate it, surgical sympathectomy may be considered.

DRUG THERAPY. Sympathomimetic drugs such as Etamon and Priscoline can be used to support the other measures.

CORTISONE. The use of cortisone in

relatively small dosage is effective in this disorder when primary conditions do not contraindicate. The cortisone relieves the pain and improves muscle function, counteracting the sympathetic upset. It may be started with 5 mg tablets and the patient carried on this as a maintenance dose for two to three weeks. As with the other methods of treatment, treatment of the primary cause and physiotherapy to the part are applied at the same time.

TREATMENT SUMMARY FOR SHOULDER AND RADIATING PAIN

Cervical Root Syndrome

1. Recognize the common cause as intraforaminal compression but remember that more serious lesions like tumors are possible.

2. Remember special methods of investigation: oblique x-rays, contrast studies, cerebrospinal fluid analysis.

3. Excise tumors, but treat other lesions conservatively, as a rule.

4. Apply traction by hospital or home apparatus.

5. Follow with a plaster collar or light chin splint if necessary.

6. Instruct patient in proper sleeping routine, with a small pillow and firm bed.

7. Cases unrelieved by conservative means are few, but in these few, cervical laminectomy or foraminal decompression is indicated.

Cervical Ribs

1. Recognize this lesion by the neurovascular character of symptoms, often bilateral, and the typical x-rays.

2. Try a conservative program of exercises first; avoid irritating positions and occupational strain.

3. In patients with persistent symptoms, do scalenotomy with or without resection of the rib, depending upon the condition found at operation.

4. Remember that vascular anomalies frequently accompany the rib disturbance and unusual formations may be encountered at operation.

Scalene Syndrome

1. Remember this possibility when symptoms and signs are suggestive of a cervical rib but x-rays are negative.

2. Special signs of scalene irritability include local tenderness and reproduction of symptoms on tilting head away from the sore side. These are relieved by local anesthetic infiltration.

3. Try a conservative regime first, and if not successful do a scalenotomy.

Clavipectoral Compression Syndromes

1. Think of this group of disorders as an explanation for cases not fitting well into cervical rib or scalene categories.

2. Recognize the common pattern of neurovascular radiating discomfort of moderate severity and then consider the subgroups of costoclavicular, postural, hyperabduction and nocturnal disorders.

3. *Costoclavicular Lesions.* Prevent irritating activities, improve muscle tone and power of suspensory group. Eradicate obvious structural abnormalities of clavicle.

4. *Postural Group.* In the acute phase, use sling support for both arms, rest and physiotherapy. Improve general systemic health. Treat any obvious irritating lesion like trapezius paralysis.

5. *Hyperabduction Syndrome.* Think of this disorder in young, active men of stocky stature who perform heavy labor. Correct the work or recreational habit that initiates the symptoms, usually unaccustomed or excessive hyperabduction. Cut pectoralis minor in refractive cases.

6. *Sleep Disturbances.* This common complaint is often initiated by a change in sleeping position or surroundings. Break the habit of compressing the shoulder or upper arm region during sleep.

Shoulder-Hand Syndromes

1. Recognize this as a symptom complex that may be started by many disorders; trauma, cardiac and cerebral disturbances are the commonest.

2. Treat the primary disorder appropriately.

3. Treat the sympathetic upset by stellate blocks or sympathomimetic drugs.

4. Give cortisone in relatively low dosage when there are no systemic contraindications.

5. Good physiotherapy to both shoulder and hand should accompany all measures.

Tests for Shoulder and Radiating Pain

Discs

Tilting head and neck to the painful side produces pain.

Scalenus anticus

Tilting head and neck away from painful side produces pain.

Costoclavicular test

Backward and downward pressure on shoulders produces discomfort.

Hyperabduction syndrome

Abducted position of the arm reproduces the discomfort and the obliteration of radial pulse; these are relieved by the arm hanging down.

CERVICAL FORAMINA STENOSES

The three foramina of the cervical spine, its nerve roots and the vertebral artery may become obstructed partly or completely by exostoses. For many years these changes were regarded as completely innocuous, but more recent assessment has shown that this is not so.

Irregular bony overgrowth may develop as a degenerative change, as the result of metabolic abnormalities, as congenital aberrations, from trauma or from a combination of these disturbances. Depending on the location, size and contour, symptoms run the full gamut from headache to paraplegia. The vital contents of these foramina of the spinal cord, nerve roots or artery may be seriously involved by the resulting distortion when there is added cervical spine motion on either a natural or pathological basis.

Many factors add to the propensity for foraminal encroachment, and none of the major foramina are immune to these influences. The site, extent and rapidity of formation comprise one segment of the cause while the other irritant is the movement of the cervical spine and its segments. Variants of location include site and level; variants of severity include local and systemic disease; variants of progression include trauma, metabolic aberrations and degenerative processes. (See also Chapter XV.)

HISTORICAL DEVELOPMENT

Parts of this general entity have been identified and the process recognized principally in relation to cervical nerve root pressure. From this has gradually developed the realization that the spinal cord may also be involved in almost identical processes, and it has been a natural corollary to appreciate that the vertebral artery may also be afflicted.

In 1943 Simms and Murphy reported the surgical treatment of cervical disc protrusion causing nerve root compression. In 1892 Gowers had alluded to vertical body changes in rheumatoid arthritis as potential cord irritants. More recently Stookey, Elsberg and

Buoy identified these changes as chondromas and presented meticulous studies of their neurosurgical management. Frykholm described changes of this nature in 1951 and presented foraminotomy as a solution. A monumental presentation by Keys and Compere more accurately interpreted the primary pathology of these lesions, relating them to intervertebral disc distortion. Bain and associates in 1951 and 1954 reported extensively on clinical spondylosis, and more recently Brain and Wilkinson have contributed excellent monographs including reference to the vertebral foramen complications involving the vertebral artery.

Basic pathological changes are common to all three of the major foramina, but the relative extent of involvement in each instance may produce a completely different syndrome so that from a practical standpoint it seems reasonable to refer to the general process as "foraminosis" and then elucidate the common changes relative to the vertebral canal, nerve root canal or vertebral artery foramen.

VERTEBRAL FORAMINOSIS

Osteophyte formation on the margin of the vertebral bodies is an accepted development with increasing age. These changes so commonly seen in x-rays may never be the source of clinical disturbance, but a variety of factors imposed after they have developed may usher in a clinical state. The cervical cord is able to adapt profoundly to encroachment on the foramen, but should the canal be smaller than normal the developing ridge or bar can encroach abnormally and cause spinal cord pressure.

In this connection the significance of the width of the vertebral foramen has been appreciated and careful studies carried out estimating the normal size. The spinal cord has considerable leeway for displacement. The average segmental dimension has been estimated at 17 mm. and the average anteroposterior dimension of the cord as 10 mm. Those patients presenting symptoms of myelopathy have been estimated to have an anteroposterior measurement of 14 mm. (Payne and Spillane, 1957). The critical measurement has been estimated by Brain Wilkinson at 11 mm. If the canal measurement is 11 mm. or less, encroachment on the cord is possible.

Stenosis of the cervical canal of sufficient

severity to produce neural signs and symptoms is encountered in a variety of states, the commonest entities including degenerative changes, rheumatoid disease, congenital abnormalities, Strümpell-Marie spondylitis, Paget's disease and disc protrusions.

Clinical manifestations

Regardless of the precipitating entity a common picture may be recognized featuring profound neurological disturbance. Some variations according to the individaul disturbance then may also be identified.

The outstanding feature is the creeping or insidious onset of symptoms which for some time may not be identified as coming from cervical cord involvement. Weakness in the lower limbs and a creeping spasticity which gradually interferes profoundly with gait are salient findings.

In contrast, sensory changes are sparse. A sign of importance is the thermite sign, a test in which passive flexion of the neck initiates a lighteninglike pain through the spine. A startling finding is that the structural changes can progress to the point where there is a complete block in the myelogram and yet there may be relatively little clinical change. In many instances upper limb symptoms are present, but in the entity under discussion, vertebral canal spondylosis, these are of secondary prominence; the two conditions can coexist in varying degrees. Trauma often precipitates the clinical picture and may incite an acute reaction or be only an insult that speeds changes to a climax one or two years later.

Myelography is essential to identify the lesion, and electromyography is extremely helpful in depicting the complete pattern of the neural involvement. It also assists considerably in sorting the cord and root involvement. (See also Figure 15–22.)

The changes as a whole are less severe than cord compression due to tumor and differ particularly in not having the profound sensory loss or interference with sphincters except in the very late stages.

Strümpell-Marie Spondylitis

Ankylosing spondylitis predisposes to a type of cervical instability which encroaches upon the vertebral canal, particularly at the level of the atlantoaxial joint. Subluxation of the atlas on the axis is now recognized as a frequent complication of this disease and may lead to significant cord signs. Stabilization of C.1 and C.2 has become the treatment of choice.

Rheumatoid Arthritis

When the cervical spine is involved in rheumatoid arthritis, subluxation of the vertebral bodies may develop at various levels. Narrowing of the interbody space and osteophyte formation contribute to possible foraminal encroachment.

Congenital Anomalies

A variety of congenital anomalies may progress so as to encroach upon the spinal canal. A common vertebral body anomaly, fusion of two or more adjacent vertebrae, may constitute a mechanical disturbance as aging progresses. Coalescence of the vertebral bodies focuses greater motion at the mobile level above and below the fused area and enhances wear and tear changes. In most instances symptoms do not arise from such a development, but it can happen that the addition of trauma or systemic disease to this state may favor vertebral foramina encroachment.

References

Amick, L. D., et al.: The holistic approach to the shoulder-hand syndrome. Southern Med. J. *59*:161–167, 1966.

Baer, R. D.: Shoulder-hand syndrome: Its recognition and management. Southern Med. J. *59*:790–794, 1966.

Bailey, R. W., and Badgeley, C. E.: Stabilization of the cervical spine by anterior fusion. J. Bone Joint Surgery, *42A*:565–594, 1960.

Bielecki, A., et al.: A case of cervical rib with compression of the neurovascular bundle of the right arm. Chir. Narzad. Ruchu Orthop. Pol. *30*:405–409, 1965.

Bozyk, Z.: Shoulder-hand syndrome in patients with antecedent myocardial infarctions. Reumatologia (Warsz.) *6*:103–106, 1968.

British Association of Physical Medicine: Pain in the neck and arm: A multicentre trial of the effects of physiotherapy. Brit. Med. J. *5482*:253–258, 1966.

Cailliet, R.: Pain in neck and arm. Diagnosis by history and examination. Calif. Med. *108*:99–103, 1968.

Cailliet, R.: The diagnosis of neck and arm pain by examination. Illinois Med. J. *133*:277–288, 1968.

Cinquegrana, O. D.: Chronic cervical radiculitis and its relationship to "chronic bursitis." Amer. J. Phys. Med. *47*:23–30, 1968.

Claessens, H., et al.: Vasculo-nervous reflex changes in the upper limb. J. Belg. Rhum. Med. Phys. *20*:83–88, 1965.

Cloward, R. B.: The anterior approach for ruptured cervical disks. J. Neurosurg. *15*:602–617, 1958.

Connolly, E. S., et al.: Clinical evaluation of anterior

cervical fusion for degenerative disc disease. J. Neurosurg. *23*:431–437, 1965.

De Villiers, J. C.: A brachiocephalic vascular syndrome associated with cervical rib. Brit. Med. J. *5506*:140–143, 1966.

Duplay, S.: On scapulohumeral periarthritis. Med. Press *69*:571–573, 1900.

Freiberg, J. A.: The scalenus anterior muscle in relation to shoulder and arm pain. J. Bone Joint Surg. *20*:860, 1938.

Friedenberg, Z. B., Edeiken, J., Spencer, H. N., and Tolentino, S. C.: Degenerative changes in the cervical spine. J. Bone Joint Surg. *41A*:61–70, 1959.

Hadley, L. A.: The co-vertebral articulations and cervical foramen encroachment. J. Bone Joint Surg. *39A*:910–920, 1957.

Hantz, E., et al.: Bilateral cervical rib syndrome complicated by osteolysis of the distal phalanges. Bull. Soc. Chir. Paris *56*:38–43, 1966.

Harris, J. D., et al.: Vascular complications of cervical ribs. Aust. New. Zeal. J. Surg. *34*:269–274, 1965.

Howard, L. G.: Neck and shoulder pain syndromes. Med. Clin. N. Amer. September, 1952, pp. 1289–1307.

Hunt, J. C., et al.: A convalescent cervical collar. Amer. J. Orthop. *7*:109, 1965.

Kirkaldy-Willis, W. H., et al.: Surgical approaches to the anterior elements of the spine: Indications and techniques. Canad. J. Surg. *9*:294–308, 1966.

Korst, J. K., van der, et al.: Phenobarbital and the shoulder-hand syndrome. Ann. Rheum. Dis. *25*:553–555, 1966.

Kosina, W., et al.: Neurological disorders and radiological diagnosis of developmental abnormalities of the cervical spine. Rheumatologia (Warsz.) *3*:135–145, 1965.

Kucik-Scherffowa, Z., et al.: Three cases of hand-shoulder syndrome with degenerative changes of the cervical spine. Wiad. Lek. *19*:143–147, 1966.

Laurin, C. A.: Cervical traction at home. Un. Med. Canada *95*:80–83, 1966.

Lippman, R. K.: Frozen shoulder: bicipital tenosynovitis. Arch. Surg. *47*:283–296, 1943.

Maldyk, H., et al.: The cases of shoulder-hand syndrome treated satisfactorily with griseofulvin. Rheumatologia (Warsz.) *4*:97–101, 1966.

Mayfield, F. H.: Cervical spondylosis. Observations based on surgical treatment of 400 patients. Postgrad. Med. *38*:345–357, 1965.

McLaughlin, H. L.: On the "frozen" shoulder. Bull. Hosp. Joint Dis. *12*(No. 2):383–393, 1951.

McMillan, J. A.: Therapeutic exercises for shoulder disabilities. Phys. Ther. *46*:1052–1059, 1966.

McRae, D. L.: The cervical spine and neurologic disease. Radiol. Clin. N. Amer. *4*:145–158, 1966.

Michelsen, J. J., and Mixter, W. J.: Pain and disability of shoulder and arm due to herniation of the nucleus pulposus of cervical intervertebral disks. New Eng. J. Med. *231*:279–287, 1944.

Murphey, F., et al.: Ruptured cervical disc. Experience with 250 cases. Amer. Surg. *32*:83–88, 1966.

Neviaser, J. S.: Adhesive capsulitis of the shoulder. A study of the pathological findings in periarthritis of the shoulder. J. Bone Joint Surg. *27*:211–222, 1945.

Neviaser, J. S.: Adhesive capsulitis of the shoulder. Instructional course lectures of the American Academy of Orthopedic Surgeons. Vol. VI, 1949, pp. 281–291.

Robinson, R. A., and Smith, G. W.: Antero-lateral cervical disc removal and interbody fusion for cervical disc syndrome. Bull. Johns Hopkins Hosp. *96*:223–224, 1955.

Robinson, R. A., Walker, A. E., Ferlic, D. C., and Wiecking, D. K.: The results of anterior interbody fusion of the cervical spine. J. Bone Joint Surg. *44A*:1569–1587, 1962.

Roos, D. B., et al.: Thoracic outlet syndrome. Arch. Surg. (Chicago) *93*:71–74, 1966.

Rosenberg, J. C.: Arteriographic demonstration of compression syndromes of the thoracic outlet. Southern Med. J. *59*:400–403, 1966.

Rubin, D.: An exercise program for shoulder disability. Calif. Med. *106*:39–43, 1967.

Saadi, M. H.: Unilateral cervical rib with exostosis of the first rib and pseudoarthrosis. Brit. J. Clin. Pract. *20*:93, 1966.

Scoville, W. B., et al.: Lateral rupture of cervical intervertebral discs. Postgrad. Med. *39*:174–180, 1966.

Scoville, W. B.: Types of cervical disc lesions and their surgical approaches. J.A.M.A. *196*:479–481, 1966.

Servelle, M.: The thoracic approach in vascular complications of cervical ribs. Ann. Chir. Thorac. Cardiov. *5*:692–695, 1966.

Simmons, E. H., and Bhalla, S. K.: Anterior cervical discectomy and fusion. A clinical and biomechanical study with 8 year follow-up. J. Bone Joint Surg. *51B*:225–236, 1969.

Smith, G. W., and Robinson, R. A.: The treatment of cervical spine disorders by anterior removal of the intervertebral disc and interbody fusion. J. Bone Joint Surg. *40A*:607–624, 1958.

Shenkin, H. A., et al.: Scalenotomy in patients with and without cervical ribs. Analysis of surgical results. Arch. Surg. (Chicago) *87*:892–896, 1963.

Steinbrocker, O.: The shoulder-hand syndrome: Present perspective. Arch. Phys. Med. *49*:388–395, 1968.

Ware, C.: Cervical dumb-bell neurilemoma. Proc. Roy. Soc. Med. *59*:425, 1966.

Wright, I. S., et al.: The subclavian steal and other shoulder girdle syndromes. Trans. Amer. Clin. Climat. Ass. *76*:13–25, 1964.

Wright, V.: The shoulder-hand syndrome. Rep. Rheum. Dis. *24*:1–2, 1966.

TRAUMA TO THE NECK AND SHOULDER

Chapter X

INDUSTRIAL INJURIES

The many facets of the industrial accident warrant special attention to injuries sustained by workmen. The workman's accident so often menaces his earning capacity that there always is a greater element of fear to overcome. Because his limbs are so frequently his tools, it is mandatory that the most skilful reconstruction possible be obtained. After this has been done, more particular attention to relearning of limb action is essential because of his special needs. Finally, recognition of all the problems involved is essential, with attention being given to the morale and the mental trauma as well as the injured limb. Truly, we must be physicians of the psyche as well as the body to do the best for the workman.

INJURY MECHANISMS COMMON OR PECULIAR TO INDUSTRY

Consideration of the way in which the workman sustained injury not only provides a lead as to the structures which may be involved, but frequently allows a quick classification of disturbances. There are also special properties of the injury mechanisms as related to the neck and shoulder which merit study not only of the lesion but also of its extent and of possible complications. Analysis of the injury mechanism lends itself to consideration under two main headings, those lesions which result from primary action of the body, so-called direct injuries, and those lesions which are afflicted primarily as a result of some external force working on the inactive body.

PRIMARY OR DIRECT INJURY MECHANISM

Stumbles. The workman stumbles because some unprepared for obstacle is encountered and he does not have time to protect his body adequately. It may be a protruding beam at the head or shoulder level or a carelessly placed object at toe level. He may fall on the shoulder point or on the shoulder-neck angle. In one instance he damages the head of the humerus cuff mechanism; in the other he may stretch the brachial plexus. The element of unpreparedness usually means a more severe injury. If he takes his weight or the brunt of the fall is borne on the point of his shoulder, he may so stretch his acromiomastoid dimension that the brachial plexus is implicated. If the shoulder is well padded, some cushioning is obtained and the point of the shoulder bears the brunt so that he may avulse a small portion of the tuberosity of the humerus or split the insertion of the rotator cuff.

If purely local discomfort and impairment

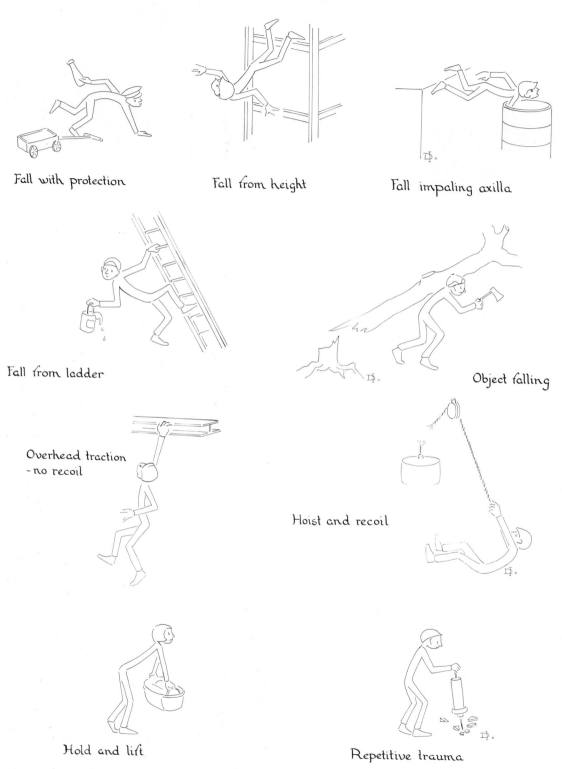

Fall with protection

Fall from height

Fall impaling axilla

Fall from ladder

Object falling

Overhead traction - no recoil

Hoist and recoil

Hold and lift

Repetitive trauma

Figure 10–1   Some common injury mechanisms in industry.

ensue, there has been only a bruising of the tissues involved. Rapid recovery apart from local tenderness is the rule. When there is involvement of other elements in the shoulder-neck complex, evidenced by weakness in lifting the arm, more than simple contusion of the tissues has occurred and investigation of the cuff, or plexus, is required.

Falls. Most falls involve some element of preparedness so that, in addition to possible local contusion, there is included the element of damage to the lever which is brought into action to protect the body in the fall. In the case of the shoulder-neck region, the usual protecting mechanism is the outstretched arm, either at the side or at the front of the body. Frequently the protecting lever bears the brunt and suffers most damage. Fracture of the surgical neck of the humerus or of the clavicle, for example, may result when the force has been precipitous. When it has been less severe, it means that the soft tissues have accepted the brunt of the insult and that these may be damaged. In the case of the shoulder, it is the superior and anterior capsule which is most often implicated.

Slips. The action of slipping involves body imbalance which most often brings the body into the extension phase because the slipping force propels the lower part forward and the upper portion of the body backward. As related to the shoulder-neck region, the common performance is a fall with the arm and hand stretched backward to protect the head from striking the ground. Again, when the forces involved are of sufficient severity, the hard structures may give way, but often the soft parts bear the brunt. Such a mechanism affects the anterior portion of the shoulder, the capsular zone, the related bicipital zone and sometimes the neurovascular bundle.

APPLICATION OF DIRECT FORCE

Falling Objects from Above. The neck and the shoulder are prime targets for this type of injury. A falling object may hit the head and upper portion of the neck before it slides off the shoulder. Often the workman has some warning, perhaps just enough to allow him to flex his head and neck a little so that the brunt of the falling object is taken directly between the shoulder and neck as he flees from the dropping object.

The point of impact often governs the damage which ensues. If the object lands directly on the point of the shoulder, the result is a spreading of the acromiomastoid dimension and possible serious involvement of the brachial plexus. If the blow lands a little more posteriorly, these structures escape and the stress is much less of stretch and more of contusion, so that a fracture of the spine of the scapula or posterior spinous processes of the cervical spine may result. Many combinations of damage are possible, but the pattern of injury involving the posterior neck-scapular region by flexion and flight is the same.

Machinery Injuries. The hazards of multiple wheel and belt connections in factories are well known. For years they have been protected by guards, but it can still happen that the upper limb of a workman is caught in a belt or a whirling wheel. A two-fold application of force results: there is the damage which occurs directly to the part which is caught in the belt and, secondly, the damage which results from the traction applied to the limb as a whole. The first often produces a fracture of both bones of the forearm or the humerus. The second frequently involves the neurovascular bundle at the root of the limb.

Cutting and Crushing Tools. The direct application of cutting forces produces obvious damage to the structures beneath the area involved. However, a sliding or crushing force may have an oblique element which distorts and damages tissue apart from the point of direct impact. A heavy box sliding down from the point of the shoulder may so stick to the skin or dig into the tissues that it avulses muscle, tendon or nerve beneath in a sliding type of crush.

Pneumatic Tools. The constant use of high pressure pneumatic drills has long been recognized as a source of upper limb damage. In this instance it is not the initial episode but the summation of repeated minor or micro trauma which eventually causes damage. Most of the time it is the hand zone or the elbow which is affected, but force can be transmitted to the shoulder or the cervical spine zones. In a not so young workman, for example, the repeated use of pneumatic tools may progressively implicate zones susceptible to degeneration, such as the cervical intervertebral discs. The initial warning is neck stiffness, but this may be followed by more specific signs of nerve root irritation as the force irritation continues.

Electric Shock. Although not a common

mechanism of injury, there are some specific considerations as related to the shoulder and neck. Most frequently the application of the excess current comes through the hand or upper extremity and this zone bears the brunt. The convulsive muscle contraction and reaction which follow a severe electric shock can dislocate the shoulder. The convulsion-like seizure can also implicate the cervical spine, precipitating nerve root syndromes.

COMMON NECK INJURIES

ACUTE NECK STRAIN

Only the most minor type of neck disturbances are considered under this heading. They are seen more commonly in the age group below 45. Typically the patient is seized with acute pain in the neck while straightening from a forward bent or slightly forward and rotated position. This often happens in straightening up from bending beneath a desk or workbench. The patient holds his neck rigidly, but in the forward bent position. Tenderness can be elicited over the erector spinae on both sides, usually at the midlevel, and in neck motion both rotation and flexion-extension are implicated.

As a rule, such an episode results from a catching of one of the apophyseal joints and pinching of a piece of synovium. The condition is effectively treated by cervical traction with the patient recumbent. Gentle manual traction will usually relieve the condition dramatically, but when this is not available, halter traction using 10 to 15 pounds for 15 to 20 minutes can be used. This is followed by massage and application of deep heat. The symptoms persist for a matter of days and the program of local treatment should be supported by administration of muscle relaxants or some form of anti-inflammatory drug, if this is tolerated. In the older age group the onset is less acute and the course somewhat more chronic. Longer irritation stems from the reaction, implicating the neurocentral joints rather than the apophyseal joints above. Disc degeneration may help to precipitate irritation of these accessory joints.

The usual complaint is of neck soreness, again following a forward twisting motion, followed during the next several days by persistent stiffness rather than acute "locking" of the neck. X-ray investigation identifies already established interbody changes, suggesting the source of the acute symptoms. Manual manipulation or traction is not likely to help this less acute lesion, but recurrent halter traction with heat, systemic medication and avoidance of further similar irritating motions does bring this episode under control.

ACUTE TORTICOLLIS

A somewhat different lesion from the acute neck strain is that described as acute wry neck. This condition arises from another type of injury in that it is a stretching of both the neck and the shoulder girdle, in opposite directions, rather than simple neck twist. A twisting and turning action of the neck accompanied by a stretching outward or sideways of the arm focuses stress to the medial shoulder-neck angle, sometimes stretching ligamentous or muscle attachments. The chin and head are held away from the side of the injury in the wry neck position. Marked muscle spasm is present, and a point of quite definite maximum tenderness in the shoulder-neck zone can be identified.

Manual manipulation is not much help to this lesion. Halter traction assists but does so from the standpoint of neutralizing the muscle spasm rather than correcting any primary alteration of the neck contents. Therefore, it should be relatively light, with less weight being used than in the more acute flexion strain. The condition comes under control with the application of a cervical collar, systemic medication and physiotherapy, including heat and massage. If an acutely tender point is identified, injection with a local anesthetic, or superficial skin analgesia with a topical freezing agent, is effective.

NECK SPRAIN OR FLEXION INJURY

Under this heading are considered entities of deeper severity and greater significance than the so-called neck strain. We consider a strain as a reaction to overuse of a muscle or excess stress placed upon a ligament. Sprain, in comparison, is the reaction from the taking of a joint beyond its normal range of motion with resultant reaction set up in the retaining structures. In the neck this often results from so-called indirect or passive injuries, that is, the application of force apart from purely voluntary acts. In contrast, most neck strains implicate a voluntary mechanism only. The notorious whiplash injury is an indirect or passive type of lesion in that force is applied apart from the voluntary range of action of the neck.

Neck sprain chiefly involves the interspinous elements because these are the farthest away from the common fulcrum of motion, so that greater leverage is applied to these than other cervical structures. The blow on the back of the head or neck, forcing it forward, bends the neck at its usual fulcrum, but the transmission of the force will implicate the structures at the end of the posterior lever more than those in the center. The workman rising suddenly from a crouched position and hitting the back of the head unexpectedly on an overhanging object sustains this type of flexion injury.

Examination of a patient with this type of injury shows local tenderness in the midcervical region; he is holding his head and neck quite stiffly, but in the extended, in contrast to the forward flexed, position. Frequently the point of maximum tenderness can be identified directly between the posterior spinous processes of C.6 and C.7. Treatment includes local injection of the damaged ligament, application of a cervical collar and adequate systemic medication. Traction or manipulation is of no help in this type of injury. A light fabric type of collar is usually best, but the patient will need to wear it for six to eight weeks. A more severe form of this flexion injury is one in which the force has been of sufficient severity to pull off a portion of the posterior spinous process. In place of the interspinous ligaments giving way, a portion of the tip of the spinous process can be avulsed. When this has happened, the initial management is the same, but the collar is worn for a period of 12 weeks. Delayed or nonunion of the avulsed piece is common and when this occurs, it should be removed surgically. The application of flexion trauma may be of much greater severity, resulting in more serious bone and joint abnormalities, which are considered now.

ROTATORY INJURIES

Severe rotatory injuries are not common in industry because they usually occur when rotatory stress is applied externally, as in a football tackle, rather than from voluntary action of neck structures.

Rotatory Sprain. Active and violent rotation of the head and neck can result in a sprain, with stretching or partial tearing of the ligaments holding the apophyseal joints. Severe muscle spasm results in a pulling of the head toward the involved side, which is in direct contrast to the so-called wry neck, in which the head and neck are tilted away from the side which is involved. Other differences of this injury are the point of maximum tenderness, which is much nearer the back and implicates the cervical spine rather than the shoulder-neck angle.

Light cervical traction followed by the application of a soft collar, systemic medication and rest of the involved area bring this injury under control.

APOPHYSEAL SUBLUXATION

When sufficient force is applied, the articular process may slide partially off and become locked in this position. If this occurs, the head and neck are locked in a position turned to the opposite side. The state of subluxation is recognized by the more powerful forces which were involved initially, the greater rigidity of the head and neck, the point of tenderness related to the cervical spine posterolaterally and the persistence of these changes.

Traction is essential to alleviate this condition, preferably the gradual application of halter traction. The patient should be in bed with the traction applied continually or as it may be tolerated at intervals until the luxation is overcome. Sedation and systemic medication, followed by the application of a firm collar, are required. The immobilization should be continued for 12 weeks to allow periarticular ligaments to heal as much as possible.

ATLANTOAXIAL SPRAIN

A less common lesion may be recognized which is characterized by suboccipital pain and restricted rotation of the head and the neck; bending, however, is not implicated.

Ordinarily the atlanto-occipital and atlanto-axial articulations have such powerful ligamentous protection so that luxation or derangement, apart from the application of strong external force, does not occur. However, in the older workman in whom there may already be some existing articular irregularity, this type of sprain may occur. The lesion is identified by the position of the pain, the local tenderness related to the upper portion of the cervical spine, and the rotatory restriction of motion rather than pain on flexion or extension. X-ray examination shows some already existing irregularity.

Halter traction followed by the application of a soft collar and the continued use of the collar during sleep is required. A program of physiotherapy, including deep heat, and systemic medication are added as the acute reaction subsides.

EXTENSOR INJURIES

The application of backward force on a passive basis is much more frequent in athletics than it is in industry. Powerful backward push strains the anterior attachments of the vertebral bodies and the anterior longitudinal ligament. If this force is continued, extremely serious involvement of the cord will result from dislodgement of the body from its anterior anchorage.

The common episode in the workman results from slipping down a step or short depth and striking the chin or head forcibly so that the neck is slipped backward. The structures at the anterior aspect of the neck are put on tension, particularly the anterior longitudinal ligament. This ligament resists more rigidly than the soft substance of the viscera and vessels, which would give way before such a force. The attachment of the ligament to the top of the respective bodies may be avulsed, carrying a small spicule of bone with it. In older workmen, whose cervical spines are already the seat of osteophytic formation, the frequent lesion is a fracture of an osteophyte.

The injury is recognized primarily from the description of the damaging force. There is considerable muscle spasm at the side of the neck, anterior tenderness and extreme discomfort on lifting the head and neck backward.

The injury is treated by immobilization in slight flexion with a cervical collar and a soft collar at night for a period of eight to ten weeks. At least this length of time is required for adequate healing in this type of injury. The more severe and extremely serious sequelae of violent extensor injury are considered under fractures and dislocations of the cervical spine.

ACUTE EXTRUDED CERVICAL INTERVERTEBRAL DISC

Workmen seldom have acute nuclear extrusion in the cervical region in contrast to the extremely vulnerable lumbar zone. When it occurs, a pertinent history of injury is obtained, most often a drop or fall from a height so that there has been application of a jarring force in the vertical position. In contrast to the lumbar area, where heavy lifts and extension action from the forward bent position are the sources of annulus rupture, the common protrusion in the neck is to the lateral side. When this develops, there is much more likelihood of implication of a nerve root than is the case in the lumbar region.

Neck pain and stiffness result, but very quickly these are overshadowed by pain radiating to the shoulder and down the arm to the hand. The feature of these lesions is the burning, tingling pain below the elbow. The precise distribution of the dominant pain will vary according to the level which is involved. The acute lesions occur much more frequently between C.5–C.6 and C.6–C.7, so that the clinical distribution varies. Persistent shoulder pain unrelated to shoulder movement, weakness of the deltoid, sensory changes over the lateral aspect of the arm and alteration of the biceps jerk as compared with the opposite side implicate the fifth cervical root.

Involvement of the sixth cervical root favors atrophy of the upper arm, with weakness of pectorals, biceps and triceps and hypesthesia along the lateral aspect of the arm and forearm as far as the thumb. Either or both biceps and triceps reflexes may be altered. Involvement of the seventh root is usually indicated by more precise hypesthesia and subjective numbness in the thumb and index finger, weakness and wasting of the triceps, alteration of the triceps reflex and, sometimes, by weakness in the extensors of the wrist.

These lesions are treated by cervical traction, application of a cervical collar, systemic medication and adequate sedation. This should be preceded by contrast studies of the cervical spine, which will assist in determining whether an anterior or posterior approach to the interbody area should be carried out if surgery becomes necessary. When there is evidence of an extensive extrusion, particularly if it has been large enough to implicate the spinal cord in the midline, posterior decompression is probably preferable. In the common lesion the trend is to approach it from the anterior aspect. In contrast to lesions in the lumbar spine, the extruded disc material does not often pass up or down from its site of extrusion through the posterior longitudinal ligament. For this reason it often is feasible to "fish it out," as it were, from an anterior approach. Sometimes this can be accomplished with greater delicacy and more finesse, producing less trauma to the cervical cord than is the case with the posterior approach.

In the lumbar spine adequate space exists following laminectomy to lift the spinal cord to one side and deal with the extrusion without embarrassing the dural contents. Such is not the case in the cervical spine, where the cord occupies a relatively much larger space within the canal. Greater traction and pressure on the cord are necessary and, hence, there is greater possibility of damage. These considerations favor the anterior approach.

A further reason for dealing with these lesions from the front is that interbody stabilization may be carried out effectively at the same time and with ease. The standard procedure is to insert a small corticocancellous graft in such a way that it can be locked in place between the intervertebral bodies. A period of immobilization in a cervical collar will firmly stabilize the involved areas. (See Chapter XVI for detailed operative technique.)

SUBACUTE OR CHRONIC CERVICAL DISC INJURY

A much more common entity resulting in the gradual development of neck, shoulder and radiating pain occurs from degenerative disc disease without actual nuclear protrusion. In industry the older workman is a frequent sufferer from this disturbance. The relationship of the accident at work usually is that some episode of more than usual severity, such as a fall, stumble or slip, jerks the neck, thereby initiating this whole group of signs and symptoms. The underlying pathology is a loss of the normal disc turgidity followed by bony proliferation at the periphery, which favors a foraminal encroachment on the nerve roots. In contrast with the lumbar region, the cervical roots have much less reserve space in the foramen with which to shift and accommodate to any intrusion of the nucleus, so that impingement can develop from a much smaller bony change.

Injury frequently precipitates the syndrome and commonly it is a complaint of burning, tingling or clumsiness in the hand, particularly the thumb and index finger, that is first noted. Some general neck stiffness and shoulder discomfort may precede this, but the persistent element usually is related to the hand.

The dominating discomfort is the radiating pain, but because of the chronicity and the innate, often slow-developing nature of the lesion, a whole group of secondary phenomena, particularly a referred type of pain, is associated with this lesion. It is the development of these secondary pain patterns that often makes the diagnosis difficult or the recognition of the true source of the primary state obscure. Aching pain in the shoulder, pain between the scapulae and sometimes headache or occipital discomfort are associated. Areas as far away as the face, temporal zone and even the eye have been implicated in this process. The discomfort in these areas is unaccompanied by motor and sensory changes, and it is largely a subjective burning, tingling or numbness that is identified.

The most effective treatment for this state is a program of cervical traction in the slightly flexed position with the neck then immobilized in a properly fitting collar between the periods of traction. If relief is not obtained from the radiating symptoms within a short while, the traction should not be persisted with; the emphasis should be shifted to more complete immobilization of the neck. Physiotherapeutic measures assist considerably. Deep heat, ultrasound and cervical muscle massage should accompany the traction-rest program as required. Adequate sedation, particularly for rest at night, and use of a soft collar or special cervical pillow followed by a program of systemic medication, such as phenylbutazone, are included in the routine.

In the young middle-aged workman in whom these symptoms develop and are unrelieved by conservative treatment, careful identification of the levels involved is required by contrast studies, sometimes assisted by discography. Anterior interbody fusion with removal of the degenerated disc is then the procedure of choice (see Chapter XVI).

REFERENCE

Elson, R. A.: Costal chondritis. J. Bone Joint Surg. 47B:94–99, 1965.

Chapter XI

ATHLETIC INJURIES

Interest in athletic injuries as a separate group of lesions has gradually come to the fore because of the special considerations surrounding the management of disorders suffered in sports. Athletic injuries differ profoundly from those received under other conditions. Differences can be identified not only in the type of injury and the mechanism by which this is produced, but also in the participants. The responsibilities entailed in handling these incidents have varied. For years the goal of treating the injured athlete was to keep him playing regardless of the precise pathological state. All this has changed now, with the increase in knowledge, and better care that can be provided for the sports participant.

The enlightened approach involves emphasis on prevention as well as on treatment. The goal is complete recovery because, if this is not attained, the patient may no longer be an athlete. The significance of professional sports has also increased; the spread of spectator interest in professional football, basketball and hockey has been tremendous, but probably has been even further outpaced by the increased number of individuals who now participate in sports.

Interest at the amateur level in our schools has broadened, and good programs of athletic development now begin at an early age; organized sports have come to be recognized as important ingredients of a comprehensive education.

Athletes differ in several ways. As a rule, they are in first class physical condition, they are young and they have tissues that heal readily. Perhaps the most important difference is the tremendous incentive to get well and to make the injured part not only perform a job but do it as well as before the injury.

PREVENTION OF INJURIES ABOUT THE SHOULDER-NECK REGION

The program of supervision of injuries sustained in sports now includes emphasis on conditioning programs and provision of proper protective equipment.

CONDITIONING PROGRAM

The concepts of total body conditioning are accepted but, in addition, now embrace exercises and training to improve specific areas. Of necessity, certain sports place more strain on some regions than others. The throwing arm of the pitcher or passer merits very special consideration. The swing of the golfer is absolutely vital, and in a professional is the basis of his livelihood.

The program of regional conditioning is thought of principally in terms of sports like football and hockey where it is aimed at producing sufficient strength and basic control to ward off injury. A much more specific program is required for the athlete such as a baseball player who has to use the shoulder, for the limb constitutes the vital offensive entity. For this reason, no across-the-board group of exercises can be specified, and it is best to consider special problems in discussions of the individual sports.

PROVISION OF PROTECTION

Head gear, neck guards and shoulder pads constitute a front line protection against injuries in this area. Many improvements have occurred in the production of these appliances, but they are principally of a defensive nature. The discus thrower, the tennis player and the shot putter have equally important needs, but these are met by proper management of the act and the material used, rather than defensive protection.

Competitive sport now involves such a broad spectrum of skilled activities that it has seemed best to consider the common injuries in discussions of the various sports. In considering activities which involve the shoulder-neck region, it is possible to divide them into two broad groups, the throwing sports and the body contact sports.

INJURIES IN THE THROWING SPORTS

The contribution of the shoulder has often been taken for granted in throwing sports, in which it really has a particularly important function. In these activities emphasis has often been focused at the opposite end of the limb, with attention paid to the grip of the ball or the racket or the stance during the delivery phase of an action rather than to the shoulder, which is the fulcrum and base of the whole act.

Virtually all games involve a degree of throwing, but the act dominates baseball, softball, football and bowling. In less strenuous but highly scientific and meticulously precise forms of sport such as golf, the shoulder also has a critical role. In sports like discus throwing, shot putting and hammer and javelin throwing great stress is again focused on the forequarter zone. Basketball involves a throwing action, but it is a somewhat different maneuver from the others. Such sports as horseshoe pitching, bowling and even darts implicate the shoulder in such a fashion that its injury or abuse may easily mar performance. In order to understand athletic injuries in the throwing sports properly, the throwing mechanism should be precisely understood. By and large, the neck does not play an important role in these endeavors, so that attention is focused on the shoulder girdle and the way it functions.

MECHANISM OF THE THROWING ACT

Throwing is a beautifully coordinated act that may involve the whole body, as in the hammer throw, or only the wrist and the fingers, as in the flip shot of a basketball through the hoop. Since the act involves the transfer of momentum from the body to the object to be propelled, the heavier the object, the more use of the body that is required. Arm, shoulder and trunk come into play to overcome the inertia of the object. When it is desired to add speed and distance, as in propelling a light object such as a baseball, more segments are successively brought into play and are coordinated throughout the act.

In all throwing or swinging activities involving the upper limb, two principles or distinct contributions of the region may be identified. The shoulder girdle first acts as a base or platform for the arm to be used as a lever. Secondly, a portion of it then serves as a fulcrum on which the whole lever of the arm may be swung (Fig. 11–1). The combination of the platform as a base for the take-off or fling of the arm has been likened to the handle of a whip in the whiplash action. The fulcrum not only allows the swinging motion but affords a zone for direction and control to be inserted at the base of the lever, setting the stage for finer and more intricate influence at the end of the lever by the fingers. The finest elements of control are contributed at the ends of the lever, either at the shoulder or at the fingertips. The portion of the arm in between is really a lengthening and shortening mechanism which serves as a means of adding momentum under control.

The coordinated act involves foot work, leg action, hip motion and trunk rotation

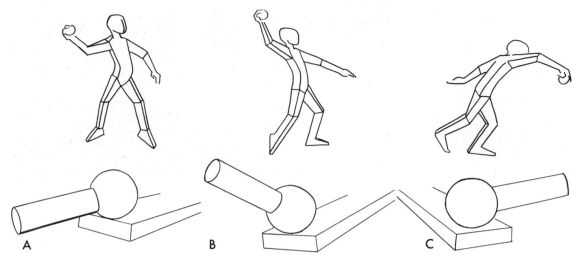

Figure 11–1 Basic functions of the shoulder in throwing: *A*, platform; *B*, fulcrum; *C*, follow-through.

plus some action of the opposite arm (Fig. 11–2). Some momentum is gained on the initial act of the throw by taking a few steps or a hop forward or sometimes by elevating the leg opposite the throwing arm. This forward motion is then enhanced by a twist of the trunk away from the throwing arm. This "step and twist" phase is also used to align the direction of the throw. As this motion flows from legs to hip to trunk, the shoulder falls into the swing and winds up for the flail motion of arm and forearm; the momentum is increased by the follow-through extension of the elbow and finally passes out through the forearm and fingers.

Mechanism of the Shoulder in Throwing. The act of clasping an object with the hand leads to extension of the wrist, supination of the forearm and internal rotation of the shoulder. From this position the upper arm is extended, abducted and rotated externally, which brings the extended wrist and elbow above the head preparatory to the powerful flexion flail of the follow-through motion (Fig. 11–3). Two separate sets of muscle motors may be identified in each phase of the complete act: the coarse heavy group of "external muscles" such as the deltoid, the pectorals, the biceps and the triceps, and the finer internal group made up of the rotators, supraspinatus, infraspinatus and subscapularis.

During the preparatory or "handle" phase, the posterior and the middle fibers of the deltoid along with the triceps provide the "coarse" action while the spinati produce the external rotation. In the normal shoulder little dysfunction develops during this phase

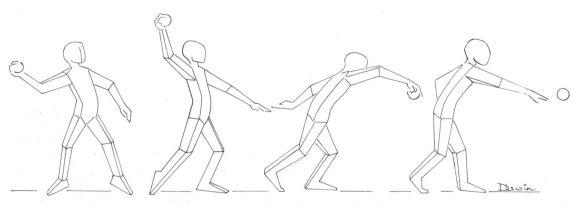

Figure 11–2 Body mechanism in throwing.

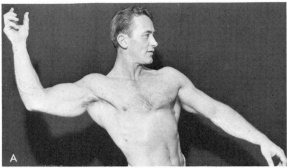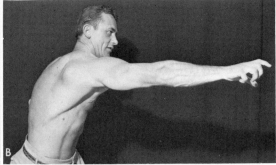

Figure 11–3   Upper limb action in throwing.

and not many derangements occur. However, difficulty arises if there has been any previous damage to the vital rotator cuff. Few injuries affect the coarse or heavy muscles participating in this act, but if the cuff has been stretched or roughened, obstruction will hamper the external rotation so that the preparatory phase of an overhand delivery is seriously interfered with. The thrower with a roughened or irritated cuff cannot or will not, because of pain, rotate the head of the humerus as far externally as he should. The result is that his wind-up is cut short and the force of his delivery phase is diminished. Minor changes or roughening in the cuff lead to discomfort right at the end of the backward external swing of the wind-up. Sometimes this is not apparent during the preliminary or warm-up phase and sometimes, once the muscle action is going smoothly, the player may be able to control the external rotation, stopping it just short of the painful arc. When this happens, there may be only a small amount of interference with the external rotation, but it may be enough to mar the performance and jeopardize effectiveness.

Sometimes so much leverage is applied during the external rotation swing that the head of the humerus impinges repeatedly against the glenoid posteriorly, producing a crease in the humeral head. When this is continued, an element of "rocking" motion develops and this frays the cuff and roughens or creases the humeral head.

The forward flexion or initial phase of the follow-through is a powerful maneuver and the more severe and acute injuries occur during this phase. These actions are motored by the anterior deltoid and pectorals which pull strongly downward and forward on the head of the humerus, aided by the internal rotators of the cuff group.

The final segment of the act is the braking of the follow-through flail. When power and force are developed in a pitch, there is a tremendous drag or pull on the head of the humerus to prevent its being pulled away from the glenoid as the extremity is flung with all momentum possible; this stretches the casing which keeps the head of the humerus in the glenoid. The stress is focused at the capsule and its covering, which are attached principally to the glenoid posteriorly. The pull strains the periosteal tendinous union, leading to a heaped-up marginal type of lipping or bone formation. The changes are seen much more frequently in a hallux rigidus, where lipping of the dorsal surface of the head of the metatarsal is encountered. These periosteal pieces may be dislodged by further stress introducing an acute phase of disability.

DIAGNOSIS AND INVESTIGATION OF THROWING INJURIES

When the throwing mechanism is understood and the specific function of the vulnerable structures is correlated properly, the diagnosis of the likely abnormalities is straightforward. The history along with systematic examination and testing of the shoulder structures usually pinpoints the source of trouble. Some special aspects in this routine may be emphasized. The time in the throwing act that maximum pain occurs is significant. Constant pain at the start of the delivery usually means well established change due to wearing or roughening of the head of the humerus from leverage on the posterior glenoid. Discomfort at the end of the pitch, in contrast, generally indicates capsular or soft tissue damage that is more likely to be recent and superficial. Pain posteriorly and inferiorly in the follow-through mechanism implicates the long head of the triceps and related structures at the postero-inferior margin of the glenoid. Sharp localized discomfort midway in the delivery indicates irritation of the midzone of the cuff and subacromial bursa. Precise localization of the points of tenderness is important. It matters a good deal whether tenderness is over the supraspinatus insertion or whether it is directly at the front of the joint, which would implicate the anterior capsule and subscapularis. The relationship of a tender area to the position of relative rotation is also significant. Is it necessary to rotate the head of the humerus internally to localize a tender zone at the back of the head or to feel a linear defect? Is the zone of tenderness more medial and inferior and related to the origin of the long head of the triceps rather than the head of the humerus? Is it constant and not altered by rotating the head of the humerus?

Good x-rays should be taken of the shoulder, including views in external and internal rotation, supero-inferior views, views of the acromioclavicular joint, bicipital groove and special glenoid labrum view. The one form of special investigation that should be kept in mind is the use of contrast studies. Arthrography has proved to be the most reliable means available of diagnosing internal derangements of the shoulder.

Throwing can be so strenuous that it can produce a full thickness tear of the cuff and, although this is not common, it must be kept in mind. Smaller tears and incomplete defects are more common. The more frequently encountered lesion is a partial tear of the cuff in which a few fibers of the deep layers are avulsed from the tuberosity. The arthrogram can show this defect, which often is an explanation for persistent or recurrent pain on throwing.

BASEBALL INJURIES

Baseball is the major throwing sport, and injuries to players are many and varied. Two types of injuries may be identified, an acute group consisting largely of soft tissue irritations, and a chronic or recurrent collection in which more permanent structural change occurs, causing repeated trouble.

Soft Tissue Baseball Injuries. By far the commonest injury is a partial tear of one of the muscle attachments about the shoulder. The vulnerable area is the posterolateral anchoring zone that bears the brunt of the follow-through of the delivery. Tearing and avulsion of a few fibers in this area can result from an uncontrolled "hard pitch." Repeated throwing then keeps these fibers avulsed and they fail to heal. If the shoulder is rested adequately at the first indication of injury, the muscle tear will heal. Recurrent strains initiate a periosteal reaction at the osseotendinous junction; minute streaks of calcium appear in the early stages, to be followed in later stages by frank osteophyte formation.

Recurrent Injuries. The real problems are the recurrent or repeated disturbances. Almost always these are based on a demonstrable structural change.

POSTERIOR OSTEOPHYTES. Extensive osteophyte formation related to the triceps on the posterior capsule is a common lesion. Recurrent stretching trauma produces minute osseotendinous ossification that often becomes enlarged and increased with continued stress. Spur-like formation then develops, spreading from the region of the triceps attachment along the posterior aspect of the capsule (Fig. 11–4). Sometimes fragments of these spurs are dislodged and come to lie inside the joint, eventually constituting loose bodies.

In some instances the joint needs to be explored. The posterior aspect is exposed and the fragments are excised. This may be done with a minimum disturbance of muscles and capsule, favoring a good result. If extensive dissection and disruption of muscles is carried out during the exposure, the chances of returning the shoulder to a full time pitching responsibility are greatly decreased. Fortunately, in throwing the usual injury is a partial avulsion of some of the deep cuff fibers.

CUFF TEARS. A partial avulsion or roughening of some of the fibers in the deep aspect of the cuff is not uncommon. A degree of healing will occur with rest for a period of four to six weeks, but if hard throwing is started too soon, the scar will break down again. When the discomfort is prominent during the middle phase of pitching rather than during the wind-up or follow-through, the irritation is likely to be in the rotator cuff. Sometimes, after the initial lesion has healed, irregularity of the cuff will stir up a subacromial bursitis, but this responds quickly to simple conservative therapy. The regimen should include a period of rest, a

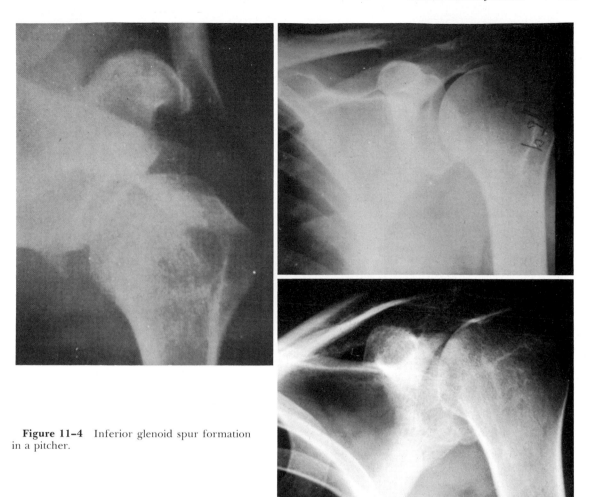

Figure 11–4 Inferior glenoid spur formation in a pitcher.

period of skillful physiotherapy and systemic administration of phenylbutazone. Full thickness cuff ruptures also occur in shoulders used for hard throwing. Players such as catchers and shortstops, in contrast to pitchers, need a maximum stress or a quick powerful wind-up to deliver a fast throw in a hurry. Stress in these circumstances is borne by the antero-inferior capsule, which may rupture as in acute subluxation of the shoulder. In some instances massive avulsion occurs, requiring precise surgical reconstruction.

New studies on the lubrication mechanism of the shoulder joint have been carried out with the aid of contrast studies and motion studies (Fig. 11–5). In the throwing act, as the arm is abducted and externally rotated, it can be seen that a major amount of joint lubricant flows to the inferior aspect of the joint and this zone becomes filled. At the same time nearly all the lubricant is drained out of the superior aspect of the joint, so that during the act of impingement on the cortico-acromial arch there appears to be a minimal amount of lubricant working. As the arm comes down to the side in the follow-through act, fluid can be seen to move from the inferior recess, the upper of the head of the humerus, bathing the upper aspect. Possibly this diminution in the amount of lubrication at a critical point favors wear and tear changes in this zone to a greater degree than in other areas which appear to be more evenly lubricated.

POSTERIOR ARTICULAR CHANGES. The postero-inferior aspect of the joint, the lower margin of the glenoid and the adjacent area of the head of the humerus bear the brunt of wear and tear changes of prolonged use. Some of this develops from continued pressure in the wind-up, where the head of the humerus rocks against the glenoid. To this is added the stretching stress of the

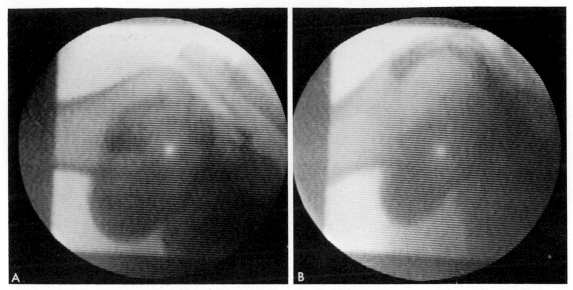

Figure 11–5 Arthrograms in throwing. *A,* In the wind-up phase dye and lubricant accumulate inferiorly, with little dye over the upper end of the humerus. *B,* At the end of delivery, with the arm at the side, more fluid flows over the upper surface of the humerus.

anchoring function of the capsule which comes into play in the follow-through braking motion. Sometimes a groove is produced on the posterior aspect of the head, something like that seen in recurrent dislocation of the shoulder, but in a slightly more inferior position.

Roughening of the articular cartilage with chipping and fragmentation is the usual sequel. The osteophyte may have sufficient vitality to remain anchored, but as it grows, further uncontrolled pressure may snap it, increasing the friction distortion considerably. The final picture is one of a typical posttraumatic osteoarthritis. Under these circumstances operative treatment may be the only solution, but it is difficult to produce a shoulder effective for heavy activity. The major hope lies in the disturbance's being sufficiently localized that a precise local debridement may be carried out without much tissue disruption.

FOOTBALL PASSING INJURIES

Football is basically thought of as a body contact sport, and injuries result from the mechanism of the contact. However, considerable throwing is involved and this is of a different nature from that used in playing baseball. The basic mechanism is the same, but there are significant differences in the overall act that influence the type of

injury that may occur. The wind-up is less extensive, the forward fling is shorter, and the follow-through is in a different arc and not so powerful. The football is a heavier and bulkier object so that, to a degree, there is a forward pushing element in this propelling act rather than a wholly flinging motion as in the case of a baseball (Fig. 11–6). The football passer takes his arm into a position that is vulnerable to a severe contusion type of strain. The passer often is hit in the act of throwing, so that force is applied to the upper arm just as it is going through the initial phase of the throwing motion. There is added to this a blocking or contusion element which leads to a bruising and tearing of muscles as well as some force of avulsion. It is usually the posterior aspect of the shoulder, particularly the quadrilateral space, which is implicated.

The contusion type of sprain occurring in an area with a copious blood supply and a large plexus of veins favors myositis ossificans. Football passers often develop large zones of calcific plaques implicating the posteroinferior aspect of the shoulder.

SHOULDER INJURIES IN GOLF

Shoulder action contributes significantly to the golf swing. In contrast to the throwing act, tremendous power of swing is developed from a stationary stance so that body weight

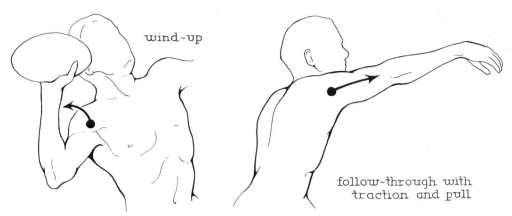

wind-up

follow-through with
traction and pull

Figure 11–6 Shoulder action in passing. Greater stability is required in this act because of the pushing element in the throw.

follow-through implicates particularly the upper half of the body. The initiation of the swing phases into extensor action and abduction, with maximum stress focused at the horizontal or above the horizontal level. This is in marked contrast to the throwing act. The golf swing involves a beginning synchronous action of both shoulders, with a counterpull developing in the shoulder toward which the swing is completed. The significant element is that the crucial application of force and swing comes at the horizontal level, or in traveling toward it.

The back swing is initiated by the muscles of the arms and shoulders. The club is swung upward and backward with the head held as nearly in the line of flight as possible, until the rotation of the body carries it back and inside. The completion of the back swing lifts the shoulder above a right angle. The wind-up in the case of the golf swing is taken through the body; in baseball the wind-up is in the limb. As the swing is continued, the club retraces the path of the back swing. The completion of the follow-through then brings the club back over the shoulder. For the most part, it is the large muscles about the shoulder which are involved, such as the pectoralis major, deltoid, coracobrachialis and triceps. The rotators play a less significant role than in the case of the baseball pitcher because of less need for finite control at the end of the swing. The implication of the heavy muscles about the shoulder, inluding trapezius and latissimus, focuses stress on the girdle as a whole rather than on the glenohumeral joint. Because of the force disposition from back swing to percussion point to follow-through, there is

primarily the transmission of force in the coronal plane of the body. The maximum effect of this is focused at the horizontal level.

Acromioclavicular Lesions. The commonest chronic golfing disorder about the shoulder implicates the acromioclavicular joint. This is because the disposition of the swing focuses stress at a horizontal level from the position of abduction and extension to abduction and flexion across the chest. In the case of the right-handed golfer, there is added to the act of propulsive effort of the right shoulder zone, the pull of the follow-through from the opposite side, which reaches its maximum at a horizontal level. Minor disturbances are alleviated by a period of rest, Novocain and steroid injection of the joint, and systemic medication. The lesion can be identified by a point of maximum tenderness over the acromioclavicular joint and reproduction of the discomfort by swinging the arm across the chest at the horizontal level.

Soft Tissue Injuries. Mild muscle irritations or traumatic tendinitis also occur, usually from forcing the back swing so that the head of the humerus rocks in the glenoid, putting traction stress on the capsule. In contrast to baseball, extensive glenohumeral changes are not encountered but superficial tears in the cuff may occur.

A point of particular importance to remember is that the golfer may have hurt his shoulder in some other activity, apart from his golfing exercise. Just like anybody else, he may slip and fall, taking his weight on the outstretched arm and traumatizing the capsule or long head of the biceps. The discomfort may come to light, or come into clinical focus, when he starts swinging a golf club. A small tear in the capsule can crop up as persistent pain, particularly in the back swing. Tenderness will be identified anteriorly, related to glenohumeral action; contrast studies are essential in those with persistent complaints not responding to conservative treatment. These should be managed just as such lesions are elsewhere, with an initial program of conservative treatment. The telltale sign, however, is the persistence of symptoms and the failure of response to conservative management over a reasonable period. When this occurs, more careful scrutiny should be carried out, including contrast studies.

Surgical treatment of the golfer's shoulder is extremely successful. In most instances, when the lesion is accurately identified, surgical reconstruction allows the golfer to return to his previous activity without jeopardizing his peak form.

HEAVY THROWING SPORTS AND FIELD EVENTS

Included in this group are activities such as discus throwing, shot putting and javelin throwing.

The propelling mechanism in these sports implicates the shoulder in a fashion quite different from baseball or golf, and acute episodes are the more frequent source of injury rather than chronic disabling entities. The mechanism of the throw places tremendous traction and pull on the follow-through phase, affecting principally the large anchoring muscles about the shoulder. Certain lesions are peculiar to these sports.

Interscapular Muscle Tears. The pull of the heavy weight places stress on the anchoring structures, and occasionally muscle tears occur in the interscapular zone. An area of tenderness and swelling localized to this region can be identified. The injury is treated successfully by local anesthetic blocks, physiotherapy, a period of rest and systemic medication.

Scapulocostal Injuries. Javelin throwers are subject to recurrent attacks of sharp discomfort related to the medial border of the scapula. Recurrent minute muscle tears occur, and with slow healing a tendinitis develops. Zones of tenderness related to

the medial border of the scapula accompanied by considerable crepitus can be identified. If untreated, the complaint tends to become chronic and may be aggravated by cervical spine action as well.

In the initial acute stage the shoulder girdle should be immobilized in a figure-of-eight shoulder strap splint for two weeks, followed by gradual use, physiotherapy and systemic medication.

BOWLING, CURLING, SOFTBALL

These activities are linked by a common mechanism in that the shoulder action involves underarm pitching action. This largely flexion delivery focuses stress on the anterior aspect of the shoulder, and the typical disturbances appear to be quite different from those acquired in sports using overhand delivery. The structures that are involved are principally the anterior capsule and the bicipital apparatus. The biceps is particularly vulnerable because the forearm action further increases tension and stress on the biceps in the motion of supination. A jerking type of delivery or a slipping of the ball from the hand favors uncontrolled stretch focused on the anterior aspect of the shoulders. The strong internal rotation with flexion stretches the long head of the biceps in its groove. Such acts irritate the bicipital sheath and initiate tenosynovitis or even a fraying of the capsular structure if the act is repetitive.

Bicipital Tendinitis. Sometimes it is an unusually forceful supination strain that is the irritant. In all underhand deliveries there is a supination-flexion element; it is the supination that may be taken beyond the normal range. When this is coupled with arm and forearm flexion, it may spring the intertubercular fibers, anchoring the long head of the biceps in the humerus and allowing it to swing more freely in its trough. When extreme force has been used, the tendon may slip right out of the groove, leaving a slipping biceps tendon.

In its initial stages this lesion is cured by rest and avoidance of the irritating activity. When the force has been sufficient to weaken the intertubercular fibers, allowing the tendon to slip, operative repair is the cure. If the intertubercular fibers are properly restored, a full return of function may be anticipated. This is not a disabling procedure and can be accomplished without jeopardizing important structures.

INJURIES IN BODY CONTACT SPORTS

Many serious injuries occur in the heavy body contact activities such as football, hockey, basketball and soccer.

MECHANISM OF INJURY

In these sports the cause of the injury is quite apparent, and one does not have to look for an intricate explanation. The commonest offending act is application of a heavy force from the side, a sideways fall on the shoulder, a rugged block or a heavy boarding action. The back and the front of the shoulder-neck region may be well protected, but it is application of force from the side that often is damaging. When contact with the lateral aspect of the shoulder is unobstructed, the brunt is transferred to the suspensory mechanism of the clavicle. Force may be dissipated at the acromioclavicular junction or along the shaft of the clavicle, or it may penetrate deeply and implicate the suspensory ligaments. The angle and level of application, the degree of violence, and the instrument involved control the damage that results. Unprotected falls or sideways contacts in the coronal plane nearly always implicate the acromioclavicular mechanism. Recurrent minor episodes then serve as a constant irritant to this joint. Instantaneous application of violent force is more likely to shatter the bony strut of the clavicle without the force being dissipated in the suspensory mechanism. In this way the strut crumples under the impact.

When force is applied in a more downward direction, but is not of shattering dimensions, the suspensory ligaments bear the brunt and may give way, allowing dislocation of the acromioclavicular joint. In assessing the damage roentgenologically, views of the opposite joint should be made for the sake of comparison.

Severe soft tissue injuries are encountered in the body contact sports, and almost all the fractures and dislocations implicating the shoulder girdle are derived from these activities. Dislocations of the glenohumeral joint, subluxation of the joint and recurrent dislocations are common in these sports.

INVESTIGATION AND DIAGNOSIS OF CONTACT SPORT INJURIES

The neck and shoulder region is a critical area, and all injuries in this region require special attention and investigation.

On the Field Investigation. The trainer is the one who gets to see injuries first in most team activities, so he should not only work closely with the team physician but have a good working knowledge of the principles of this region particularly. He receives the most accurate description of what has happened, how the injury occurred and how much force or how many bodies were involved. When there is the slightest suggestion of involvement beyond the superficial tissues, the doctor should be brought on the field before the patient is moved. The most critical area is the neck, and if there is any question of a neck lesion, the patient should be moved on a stretcher on his back, with the head sandbagged or held carefully; any complaint involving the neck demands that the player be taken completely off the field and a meticulous examination carried out. If he is lying prone he must not be allowed to sit up; if he is sitting or standing, the head must be supported in extension as he leaves the playing area.

When the shoulder is obviously deformed, the patient should also be put on a stretcher because then the body and the stretcher effectively splint the whole area comfortably to allow transportation.

Hospital Investigation. The place to examine and assess these patients properly, when suspicions have been aroused of a serious injury or there is obvious deformity, is in the hospital, not the dressing room. Only preliminary assessment should be made until the patient is in a place where everything necessary for his care can be provided instantly. When the dressing room assessment indicates that there has not been implication of the deep structures, bones, joints or nerves, preliminary care can be carried out. When the lesion implicates these categories, the patient should be taken to the hospital.

Clinical Assessment. The neck should be assessed initially with particular attention being paid to any sharply localized tenderness, fear of motion, stiffness or fixed deformity. When any of these are present, an x-ray should be taken immediately with the head and neck carefully protected, preferably in a chin halter with gentle traction in extension. Attention is paid to the shoulder after neck complications are ruled out.

ACUTE SOFT TISSUE INJURIES

Acute Anterior Sprain of Shoulder. The area about the shoulder susceptible to soft tissue injuries in contact sports is the antero-inferior aspect. This is because the axillary zone is opened up in abduction and external rotation so that considerable force may be applied directly to the axilla or on the lever of the arm, with force transmitted to the anterior capsular elements. A hard driving helmet, knee or shoulder can implicate the axillary region, or the abducted externally rotated arm may be forced backward in the attempt to tackle an on-rushing runner.

Impacts like this stretch the subscapularis and anterior capsular region. It may be of sufficient severity to luxate the head of the humerus or tear the muscle completely (Fig. 11–7).

In such injuries the patient has immediate pain on the anterior aspect, and a zone of definite tenderness can be identified which becomes more apparent when the examining fingers are placed in the axilla and pushed upward and inward. Considerable swelling often ensues; there is weakness on internal rotation and forward flexion of the humerus in the glenoid.

TREATMENT. The injury is treated conservatively by immobilization in a sling or body swathe for four weeks.

Upon occasion, definite anterior luxation will persist and can be identified by lateral views showing the relation of the head of the humerus to the glenoid. Contrast studies will identify the continuity of the anterior capsule and its relationship to the glenoid. When a defect can be demonstrated, surgical repair with reattachment of the anterior capsule, as in a recurrent dislocation, is required.

Ruptures of the Rotator Cuff. Acute rupture of the superior rotator cuff in the young athlete is rare, unless there has been a fracture of the greater tuberosity. It can happen that strain so placed, carrying the arm into abduction passively and yet preventing external rotation, avulses the greater tuberosity, carrying with it a piece of the rotator cuff. Surgical treatment is required for this injury when there is visible displacement.

Football and hockey rarely produce acute cuff ruptures because the tendons at this age are strong and minimal degenerative changes have set in.

Bicipital Injuries. Disturbances of the bicipital mechanism are not so frequent in body contact activities as in the throwing sports. Three primary entities of bicipital disturbances, however, may be encountered: bicipital tenosynovitis, bicipital luxation, and rupture of the long head of biceps tendon.

BICIPITAL TENOSYNOVITIS. Traumatic tendinitis implicating the biceps tendon is occasionally seen. As a rule, the disturbance implicates the upper portion of the tendon close to the intertubercular zone. The ante-

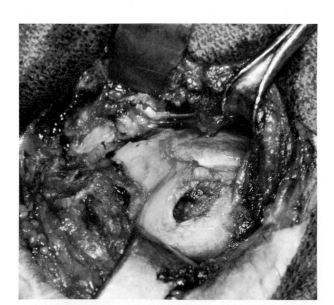

Figure 11–7 Acute rupture of the anterior capsule in a young athlete.

rior aspect of the shoulder is exposed in line blocking, body checking and boarding activities so that it can be implicated in a contusion type of disturbance. It is really a crushing type of injury which occurs rather than the chronic irritating mechanism commonly seen in other sports. Contusion causes a degree of fraying of the tendon, and a friction type of synovial reaction develops implicating the length of the tendon in the groove. Treatment as for a contusion elsewhere is all that is required, with rest, systemic phenylbutazone and gradual resumption of activities.

SUBLUXATION OF BICEPS TENDON. Contusion type of trauma may so implicate the bicipital mechanism when there is a congenitally shallow groove in the humerus that the tendon may burst its intertubercular fibers. Almost always this develops where there is a large tendon with a shallow groove. Football passers sometimes suffer this injury because the abducted externally rotated arm may be struck forcibly while the player is in the act of passing, thereby throwing sudden stress on the intertubercular zone, and the tendon may jump from the groove.

If the fibers are sprained, rest and treatment as for a tenosynovitis will suffice. If a frank rupture is suspected, surgical repair is required (Fig. 11–8). The dislocation of the tendon can be identified on clinical examination by feeling the tendon slip from its groove on passive external rotation in the horizontal position. It is an extremely painful episode, with the discomfort localized in the anterior shoulder.

ACUTE RUPTURE OF LONG HEAD OF BICEPS. Rupture of the long head, like rotator cuff injuries, is not frequent in this group of patients because of the minimal degenerative changes. Severe contusions of the muscle belly and avulsion at the musculotendinous juncture may occur. These are usually also a contusion or crushing type of traction injury rather than rupture of the tendon in the groove.

Treatment. This is a significant injury in an athlete and should be treated by surgical means (Fig. 11–9). The earlier it is carried out, the better, because delay militates considerably against a successful result. The tendon should be transferred to the coracoid and plicated to the short head, or fastened to the coracoid if sufficient length of long head tendon remains. Unless this is done, considerable power of flexion at the shoulder will be lost and there will be a decrease in flexion and supination of the forearm. The operation of tacking the long head of the tendon to the groove is inadequate because this tendon then no longer plays across the shoulder joint and the flexion contribution is entirely lost. So significant is this action that if insufficient length of tendon remains, an effort should be made to use a strip of fascia from the thigh, imbricating it into the proximal portion of the muscle and then attaching it to the short head and coracoid.

BONE AND JOINT INJURIES

Included in this group are acromioclavicular dislocation, fractures of the clavicle, ruptures of the suspensory ligaments, dislocations of the glenohumeral joint and dislocations of the sternoclavicular joint. Fractures of the scapula and upper end of the humerus may also be encountered, but these are unusual.

Acromioclavicular Injuries. Perhaps the commonest injury about the shoulder in athletes is some damage to the acromioclavicular joint. This may be a subluxation, a dislocation, or a dislocation with rupture of the suspensory ligaments. In sorting out these injuries it is desirable to discuss these three separate phases of involvement. Force in the coronal plane of the body is involved in many positions and activities of body contact sports. Application of force to the lateral aspect of the humerus results in transfer through the suspensory ligaments, the acromioclavicular joint and the clavicle to the sternoclavicular joint and central portion of the body. The myriad patterns of such force

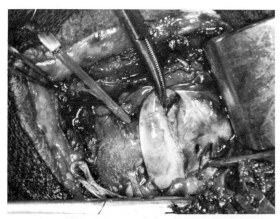

Figure 11–8 Subluxation of the biceps tendon.

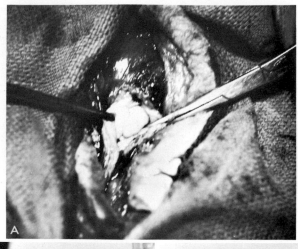

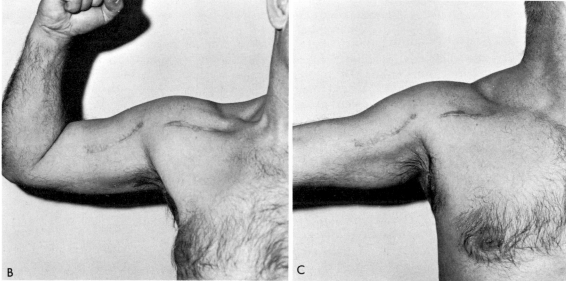

Figure 11-9 Rupture of the long head of the biceps. *A,* Incised lesion. *B* and *C,* Incisions and healing following transfer to the coracoid process after surgical repair.

application explain the frequency of these injuries. Opposing players, the ground, the ice, the boards may all be used as a bouncing post by the player who instinctively turns to avoid head-on application of force.

ACUTE SPRAIN OR ACROMIOCLAVICULAR SUBLUXATION. In such an injury some stretching or tearing of the acromioclavicular ligaments has occurred. Tenderness over the acromioclavicular joint, but not necessarily extensive mobility of the clavicle, can be demonstrated. Possibly on pressure the clavicle appears to ride down a little farther than normal, but the gross relationships of the joint are rarely distorted.

Treatment. The arm should be kept in a sling or strapped to the side, preferably with adhesive strapping applied with the fulcrum over the middle or inner third; lifting the arm in the region of the elbow is also desirable. A useful clavicular sling is one which lifts the humerus by pressure through forearm and elbow with a strap placed more medially over the clavicle so that, when tightened, there is upward pull on the acromion and downward pull on the clavicle. The lesion requires four to six weeks to heal satisfactorily. This program is supported by local anesthetic block and systemic medication. The active treatment program is followed by the gradual resumption of activity with avoidance of further similar stress.

DISLOCATION OF THE ACROMIOCLAVICULAR JOINT. When true laxity of the clavicle on

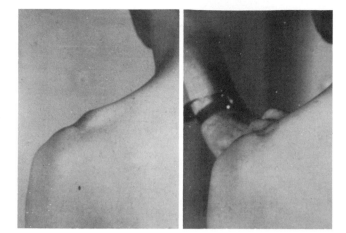

Figure 11–10   Dislocation of acromioclavicular joint.

the acromion can be identified, much more extensive injury has occurred. The horizontal fibers extending across the superior aspect of the joint have been ruptured, and the coracoclavicular or suspensory ligament has been stretched, allowing upward displacement of the clavicle and a downward and lateral displacement of the acromion (Fig. 11–10).

Treatment.   This is a significant injury and by far the best management, particularly in an athlete, is some form of internal fixation. It is preferable to do this under a general anesthetic, inserting wires or a threaded wire through the acromion into the clavicle in the reduced position. Fixation is carried out for a minimum of six weeks and is followed by a program of rehabilitation and gradual use.

DISLOCATION WITH RUPTURE OF SUSPENSORY LIGAMENTS.   This is an extremely disabling injury, the severity of which is often unrecognized. The typical finding is frank upward displacement of the clavicle at least the distance of the clavicular thickness, along with some dropping downward and forward of the acromion so that the acromioclavicular joint dimension is grossly widened (Fig. 11–11). The distance between the clavicle and the coracoid also is greater on the injured side than when compared with the uninjured side. In such a lesion it is not enough to restore the acromioclavicular relationship; the suspensory ligament must also be repaired. If there is strong suspicion but some uncertainty concerning this injury, the patient should be examined under anesthesia. When the patient relaxes, the clear nature and the extent of the lesion im-

mediately become apparent. The acromion and the shoulder will drop downward and forward to a surprising degree, leaving no doubt that the suspensory mechanism has been torn. Sometimes it is sufficient to take x-rays of the weighted shoulder, but this is not so complete as an assessment under anesthesia.

Treatment.   By far the most satisfactory solution is open reduction and repair of the ligaments. Reduction of the clavicle is main-

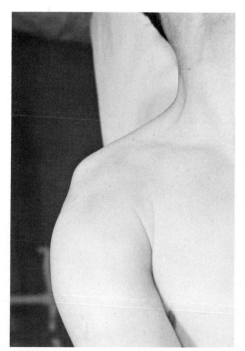

Figure 11–11   Dislocation with rupture of suspensory ligaments.

tained by the insertion of pin fixation. In some instances it is possible to sew the coranoid and trapezoid ligaments together adequately once the dislocation has been reduced. In most instances it is preferable to restore the ligament by insertion of a new fascial band from the acromion across the clavicle and into the spine of the scapula. Restoration in this fashion does more to restore the acromioclavicular relationship to normal than merely attaching the coracoid to the clavicle. When viewed from above, the normal relationship can be seen to be restored by this maneuver. (The operative technique is discussed in Chapter XIII.)

RECURRENT ACROMIOCLAVICULAR SUB-LUXATION OR INTERNAL DERANGEMENT OF THE ACROMIOCLAVICULAR JOINT. In young athletes, especially teen-agers, a somewhat uncommon entity may be encountered in the form of an internal derangement of the acromioclavicular joint. Young athletes sustaining repeated sagittal injuries may damage the small intra-articular disc within the acromioclavicular joint (Fig. 11–12).

Typically the patients complain of pain in the shoulder and a catching sensation in certain motions, particularly abduction and flexion. They are not able to locate the source of the clicking action precisely since it is not a consistent result of movement of the arm.

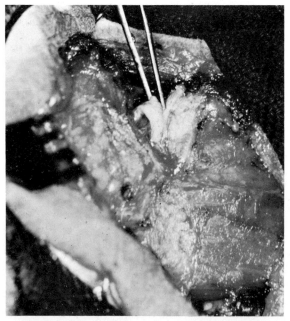

Figure 11–12 Rupture of the intra-articular disc in the acromioclavicular joint.

On examination tenderness can be identified related to the acromioclavicular joint, and as the patient lifts his arm into abduction and then across the joint flexion, the discomfort of which he has been conscious may be produced. At the same time a minimal degree of subluxation or incongruity of the acromioclavicular joint margins can be identified. A further test is to manually shift the acromion on the clavicle, holding one bone in each hand. This frequently produces the clicking sensation and the pain of which the patient has been complaining.

Fractures of the Clavicle. Particular attention is required for clavicular injuries, especially in professional athletes, because unsatisfactory treatment will so often permanently mar performance or interfere with earning a livelihood. As a rule, some form of rigid internal fixation is required, and if there is much comminution, the fragments should be replaced accurately at open reduction and suitably held.

FRACTURES OF THE OUTER THIRD OF THE CLAVICLE. Two separate types of injury of importance in this zone may be recognized: (1) The first is a splintered type of injury sustained from direct violence which cracks the outer third of the clavicle, distorting the acromioclavicular relationship. When there is significant displacement, implication of the joint is inevitable and eventual acromioclavicular arthritis can be anticipated. When the joint has been involved, resection of the outer half inch of the clavicle, really an acromioclavicular arthroplasty, is highly desirable. (2) Fracture through the distal or lateral one inch of the clavicle may be of the same proportions or configuration as a rupture of the suspensory ligament in that the medial fragment is displaced upward and the lateral fragment is displaced downward. This is a serious injury and also requires open reduction and internal fixation. The suspensory ligament should be inspected at operation after the fracture has been accurately reduced and transfixed. If the ligament has been damaged, it should be reconstructed or repaired (see Chapter XIII).

FRACTURES OF THE MIDDLE THIRD OF THE CLAVICLE. Similar considerations apply to this fracture, no matter what type of patient is involved, but the dictum of extremely accurate reposition holds particularly in athletes. By far the most satisfactory treatment is open reduction and internal fixation. Fixation can be obtained by a threaded wire inserted through the medial fragment and then out through the lateral end. If a threaded wire is not used, the end of the wire should be turned so that it cannot wander. In some instances an extremely useful form of internal fixation is a Knowles pin. The pin may be inserted in such a fashion that rigid internal fixation is provided and it may be left in situ.

FRACTURES OF THE INNER THIRD OF THE CLAVICLE. Fractures of the inner third are rare in athletic activities, since they usually result from an extremely severe overhead crushing type of trauma. Neurovascular complications are frequent and often overshadow the bone injury. Occasionally an oblique fracture at the sternal end will occur, which is really a part of subluxation. Conservative methods, as a rule, provide satisfactory results unless there has been significant displacement. If a fragment is widely separated, excision is desirable.

RETROSTERNAL DISLOCATIONS. A more serious dislocation develops if the clavicle is shoved behind the sternum. If such an injury is seen shortly after the episode, the clavicle may be gently elevated into place by grasping the medial third with the fingers and pulling upward and laterally.

Special care must be taken in such reduction if implication of retrosternal structures is apparent. In some instances, as advocated by De Palma, a towel clip may be used to grasp the tubular area for proper purchase to lift the clavicle slowly and carefully into its notch. In easy standing dislocations of this type, fascial repair which resects a figure-of-eight sling through the clavicle and into the sternum should be added to maintain stability.

STERNOCLAVICULAR INJURIES. Powerful force applied in the coronal plane may implicate the medial end of the strut when there is added a somewhat oblique or downward pressure from behind. The medial end of the clavicle may jump upward, or if the blow is from the front, it may be forced retrosternally and then ride superiorly or inferiorly.

Treatment. Closed reduction of the uncomplicated anterior dislocation can be accomplished in the early postinjury period by backward pressure on the shoulder and pressure over the medial end of the clavicle. In longer standing injuries open reduction is required. Under these circumstances there is often a tendency for the medial end not to sit securely in the notch, and the ease with which the dislocation may recur is apparent. Under these circumstances fascial repair of the capsular ligaments and costoclavicular band is carried out (see Chapter XIII).

Fractures of the Acromion. Mention is made of this injury here so that it will be kept in mind in the investigation of athletic injuries about the shoulder. It usually results from a contusion type of trauma, with a heavy body falling on the superior aspect. Commonly it is a crack or almost a greenstick type of injury without extensive displacement. Conservative measures suffice, as a rule. If the lateral end has been bent down, it may be pried into quite accurate alignment by manipulation under a general anesthetic without open reduction. The fracture will heal if the arm is immobilized in a body swathe, but most of these patients are much more comfortable in a properly applied shoulder spica that is worn for six weeks. When this extensive immobilization is employed in an athlete, however, a vigorous program of rehabilitation is essential afterward.

Rarely, a fracture of the acromion displays considerable displacement. When this is the case, open reduction can be carried out, with internal fixation by a circular wire loop or a single small Knowles pin. Little reaction ensues from such an open reduction, and the injury heals rapidly.

Fractures of the Body of the Scapula. Occasionally contusion injuries break the body of the scapula. These lesions may be treated conservatively with immobilization in a sling or body swathe for six weeks.

Dislocation and Subluxation of the Glenohumeral Joint. Body contact sports produce more dislocations of the shoulder than any other activity. All the common and uncommon varieties of subluxation and dislocation can be encountered in sports (Fig. 11–13). This includes simple anterior dislocation, anteroposterior subluxation, posterior dislocation, inferior dislocation, recurrent anterior dislocation and recurrent posterior dislocation. The management of all the various phases of these injuries is the same in athletes as in others and has been considered extensively in Chapter XIII, Fractures and Dislocations. The one consideration with regard to the athlete which is different is the patient's enthusiastic desire to have as complete a return of function as quickly as possible.

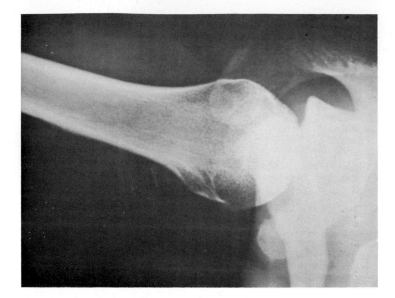

Figure 11–13 Recurrent subluxation of the shoulder in an athlete.

In the initial anterior dislocation the arm should be kept in a sling at the side for at least six weeks. This should be followed by a skillfully paced program of resumption of function carried to a point at which a full range of motion is obtained, so that there is no limiting rotatory deficiency to mar performance. In recurrent dislocation it is strongly recommended that surgical repair be carried out at an early date. The question often comes up of how long the athlete should be kept out of active participation after the initial dislocation. The author believes that the shoulder should be protected for six weeks under these circumstances, and most of the time this means he cannot play until the following season. If it is a recurring episode, the second or third dislocation should be treated operatively.

The prime reasons for conservatism are, first, to complete healing as securely as possible, thereby avoiding recurrence. Second, a shoulder so insulted is in poor condition to withstand a further episode which may, this time, be of more severe proportions; for example, complicated by a stretch lesion of the axillary nerve and resultant deltoid paralysis.

NECK INJURIES IN SPORTS

Body contact sports are a potential source of neck injuries and some may be extremely serious. Because of this, a word regarding emergency handling is essential when a neck injury is suspected. The time for the most critical precautions may occur directly on the playing field, so that it behooves trainers and handlers in particular to have some special knowledge of the seriousness of neck injuries. As a rule, it is the trainer who reaches the injured player first, and he should be taught that if there are symptoms suggestive of neck involvement, the patient should not be moved nor should there be any effort to disturb him until the physician has come on the field. It takes but a short time to determine whether there has been a serious accident with cord involvement. The patient should be moved to a stretcher, with special care being taken in placing him on the stretcher to prevent significant excursion of the neck. Preferably he should be put on his back, with the neck held in the midposition by an attendant.

Once the player is in the dressing room, the physician can make a more detailed examination and decide whether the injury has penetrated to deep structures.

Particular care must be taken to prevent the patient from sitting up, or allowing handlers, technicians or anyone else to raise the patient into the sitting position. Once the degree of severity has been identified by physical examination and, if deemed necessary, X-ray examination, proper management may be instituted. The collection of neck injuries may best be considered according to the depth of injury, whether it has been confined to the soft tissues only or whether bone or joint involvement has occurred.

SOFT TISSUE INJURIES

Contusions of the Neck. As a mobile zone the neck is relatively unprotected, so that in athletic activities, particularly body contact sports, it remains a vulnerable zone.

Blows from the Front. As a rule, the vital larynx and trachea are protected by the instinctive lowering of the head, but this does not always protect the throat zone. Sharp blows may interfere with breathing and speech. Spasm of the larynx may leave the player speechless and extremely short of breath. The combination of difficulty in breathing and momentary loss of speech is a frightening one. Fractures of the trachea, thyroid cartilage or hyoid can happen, but they are rare in young athletes.

If the symptoms persist, the patient should be taken to a hospital at once, put at complete rest and given oxygen; appropriate investigation of the neck structures should then be carried out. In by far the majority of cases, it is only a stunning or bruising with transient interruption of functions that results, and the player recovers quickly.

When some doubt exists as to the state of the vital structures, continued supervision in the hospital where suction and oxygen therapy are available is essential. The neck should be splinted with a soft collar and activities resumed very gradually.

Blows from the Back. Direct contusion of the back of the neck produces bruising of the muscles, sometimes hematoma formation and, rarely, a splintering of the spinous processes. In the acute stage, freezing to a very superficial degree of the overlying painful skin area produces immediate relief and relaxes the muscle spasm. This should be followed by physiotherapy and the application of a light fabric collar until the soreness has subsided.

Lateral Contusions. The side of the neck is much better protected than the back, but direct blows here may produce an additional element of discomfort from trauma to the brachial plexus. In addition to the usual muscle bruising syndrome, the patient may experience the feeling of burning numbness and shock-like extension down the arm. The arm may momentarily be numbed, and he will be unable to move it. As a rule, over a period of mere seconds he is once again able to shrug, lift and use it, and the unpleasant sensation disappears. Should there be a persistence of the paresthesia, more extensive investigation is required. When only muscles are involved, the contusion is handled in the same fashion as those sustained from the posterior aspect.

Neck Sprain. Precise separation of the various degrees of soft tissue insult is difficult since one tends to merge into another. The common ligamentous injury in the neck which may be called a sprain is involvement of the posterior elements, the interspinous ligaments and the ligamentum nuchae. The commonest and severest insult is a flexion type of injury with the force so applied that the posterior spinous elements are torn apart. Various degrees of this force, in turn, implicate the apophyseal joint structures which then, with a further continuation of the force, may separate the articular processes and shift the vertebral bodies forward.

The common injury is contained within the posterior elements. Following the forward flexion strain, the neck has a lax feeling, and quite definite posterior tenderness can be identified, usually related to one set of posterior spinous processes. Shortly all the erector spinae muscles become spastic, and the patient holds his neck rigidly, being unwilling to allow it to bend forward.

In the acute phase, if a precise point of ligamentous separation can be identified, it should be injected with a local anesthetic and a soft cervical collar applied. The neck is kept at rest, both night and day, for a period of six weeks until the ligament has healed.

When the force has been of sufficient severity to avulse the spinous processes, the most satisfactory management is surgical excision. Failure of an avulsed process to unite is common, so that all these injuries should be x-rayed and the depth of the damage identified as accurately as possible (see Chapter XIII).

BONE AND JOINT INJURIES

Sprain Subluxation. When the flexion force has been of sufficient severity to extend to the articular elements, some luxation of the facets occurs. This may be enough to allow complete sliding forward of one vertebral body or merely a loosening with some instability. In the absence of obvious alteration in the alignment of the articular processes, the injury just appears as a very bad sprain. Extreme spasticity of the muscles, almost a rigidity, results, and there is so much pain that it is difficult to identify a precise level. X-ray examination will show a straight spine and sometimes sufficient spasm to reverse the normal curve (Fig. 11–14). Careful flexion and extension films may suggest the level of luxation but, as a rule, this is difficult to pick out. It usually is quite apparent from the local findings that much more than a tear of an interspinous element has occurred (Fig. 11–15). The neck must be put at rest, initially in light cervical traction in the midposition, followed by the application of a plaster collar. The ordinary soft cervical or other mechanical collars are inadequate in an injury of this severity. Eight to ten weeks is required for satisfactory healing and stability following this type of injury.

In some instances the aftermath of subluxation is a posttraumatic arthritis and chronic instability which requires bony stabilization. Cervical subluxations are often

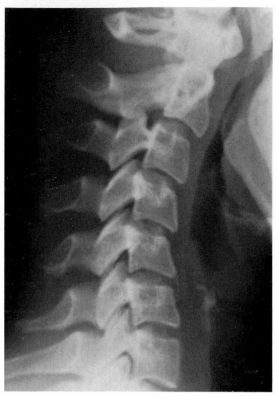

Figure 11–15 Subluxation at C.4–5 indicating ligamentous damage.

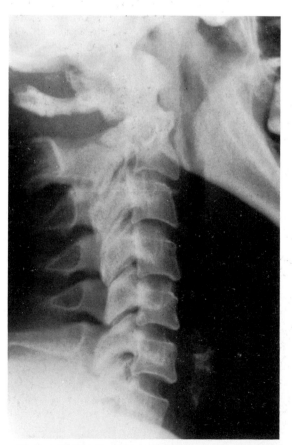

Figure 11–14 Straight spine due to muscle spasm in cervical subluxation.

overlooked, and it is not until the chronicity of symptoms demands more careful investigation that the true identity is revealed.

Rotatory Subluxation. The extreme mobility of the neck makes it vulnerable to twisting injuries also. The common injury is a forcible turning of the head and neck beyond the normal range. Normally the head and neck can rotate through 120 degrees, or 60 degrees on either side of the neutral frontal plane. Some elements of flexion stress are involved in this as well as the pure rotation, but the damaging element is the excess rotation.

Many degrees of this injury can be identified, but the significant ones are those in which the force has been sufficient to implicate the capsular structures, stretching and tearing the ligaments of the apophyseal joint.

The nature of these injuries is identified by the production of pain on the reproduction of the rotatory stress. A point of tenderness over the involved joint can be identified on the side of the neck opposite to the one to which the head and neck are turned. Most often this constitutes a true sprain without any persistent dislocation of the articular facets. Following the initial acute stage, there is a tendency for the patient to protect the side on which the sprain has occurred, so that he tends to tilt the head and neck toward that side but does not rotate the chin significantly (Fig. 11–16). There is an element of flexion in this, since it is in this position that he is best able to protect the joint. Initially this may look like a wry neck or torticollis, but it is quite different; the torticollis is a sprain or strain of the sternomastoid rather than the apophyseal joints. These injuries require careful treatment, which includes gentle traction, deep heat to relax the muscle spasm and muscular relaxants, followed by the application of a soft collar. The ligamentous injuries require four to six weeks for satisfactory healing and the player should not be in competition before that time. It is permissible for him to participate in practice, but only if he is wearing a protective collar. (See also Figure 12–5.)

DISLOCATIONS

Bilateral Rotatory Dislocation. Severe rotatory force continuing beyond the level of simple sprain of the joints and ligaments may progress to true dislocation as an apophyseal joint slides off, becoming locked in this position.

In the rotatory dislocation the displacement has little of the flexion element, which separates it from the bilateral dislocation. The head and neck are twisted to the opposite side, allowing the articular process to slip off on the involved side (Fig. 11–17). This force may be extended to the opposite side, so that there is some chipping or fracturing of the articular process on the side away from the dislocation.

These injuries are serious and require immediate hospitalization. Cervical traction, usually by the halter method, is applied, and muscle relaxants and adequate sedation are given. In the initial stages the carefully controlled intravenous injection of a relaxant is extremely helpful in allowing quick and painless reduction of the dislocation. Following reduction of the luxation, the head is immobilized in a Minerva jacket for eight to ten weeks.

As a rule, with adequate relaxation, both the subluxation and the rotatory dislocation will be reduced satisfactorily. Occasionally this is not so, particularly when the injury has not been identified at an early stage. Those skilled in the management of these injuries may attempt gentle manual traction

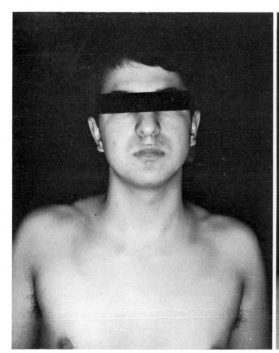
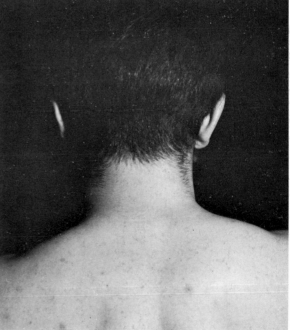

Figure 11–16 Rotatory sprain of the cervical spine. There is a barely perceptible tilt of the head to one side with a little rotation of the chin.

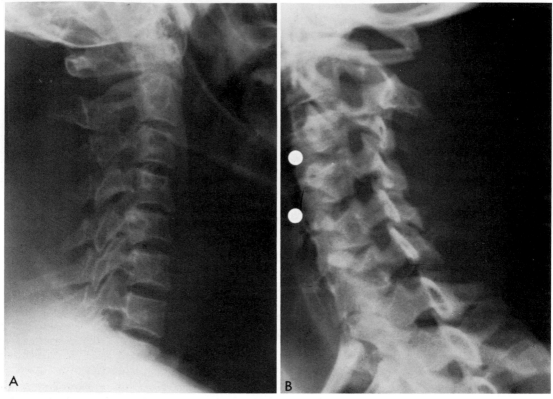

Figure 11–17 Rotatory subluxation of the cervical spine. *A*, Routine lateral view does not show extensive displacement. *B*, Oblique view shows the true state with C.6–C.7 facets locked out of alignment.

under anesthesia. The head is gently flexed and rotated in the direction to increase the deformity until the facet is unlocked. At the same time as the neck is flexed, traction is increased and the head is carefully turned and tilted toward the injured side. Once the facets have become unlocked, the head is tilted away from the lesion and the chin then rotated toward the side of the lesion. The neck is then pulled into gentle extension to maintain the reduction. If there is any obstruction in the last maneuver or any resistance to the gentle extension, then the facet has not become unlocked. Repeated attempts to obtain reduction by closed manipulation are to be condemned, and there is some question whether it should be attempted if the lesion is even of several days' duration. Operative reduction can be accomplished without the risk of cord damage and is probably the preferable maneuver if traction and proper muscle relaxation and sedation are unsuccessful As a rule, once these dislocations are reduced, they are stable, so that internal fixation or stabilization is not often so necessary as in the more serious forward bilateral dislocations (see Chapter XIII).

Hyperextension Subluxation Dislocation. Football injuries are the common source of these lesions. Violent application of force to the face, jaw and head can result in forced extension injuries which can be of sufficient severity to produce subluxation or dislocation.

One of the more serious aspects of these injuries was once caused by the type of helmet that was used. For a time the football helmet had a hard edge at the back on which there was little padding. When the neck was pulled or bent backward forcibly, this could dig into the back and with the spinous processes serving as a fulcrum, produce complete dislocation, sometimes with cord severance. The covering of the back of the helmet with a soft material has altered this situation so that the leverage force can no longer be brought into action, thereby removing this grave danger.

As in the flexion injuries, various degrees

of the extensor stretching damage can be identified. When the head and neck are forced backward, the posterior spinous processes impinge as the force is continued and eventually may break on each other. Sometimes the leverage is applied in such a way that the spinous process does not give way, forcing greater pressure on the cord elements anteriorly, and the cord may be sheared directly across.

Anterior Longitudinal Ligament Strain. Perhaps the mildest form of this extensor injury results in a stretching or tearing of the anterior longitudinal ligament. The injury is recognized by reproduction of the pain or extension and anterior tenderness. Often a small detached fragment from the anterior aspect may be identified in a lateral x-ray.

These injuries should be treated by traction in the prone position with sufficient weight being used to hold the head steady without distraction of the articular elements. The traction will be most comfortable with the head flexed slightly. Following subsidence of the initial muscle spasm, a cervical collar (preferably of firm felt) is applied; this keeps the head and neck in gentle flexion rather than extension. Most of these injuries heal satisfactorily, and surgical measures are not required.

Posterior Dislocation. The extreme form of extensor injury is followed by posterior dislocation or subluxation of one body on the other. This is an extremely serious injury and quite often is followed by complete cord paralysis. Transient cord and nerve root symptoms may occur without extensive posterior displacement of the vertebral bodies, but this is one of the most dangerous injuries in the neck. Extensive ligamentous rupture may occur with sufficient displacement of the bodies for the damage to be identified in the x-rays. Even minute posterior subluxation should be interpreted as having caused extensive ligamentous damage and should be treated by plaster immobilization for eight to ten weeks to allow adequate healing. In some instances the persistence of root symptoms, which indicates damage to the interbody structures favoring interbody instability, will require stabilization, preferably by the anterior route.

Fracture Dislocation. When the force has been of massive proportions or the mechanical application of great severity, fracture dislocation may result from either the flexion or extension type of application.

This is an extremely serious lesion and is almost always accompanied by cord damage, sometimes causing complete quadriplegia. All these are serious injuries and are not often encountered in sports, so that they are more appropriately considered under the discussion of fractures and dislocations in Chapter XIII.

Fractures of the Cervical Spine. Penetration of force to the bony structures of sufficient severity to produce fracture is not common in body contact or throwing sports. In some instances fractures occur in the lateral mass that are difficult to identify by routine x-ray. Laminograms should always be carried out on any zone in which persistent tenderness and reduced motion are apparent.

DIVING INJURIES

The most serious injuries of all involve diving accidents, although this rarely happens as a part of competitive sport. Normally in diving the head precedes the body into the water. This is followed by flexion of the spine and head, with continuation of the flexion force to the rest of the thoracic and lumbar spine. Added impetus is given to the dive by the springboard or by the height from which the dive is made, and a voluntary hurtling force is added, which makes the body contact with another surface one of much greater force than in ordinary falls or tumbles.

Diving into shallow water, carelessly heading into a pool which has been emptied or diving into unknown waters is the usual source of these tragedies. It is extremely rare for serious accidents to occur under normal conditions. Almost all these injuries are severe compression flexion injuries that produce compression fractures of the cervical spine or more serious fracture dislocations. When any of these lesions occur, extensive cord damage is possible and the management of the injury dictates attention to the preservation of life first because of possible interference with the vital centers. It is the disruption of the bulbar control which causes the fatalities, so that if at all feasible, this needs to be brought under control first. Resuscitation, tracheostomy and artificial breathing apparatus may all be required in treatment of extensive cord damage. Anyone with such an injury should have the head and neck held in the midposition to avoid increasing any cord damage already present. A skeletal traction is applied before any further treatment is given.

Compression Fractures Only. The average compression fracture can be treated by skeletal traction for a period of one to two weeks and should be followed by the application of a Minerva jacket. Manipulation or surgical treatment is not required unless there are associated neurological changes. However, if neurological abnormalities improve in a matter of days, surgical treatment is not necessary. The Minerva jacket is worn for 12 to 16 weeks.

Fractures with Cord or Nerve Root Involvement. Fractures of the articular processes and laminae or pedicles may complicate the compression injury, producing neurological changes. The initial management is with a period of cervical traction, but if the initial neurological abnormalities have not decreased at the end of two weeks, laminectomy should be carried out. The need for surgical intervention is not nearly so great when there has been no dislocation.

Cervical Dislocation and Fracture Dislocations. Following satisfactory handling during the acute postinjury phase, the traction is increased from 12-15 to 25-30 pounds to restore the dislocation. Frequent x-ray examinations, usually simple lateral plates, are taken to judge the effectiveness of the traction and the likelihood of reduction by closed means. If reduction is not obtained over a period of three to four days, or if there is any suggestion of neurological defect still present or increasing, open reduction should be carried out.

The reduction is carried out with the traction in place. Care is taken in administration of the anesthetic to prevent application of any extension force which could damage the cord.

Fracture dislocations require some form of internal fixation. If the reduction seems stable, wire fixation may be used; if there is any question about the stability, arthrodesis should be done at the same time, providing the patient's condition will permit. Skeletal traction is continued postoperatively, and when the patient's condition permits, the Minerva jacket is applied and left in place for four months. Weight bearing in the plaster is not allowed for eight to ten weeks after operation, and the patient uses a cervical collar for a further three to four months following removal of the Minerva jacket. The

"halo" apparatus may be used in preference to skeletal traction.

Injuries of the Atlas. Fractures or fracture dislocations of the atlas are primarily treated conservatively, with use of skeletal traction. When there is an increase in neurological changes, laminectomy and stabilization are required. In some instances the fractures heal with instability, necessitating occipitocervical arthrodesis.

FRACTURES OF THE AXIS. Fractures of the odontoid are not uncommon and frequently are accompanied by dislocation of the atlas so that there may be serious cord involvement. These injuries are also treated conservatively, with the application of skeletal traction maintaining the head in the midposition. Repeated x-ray examination is carried out to judge the appropriate weight required. Attention is paid to keeping the head and neck in the midline to favor early union of the odontoid. Many of these fractures heal well without serious residual symptoms. If the fracture appears stabilized in position at the end of six to eight weeks, a Minerva jacket may be carefully applied and left in place until union has occurred. Sometimes this requires longer than the usual 12 weeks, four to six months being necessary. Failure of union of the odontoid leaves a precariously unstable cervical spine and requires occipito-atlanto-axial stabilization.

The techniques of open reduction of the cervical spine and stabilization are delicate and difficult and should be carried out only by the experienced orthopedist. When there are signs of extensive cord involvement, management of the case should be a team effort, and should include a neurosurgeon. For the technical details of these procedures, the reader is referred to the pioneer works of W. A. Rogers, W. E. Gallie, and Robinson and Southwick.

Occipitocervical Arthrodesis. Posttraumatic instability of the occipito-atlanto-axial articulation comprises the most frequent indication for occipitocervical arthrodesis (Fig. 11–18). In most instances at least transient neurological changes involving both the upper and the lower limbs are present. These include ataxia, spasticity, some cervical nerve signs and posterior columnar involvement.

Similar disturbances arise in platybasia with foramen magnum cord compression and in rheumatoid arthritis with atlantoaxial subluxation. The problem may be complicated acutely by the necessity for

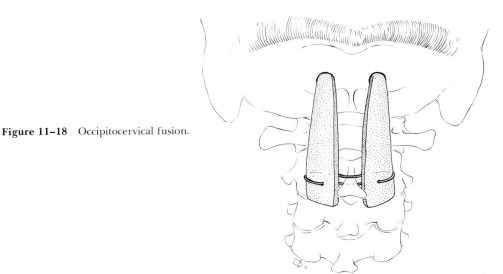

Figure 11–18   Occipitocervical fusion.

decompression laminectomy to relieve cord disturbance.

TECHNIQUE.   Certain preparatory precautions are mandatory and vary with the severity of the neurological complications. Skull tong traction is applied and a cerebellar head rest are used to maintain stability during the operation.

A 6- to 8-inch longitudinal incision is made distally from the external occipital protuberance. Using the electric knife, the muscles and nerves are detached from occiput to C.3 and C.4, including a portion of the upper laminal and cortex processes. The occipital bone is excised below the occiput.

Various methods of preparing a bed for grafts have been developed. The principle is to expose an area of the occiput below the nuchal line, then drill holes in the occiput. Grafts are fixed with wire around the posterior spines or around the arch of the atlas.

Cancellous bone chips are packed about the area, with the iliac crest used as the donor site.

Postoperatively, skeletal traction is retained and the patient is treated on a Stryker or other turning frame for four to six weeks. A prepared neck-chest brace is then applied and fixation is continued for six months.

REFERENCES

Allman, F. L., Jr.: Fractures and ligamentous injuries of the clavicle and its articulation. J. Bone Joint Surg. *49A*:1502–1510, 1967.

Blazina, M. E.: Shoulder injuries in athletics. J. Amer. Coll. Health. Ass. *15*:143–145, 1966.

Coughlin, E. J., et al.: Management of shoulder injuries in sport. Conn. Med. *29*:723–727, 1965.

Drill, F. E.: Injuries of the shoulder in athletes. Minn. Med. *48*:1665–1667, 1965.

Gal, A. J.: Severe cervical spine injuries. Trauma *5*:379–385, 1965.

Hoyt, W. A., Jr.: Etiology of shoulder injuries in athletes. J. Bone Joint Surg. *49A*:755–766, 1967.

Melvin, W. J., et al.: The role of the faceguard in the production of flexion injuries to the cervical spine in football. Canad. Med. Ass. J. *93*:1110–1117, 1965.

Peltokallio, P.: Typical joint injuries of the throwing hand in Finnish baseball players. J. Sport Med. *3*:229–235, 1963.

Pictrowski, W.: Diving injuries of the cervical vertebrae. Langenbeck Arch. Klin. Chir. *313*:575–579, 1965.

Quigley, T. B.: Injuries to the acromioclavicular and sternoclavicular joints sustained in athletics. Surg. Clin. N. Amer. *43*:1551–1554, 1963.

Schinbein, J. E.: Athletic injuries. Med. Serv. J. Canada *19*:881–887, 1963.

Symposium on Sports Medicine, American Academy of Orthopedic Surgeons. St. Louis, The C. V. Mosby Co., 1969.

Warrick, G. K.: Posterior dislocation of the shoulder joint. Brit. J. Radiol. *38*:758–761, 1965.

Weseley, W. S., and Barenfeld, F. A.: Ball thrower's fracture of the humerus. Six case reports. Clin. Orthop. *64*:153–156, 1969.

Chapter XII

AUTOMOBILE INJURIES

Automobile injuries have become the most serious public health problem on the American continent. The "war" on the highways in a single year produces a casualty list of 50,000 dead, 3,500,000 injuries and billions of dollars in property damage. No further reasons need to be documented for presenting a separate consideration of this aspect of trauma. The neck and shoulder region are prominently involved in the injury processes.

Extensive new legislation and new programs of investigation, dealing with drivers, highways and the automobile itself, have been introduced. Losses resulting from highway accidents in one year have resulted in a greater dollar cost than is required to wage the combat in Vietnam for the same period. Figures presented by the National Safety Council show that in one year traffic accidents kill 50,000 people in the United States as compared to battle casualties of 6000 to 7000. This represents a stark presentation of the problem.

MECHANISMS OF INJURY

The manner in which people are injured in car accidents has become of extensive scientific interest. New emphasis has been focused by governing authorities on ways and means of preventing accidents, and this has led to improved car construction, better highways and stricter assessment and control of the driver. The serious injuries can be minimized by improved steering columns, instrument panels, dashboards, seat contours, and shoulder and body harnesses, but the ultimate dimension remains the driver's control of his vehicle. The design of seats with headrests represents a significant step toward minimizing neck injuries. Bucket seats and shoulder harnesses are deterrents to body commotion and, therefore, of similar assistance.

An analysis of the mechanism of injury has an important place in the precise diagnosis and therapeutic management of all these problems. The rear end collision is a common problem but it is ironical that it is the vehicle that is struck rather than the one striking in which the occupants receive injuries of more widespread medicolegal, time-consuming interest than of pathological severity (Fig. 12–1). In contrast, the striking vehicle is the one in which the occupants may have the most severe injuries, and yet this contributor to the impact is less likely to become of medicolegal significance. These contrasting

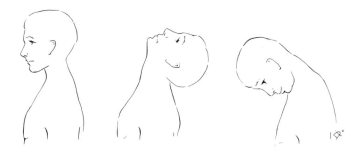

Figure 12–1 Extension-flexion injury.

states highlight two dominant injury processes: an extension-flexion trauma to the neck, and a predominantly flexion-extension process—one an injury of acceleration and the other an injury of deceleration (Fig. 12–1).

INJURY PATTERNS OF REAR END COLLISIONS

EXTENSION-FLEXION PATTERN OF DIRECT REAR END IMPACT

The impact of the vehicle striking from behind thrusts the seated lower portion of the body forward and tilts the unsupported head backward (Fig. 12–2 A); the head (weighing approximately 10 pounds) as a posterior swinging force strongly extends the neck. The second phase is a decelerating or arresting one, throwing the weighted neck forward. The force of the impact governs the backward phase but it does not necessarily control the forward phase. The weight of the car being struck, the position of the body on the seat (driver or passenger), the time of braking application and additional braking forces (backward, forward impact) influence the secondary phase (Fig. 12–2 B).

The involved tissues are damaged by two phases, since changes both at the front and the back of the neck are encountered. The sites of likely tissue damage will then vary to a considerable degree according to the influencing factors. The backward swing may be so free that the head hits the back of the seat. The forward swing may be stopped by the patient's muscle contractions or by his striking some part of the vehicle in front. In the case of the driver, the steering wheel provides protection, limiting the forward excursion significantly. In the case of the passenger at his side, the sweep before contact-producing injury is much greater, extending to the dashboard or the windshield in front.

The primary or extensor phase tenses all structures in front of the sagittal fulcrum of the cervical spine (Fig. 12–2 A). The varying position of the fulcrum from the base of the skull to the cervicothoracic junction explains to a considerable degree the localization of many tissue changes resulting from the whip or extension phase of whiplash. The structures sustaining the stress in front of the sagittal fulcrum then include the strap muscles, trachea, esophagus, anterior longitudinal ligament and vertebral body. As this force is continued, compression then falls on the apophyseal joint and lateral masses, and with extreme application of force, the spinal cord can be involved.

In the secondary or flexion phase, structures behind the fulcrum are implicated, including laminae, interlaminar ligaments, interspinous ligaments, spinous processes and ligamentum nuchae (Fig. 12–2B). Nature has provided protective zones for the soft neural tissue and the consistency itself allows a degree of flexibility that is a further protection. The dura mater and cord linings along with the space within the spinal column act as zones of cushioning. In a similar way the nerve roots are snubbed by an enveloping sheath as they extend through the intervertebral foramen. Sufficient space and leeway are available that direct damage to these structures, apart from overpowering force, is not likely to occur, but they may be implicated in secondary reactions initiated by the injury process. In the latter or flexion phase the main zones of protection are: (1) ligamentum nuchae and erector spinae muscles, (2) ligaments about the apophyseal joints, and (3) vertebral bodies and interbody elements. To some degree the recognition of these zones of defense serves as a practical classification for the types and degrees of injuries which are encountered. The infinite

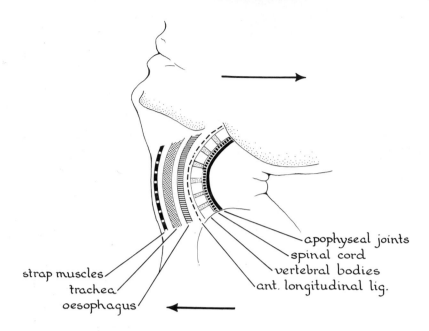

WHIPLASH - POSTERIOR SWING ACCELERATION

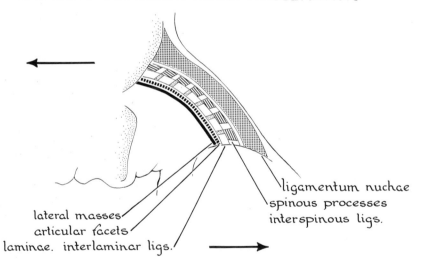

WHIPLASH - FORWARD SWING - DECELERATION

Figure 12–2 Structures involved in reaction to rear end collision. *A,* Primary extension phase. *B,* Secondary or flexion phase.

number of force applications along with the varying severity make precise identification of the changes difficult, but some appreciation of the tissue response to the force is helpful. The large majority of these injuries implicate soft tissues only, and when there is severe bone and joint involvement, it is usually the result of overwhelming force.

In interpreting the site of tissue change it is important to remember that the neck extension-flexion, although it is usually depicted as a free swinging action, is actually a compound movement including a sliding or gliding element. The shape and structure of the bones make this the only way in which these bones may move, one on another (Fig.

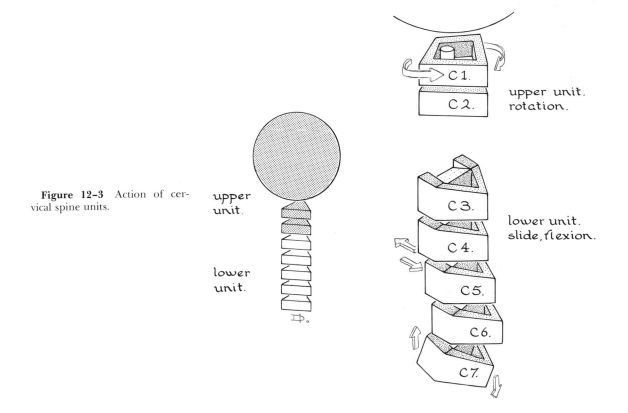

Figure 12-3 Action of cervical spine units.

upper unit.

lower unit.

upper unit. rotation.

lower unit. slide, flexion.

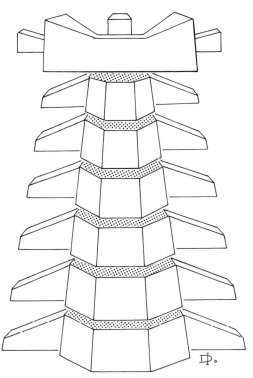

Figure 12-4 Cervical vertebrae. Note wide angle atlas and progressive increase in size of the remaining vertebrae to C.7.

12–3). It is the summation in the gliding arc that makes it look like a swinging arc.

There are some further structural properties related to the cervical spine that are of importance in swinging types of trauma. The size and shape of the vertebral bodies vary (from the smallest to the largest) from above downward, so that greater damage can be caused to the more delicate upper segments than the more sturdily constructed lower ones. As one looks at the cervical spine from the front, the gradation in size is pyramid fashion from the top to the bottom (Fig. 12–4). Similarly, the posterior outrigging cervical spines provide a natural zone of protective restriction of motion at the bottom because of impingement; the longer the lever, the greater the protection, so that once again the lower portion is better buttressed. The area of C.4–C.5, with a smaller posterior spinous process, exhibits the greatest range of motion.

A further structural element of importance is that in extension, as the spine shifts backward, there is very little obstruction to the posterior gliding swing. It depends almost entirely upon the security of the ligamentous attachments, including the longitudinal ligaments and interbody mechanism of anulus and disc. The central nucleus does not contribute to braking action because of its innate function in providing a rolling, gliding motion. However, the ligaments and anulus are so constructed and attached that they do provide a strong braking force.

TANGENTIAL AND TORSION INJURIES

Many accidents occur in which the application of force is from the side, and this constitutes a significant variation. One of the important facets of so-called sidelash is that some of the stress from such an impact is converted into a torsion or tangential element because the cervical spine is so constructed that a degree of rotatory reaction ensues from sidewise force application (Fig. 12–5). Furthermore, the angle of application is likely to be at a variant from the center, in contrast to rear end collisions where the force application is so often directly in an anteroposterior direction. Somewhat similar considerations apply in a rear end collision in which the occupant's head and neck or body are in a partially turned position. The result is that the stretching forces fall on structures already under a degree of tension. With the head and neck turned in one direction, some stress is already on the periarticular ligaments (Fig. 12–5*A*). When additional force of an unexpected nature is applied, it catches these elements already on the stretch and there is likelihood of damage to other areas of the vertebra.

COMPOUND IMPACTS

A frequent further force to be assimilated is that, in addition to the rear end impact, the struck vehicle may collide with another obstacle in front. This mechanism adds a further element in that there is an accentuation of the already started phase of braking and accentuation of the flexion-deceleration element. In some instances a third phase of forced extension ensues. The effect of these forces is to magnify the damage, particularly as applied to the posterior soft tissues. The variations of tissue damage that result from these mechanisms are infinite, but for practical purposes, they may be considered under four main headings: (1) soft tissue injuries,

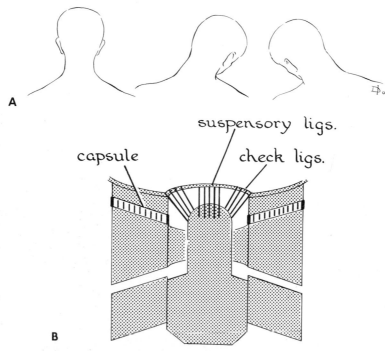

Figure 12–5 *A*, Motion of head in side lash. *B*, Ligaments limiting rotation at occipitocervical junction.

(2) nerve root implications, (3) aggravation of pre-existing pathological changes, and (4) fractures and dislocations.

Soft Tissue Injuries

The effects of extension-flexion and flexion-deceleration forces may be entirely confined to the soft tissues producing: (1) musculoligamentous injuries, (2) ligamentum nuchae injuries, or (3) torsion and combination injuries.

Musculoligamentous Tears. The commonest result of a rear end jolt is stress diffused through the soft tissues, extending to structures both at the front and the back of the sagittal fulcrum. The normal extension-flexion range is through 90 degrees, 45 degrees in extension and 45 degrees in forward flexion from the midline. The impact from behind throws the neck through an increased range posteriorly; as much as a further 45 degrees may result from a rear end impact, focusing a wrenching stress on soft tissue attachments. The anterior longitudinal ligament bears the brunt of this extensor stress, but as the force penetrates, extension occurs to involve the strap muscles at the front of the neck, the prevertebral fascia, longus capitis and longus colli muscles and trachea. The braking action is effected by the ligamentum nuchae, the interspinous ligaments and the capsular ligaments about the apophyseal joints. Since s~~o~~ force applications are directly ~~in~~ posterior direction, the apophy~~seal~~ not play so important a part as ~~the~~ ligamentous structures (Figs. 12~~·~~

RADIOLOGICAL FINDINGS. Proper x-ray examination and interpretation is of considerable importance in all such injuries. Good films are essential and special views are often required. In patients with significant signs and symptoms, repeat films should be carried out at 6- and 12-week intervals because of the difficulty in identifying many of the so-called occult fractures. The standard assessment radiologically should include an anteroposterior view supine, odontoid process (open mouth), lateral views in neutral maximum flexion and maximum extension, and right and left oblique views of the foramina. Two further views are extremely useful also, a caudal view of the foramen magnum and a "facet" view which is a 30 degree angled anteroposterior view (see Chapter IV).

As indicated by Zatzkin, the assessment of these views allows identification of certain precise changes resulting from whiplash trauma. The findings of significance then include: (1) loss of normal cervical lordosis, (2) decrease in flexion range, (3) a rigid spine with loss of both flexion and extension, (4) narrowing of interbody space in association with evidence of extreme spasm, (5) addi-

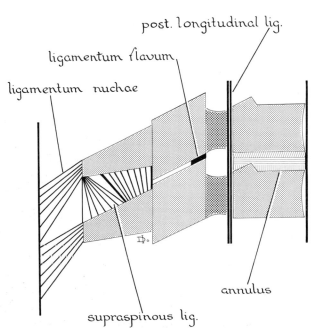

Figure 12–6 Ligamentous layers of cervical spine involved in whiplash injuries.

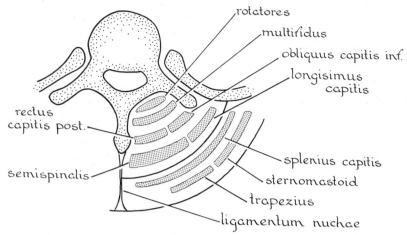

Figure 12–7 Six layers of muscles pad cervical region, all with firm bone attachment.

tional lateral curvature of the spine, and (6) alteration of what appear as pre-existing changes such as fractured spurs or displacement producing foraminal encroachment.

CLINICAL PICTURE. The onset of symptoms shows considerable variation, but the most frequent story is of some immediate soreness, followed in a matter of hours by neck stiffness and headache. Commonly, the following day all these have increased, particularly the stiffness. From then on the patient may become conscious of more widespread symptoms.

Neck Pain. Discomfort at the back of the neck, at the sides or at the front, frequently extending to the shoulder-neck angle, is common. It is aggravated by motion and minimized by keeping the neck still. Some extension may be present to the anterior chest or to the area between the scapulae posteriorly. Initially the discomfort is diffuse, but over a period of about 72 hours it commonly settles into a more discrete pattern.

Headache. Extension of the pain up the back of the neck to the suboccipital, occipital and parietal zones is frequent. As a rule, it involves both sides of the head to start with, but subsequently may localize to one side. There may be a pattern of direct extension from the suboccipital region, or some soreness in this area associated with frontal headache or forehead discomfort. It is usual for the pure headache element to shortly become intermittent, with the frequency of the headaches decreasing progressively over a period of months. The acute soreness that accompanies the headache subsides fairly quickly.

A group of patients may be identified who have a more persistent and somewhat different form of headache. These patients complain of suboccipital discomfort on one side or the other which is of greater severity and frequently extends up the back of the neck to the vertex and frontal region. This pain is in addition to the generalized neck ache and headache. This discomfort is present intermittently, occurring in somewhat spasmodic fashion, and, with increase in the severity, appears to involve both sides. Manipulation of the greater occipital nerve area initiates the discomfort; sometimes extension with lateral bending toward the side of the pain also aggravates it. In some instances a zone of hyperesthesia corresponding to the distribution of the greater occipital nerve can be identified.

F. H. Mayfield has called attention to the vulnerability of the entire second nerve root, which supplies sensation to most of the scalp. He has suggested that as the nerve emerges from between the laminae of C.1 and C.2, it may be more vulnerable to extension-flexion trauma than the other roots (Fig. 12–8).

The author has found local injection and alcohol block of the greater occipital nerve to be helpful both in decreasing symptoms and in identifying the source of this extra discomfort. Mayfield, on the basis of extensive experience, has advocated section of the entire second nerve root through a midline incision, identifying the nerve as it passes upward from between the laminae of C.1 and C.2. The nerve is sectioned, but not avulsed, at this point. However, complete relief of

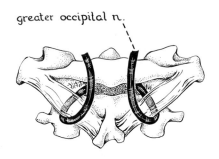

greater occipital n.

Course and relations of greater occipital nerve

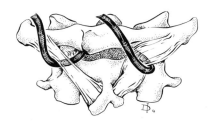

Potential stress in injury process

Figure 12-8 Course and relations of greater occipital nerve.

pain has not been noted in more than 50 per cent of the patients so handled. The author's colleague, Dr. J. C. Colwill, has reported similar success through avulsion of the greater occipital nerve using the technique described (Fig. 12-9).

Limitation of Motion. Stiffness of the neck is the commonest sensation, and it sometimes antedates neck ache, but in all except the more extensive injuries it progressively subsides until, at the end of a week, only a portion of any given range of motion is implicated. It is usual for the stiffness to be much more apparent for several days following the injury in the straightforward anteroposterior type of injury, reaching a maximum at about a week or ten days and then gradually subsiding.

Cerebral Symptoms. Many whiplash incidents are followed by mental upset of varying degrees. Often this reaction is considerably out of proportion to the violence involved in the impact. Female patients complain more often of these changes, but this is not always so. The symptoms include headache, dizziness, difficulty in remembering and concentrating, emotional lability, fatigue and generalized weakness.

Much of such reaction is understandable, because the episode can be a very upsetting one owing to its total unexpectedness and the lack of preparation. The average patient going to the hospital for the treatment of other lesions has had a considerable period of preparation and emotional adjustment that is a steadying factor, but such adjustment is entirely lacking in these injuries. Variable instability is apparent in patients requiring emergency surgery, such as having a fractured wrist set, but their calmness and control is often in marked contrast to the befuddled and distraught condition of the individual who suddenly finds himself in the emergency treatment room of a hospital following a rear end collision.

The absence of serious structural change should not be interpreted as a lessening factor of such an individual's upset. Many aspects of the episode—fear, unpreparedness, concern over property, injury to others —are all legitimate irritants in addition to the unexpected physical insult. Of further constant significance is the fact that the patient is usually completely innocent of misjudgment or mismanagement and yet, while law-abidingly minding his own business, he has been unceremoniously upset.

Although it is proper to recognize that these symptoms are legitimate results of the accident and that they may last for a reasonable period of time, it is also correct to interpret their progress in the light of known healing processes under other circumstances. There are established ranges of time in which such abnormalities arising from other sources usually quiet down and the reaction subsides. This means that disproportionate prolongation of these complaints may be unreasonable. Similarly, permanent or likely residual effects may be properly gauged in light of the known results of similar upsets in other phases of disease. These experiences serve as a baseline for assessment of disability in these injuries. Occasionally, emotional upset is prolonged, necessitating neuropsychiatric assessment.

Dizziness. Transient subjective giddiness or dizziness is common, but usually passes off in a matter of days. Persistent vertigo may be due to labyrinthine irritation or to vertebral basilar ischemia when there are extensive spondylitic changes and atheromatous changes in the vertebral arteries. True labyrinthine damage can be identified by special studies that compare responses to body rotation and to head rotation alone.

Tinnitus and hearing deficiency may also

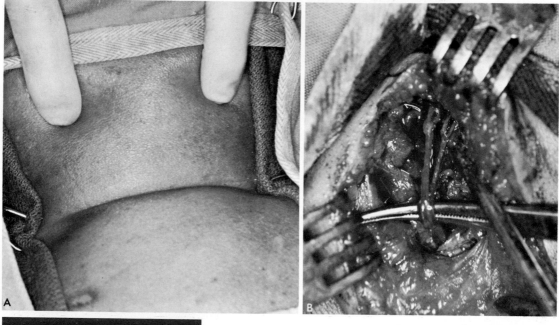

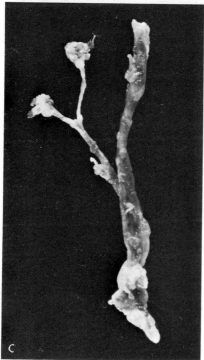

Figure 12–9 Resection of occipital nerve. *A*, Operative field. *B*, Exposure and removal of nerve. *C*, Specimen of nerve resected.

be present when the force has damaged the labyrinth.

Persistent attacks of vertigo related to sudden head and neck motion can stem from disturbance of the vertebral basilar artery system. Atheromatous changes in these vessels are the predisposing elements, but it is assumed that any spondylosis may involve the vertebral arteries' course, and when trauma is added to such a system, these attacks are possible.

Ocular Lesions. When the body has been subjected to considerable violence, the commotion can reasonably involve the ocular apparatus. Horwich and Kasner have studied these changes carefully; they include transient diplopia, eyeball ache and difficulty in focusing on near objects. As a rule, they are transient.

Vasomotor Upset. Concussion of vital centers and cerebral ganglia has been postulated as the source of vasomotor changes that occur in some of these patients. Cold and sweating hands and feet may be present for a matter of weeks. However, persistence of such problems is not likely from this mechanism; if they do persist, other explanations should be sought.

Difficulty in Swallowing. The posterior swing of the neck may reasonably implicate the anterior structures, sometimes tearing strap muscles and irritating the trachea. Tearing of the anterior longitudinal ligament may be followed by a retropharyngeal hematoma of considerable size, which will contribute hoarseness and huskiness as well as difficulty in swallowing for some time.

Chest Pain. A few days following the injury many patients mention discomfort in the anterior chest that is aggravated by breathing. In some instances, this is the result of direct contact of the chest with a hard object in the flexion or secondary phase of the injury; in others it is a referred pain and is due to transient nerve root involvement. These changes are more likely to be present when there is extensive spondylosis, to which has been added the extension-flexion injury.

TREATMENT. The usual management of these patients is initiated in the emergency treatment room of the hospital, where x-rays are carried out, sedation is provided and if possible, the patient is returned to the care of his personal physician. Their further management includes the following:

Splinting. These are painful lesions, and some form of cervical immobilization is usually required for a period of weeks. A firm splint by day and a soft collar by night works best. Immobilization is continued as long as muscle spasm is present. A contour pillow is recommended after the night splint is discarded, often being used for a matter of months.

Traction and Physiotherapy. The patients with persistent radiating pain benefit particularly from cervical traction, but other forms of physiotherapy are beneficial in the routine and less extensive injury. This should start in the physiotherapy department; if traction is being used, it may gradually become a home treatment under instruction

by the physiotherapist. Other modalities to decrease the muscle spasm include massage, heat, deep heat and sometimes, in the very acute stage, ice. Other measures may be applied at the physiotherapist's discretion.

Medication. Mild medication, both daily and at night, is needed in the immediate postinjury period. Anti-inflammatory drugs such as phenylbutazone materially decrease tissue reaction; in addition, some light sedation for pain relief should be provided.

Injection of Trigger Areas. One of the most effective aids beyond the immediate injury period is the local infiltration of residual trigger zones. In the soft tissue injuries these are commonly related to the suboccipital area, where particularly tender zones on one or other side may be identified. A local anesthetic is injected, sometimes with the addition of a small amount of absolute alcohol; about 1 cc of alcohol in 5 cc of 2 percent anesthetic solution is extremely effective.

Surgical Measures. Definitive surgical measures are not required in the injuries in which the symptoms are confined to soft tissues, but in other degrees of this injury, such as ligamentum nuchae injuries with fracture of spinous process, excision of the avulsed spinous process may be required, and sometimes section of the greater occipital nerve is necessary. In the more severe form with persistent nerve root pressure, discotomy and anterior interbody fusion may be needed, but all these surgical measures are discussed under the headings of more extensive pathology.

Ligamentum Nuchae Injuries. A more severe degree of soft tissue damage is separated from the general extension-flexion injuries wherein more force has been applied and has been of sufficient severity to produce either minute tears in the ligamentum nuchae or other lesions of the posterior spinous processes. In the forward or flexion swing of the whiplash, the principal force is focused at the top and bottom of the neck, representing the points of anchorage of the ligamentum nuchae (Fig. 12–10). In most instances greater pull is focused in the suboccipital zone, so that there is avulsion of the inserting fibers in this region. Clinically this is demonstrated by points of maximum tenderness in the suboccipital zone at the tendon-bone junction and by the persistence of soreness over the individual posterior spinous process tips. The opposite end of the liga-

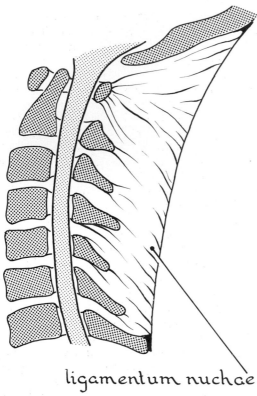

Figure 12-10 Ligamentum nuchae and its anchoring points.

that the car has hit the patient's vehicle or to the patient's being turned to one side or the other at the moment of a rear end impact, is focused on the periarticular structures because these are the main zone of resistance to such a force mechanism. Commonly the force penetrates to a deeper level because there is lack of the protecting element from the strong longitudinal ligaments that guard the front and the back.

Characteristically these patients complain of soreness at the side of the neck and have considerable restriction in rotatory motion. The pain lasts for a long period of time, and they are likely to retain some rotatory limitation for a matter of months. In many of these patients occult fractures occur, implicating the lateral masses related to the articular processes, so that recheck x-rays should be done at six and 12 weeks. These patients also benefit from traction therapy but require the application of a brace for a longer period than do those with routine anteroposterior injuries.

NERVE ROOT INJURIES

Separate consideration must be given to those patients who present clear-cut signs

mentum nuchae attachment is to the spine of C.7, and it also sustains considerable avulsing stress. The intervening posterior spinous processes have less secure attachments to the heavy central strand of the ligamentum nuchae, so that it is at either end that the ligament damage principally accumulates. The force applied may be sufficiently severe to pull off the tip of the spinous process of C.7, somewhat similar to the clay shoveler's injury (Fig. 12-11).

TREATMENT. These injuries respond to the same modalities as the musculoligamentous injuries, but more frequently require local injection of the trigger points or zones of ligamentous avulsion. A longer period of fixation in a splint and more extensive physiotherapy and systemic medication is the rule.

Torsion Injuries. The group of injuries in which application of force is from the side is considered separately because of additional symptoms which these patients commonly have. The oblique application of the force, whether it be due to the angle

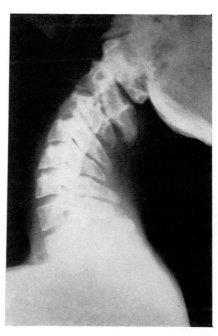

Figure 12-11 Avulsion of spinous process of C.7 in flexion-extension injury.

implicating nerve roots in addition to the symptoms presented above relative to soft tissue injuries. Two distinct phases may be identified, the acute and the chronic.

Acute or Transient Nerve Root Pressure

The acute injury is the one of greater concern because it is more precisely related to the incident in question. The chronic lesion is perhaps more often an aggravation of a pre-existing state, and nerve root irritation develops in a spine already the seat of degenerative changes, but which has been further insulted by this accident.

Following what is usually quite sharp extension-flexion trauma, the patient experiences pain extending from the neck to the shoulder and down the arm to the hand and fingers. This pain has a burning or shooting quality and is accompanied by a sensation of numbness and tingling. Quite precise localization in the hand is much more characteristic of root involvement than is the complaint of a general whole hand involvement. Sometimes a period of stiffness in the neck precedes the onset of radiating symptoms, but often the patient continues to experience this lancinating discomfort which was noticed a matter of minutes after the accident. Commonly there is extension of pain to the interscapular area and to the front of the chest. All elements are aggravated by cervical spine motion and are accentuated by vertical compression of the head on the neck. Similarly, bending toward the side of the pain accentuates it, but bending to the opposite side tends to diminish it.

Transient nerve root symptoms are common in extension-flexion injuries. Numbness and tingling may be experienced for a matter of days and then subside completely. It is in those patients in whom the radiating discomfort persists and ultimately becomes the dominating complaint that the nerve root has been compressed, possibly by disc herniation rather than simple jarring. In analyzing extension-flexion injuries, the mechanism suggests that it is in those instances in which the second phase, the forward flexion phase, is powerful that nuclear herniation is likely to be sustained. Nuclear herniation to produce nerve root symptoms must be posterior, but it requires considerable force to do this because of the double layer protection of the posterior

longitudinal ligament. In contrast to injuries in the lumbar spine, in which the ligament is, comparatively, not so thickly protective, the squeezing of nuclear tissue is not so apt to occur. Severe extension force, while it will implicate the nucleus, would favor anterior herniation; it is felt that a loosening of the anterior longitudinal ligament from the compressed disc pressure is common, but rupture is still prevented by the ligament's strength. A further protective mechanism is that the fulcrum, of bend or glide, of one body on the other in the interbody area, lies farther posteriorly than in the lumbar region.

Where there is involvement of nerve roots, alteration in biceps and triceps jerks, weakness in these muscles and sensory changes in the hand can be demarcated. In most instances it is a subjective change that is retained, usually in the thumb or index finger or the second and third fingers.

Treatment. Such patients are significantly disabled and have difficulty carrying on their work. Application of a properly fitted cervical splint is required, along with daily cervical traction. The amount and length of traction depend upon the size of the patient and are an individual response. In most instances traction for 15 to 20 minutes, using 5 to 12 lbs, is sufficient to relieve the radiating discomfort. Traction must be applied in a slightly flexed position, with the amount and the length of application guided by the relief attained by the patient. The patient can be taught to use a cervical halter at home in most cases and to increase the period of traction himself. The cervical collar needs to be worn for three months and, during the acute stages, should be replaced at night by a light felt collar.

SURGICAL TREATMENT. Not many of these acute episodes require surgical treatment, and it is usual for the radiating symptoms to be relieved by conservative measures. In some instances stiffness and cervical discomfort persist for a matter of months. The neck pain will gradually subside also, and its persistence does not, as a rule, constitute an indication for surgical treatment.

In those instances in which the radiating pain persists for a period of six months, there will usually also be persistence of sensory changes and some motor weakness. The motor weakness may take the form of atrophy of the upper arm, with weakness in either of the anterior or posterior groups or atrophy of the intrinsic muscles of the hand. When this occurs, discotomy and interbody fusion by the anterior approach is the treatment of choice (see Chapter XVI).

Persistent or Chronic Nerve Root Pressure

In contrast to the acute episode just described, the chronic lesion is evidenced by a more gradual onset of the radiating discomfort, sometimes a matter of weeks or months after the inciting trauma. Under these circumstances there have nearly always been pre-existing interbody or foraminal changes to which a new insult has been added. Sometimes a history is obtained of frank pre-existing nerve root involvement. The signs and symptoms are the same as in the acute episode, but take longer to develop. As a rule, this occurs in the older age group, patients in the fifth and sixth decades. Because of the chronicity of their complaints they are usually controlled by conservative measures; it is reasonable to persist with conservative management for a longer period than in the acute episode. In those instances in which there has been a pre-existing nerve root irritation, surgical treatment may be necessary, provided the patient is not too old for such a procedure.

Injury Added to Previous Pathology

Separate consideration of the effects of new injury to a neck already the seat of degenerative changes is necessary for many reasons. After age 50 most cervical spines show radiological evidence of wear and tear, so that the pattern of symptoms may follow a previous course or be significantly influenced by these changes in addition to the per se effects of the new insult. Such changes modify impairment, length of disability, treatment and degree of legal responsibility. The states to be evaluated include: (1) vertebral body changes, and (2) interbody and foraminal changes.

Vertebral Body Changes. Some degree of cervical spondylosis is present in well over 50 per cent of the population over 50 years of age. Commonly these changes are osteophytes on the vertebral borders, projecting anteriorly and posteriorly. These changes decrease flexibility of the neck, so that bony resistance to the shock of injury is encountered earlier and to a greater degree

than in undamaged spines in which the soft tissue resistance is more prominent. The likelihood of fracture, then, is increased. Fracture of the anterior spur results from predominantly extensor force with avulsion of the posterior edges occurring from the flexion stress. The cracked osteophyte needs to be differentiated from congenital and developmental changes such as an intercalary bone. This is accomplished by recognition of an oblique defect of the margin with a smoother contour in contrast to the sharp protruding spur that has been broken. All such changes indicate more extensive injury and the likelihood of longer impairment.

In spines such as this the application of torsion or tangential force is also more likely to produce bone damage. The general loss of resiliency adds to the resistance of the sidelash thrust, and the joints of Lushka also serve as a deterrent to lateral displacement. In this age group spur formation and trauma to this projection will be greater (Fig. 12–12).

Interbody and Foraminal Changes. Degenerative changes implicate the foramina also and are a composite result of disc thinning, marginal osteophyte formation and joint changes. A study has indicated that changes at C.5 and C.6 and C.6–C.7 level are present in over 50 per cent of patients over 40 years of age. Fractures of the uncinate processes may create osteophytes that will encroach on the foramina and, hence, may implicate the nerve roots. Ruth Jackson has called attention to the protected course which the cervical nerve roots run as they extend from the spinal cord downward and laterally. They lie over the central portion of the vertebral body, and it is not until they reach the foramen zone that they become related to the disc spaces. In this anatomical pattern lies the explanation for the type of neurological changes frequently seen in extreme spondylosis (Fig. 12–13). The intervertebral body reaction, with the lipping and spondylosis, may implicate the spinal cord, with a myelopathic process developing more extensively than root irritation.

Fractures of the uncinate processes can be shown only by very careful examination. Sometimes x-rays repeated at eight to ten weeks after an injury are necessary to identify changes suggestive of fracture healing of one of these spurs (Fig. 12–14).

In patients in whom no fracture is seen, the narrowed foramen is still more likely to

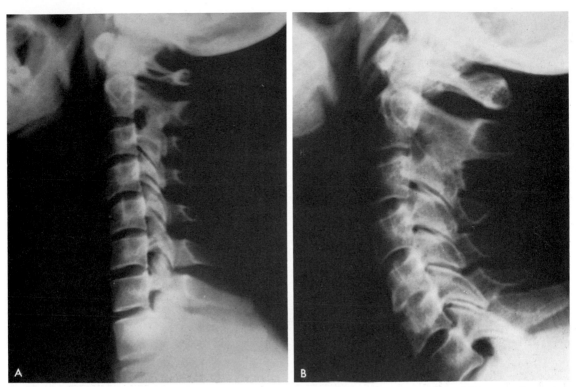

Figure 12–12 Interbody narrowing accentuated following whiplash injury. *A,* At time of injury. *B,* Four years later.

produce nerve root irritation than is the case with the normal spine. The spurs that are visualized in the foramen on the anterior aspect result from uncinate process distortion; on the posterior aspect they are the curled-in edges of the inferior articular process of the corresponding apophyseal

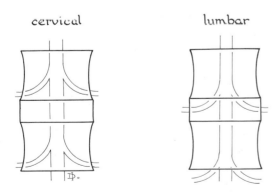

Nerve root relationship to disc level

Figure 12–13 The level at which the nerve roots arise from the spinal cord is slightly above the annulus in the cervical area as compared to a lower level in the lumbar region.

joint. Since some increase in the size of the foramen occurs from above downward, the constriction from these changes is likely to be greatest at the C.4–C.5 and C.5–C.6 level, rather than at the C.7 to T.1 levels.

TREATMENT. Stiffness, neck ache and headache last longer in these patients and there is greater likelihood of nerve root irritation. A firm cervical brace, preferably of the Plexiglass type, is required because a soft collar does not provide sufficient immobilization (Fig. 12–15). Sometimes plaster immobilization is required. More sedation is necessary, as well as muscle relaxants and anti-inflammatory drugs.

Physiotherapy is given after the acute reaction has subsided, and the judicious application of traction is necessary if there are persistent root symptoms. In some instances traction may aggravate the discomfort and, for this reason, it should be initiated gradually and with careful adjustment of the amount of weight that can be tolerated. When the traction cannot be accepted, more secure immobilization for a prolonged period is required.

A large number of these patients may be candidates for discotomy and anterior inter-

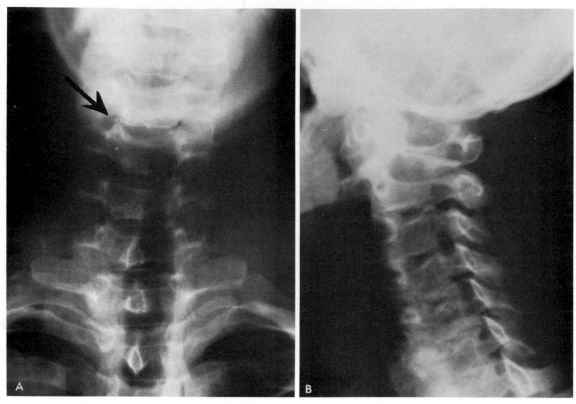

Figure 12-14 Fracture through the spur of uncinate process.

body fusion because of persistent root symptoms. When the clinical state embraces pain and sensory changes only without motor or reflex signs, there is a good possibility of subsidence over a period of four to six months without surgical treatment. When the symptoms persist and signs of motor involvement develop, with either definite weakness and atrophy or consistent electromyographic evidence of denervation, stabilization should be carried out if there are no general systemic deterrents or contraindications (see Chapter XVI).

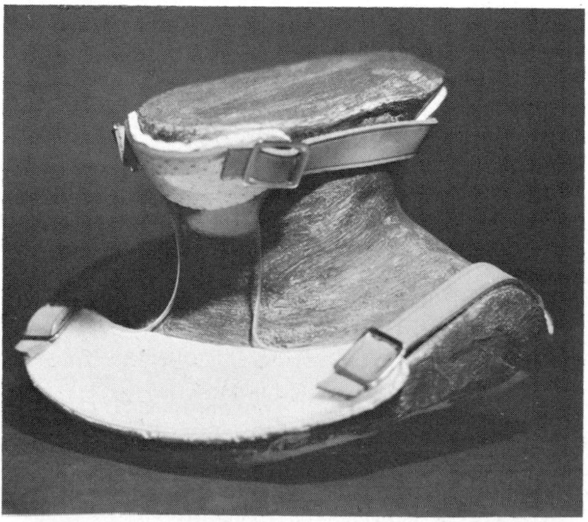

Fractures and Dislocations in Whiplash Injuries

Rear end collisions have resulted in a number of difficult to define and less obvious bone and joint injuries which require special consideration. These "occult" fractures are quite apart from the more severe and quite obvious fractures and dislocation of the cervical spine which have been considered elsewhere and which require the same management as similar lesions sustained under any circumstances. As one investigates the effect of rear end collisions, a greater number of these occult injuries come to light.

Subluxations. Severe extension-flexion episodes may so damage supporting ligaments that distraction or malalignment which is just short of a dislocation results. In some

Figure 12-15 Plexiglas collar for cervical fixation.

instances, perhaps, there has been momentary dislocation and immediate reduction. The result is abnormal laxity at one level, usually in the midspine, and this can be demonstrated radiologically.

Such patients have more acute and persistent local tenderness, frank muscle spasms, more pronounced and persistent headache and greater restriction of spine motion. The older patients who already have degenerative changes are prone to develop radiating symptoms if the subluxation type of injury has occurred. The luxation may be either anterior or posterior, depending upon the preponderance of force application.

When such injuries are suspected, flexion and extension films are done with caution. The maximum change tends to be focused at one level, where there is a sharp angulation of the usually smooth line of projection of anterior and posterior vertebral body margins. The subluxation, when identified, calls for immobilization for a period of at least three months (Fig. 12–16).

Dislocation. The force may be severe enough to allow forward slipping of an inferior or a subjacent superior facet to a degree that it locks in this position (Fig. 12–17).

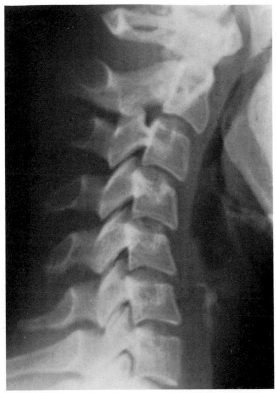

Figure 12–16 Subluxation at C.4 and C.5, indicating ligamentous damage.

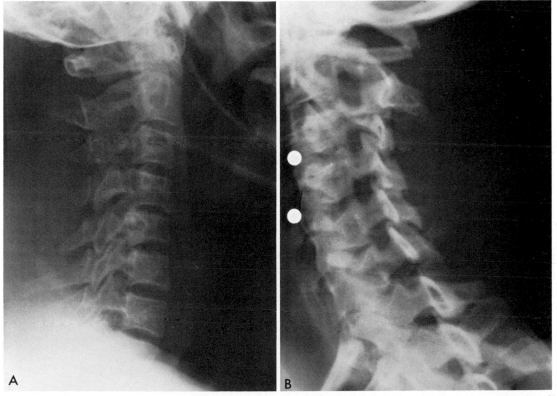

Figure 12–17 Rotatory subluxation of the cervical spine. *A,* Routine lateral view does not show extensive displacement. *B,* Oblique view shows the true state with C.6–C.7 facets locked out of alignment.

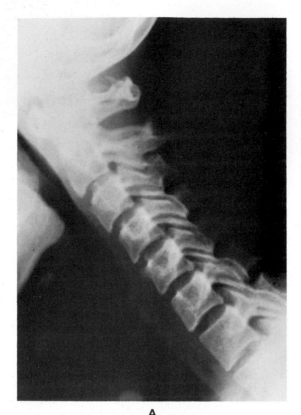

A

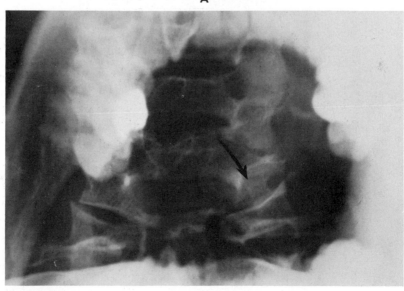

B

Figure 12-18   Occult or hidden fracture. *A,* Not visible in routine view. *B,* Special view necessary to demonstrate it.

Sometimes there is an associated compression fracture of the lower vertebral body. When it is an extensor injury, force may extend to the arch and fracture it. Rotatory dislocations are more commonly seen in other injuries and have been considered in Chapter XVI, Fractures and Dislocations.

Lateral Mass or Occult Fractures. Torsion strain from lateral force application is a common complication of these injuries. When a car is struck broadside or when at the moment of impact the passenger is turned sideways, the head and neck are bent laterally in addition to receiving an element of extensor-flexion injury. Under these circumstances fracture in the lateral mass or the intra-articular zones may result. The uncinate process may also be broken.

Such damage should be suspected from a history of this type of injury in which there is persistent tenderness of the lateral aspect of the neck, pain on lateral flexion and often spasm of the lateral muscles.

Special x-rays to show the posterior elements of the arch and articular processes should be done in such patients. When signs and symptoms persist, x-rays should be repeated in eight to ten weeks because the healing process about an occult fracture can often then be seen (Fig. 12–18).

Upper Segment Occipito-Axis Atlas Injuries. Maximum application of force tends to be focused on the central and lower area of the neck in these particular injuries, but the upper unit may also be implicated.

ATLAS FRACTURES. Sufficient force may be generated in a projectile fashion to produce vertical compression on the top of the head which is severe enough to fracture the lateral mass of the atlas (Fig. 12–19). Cord symptoms are frequent, requiring skull traction, application of halo fixation or a Minerva jacket until the fracture is healed. A firm cervical splint is worn for a further four to six months.

Fracture of the posterior arch of the atlas may occur but usually results from injuries received under different circumstances and has been considered in the chapter on fractures and dislocations.

AXIS FRACTURES. Fracture of the odontoid is usually not encountered unless there has been considerable force of a projectile nature. The hurtling of the body out of the car, for example, may involve the cervico-thoracic or occipitocervical zone in such a fashion that the odontoid is fractured at its

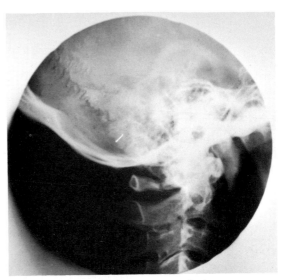

Figure 12–19 Fracture of atlas.

base. The management of these injuries has been considered in the previous section on fractures and dislocations.

Lateral Mass and Processes of Axis. The body and articular elements may be fractured as the result of severe trauma involving a direct contact force on the upper segment, such as the head striking the windshield or the roof. Skeletal traction, followed by plaster fixation for a period of four to six months, is required.

POSTERIOR SPINOUS PROCESS FRACTURE. When the flexion element of the extension-flexion mechanism is severe, sufficient pull may be exerted on the base of the ligamentum nuchae to avulse the posterior spinous process of C.7. The management of this particular fracture has been considered under ligamentum nuchae injuries. When local tenderness persists and is accompanied by pain, excision of the detached fragment and repair of the defect is indicated. (See the discussion of ligamentum nuchae injuries.)

REFERENCES

Abbott, K. H.: Anterior cervical disc removal and interbody fusion. A preliminary review of 101 patients followed for one to three years. Bull. Los Angeles Neurol. Soc. *28*:251–259, 1963.

Aufranc, O. E., et al.: Comminuted fracture dislocation of the proximal humerus. J.A.M.A. *195*:770–773, 1966.

Cameron, B. M.: Cervical spine sprain headache. Amer. J. Orthop. *6*:9, 1964.

Cave, E. F.: Immediate fracture management. Surg. Clin. N. Amer. *46*:771–788, 1966.

Colwill, J. C.: Personal communication, 1969.

Gal, A.: Severe cervical spine injuries. J. Trauma *5*:379–385, 1965.

Gissane, W.: The causes and the prevention of neck injuries to car occupants. Ann. Roy. Coll. Surg. *39*:161–163, 1966.

Gjores, J. E., et al.: Prognosis in primary dislocations of the shoulder. Acta Chir. Scand. *129*:468–470, 1965.

Halliday, D. R., et al.: Torn cervical ligaments; Necropsy examination of the normal cervical region of the spinal column. J. Trauma *4*:219–232, 1964.

Horwich, H., and Kasner, D.: The effect of whiplash injuries on ocular functions. Southern Med. J. *55*:69, 1962.

Howard, F. M., et al.: Injuries to the clavicle with neurovascular complications. A study of 14 cases. J. Bone Joint Surg. (Amer) *47*:1335–1346, 1965.

Jackson, R.: The Cervical Syndrome. Springfield, Illinois, Charles C Thomas, 1966.

Jung, A., et al.: The auricular disorders of unco-vertebral cervical arthrosis. Their treatment by uncusectomy and decompression of the vertebral artery in 15 cases. Ann. Chir. *20*:181–194, 1966.

Kahn, E. A., et al.: Acute injuries of the cervical spine. Postgrad. Med. *39*:37–44, 1966.

Kline, D. G.: Atlanto-axial dislocation simulating a head injury: Hypoplasia of the odontoid. Case report. J. Neurosurg. *24*:1013–1016, 1966.

Maurer, W., et al.: A skull holder with interchangeable security pins in the treatment of recent cervico-vertebral injuries. Chirurg. *36*:324, 1965.

Mayfield, F. H.: Clinical Neurosurgery. New York, 1954. Symposium on Cervical Trauma, Chapter 6, Neurological Aspects.

Meyer, R. R.: Cervical diskography. A help or hindrance in evaluating neck, shoulder, arm pain? Amer. J. Roentgen. *90*:1208–1215, 1963.

Murphey, F. , et al.: Ruptured cervical disc. Experience with 250 cases. Amer. Surg. *32*:83–88, 1966.

Sandor, F.: Diaphragmatic respiration: A sign of cervical cord lesion in the unconscious patient (horizontal paradox). Brit. Med. J. *5485*:465–466, 1966.

Schaerer, J. P.: Cervical discography and whiplash injury. Med. Trial Techn. Quart. *11*:53–68, 1965.

Zatzkin, H. R., and Kveton, F. W.: Evaluation of the cervical spine in whiplash injuries. Radiology *75*:577, 1960.

Chapter XIII

FRACTURES AND DISLOCATIONS

FRACTURES OF THE TUBEROSITIES AND THE HUMERUS

The tuberosities of the humerus may really be considered as outrigger points since they have been developed as sites of anchorage for powerful muscles that rotate the head of the humerus. Therein lies the significance of displacement of these appendages. The bony mass is not particularly important, but its potential obstruction is significant because of the interference it may produce, with the spherical head of the humerus as a blocking mechanism, or because this wrenching apart from the anchorage has removed an effective force normally applied by the tendon which it carries. Management of tuberosity fractures requires realization that their importance is far greater than a so-called chip fracture.

FRACTURES OF THE GREATER TUBEROSITY

Simple Contusion Fractures. The greater tuberosity may be splintered by application of direct force on the lateral aspect of the upper arm. The result is a crushing of the outer shell of the greater tuberosity so that several fragments are loosened at this site and along the lateral aspect of the upper end; however, they usually are not displaced, and often, because the line of the fracture is difficult to see, the fracture may be overlooked (Fig. 13–1).

TREATMENT. Such fractures heal well without significant interference with gleno-humeral function. They are mobilized in a sling or body swathe at the side for three weeks, at the end of which time active motion is initiated. One small complication may occur in that occasionally there is slight upward displacement of the greater tuberosity; if this is allowed to persist or increase, impingement on the overhanging coraco-acromial arch can result. For this reason, when there is any slight upward displacement of the separated fragment, it is best to treat this by immobilization in an abduction plaster splint for a period of four weeks and then bivalve the upper half over the arm and initiate active motion, removing the plaster at the end of a further two to four weeks.

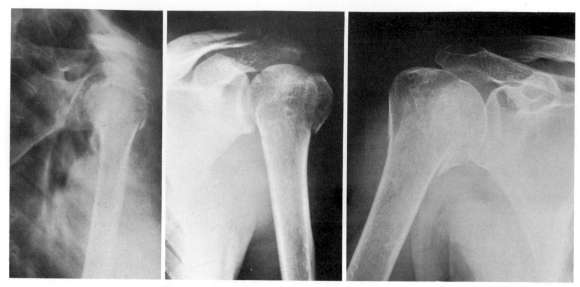

Figure 13–1 Contusion fractures of the tuberosity.

Displaced Fractures. These fractures are much more serious and, if not treated adequately, can lead to significant permanent impairment as a result of restriction of glenohumeral motion.

As a rule, a piece of tuberosity if shifted medially is pulled upward and medially, and marked tension is initiated through the rotator cuff. Displacement of a fragment from the greater tuberosity occurs in a critical zone since it constitutes potential obstruction to abduction. Furthermore, this piece often carries the anchorage of the supraspinatus with it. Confusion sometimes exists in deciding whether a zone of calcification in the x-ray represents a calcareous deposit or a small displaced piece of the tuberosity. In a fracture the fragment is clearly corticated and sharply defined and often there is apparent a small reciprocal defect in the upper end of the humerus. Calcified deposits are thinner, with less distinct edges and no tendency to cortication and they sit much more closely to the cartilage of the upper end of the humerus than does the usual fracture fragment (Fig. 13–2).

A further variant of this type of injury results from some anterior dislocations in which a piece of the greater tuberosity is knocked off the upper end of the humerus. These injuries commonly occur in a fall from a height, with the patient striking an obstacle as he drops and forcibly abducting the arm. The force of the abduction comes so quickly that he does not have time to rotate the greater tuberosity under the edge of acromion; consequently, it impinges forcibly and is knocked off.

TREATMENT. Such displaced fractures of the greater tuberosity should be treated by open reduction and accurate replacement with internal fixation. In some instances a small fragment may be excised but, as a rule, the fragments are of sufficient size and may be put back into place accurately by the use of fine wire sutures or screws.

These fractures are approached by a supero-anterior incision which lies somewhat lateral to the usual utility incision. It extends over the acromion and then distally along the direction of the fibers of the deltoid (see Chapter VIII).

FRACTURES OF THE NECK OF THE HUMERUS

Epiphyseal Injuries. The common injury in the upper end of the humerus occurring in children is a fracture or separation through the epiphysis. These injuries are seen in infants and in older children, occurring most frequently between the ages of eight and 18. The three centers of ossification appear about the third year so x-ray studies are of little help in children under three. The mechanism of injury is a fall on the point of the shoulder or a fall with the arm outstretched behind and the elbow extended. Similar damage may occur in infants from traction on the arm or pressure in the

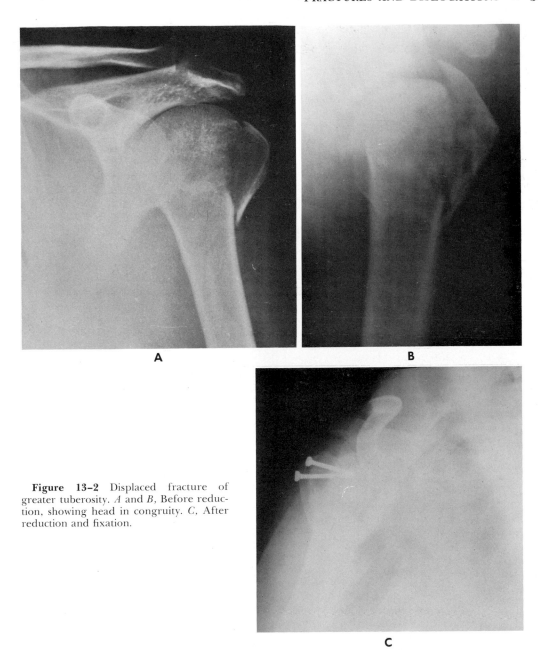

Figure 13-2 Displaced fracture of greater tuberosity. *A* and *B*, Before reduction, showing head in congruity. *C*, After reduction and fixation.

axilla. The common injury is a fracture through the epiphysis that includes a small corner of the diaphysis. The usual deformity is displacement of the upper end of the shaft anteriorly, with the head rotated into a position of flexion with the shaft. Not infrequently the periosteum is not torn completely but it is stripped up and down the shaft, leaving a tubular type of continuity of the epiphysis with the upper end of the humerus. It is probably this mechanism that explains some of the dramatic healing processes and

remodeling that go on in the upper end of the humerus after the extensive epiphyseal separations (Fig. 13-3).

In infants the diagnosis is based on decreased shoulder movement, deformity, tenderness and some shortening of the arm. Sometimes there is distortion of the anterior axillary fold. In every instance of suspected fracture both shoulders should be x-rayed. A slight variation in the position of the diaphysis as related to the glenoid on the suspected side may be all that can be seen

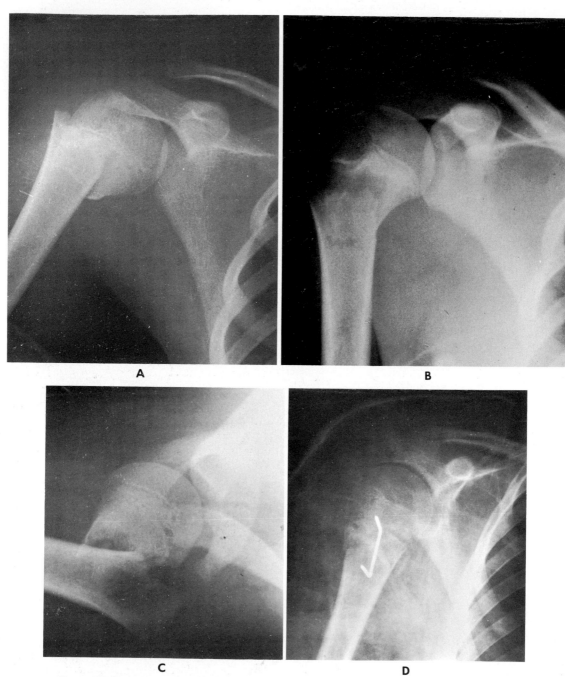

Figure 13–3 Fractures through epiphyseal plate before (*A*) and after (*B*) manipulation and closed reduction. *C* and *D*, Unstable epiphyseal fracture treated by staple fixation. (Courtesy of Dr. J. S. Neviaser.)

that is suggestive of the injury. Other varieties of the epiphyseal injury include a vertical fracture line which may proceed through the epiphysis, stopping at the epiphyseal plate, or continue, shearing off a portion of the head to the small corner of the diaphysis.

A. P. Aitken has called attention to the mechanism by which these injuries occur. The weakest link of the epiphyseal cartilage plate is at its junction with the diaphysis, where there is a zone of degenerating cartilage cells and osteoid tissue through which capillaries grow and osteoblasts appear, with the progressive absorption or replacement of cartilage by osteoid tissue. Displacement through this layer does not involve the zone of resting cells, which is at the top of the epiphyseal plate and just under the epiphysis. In this way, distortion of this layer is largely avoided so that serious deformity does not occur.

TREATMENT. The vast majority of these injuries in which displacement is not extensive can be treated by immobilization at the side in a sling with the arm bandaged to the chest wall. When there is palpable deformity, displacement is significant and this should be treated by manipulation under general anesthesia. The fingers of one hand are placed in the axilla with the thumb over the distal fragment. Pressure is exerted up and laterally with one hand and downward and inward with the thumb; at the same time the arm is gently abducted and pulled with the other hand and the fragments can be felt to slide into position. When the reduction feels secure, and it usually is because of the transverse angle of the fracture line, the arm is immobilized in a bandage at the side for a period of three weeks. When the reduction feels insecure it should be immobilized in a light plaster spica with the arm in slight forward flexion and about 45 degrees of abduction. In some instances the reduction appears unstable, and it may be necessary to immobilize the arm in flexion above the shoulder level and in full internal rotation. Rarely, in longstanding cases traction through Kushner wire in the olecranon applied in overhead fashion is carried out for a week to ten days, followed by the application of a plaster in the same position. Open reduction in these injuries is not recommended.

The question of deformity resulting from involvement of the growing centers often comes up. Remarkable ability for complete remolding even in extensive dislocation of these injuries is exhibited, particularly in young children. It is rare even in completely displaced epiphyses that significant distortion accrues, although there may be some diminution in growth. Repeated attempts at rugged manipulation are to be discouraged because many examples can be cited of fractures through the epiphysis with extensive displacement not reduced by manipulation in which the molding has progressed so effectively that no residual bowing of significance has developed.

Fractures in Adults. The surgical neck of the humerus is the most vulnerable zone in adults. The upper extremity is used as a guard to protect the body in falls, so that force is easily transmitted from the hand to the arm, with the brunt being taken at the end of the lever participating in the proximal joint. The bony configuration is such that the waistlike area just below the tuberosities, constituting the surgical neck, may be broken easily as the force is transmitted and the angulation is changed suddenly so that there is impingement of shaft or upper end of the overhanging coracoacromial arch. The angle at which this force is sustained in the shoulder region governs deformity and displacement of the fragments. If a fall is taken with the arm close to the side, force shears the head off, opening the fracture line laterally and closing it medially (Fig. 13-4). In this way the inner cortex is impacted into the base of the head, producing the so-called adduction fracture. More commonly the force is transmitted so that it reaches the upper end of the humerus with the body and the arm separating from each other. The outer angle of the fracture line is then impacted while the inner one is open. This results in the abduction type of fracture, which is the one most commonly encountered.

TREATMENT OF ADDUCTION FRACTURES. Adduction fractures are more commonly encountered in young people, and when there is obvious deformity an attempt should be made to correct it adequately. This can usually be done quite simply by manipulation under general anaesthesia. Traction and abduction disimpact the fracture, and the alignment may then be restored by a little adduction. In some instances it is necessary to abduct the arm above the right angle so that the shaft of the humerus has a lever and can use the coraco-acromial arches as a fulcrum to correct more severe deformity.

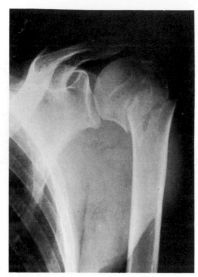

Figure 13-4   Fracture of surgical neck of humerus.

Impaction may be difficult to break down completely, and the only correction obtained then is an altering of the angle, but this is sufficient. The arm is immobilized in a shoulder spica, abducted sufficiently to correct the deformity, with care being taken to avoid traction on the nerve trunks. In elderly patients fixation with a pad in the axilla and the arm at the side may be all that is necessary. The pad should not be too thick, however, because this will accentuate adduction angulation. The upper half of the plaster spica is bivalved at the end of six weeks and assisted active motion is started. The range is gradually increased and the plaster removed at the end of another two weeks.

TREATMENT OF ABDUCTION FRACTURES. Elderly patients commonly sustain this type of fracture (Fig. 13–5). Manipulation under anesthesia is rarely necessary and the arm may be placed in a sling and bandaged to the body with a pad on the axilla. At the end of two to three weeks, depending upon the extent of the displacement, the body bandage is removed and movement is started with the arm still supported by a sling. At the end of another week the sling is discarded. Attention should be paid to the hands and fingers during the period of fixation in order to prevent the development of stiffness at the small joints. In some instances deformity is severe, and when the patient's general state permits, the fractures should be manipulated

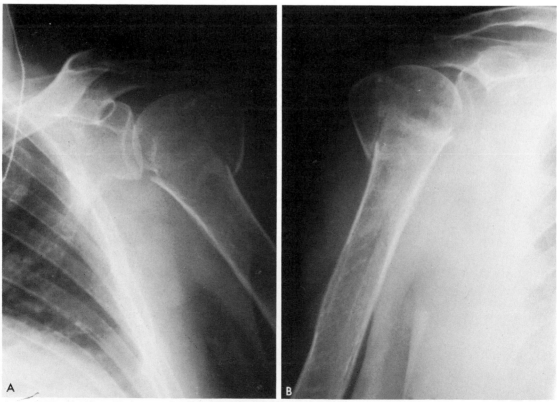

Figure 13-5   Blade plate fixation of multiple fragment fracture. (Courtesy Dr. J. S. Neviaser.)

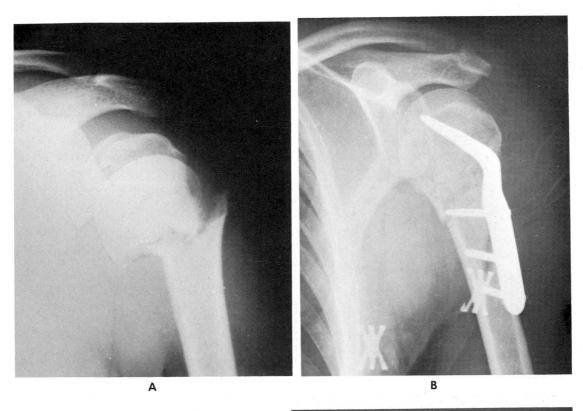

A

B

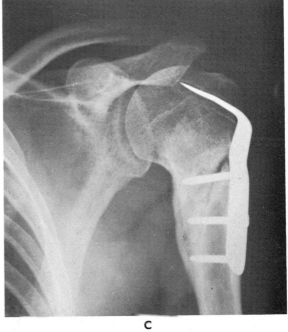

C

Figure 13–6 *A* and *B*, Blade plate fixation in high unstable fracture of humerus. *C*, Final healing.

and immobilized in a shoulder spica. The arm is adducted in this case to correct the abduction deformity and immobilized in about 50 degrees abduction.

C. S. Neer has called attention to the need for revising classification of these fractures based on the fragments involved and the displacement of these relative to the upper end of the humerus. This would include more difficult fractures and fracture dislocations which, as a rule, do not respond to previously accepted closed methods of management. In many instances, when there are two or more fragments, some form of internal fixation is desirable for the best results (Fig. 13–6). In some instances accurate position of these shell-like fragments can be retained only by the use of tied wire sutures. Fixation high in the neck is desirable in this comminution with instability, with internal fixation such as illustrated in Figure 13–7.

FRACTURE DISLOCATIONS OF THE SHOULDER

Dislocation with Fracture of Tuberosity. This injury results commonly from forcible impingement of the greater tuberosity against the acromial arch. It occurs as the arm is abducted precipitantly without external rotation above a right angle so that the tuberosity is sheared off on the arch and the head is forced downward and forward out of the glenoid (Fig. 13–8).

TREATMENT. Immediate reduction of the dislocation is essential and is accomplished by traction and levering of the head into the glenoid in the usual fashion. After this maneuver the detached fragment should be back in good position and the arm is immobilized in a bandage and sling. If it is a large fragment, a shoulder spica is applied. Extreme caution must be taken when plaster is used after a dislocation to avoid redislocation of the shoulder under the plaster. The position is checked by x-ray immediately after reduction and at one- and three-week intervals because it is possible for the head to dislocate when the spica becomes loose, causing serious pressure on the neurovascular bundle. When there is any doubt regarding the accuracy of reduction of the detached fragment, open reduction should be done. The fragment is exposed in the usual fashion and held in place by a wire suture. If there is associated damage to the cuff, this is repaired at the same time. Postoperatively, immobilization in a sling is usually all that is necessary.

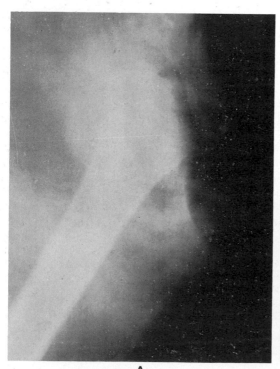
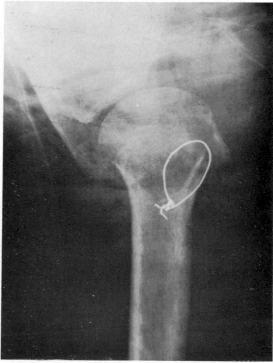

A   **B**

Figure 13–7 Example of multiple fragment displaced fracture treated by open reduction and wire fixation. (Courtesy Dr. J. S. Neviaser.)

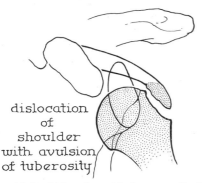

dislocation
of
shoulder
with avulsion
of tuberosity

Figure 13–8 Dislocation with fracture of tuberosity.

Gentle movements are begun as soon as the wound is healed. Fixation is not necessary longer than three to four weeks.

Impacted Fracture Dislocation. Impacted fracture dislocation is included at this point, but the major portion of the deformity is actually the fracture and the dislocation is minor. The usual configuration is a comminution of the upper end of the humerus with the head impaled on the upper end of the shaft. The head is sheared off close to its base, so that a shallow elliptical segment covered with articular cartilage remains sitting along the medial or posteromedial aspect of the neck. The dislocation is a shoving downward of the head because it sticks with the shaft as the arm is lowered to the side.

TREATMENT. This is a serious injury and the most satisfactory treatment is open reduction and internal fixation.

Technique. The joint is approached through the superior aspect, with splitting of the deltoid. Usually the head has to be fished out or pried upward to lie over the disrupted upper end of the shaft. The fragments are pieced together as well as possible. Sometimes fixation of the fragments is aided by threading the long tendon of the biceps (after Nicola) through the head. When there is extensive comminution and it is not possible to fit the fragments together satisfactorily, consideration is given to discarding the head and replacing it with a prosthesis. Any associated cuff damage needs to be repaired at the same time. The arm is immobilized in an abduction plaster or cantilever splint for a period of four weeks. At the end of three weeks the upper half is removed and assisted active movement is initiated (Fig. 13–9).

Fracture Dislocation. This injury is really a subcoracoid dislocation with a fracture through the surgical neck. In contrast to the preceding type, the dislocation is the important feature. The mechanism is one of dislocation followed by a fracture through the surgical neck as the arm is brought down to the side. The separate head then stays in the dislocated position (Fig. 13–10). This is a serious injury and on initial examination can be mistaken for a simple dislocation. X-ray examination should always be done on all suspected dislocations.

TREATMENT. Closed reduction has been recommended in the past but the maneuver of impaling the head on the upper end of the humerus is extremely difficult. The head is hard to control and it may slip back into the joint with the articular surface in contact with the upper end of the shaft. Usually this injury is much better treated by open reduction, splitting the deltoid in the direction of its fibers distal to the acromioclavicular joint. Frequently the head can be replaced accurately without opening the joint, or it may be necessary to incise the capsule anteriorly just medial to the bicipital groove to obtain accurate fixation of the head on the shaft. Fixation may then be carried out with multiple tied wire sutures or with staples such as are illustrated in Figure 13–10. The arm may be immobilized in a body swathe for a period of four weeks followed by use of a sling and initiation of exercises. If there is any question regarding the stability of the fixation, a plaster spica should be applied and removed at the end of four weeks.

Arthroplasty of the Shoulder. Severe fracture dislocation leaving a grossly disorganized joint is a common source of posttraumatic arthritis. In such a circumstance replacement arthroplasty may be indicated when age and general physical condition permit. The principle is excision of the head of the humrus and replacement with a suitable prosthesis. The condition of the rotator cuff has significant bearing on the result in shoulder arthroplasty. This is in contrast to the hip, where repair of the capsule is not an important consideration. In addition to replacement of the head, repair of the rotator cuff is frequently required. An arthrogram will indicate the state of the capsule.

Technique of Replacement Arthroplasty. The sitting shoulder position is used and the joint is approached superoanteriorly or superoposteriorly. If the cuff is intact, the author prefers to approach the joint more from the back, preserving the anterior capsule. If the latter has been torn, it is logical to proceed through the defect to replace the humeral head (see Chapter XV). The acromion is partly removed as previously described after carefully preparing an osseofascial flap for reattaching the deltoid. The capsule is incised sufficiently to allow insertion of the head. The incision is made a little medial to the tuberosity, and enough cuff is left to allow firm repair. The level of excision of the head must be done carefully. Depending upon the appliance that is to be used, the cut is made obliquely so that the head sits on the neck at the correct angle and is firmly supported. The hole for the stem should be started a little more toward the lateral cortex so that, as the appliance sinks in, some cancellous bone remains medially to support the head. If the hole is too big or too medial, the stem remains loose. A little more neck should

be resected (about one eighth of an inch) than appears necessary to allow easy passage beneath the coraco-acromial arch. The cuff is then sutured either to the prepared edge of capsule or into the tuberosity beyond the prosthesis. The security of the capsule repair governs the type of postoperative fixation. When the cuff has been little damaged, abduction traction as in cuff tears is satisfactory. If the cuff has been extensively damaged, the author prefers plaster fixation. The arm is immobilized in a shoulder spica abducted to just less than a right angle, and in a little forward flexion. This is worn for four to six weeks, at which time the arm part is bivalved and movement is started. On the basis of the progress made by the patient, the arm is transferred to a light splint and

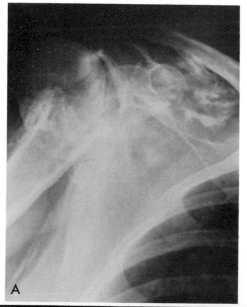

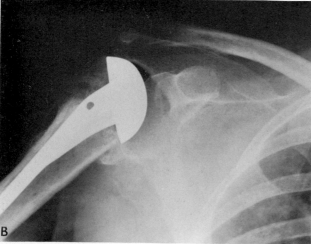

Figure 13–9 Impacted fracture dislocation. Head is in multiple fragments and best disposal is excision and replacement. *A*, Fracture dislocation. *B*, Replacement with a Neer prosthesis.

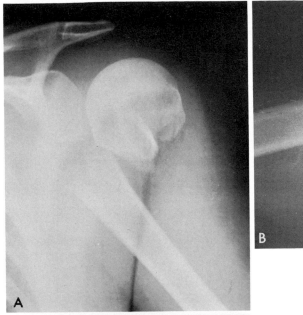

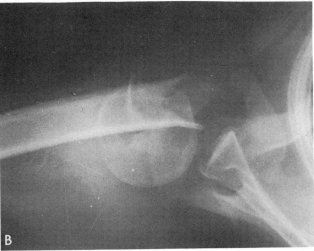

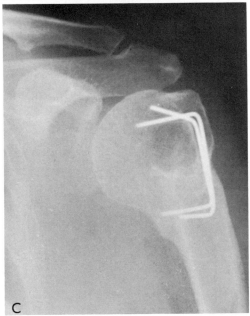

Figure 13-10 Fracture dislocations of the shoulder. *A,* Anteroposterior view. *B,* Superoinferior view. *C,* View following reduction and fixation. (Courtesy Dr. J. S. Neviaser.)

gradually lowered to the side over a further period of two to four weeks.

DISLOCATIONS OF THE SHOULDER JOINT

One of the tributes exacted for the superb mobility of the shoulder is frequent dislocation (Fig. 13-11). It is an injury of youth, in whom it occurs more often than fracture of the neck of the humerus. Solid healthy bone withstands powerful abduction twisting strain, and the weak capsule gives way. Later in life the bone is soft and the capsule contracted, so that the shaft breaks while the joint remains intact. Young adults suffer this injury often. The common accident is a fall with the arm outstretched for protection. The contribution of the elbow and body weight have been somewhat overlooked in explaining the mechanism of this injury. The essential episode is the head of the humerus being forced against the weak anterior or

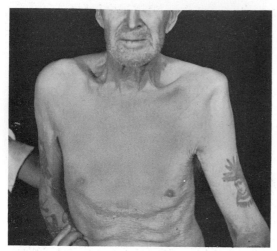

Figure 13–11 Acute anterior dislocation of the shoulder.

anteroinferior capsule. In a headlong fall the outstretched hand takes the impact with the elbow extended. As long as this relation of extension is retained, a solid strut transmits the force and the superior or postero-superior joint structures bear the brunt. In a fall the weight of the body alters this situation and as the weight is applied in full, momentary giving way or buckling of the elbow is inevitable. This breaks the solid strut and the elbow must flex, which tilts the upper end of the humerus downward and forward. As the fall continues the head slips off the glenoid rib easily. At this point the extremity is in abduction and external rotation, exposing the posterosuperior part of the humeral head to the glenoid rim, and it may be cut or creased. It is understandable that with repeated similar trauma less and less force is needed to dislocate the head. The head commonly comes to lie at the front of the glenoid, resting on the rib. Occasionally it lies higher just below the clavicle.

DIAGNOSIS OF DISLOCATION

The signs and symptoms of dislocation are characteristic. The normal rounded contour of the shoulder is replaced by a sharp, angular outline. The patient sits in pain, nursing the forearm with the elbow angled outward (Fig. 13–12). Palpation demonstrates a fossa or depression beneath the acromion where the fullness of the tuberosity should be felt. The deltoid is tense and is difficult to indent with the fingers, but just under the acromion at the posterolateral aspect there can be no

mistaking the defect. The x-ray appearance is diagnostic, but lateral views should be insisted upon in suspected dislocations. When such suspicion exists the possibility of damage to nerves and vessels should be considered automatically. The axillary nerve and posterior cord of the plexus may be stretched as the head slips from the socket. Action of deltoid and wrist extensors should be tested.

ACUTE ANTERIOR DISLOCATIONS

Treatment of Acute Dislocation. Dislocations are reduced as soon as possible. X-ray examination is done to verify the diagnosis and to rule out fracture of the neck or tuberosity.

TECHNIQUE OF REDUCING ANTERIOR DISLOCATION. The Kocher maneuver is a satisfactory method of manipulation. When it is the initial dislocation a general anesthetic or heavy sedation is usually required. There are three definite movements in the manipulation: The operator stands on the same side as the dislocation, grasping the arm at the elbow with the forearm flexed (Fig. 13–13). In *A*, traction and adduction are applied. One hand pulls downward, and the other gently lifts the elbow toward the chest. In *B*, external rotation is done with the opposite

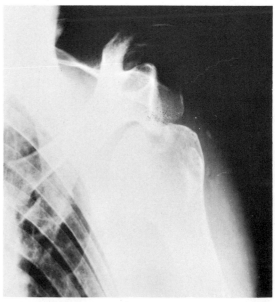

Figure 13–12 An initial dislocation of the shoulder. Note the groove in the head of the humerus and minute fragments gouged from the head.

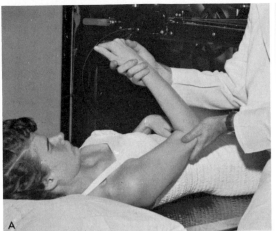

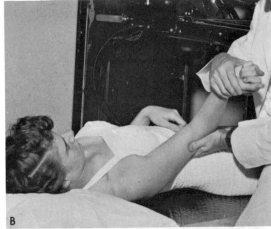

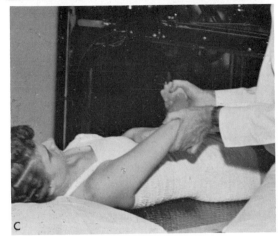

Figure 13–13 Kocher method of reducing acute anterior dislocation. *A,* Traction and adduction applied. *B,* Adduction continued with external rotation. The head is usually felt to slip back into place during this phase. *C,* Reduction completed by quick internal rotation to fix the head in place.

hand, using the forearm as a lever. The adduction and external rotation are continued gently. As the arm is carried across the chest, the head slips into the socket. At this point the third element, internal rotation, is applied to complete the reduction (Fig. 13–13, *C*). Sometimes pressure is needed on the head anteriorly to complete the reduction as the elbow is being brought across the chest. The reduction should be checked by x-ray examination and a sling applied for 14 to 21 days. Gentle movements are started at this time, but attention is paid to elbow, wrist and finger movement from the beginning. An example of deltoid paralysis following dislocation is shown in Figure 13–14.

Old Dislocation of the Shoulder

Persistent unrecognized dislocations of the shoulder crop up with unexpected frequency (Fig. 13–15). Anterior deformity is commoner, but the percentage of posterior dislocations that are overlooked is greater. In both instances, when the head has been out of the socket for a matter of weeks, the soft parts become adherent and the notch at the point of impingment of the head in the glenoid makes reduction difficult. Attempted closed reduction at this stage does more harm than good.

Unreduced Anterior and Posterior Dislocations

These injuries often come to light in a matter of weeks after an accident. At this point, pain and limitation of movement have become progressively worse. The shoulder is stiff, active and passive motion are grossly restricted, and the usual signs of anterior dislocation are present (Fig. 13–16).

Operative Technique. The shoulder is approached through an anterior incision, with deltoid fibers split as in repair for recur-

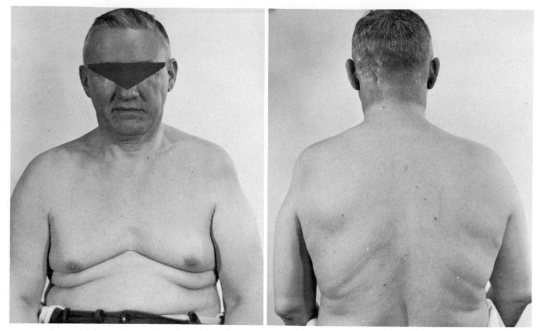

Figure 13–14 Deltoid paralysis following anterior dislocation.

rent dislocations. The capsule is exposed and loosened from the displaced head. When this has been done, reduction is usually possible; if not, the joint is opened anteriorly and the head levered back into place. As a rule, it stays in place if soft parts are adequately separated. The arm is kept in sling fixation for four to six weeks. This treatment is followered by physiotherapy (Fig. 13–16).

RECURRENT DISLOCATION OF THE SHOULDER

The purposeful evolution of the anterior appendage from static weight bearing to mobile prehension has few imperfections, but one is a susceptibility to habitual or recurrent dislocation under certain conditions. The commonest predisposition is found in

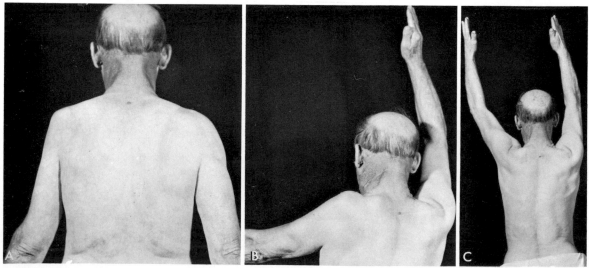

Figure 13–15 Old dislocation of shoulder. *A*, Before reduction; note flattened shoulder point. *B*, Limitation of motion before reduction. *C*, Three months after open reduction.

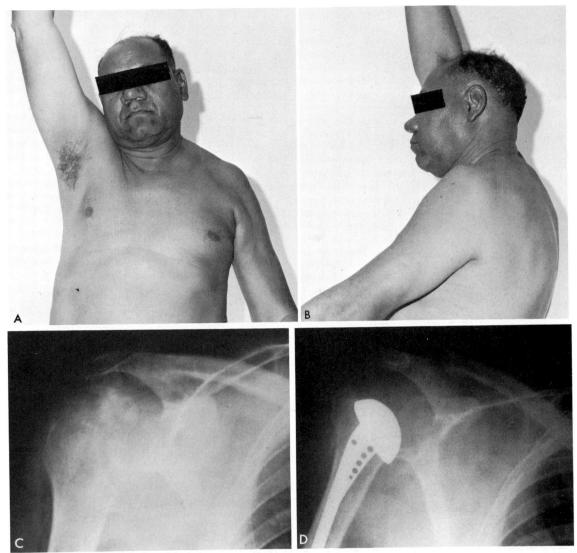

Figure 13–16 Unreduced posterior fracture dislocation treated by open reduction and replacement. *A* and *B*. Preoperative appearance. *C*, Preoperative x-ray. *D*, Postoperative x-ray.

healthy young athletes engaged in rugged activities, but it does happen in women and can happen past the age of 60. The series of dislocations starts with a fairly violent episode such as a fall or tumble, but subsequently less and less force is needed, until routine motions such as combing the hair slip the head off the glenoid rim. So much has been written on this subject that both student and practitioner may be a little bewildered. The diagnosis is straightforward and the indications for treatment clear-cut, but there are endless suggestions as to operative technique. Interest in this subject stems not from the incidence or urgency of the condition but rather from the fact it represents a classic

problem handed down as a proper challenge to those interested in reconstructive surgery.

Etiology. One of the most comprehensive considerations of this whole subject appears in the British edition of the Journal of Bone and Joint Surgery, Vol. 30, No. 1. Many pertinent observations may be drawn from this contribution. The work of Hermodsohn as translated by Moseley is a monumental one also.

In studying the origin of this condition there is a tendency to interpret some of the pathological findings as a cause when actually they are a result of a primary established state. The fundamental disturbance is a slipping of the head of the humerus off the glenoid rim, which demonstrates the natural tendency of a spinning ball to slip from a shallow saucer if control is momentarily lost. The structure of this ball and socket is such that in the dislocation the ball may be chipped or the casing torn so that it heals insecurely. When this happens the slip is easier the next time and a vicious cycle of abnormal mobility with gradual loss of control is established. Both the initial and the habitual episodes are true dislocations, and the first may lead to the second if there is sufficient critical damage and poor repair, or if the individual repeatedly exposes the shoulder to the same dislocating act. Apart from the unalterable anatomy and physiology of the shoulder, some predisposing variations and clinical states are noted as favoring habitual dislocation. The glenoids may be abnormally long, narrow and shallow. The middle glenohumeral ligament may be poorly developed, or an unduly large head may articulate within a stunted glenoid. Epileptics, as might be expected, are prone to recurrent dislocation. The lesion may be bilateral, and several members of one family may be afflicted, with very little trauma initiating the condition.

Pathological Findings. The interpretation of the cause of this disturbance is based on appreciation of the pathological changes recorded at operation and in the autopsy room. Those documented at operation are most significant, since it is possible in a measure to reproduce the dislocating act without harm and to assess the respective contribution of the various changes. The critical act is abduction, external rotation and a little extension. When this is done at operation, the head is felt to jump off the side of the glenoid; it may catch in this position. Further examination then shows changes in the head of the humerus, the capsule, the glenoid rim and labrum. There is a give and take in the incidence of damage to capsule labrum and head; they are always present in some combination, but all three may not be present in every case.

THE HEAD OF THE HUMERUS. A notch or crease is commonly found on the posterolateral surface of the head, or this zone is flatter than normal (Fig. 13–17 C). For some time this finding has been overlooked because x-rays in full internal rotation are needed for its demonstration and it is hard to see or feel at operation. One clue to its presence at operation is the jerky trajectory of the head on full external rotation. When search is

made for the defect it will be found in over 80 per cent of patients, as reported by J. C. Adams. The significance of this change is further emphasized by the observation that it is found constantly when there is no defect in the labrum; therefore, it may be interpreted as an important contributor to recurrent dislocation.

THE LABRUM. The lip of the glenoid lies in the way of the skidding head and so, as dislocation occurs, it may be detached, frayed or torn. Some damage to the labrum is found in a high percentage but often it is not sufficient to explain the dislocation; it is but a part of the problem, being combined with head and capsular changes. It can be demonstrated often at operation (Fig. 13–18). The labrum may be lifted up free from the scapula and capsule. The adjacent edge of the glenoid frequently has a palpable notch at this point as evidence of the splintering trauma of the head against the rim. The labrum may be fractured (Fig. 13–19), with a piece lying loose within the joint. It should be borne in mind that separation of the labrum may occur without any dislocation history; it is common to find it loose and frayed as a result of the wear and tear of general joint use. Abnormalities of the labrum are more easily demonstrated than those of the head and, although found frequently, are not constantly present. The author has operated upon patients in whom no significant changes in the labrum were present, but changes in capsule and head could be demonstrated.

CHANGES IN THE CAPSULE. Normally the capsule is attached firmly to the neck of the scapula but just beyond the labrum. In this middle zone it is not continuous with the labrum. In recurrent dislocation the capsule is lax and ballooned under the subscapularis. The subscapular recess is more spacious than normal. The middle glenohumeral ligament varies considerably in strength; in recurrent dislocation it is commonly weakened or poorly developed. Laxity of the capsule due to stretching and tearing with fibrotic healing reaches the point where the head is easily accommodated in the dislocated position under the subscapularis. The ballooning is well demonstrated by an arthrogram (Fig. 13–20).

Mechanism of Recurrent Dislocation. The complete mechanism includes both initial and habitual dislocations. Both are true dislocations, but changes resulting from the early episodes predispose to the recur-

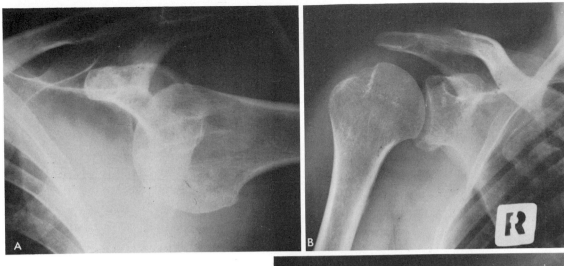

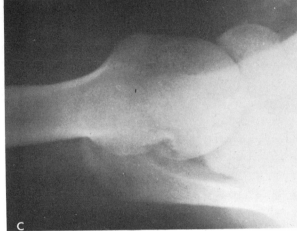

Figure 13–17 Recurrent dislocation of the shoulder. *A*, Subcoracoid position. *B*, The notch in the head demonstrated in full internal rotation. *C*, The notch shown in the posterior surface in the superoinferior view.

rent state and presumably alter the way in which dislocation occurs.

INITIAL EPISODE. The critical act is abduction, external rotation and a little extension of the arm. Force may be applied in many ways in reaching this position or after it has been taken up to complete the dislocation (Fig. 13–21).

Fall on Outstretched Arm. Force is transmitted up the arm from a forward fall, as in stubbing the toe, and has a shearing effect as it reaches the shoulder joint unless the elbow is kept rigidly extended. The forward fling of the body weight as the fall is completed buckles the elbow so that the arm is momentarily extended behind the body and the head of the humerus is thrust against the anterior edge of the glenoid, labrum and related capsular structures. The head meets the glenoid not face to face but with the angle open anteriorly so that the posterior

aspect is rotated against the glenoid face (Fig. 13–21). The amount of rotation possible by the scapula is limited in this position, and it cannot keep pace with the head going into extension so that the head is levered out at the anteroinferior margin.

It is reasonable to expect damage to the head and glenoid when force is applied in this manner. The head may be creased and the glenoid lip fractured. If the elbow flexes quickly, the force is dissipated more anteriorly and the labrum or capsule then takes the force rather than the glenoid. If moderate resistance is maintained and the force is transmitted more in extension, impingement on the rim results and, consequently, bone damage may be greater.

Forcible Movement Without Falling. A fall is not necessary to accomplish dislocation; powerful muscle contraction alone may dislocate the shoulder. Violent action such as is

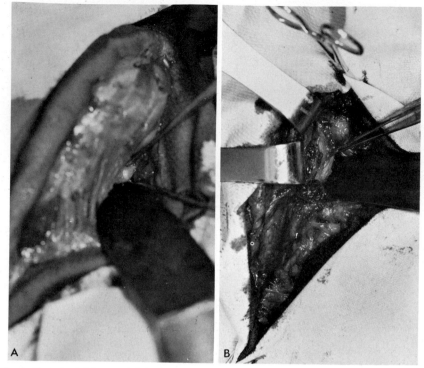

Figure 13–18 *A,* Detached labrum demonstrated at operation for recurrent dislocation of shoulder (exposure as for Gallie repair). *B,* Tear of the capsule.

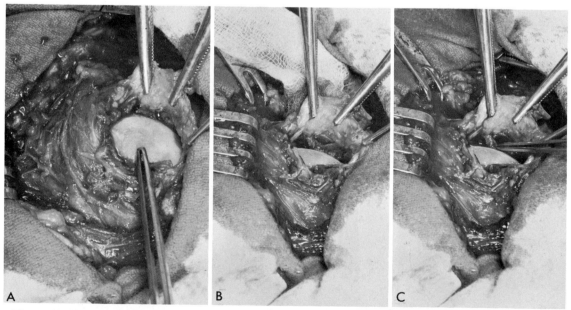

Figure 13–19 Putti-Platt exposure showing defect in the labrum. *A,* Head of humerus. *B,* Subscapularis being pulled medially. *C,* Forceps is in the defect of labral separation.

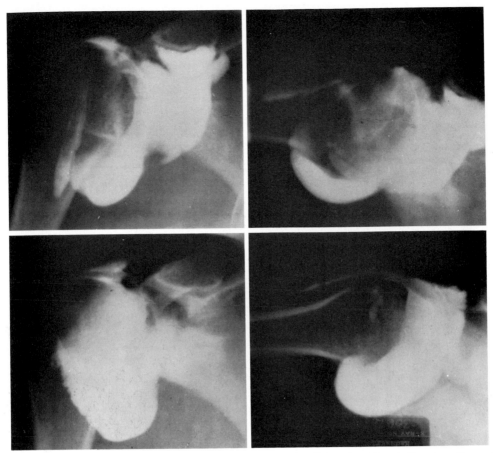

Figure 13–20 Arthrogram in a patient with recurrent anterior dislocation. Note ballooning of capsule.

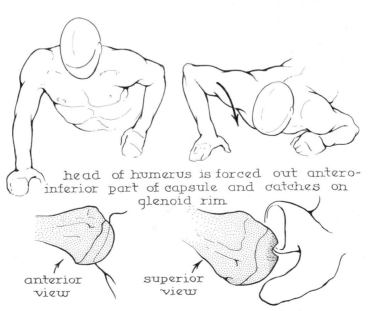

head of humerus is forced out antero-
inferior part of capsule and catches on
glenoid rim

anterior
view

superior
view

Figure 13–21 Recurrent anterior dislocation mechanism.

seen in epileptics may be cited as an example. In such a paroxysm of muscle contraction the backward flail of the arm into extreme external rotation and abduction may spin the head from the socket, rupturing the capsule. Of course, falls also contribute to dislocation in epileptics, but the crescendo of the convulsion usually occurs in the horizontal position, where internal rotation beyond body line is resisted but the backward flail of the arm, weighted by forearm and hand, is still possible. Once predisposing changes are established, uncontrolled muscle forces in subsequent attacks easily produce habitual dislocation.

Backward Falls with the Arm in Extension. When the body falls backward, the arm instinctively reaches behind to break the fall. Stress travels up the extended arm, forcing the head against the unprotected front of the joint. Dislocation may occur, but there is a difference in the damage produced. The capsule may be wrenched from its anchorage and the biceps tendon ruptured. There is less damage to glenoid and humeral head because the force is at right angles to the glenoid and the shearing stroke on the glenoid is avoided (see Fig. 3–17).

Recurrent Episodes. All recurrent dislocations start with an apparently simple dislocation, and it has not yet been possible to tell which episodes will be followed by habitual recurrence. Probably more attention to simple dislocations, careful inspection for any bone defect, or demonstration of the capsular abnormalities by arthrography will help. The amount of damage resulting from the initial dislocation appears to be the important determining factor. When there are established changes, many mechanisms operate. A defect or crease in the head

presents an obvious cleat or take-off which locks the head on the glenoid rim (Fig. 13–22). Only the muscle action of abduction and external rotation is needed to slip the head into the notch gripping the rim. Leverage of the falling arm then pries the head out of the joint. A detached labrum or lax capsule allows slack control when the arm is flailed into abduction and external rotation, and the head slips out under the subscapularis.

Successful methods of repair are based on such an interpretation of the dislocating mechanism. External rotation is limited a little; the anterior or subscapular zone of dislocation is buttressed; the labrum is reanchored and the capsule repaired; or new ligaments are fashioned across the anteroinferior aspect.

Treatment. In the beginning the dislocating episodes are incapacitating, requiring medical attention. Later, patients learn to slip the head back into the joint themselves. The designation "recurrent dislocation" should be reserved for those conditions presenting clear-cut displacement of the head. There is a condition of subluxation or lax joint which is merely a slack articulation without the history or pathological changes of true dislocation. The initial dislocation is reduced as outlined previously for simple dislocations.

The question arises as to the point at which dislocation becomes habitual. The author has classed those patients who have had three dislocations as having recurrent dislocation, and these are the ones requiring operative treatment. From this point on the disturbance is not effectively controlled by conservative measures, and patients should be advised to have the shoulder repaired. Dislocations occur with increasing ease and may happen

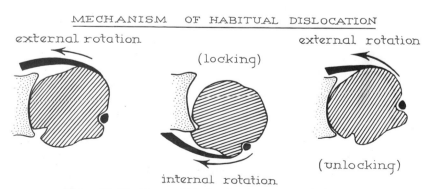

MECHANISM OF HABITUAL DISLOCATION

external rotation   (locking)   external rotation

internal rotation   (unlocking)

Figure 13–22   Humeral head action in recurrent dislocation.

in a critical situation such as swimming or climbing, jeopardizing the patient's safety.

OPERATIVE TECHNIQUES FOR REPAIR OF RECURRENT DISLOCATION Nearly one hundred different operations have been described, many with very successful results in the hands of the originator. All successful techniques take cognizance of the dominant pathological changes and, in various combinations, limit external rotation, buttress the capsule and subscapularis, or introduce new protecting ligaments. The methods of Bankart, Putti-Platt, Gallie, Nicola and Henderson, all with many modifications, have been used extensively. The most successful techniques are those of Putti-Platt, Bankart, and Gallie, which are described here.

Putti-Platt Method. The shoulder is approached through an anterior incision similar to that used in all these operations. The cephalic vein is used as a landmark. The deltoid is retracted laterally, the coracobrachialis and the short head of the biceps medially. The subscapularis then comes into view. The muscle is cut vertically about one half inch from the musculotendinous junction through the muscle fibers (see Figure 13–23). The stump is pulled laterally, exposing the anterior capsule; the capsule is repaired, and the medial portion of the subscapularis is then anchored to the humerus with the shaft in full internal rotation. The lateral stump is sutured in overlapping fashion to the medial end.

The arm is fixed in internal rotation in a sling for three to four weeks.

Bankart Technique. The principle of this operation is exposure of the capsule attachment to the glenoid from the front and repair of the detached capsule (Fig. 13–24). The joint is approached through an anterior incision. The deltoid fibers are split and retracted, and the subscapularis is exposed. The muscle is cut at the center of this tendon and retracted medially. The anteroinferior aspect of the capsule is then in view. The detached capsule or labrum is reattached to the glenoid margin. There are various methods of reanchoring the labrum and capsule. Staples may be used; fascia may be used; or holes may be drilled in the glenoid and catgut inserted. The subscapularis is then repaired and the arm kept in a sling afterward as with the Putti-Platt method.

Gallie Technique. This method was used by Dr. W. E. Gallie for 20 years and with slight modifications, has proved very satisfactory. The principle is to insert new ligaments across the anteroinferior aspect of the capsule and humerus. With a slight modification, the principle of Bankart may be embodied (Fig. 13–25).

The shoulder is approached through an anterior incision along and angled slightly at the deltopectoral groove. The fibers of the deltoid are separated, the cephalic vein is retracted medially, and the deltoid is retracted laterally. This exposes the coracoid process, the subscapular, and the upper aspect of the humerus. The lower margin of the subscapularis is then defined. A linear slit is made in the muscle about ¼ inch above the inferior aspect of the glenoid. A hole is then drilled through the neck of the scapula. A protecting retractor is used, and the hole comes out just below the spine of the scapula posteriorly. A piece of fascia is removed from the thigh 10 inches by ¾ to 1 inch. A thick knot is tied in the end. This is threaded through the hole in the scapula so that the knot impinges posteriorly, anchoring the new ligament. The fascia is then split in two and one strand is used to take a stitch through the capsule, plicating the redundant anteroinferior aspect. A knot is tied after this suture. The ligament is pulled across the anteroinferior aspect to the region of the bicipital groove. Two drill holes are inserted and connected with a curved trocar. The fascia is extracted through this and carried over to the coracoid process. A hole is drilled in the coracoid process, and the fascial strips are pulled through and tied snugly. The tension on the ligament is adjusted so that it is snug but not tight. The wound is closed in layers. The arm is in a sling and at the side for four weeks. At the end of this time, active movement is initiated.

RESULTS. The incidence of recurrence using the Gallie technique has been very low. Some slight limitation of external rotation and abduction usually results. Sometimes this is so small that only the examiner notices it and the patient is not aware of the disability. At other times a few activities may be hampered. The pitfalls in the operation are few, apart from the usual possible but unlikely operative complications. The hole in the scapula must be made low enough and the fascial strip must not be pulled too tightly or too much limitation of movement will result. The holes in the bone must be placed with care.

Text continued on page 404.

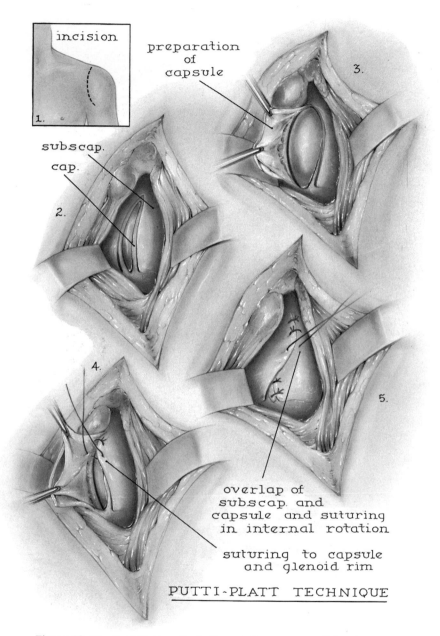

Figure 13–23 Putti-Platt method of repair for recurrent dislocation.

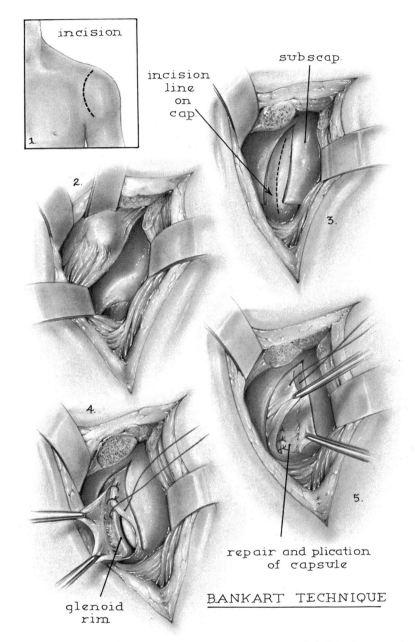

incision

1.

incision
line
on
cap.

subscap.

2.

3.

4.

5.

glenoid
rim

repair and plication
of capsule

BANKART TECHNIQUE

Figure 13–24 Bankart technique. Ingenious variations in the technique of placing the suture in the glenoid edge have been made by Eyre-Vrook and Rowe and have added to the effectiveness of this operation.

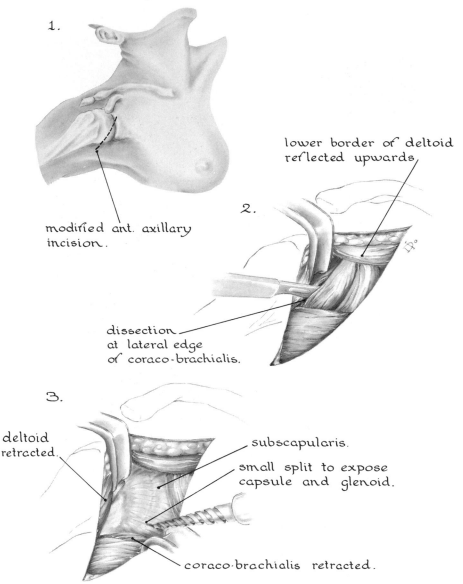

1.

lower border of deltoid
reflected upwards.

2.

modified ant. axillary
incision.

dissection
at lateral edge
of coraco-brachialis.

3.

deltoid
retracted.

subscapularis.

small split to expose
capsule and glenoid.

coraco-brachialis retracted.

Figure 13–25 Gallie technique using axillary incision. *1* and *2*, Incision exposure and placement of special retractor for insertion of the drill. *3* and *4*, Drill with special spiked point comes out posteriorly for attachment of fascia to be pulled through. *5*, Fascia is split in two and a deep stitch taken through the labrum (Bankart). The fascia is tied so that the labrum is anchored. *6*, It is then pulled over to the neck of the humerus creating strong anteroinferior ligament. The application of the fascia to the humerus may be varied according to the snugness and correction that is required. Fascia transferred to the coracoid process produces a further restricting ligament anteriorly.

4.

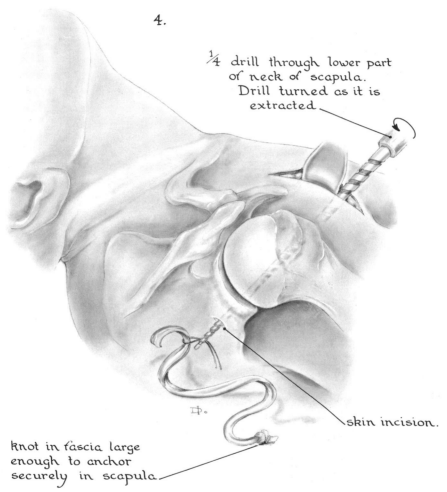

¼ drill through lower part
of neck of scapula.
Drill turned as it is
extracted

skin incision.

knot in fascia large
enough to anchor
securely in scapula

Figure 13–25 *Continued.*

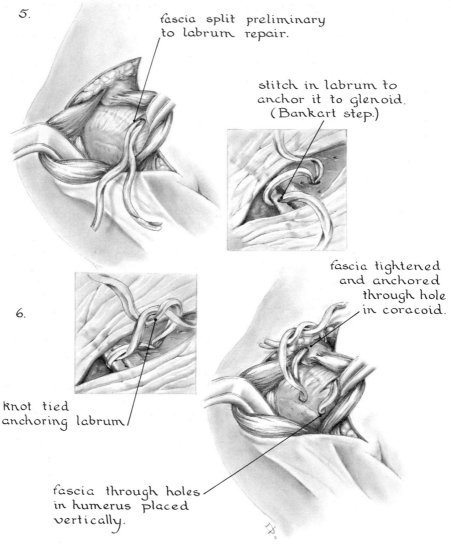

5.

fascia split preliminary
to labrum repair.

stitch in labrum to
anchor it to glenoid.
(Bankart step.)

fascia tightened
and anchored
through hole
in coracoid.

6.

knot tied
anchoring labrum

fascia through holes
in humerus placed
vertically.

Figure 13–25 *Continued.*

RECURRENT SUBLUXATION OF THE SHOULDER

The glenohumeral joint may be the seat of recurrent subluxation, a not uncommon entity quite apart from recurrent dislocation. The recent work of Blazin and Saltzman has highlighted the increasing incidence of this condition. The disturbance is most often seen in young athletes and its true nature may go unrecognized for some time. The usual history is of recurrent, painful catching episodes in the shoulder in which the patient momentarily loses control because of sudden, acute paralyzing pain. Often a sense of slipping or catching in the shoulder is described. The pain frequently extends down the whole arm so that the individual may drop or let go of an object which he is catching or holding. Strenuous activity is not necessary to cause the subluxation; often a simple forward flexion act, as for example, a young goal tender reaching forward with his stick, a quarterback starting to wind up for a pass, or a workman steadying a weight in front of him. The discomfort passes off immediately, and the patient has a sensation of something slipping back into place in the shoulder.

Often the description of these episodes is vague, the only sensation being one of sudden, acute pain followed by some general soreness but no continued apparent malfunction of the joint.

When a history such as this is presented, further careful investigation is required. Frequently on examination undue laxity may be demonstrated. The head of the humerus can be shoved forward almost half its own width. There is no true locking or dislocation and no persistence of the deformity when the episodes occur. The patient may have the feeling of fullness anteriorly, but this is not always so. Tenderness is present over the upper end of the humerus and the anterior aspect of the capsule in the acute episodes, but in the interval there may be very few signs indicative of the condition apart from laxity of the capsule.

Superoinferior x-rays should be carried out with the head of the humerus under pressure from the back and the relative laxity of the two sides compared (Fig. 13–26). No crease in the head of the humerus will be demonstrable, as is the case with recurrent dislocation (Fig. 13–27). Contrast studies are extremely helpful and show an abnormal anteroinferior ballooning of the capsule (Fig. 13–28).

Treatment. Operative measures are required to control this condition. Although the initial episodes are not so incapacitating as in a recurrent dislocation, persistence of the condition is disabling. The most satisfactory management is correction by one of the methods of repair for recurrent dislocation.

ACUTE POSTERIOR DISLOCATIONS

The head of the humerus may be dislocated posteriorly also, but this occurs with much less frequency than anterior dislocation. It results from force suddenly applied with the arm adducted and internally rotated so that the head of the humerus slips off the posterior rim of the glenoid. In this fashion the anterior aspect of the head of the humerus rests on the posterior lip of the glenoid and a crease may be formed in the head in this area that is similar to that seen in anterior dislocation but in the opposite quadrant (Fig. 13–29).

Diagnosis. The condition is seen more often in the older age group; the history is of injury followed by pain and limitation of motion. The patient may not be conscious of any deformity, but on inspection there is a posterior bulging that is obvious when the patient is viewed from the side. Anteriorly there is a fossa with a prominent coracoid process, but the head of the humerus cannot be felt in its usual position.

The true nature of the condition may not be recognized immediately because of swelling and soft tissue overlay. It is not uncommon to have the patient present some week to ten days after a fall because of the continued restriction of motion (Fig. 13–30). Superoinferior and lateral x-rays identify the lesion definitively (Fig. 13–31).

Treatment. If the dislocation has not been present for too long, closed reduction is

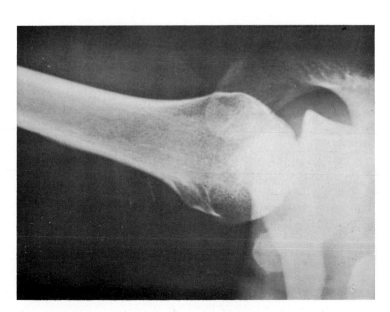

Figure 13–26 Superoinferior view of the shoulder showing subluxation.

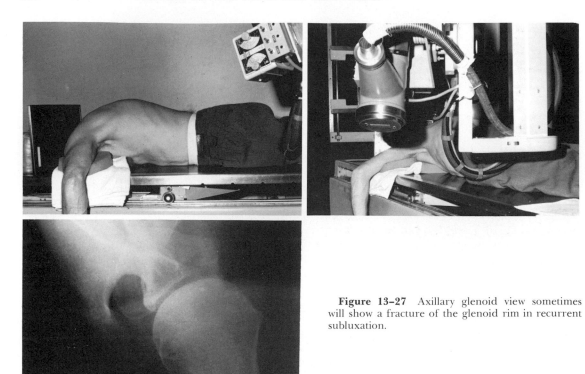

Figure 13–27 Axillary glenoid view sometimes will show a fracture of the glenoid rim in recurrent subluxation.

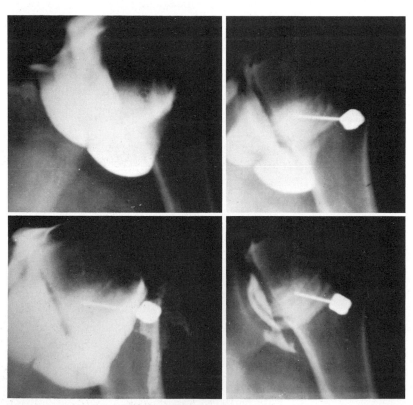

Figure 13–28 Arthrogram in recurrent subluxation of shoulder. Note ballooning of capsule anteriorly and inferiorly, which is almost as extensive as in a recurrent dislocation.

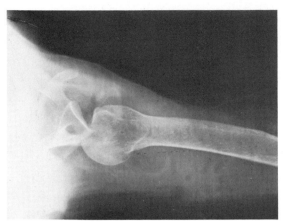

Figure 13–29 Posterior dislocation.

feasible under a general anesthetic. Traction is applied to the arm and forward pressure made on the region of the head posteriorly and, as the patient is relaxed, a gentle twisting motion will slip the head back into the socket. The arm is immobilized at the side with the arm in slight external rotation to prevent the head from slipping back off the posterior aspect of the glenoid fossa. One method of doing this is to fix a light bandage around the arm in such a fashion that it is

pulled into slight extension so that the forearm then comes to rest opposite the body; internal rotation, which may cause a recurrence of the dislocation, is then no longer possible. The fixation is maintained for four weeks and motion gradually instituted.

Unreduced Posterior Dislocation

In neglected cases closed reduction is difficult and surgical treatment is required. Once the dislocation is fixed in the unreduced position for a matter of weeks, forceful attempts at closed reduction are ineffective and may be harmful (Fig. 13–32).

Neviaser has emphasized the problems in reducing old dislocations. Considerable difficulty may be encountered in replacing the head of the humerus because of the fibrosis and shortening of muscles. The capsule becomes taut in a bowstring fashion and with the head remaining fixed against the edge of the glenoid, a notch or wedging develops in it, locking it into place.

Operative Technique. The superanterior incision is used, providing access to the top and front of the joint. The deltoid fibers are separated in the usual fashion, extending from the acromioclavicular joint distally. The coraco-acromial ligament is incised and the joint capsule exposed. An effort may be made at this point to gently lever the head of the humerus back into position, but as a rule this is unsuccessful.

An incision about 1 inch in length is made

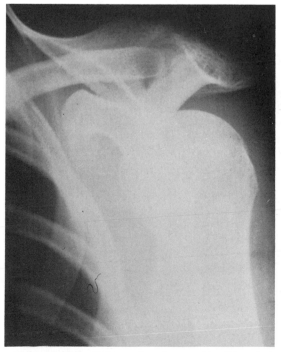

Figure 13–30 Old unreduced posterior dislocation. Note prominence of head of humerus posteriorly.

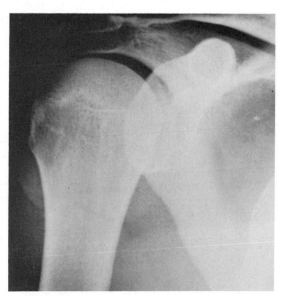

Figure 13–31 X-ray of posterior dislocation.

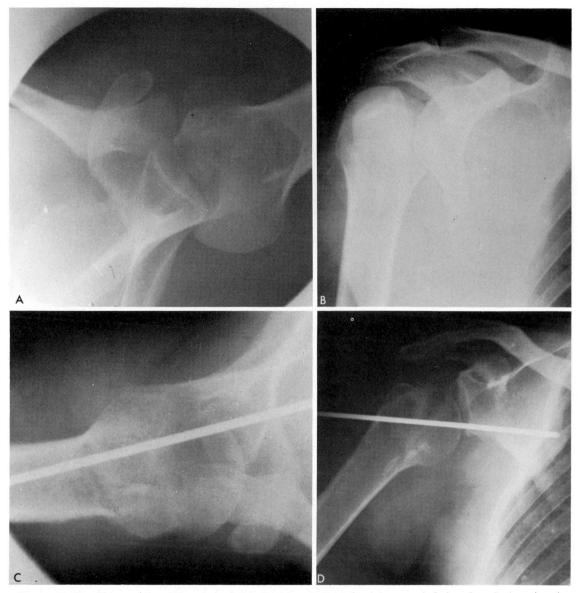

Figure 13–32 Old posterior dislocation of the shoulder. *A*, Prereduction superoinferior view. *B*, Anterior view prereduction. *C* and *D*, Postreduction with Kirschner wire to maintain reduction. (Courtesy Dr. J. S. Neviaser.)

in the superoanterior aspect of the capsule sufficient to allow a periosteal elevator to be inserted within the joint to strip the adhesions.

Some method for retaining the head of the humerus in the reduced position is necessary. If the dislocation has been accomplished without extensive soft tissue resection, a Kirschner wire may be inserted through the head into the glenoid to maintain the position and the capsule closed satisfactorily.

When more extensive exposure has been necessary, the method advocated by

McLaughlin is suggested. In this technique the tendon of the subscapularis is separated from its attachment to the humerus and then inserted into the defect in the head of the humerus caused by the dislocation. The tendon is transfixed to the bone by heavy sutures run through drill holes.

Postoperatively the arm is maintained at the side in slight external rotation in a dressing similar to that described for closed reductions. The position of slight external rotation, or one by which internal rotation is prevented, is maintained for four to six weeks.

Recurrent Posterior Dislocation

Attention is called to this entity because some confusion has surrounded its interpretation in the past. The lesion is encountered most often in children and young adults and the condition in these instances is true recurrent dislocation. It differs profoundly from the anterior counterpart in that very rarely does a specific episode of injury usher in the condition. Nearly always it is a gradual development, with the patient almost imperceptibly becoming conscious of the laxity and instability of the joint in carrying out certain motions, particularly those involving flexion of the shoulder. Such a process contrasts with anterior recurrent dislocation in which, typically, there is a single episode followed by reduction and then recurrent similar episodes, again with intervals of control. In recurrent posterior dislocation, once the abnormality is established it is a constant derangement.

Clinical Picture. The condition is encountered most often in children and young adults, and one or both shoulders may be involved. The patient becomes gradually conscious of a feeling of instability in the shoulder and has a sensation of something slipping out of place as the arm is lifted to the front. Eventually almost any act that involves flexion of the shoulder produces the uncomfortable change and the sensation of instability (Fig. 13–33). In contrast to anterior dislocation this is really a subluxation or much more gradually developing instability. When the arm hangs at the side the patient does not have a feeling of instability or subluxation, but the minute it is lifted into flexion and carried into internal rotation the posterior luxation develops. In some instances it is a developmental abnormality that gradually becomes apparent from the age of five onward. As the child matures the luxation is more noticeable, and by the age of nine or ten the condition is progressively incapacitating.

On examination the cardinal change is the prominence of the head of the humerus as the arm is lifted into forward flexion and internally rotated. This may be seen and felt. Considerable laxity of the capsule is also apparent on grasping the head of the humerus and forcibly shifting it forward and backward in the glenoid.

Radiologically little abnormality is apparent on routine films, but in the superoinferior view forced internal rotation demonstrates

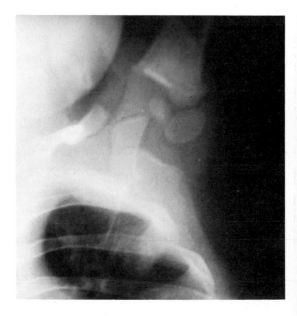

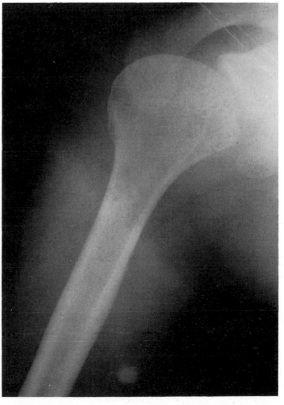

Figure 13–33 Recurrent posterior dislocation.

greater prominence of the head posteriorly than is normally encountered.

Treatment. Surgical measures are necessary to effectively correct this abnormality. In some instances the derangement does not become apparent until the late teens or early twenties; often, in girls particularly, when it is unilateral, considerable accomodation to the deformity is effected. Sometimes the voluntary control and accommodation is such that the patient feels it does not constitute a sufficient disturbance to require surgical measures. In most instances when the deformity becomes apparent at an early age, correction is required.

Many methods have been suggested. The approach favored by McLaughlin is a type of posterior bone block in which the posterior aspect of the shoulder is exposed through an oblique incision just medial to the medial border of the deltoid. The deltoid muscle is retracted superiorly and the posterior aspect of the shoulder joint exposed. An osteotomy is performed along the posterior aspect, wedging a segment of bone forward about 3/16 of an inch from the edge of the glenoid. In this defect a wedge-shaped graft cut from the iliac crest is inserted. In this fashion the posterior aspect of the glenoid is reflected in a curled fashion, anteriorly creating a buttress to block the posterior subluxation. Such a procedure may be ineffective in some patients since it does nothing to control the excessive internal rotation of the shaft of the humerus.

An alternative method is posterior capsular plication with the posterior aspect of the shoulder joint exposed in the same fashion and the capsule firmly plicated with fascia to the neck of the scapula in a fashion similar to the Bankart procedure for anterior repair.

Recurrent Posterior Dislocations in Children

The author feels that the significant abnormality of this derangement, particularly in young people, is retroversion of the head of the humerus and that, unless this is corrected, some degree of recurrent posterior luxation can be anticipated.

Osteotomy Technique. Correction of the persistent retroversion of the head of the humerus can be obtained only by a rotation osteotomy carried out just below the neck of the humerus (Fig. 13–34). The distal shaft of the humerus is carried to 20 degrees in-

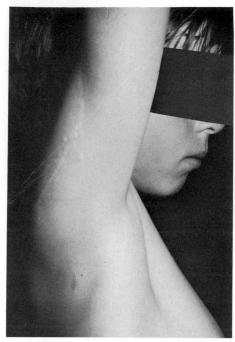

Figure 13–34 Rotation osteotomy of the humerus.

ternal rotation and fixed in this position. When this has been done the natural tendency to lift the arm in flexion then automatically turns the head of the humerus into a little external rotation, correcting the persistent retroversion.

A longitudinal incision is made anterolaterally with care being taken to preserve the circumflex nerve; the shaft of the humerus is exposed and a transverse osteotomy is performed. Fixation internally is obtained with a contact plate, and the arm is immobilized postoperatively in a shoulder spica.

In the author's hands this form of correction has given the most consistently satisfactory results. Posterior bone block and capsular fixation may be effective in minor degrees of this derangement, but in some instances are followed by recurrent luxation or undesirable intra-articular changes (Fig. 13–35).

Recurrent Posterior Dislocation in Adults

In some instances persistent symptoms of recurrent posterior dislocation do not become troublesome until adulthood. The

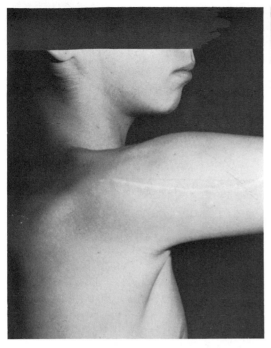

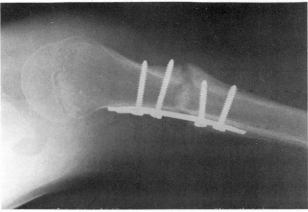

Figure 13–35. Postoperative result following rotation osteotomy. Note lack of any posterior prominence of the head of the humerus on forward flexion.

disturbance appears to involve women more than men. A degree of accommodation occurs in many instances, and the individual continues with the abnormality, feeling that it is not of sufficient severity to warrant extensive treatment. In other instances the recurrent posterior protrusion of the head of the humerus is uncomfortable, favors considerable weakness in the limb and may be accompanied by increasing pain. The author has found that a modification of the Gallie fascia technique is a relatively simple method of improving this condition.

Operative Technique (Reverse Fascial Repair). The incision and approach are carried out in the same fashion as for a Gallie repair through the anterior aspect. The fascia is anchored to the back and then brought to the front. In this instance no stitch is taken through the capsule because it is not desired to hold the humerus in internal fixation or to hamper external rotation.

A transverse hole is drilled in the neck of the humerus just below the articular surface. Through this hole the fascia is threaded first anteriorly and then taken out through the back so that when it is pulled to the front it embraces the undersurface of the head of the humerus in criss-cross fashion. As it is tensed it pulls the head of the humerus upward, snugging it against the glenoid and preventing excessive internal rotation. The fascia is then carried up to the coracoid and anchored firmly, maintaining a point of external rotation. In this fashion a checkrein is provided, limiting internal rotation and excessive flexion as the arm is lifted forward (Fig. 13–36).

Postoperatively the arm is maintained at the side in slight external rotation with the elbow pulled slightly posteriorly so that the body serves as an obstruction to internal rotation, thereby preventing tension on the new ligament. It is kept in this position for a period of four weeks and a further two weeks in a sling.

RECURRENT ANTERIOR AND POSTERIOR DISLOCATIONS

Extremely lax shoulders are encountered which present almost as examples of recurrent anterior and posterior dislocations. In some instances there is a congenital tendency toward lax joints and this mobility in the shoulder is but one evidence of a somewhat generalized tendency. The patient may present with the complaint of either anterior or posterior pain and indicate voluntarily the laxity of the capsule by subluxating at will.

Treatment. The shoulders are often pitfalls for the unwary surgeon, because operative reconstruction as for an anterior or posterior repair often materially aggravates the situation. It is not uncommon to encounter

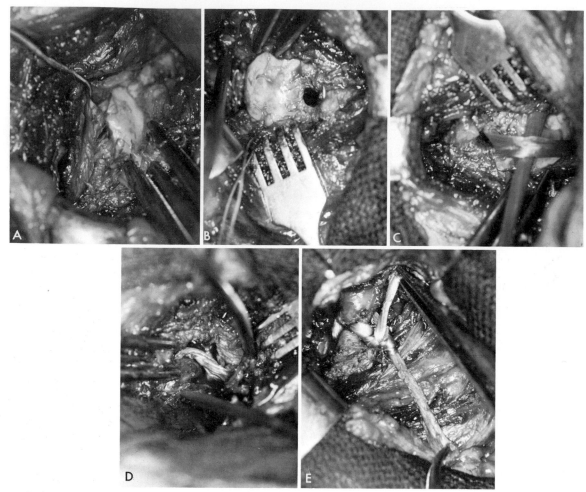

Figure 13–36 Operative technique, fascial repair of recurrent posterior dislocation in adults. *A*, Anterior pouch. Hole has been drilled in the medial glenoid margin, anchoring fascia as in anterior repair. *B*, Holes drilled at the base of the neck of the humerus ³/₄ inch apart, one hole ¹/₄ inch above and lateral to the other. The wire may be seen in place preparatory to pulling the fascia through the neck of the humerus. *C*, Fascia has been pulled through and is criss-crossed to pull the humerus toward the glenoid slightly and twisted into slight external rotation or prevent internal rotation. *D* and *E*, Fascia is pulled up and tied through a hole in the glenoid.

patients in whom multiple operations have been carried out in an attempt to balance the shoulder mechanism. The peripheral management is a conservative approach and is used with skilled physiotherapy to produce improved control by the muscles of the lax joint.

In adults habitual posterior dislocation and anterior subluxation are often controlled by appropriate exercise programs that strengthen the stabilizing muscles, both front and back. Some patients, usually women in their 20's and 30's, have habitual subluxation in which the emphasis on posterior displacement may become a problem. Under these circumstances the author has used a modified Gallie technique of fascial repair, but has changed the direction of the fascial incision so that it acts as a checkrein to full internal rotation and at the same time tightens the glenohumeral junction. The procedure is carried out through the same approach as is used for repair of anterior dislocation, with the hole being drilled through the glenoid with a special drill. The fascia is pulled through from the back and then taken directly to the space of the head of the humerus at the junction of the head and neck. At this point two holes ¹/₄ inch in diameter are drilled and so placed that they are approximately ¹/₂ inch apart, with one hole just at the rim of the articular surface and the other one ¹/₄ inch below and ¹/₂ inch lateral to this. The fascia is threaded through the hole distal from the glenoid attachment, going through from the anterior surface and being brought out through the other hole posteriorly so that the fascia criss-crosses (Fig. 13–36). The fascia is then crossed upon itself and brought out to the glenoid process where it is anchored. In this fashion a heavy fascial sling is placed in such a way that it acts as a checkrein, preventing extreme internal rotation. At the same time it snugs the head of the humerus to the glenoid, diminishing general joint laxity.

The operation leaves some slight anterior and posterior relaxation but it prevents complete subluxation in either direction, with emphasis on the limitation of internal rotation.

Postoperatively the patient is wrapped in a body swathe with the arm at the side and the elbow slightly extended to prevent extreme internal rotation. The immobilization is continued for two weeks and then the arm is placed in a sling and exercises are started.

FRACTURES OF THE CLAVICLE

The clavicle has been designated the shock absorber of the shoulder since it acts as a strut, holding the upper extremity up and out from the side. In this position it takes the brunt of force transmitted through falls in the outstretched hand or on the point of the shoulder. In most instances the force which shatters the clavicle is one which is applied from the lateral direction, transversing the width of the body.

BIRTH INJURIES

The clavicle is the bone most commonly fractured at birth. Complications of uterine presentation and unusual size and weight of the body have been the usual causes. The fracture is easily overlooked at birth but suspicion should be aroused by any abnormal contour, shortening of the neck line, or the child's inclination to use one extremity much less than the other. The mother or nurse notices that the baby cries when the affected side is handled in turning or lifting. There is considerable deformity and displacement in these fractures. Sometimes during delivery the bone is heard to crack and an x-ray then shows the fracture.

Treatment. The earlier the diagnosis is made the easier are reduction and fixation.

Callus forms rapidly and a mass of exuberant callus may be interpreted as being indicative of a more serious lesion. The fracture is handled by a flannel bandage or elastic yoke applied in figure-of-eight fashion. This is removed and reapplied every three or four days or as it becomes loose. The baby's delicate skin requires care and protection so rigid apparatus is not used as a rule. Two weeks is long enough to produce binding callus, and what appears as a gross deformity will ultimately become smooth and satisfactorily aligned.

FRACTURES IN CHILDREN

Fractures of the clavicle are common in children and nearly half occur before the age of seven. Usually it is a greenstick fracture without serious displacement. The diagnosis often is not obvious, but a history can usually be obtained. The mother has noticed that the child is crying after being picked up from a fall and that he appears hurt. The child does not use the arm naturally and cries when moving it. Examination is sometimes difficult and the child may have to be held by the parents. Investigation demonstrates a little unevenness along the upper border, but there is not the characteristic deformity or extensive displacement that is commonly seen in adults.

Treatment. The fracture is treated by reduction and fixation as in adults, but extensive physiotherapy is not needed since there is no difficulty in restoring function at this age. If displacement is minimal, a well protected plaster cross is applied. If there is any significant displacement, it is preferable to give a light anesthetia and gently lever the fragments into the position and hold them with criss-cross plaster. It is not necessary to have the accurate alignment that is sought in adults; the fracture in children heals readily and without residual deformity. Fixation is not necessary for longer than three weeks. A large massive callus may form but it fades quickly without significant sequelae.

FRACTURES IN ADULTS

The clavicle derives its name from *clavis* or key because it is double curved. This configuration plays an important part in localizing the fracture site. Fractures result from falls in which weight has been taken on the outstretched arm or on the point of the shoulder. Force tends to follow the curves, changing as the bone shape alters at the junction of outer and middle thirds. The criss-cross shape shifts from flat to cylindrical at this point too. These two properties favor force dispersal and the bone shatters in this zone, accounting for the typical localization of fractures in this region (Fig. 13–37). The usual displacement results from pull of the muscles at either end; the inner fragment is pulled up and the outer fragment downward and forward (Fig. 13–38).

Diagnosis and Treatment. There is little difficulty in diagnosing this injury. Deformity is obvious and often out of proportion to the amount of discomfort. The principles of treatment are reduction, fixation and restoration of function. No matter what form of reduction and fixation are followed, the last consideration is equally important but tends to be overlooked in many fractures. It is not good enough to have the clavicle heal solidly if the patient is left with a painful stiff shoulder or hand. The stability of the shoulder girdle is important, but the vital contribution of shoulder motion to enabling us to use our hands must always be kept in mind.

EMERGENCY TREATMENT. A triangular sling is applied to support the extremity with the elbow flexed at a right angle. The strap of the sling is carried over the opposite shoulder. If available, a cotton pad is placed in the axilla and a bandage is placed around the pad, holding the arm at the side. In all injuries to the upper extremities the function of the nerves and vessels of the hand should be established before any treatment is started. Methods of treatment available include (1) clavicular cross, (2) plaster support, (3) open reduction (medullary wires, tied wires), and (4) recumbency.

Reduction. The mechanism of injury and deformity are the clues to this method of reduction. The shoulder is lifted back and up to restore the alignment. So often the upward lift is the only effort and the need for backward pull is overlooked. Under a local anesthetic, after widely infiltrating the area, the operator gently elevates the girdle under the elbow and with the opposite hand holds the point of the shoulder backward. In this way the clavicle is molded into position by pressure on the inner fragment. Fixation is then applied. In the case of operative reduction the same maneuver of elevation and backward angulation reduces the deformity.

Fixation. Yoke Dressing. Some form of yoke dressing has been a standard method of fixation. A figure-of-eight bandage is applied about the shoulders but must be pulled tightly to exert enough leverage to retain reduction (Fig. 13–39). In many cases this must be so snug that it produces uncomfortable pressure in the axillae. If it is not snug the fracture is not held well. Frequently the bandage needs to be reapplied every four or five days and held by adhesive or it becomes loose. It is felt that this method is applicable only in patients with minimal displacement. If this type of fixation is used, plaster is preferable.

The reduction is carried out as just outlined and a bandage applied. This is then supported by a plaster dressing carried up the neck a little as a collar so that the shoulder tip is held back properly in the reduced

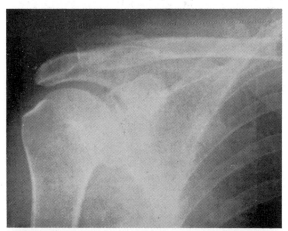
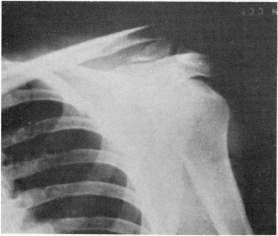

Figure 13–37 Multiple views are necessary to show some fractures of the clavicle. Fracture is not apparent here until superoinferior view is seen.

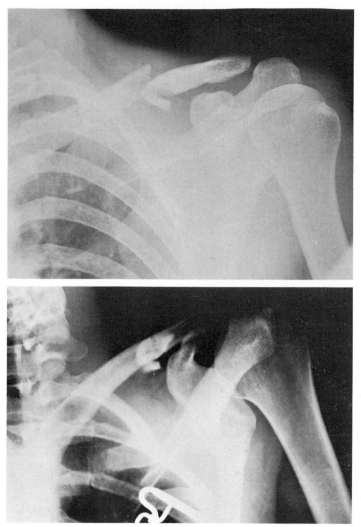

Figure 13–38   Midshaft fracture of clavicle before and after reduction using plaster platform technique.

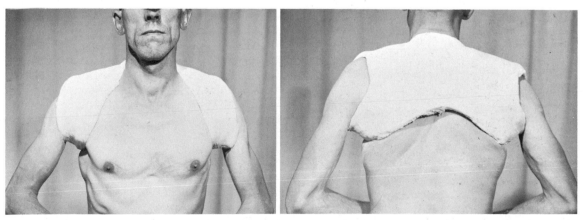

Figure 13–39   Plaster yoke dressing.

position. The fixation is left in place until the fracture is solid; in children three weeks are sufficient, but in older people four to six weeks are needed. The extent of union is judged by the patient's comfort, by lack of crepitus and by satisfactory x-ray evidence. At about four weeks the plaster dressing becomes loose and the examiner can palpate the clavicle, feeling along its length through the skin. If it can be pressed upon or gently moved without pain or crepitus, it is sufficiently firm to allow removal of the cast.

Plaster Platform. An alternative method which is useful in some cases with more severe displacement is the plaster platform. This technique is applicable when the lateral fragment is grossly depressed and there is considerable deformity. The principle is to immobilize the shoulder by fixing the arm to the body at the level of the iliac crest. In this way deformity is corrected and the clavicle is securely immobilized. Ordinary methods such as a shoulder spica do not hold the clavicle still. If a secure hold about the iliac crest is provided, it is possible to anchor the arm and forearm to it in the correct position so that the clavicle is securely fixed (Fig. 13–40).

The plaster platform is constructed by starting with a snug band of plaster applied

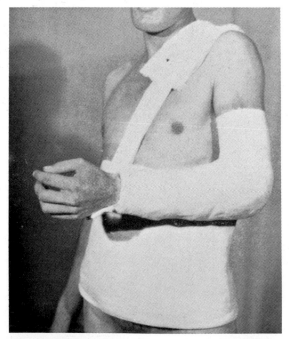

Figure 13–40 Plaster platform technique for fracture of the clavicle. Fracture shown before and after reduction as in Fig. 423.

across the iliac crest like a belt about 12 to 18 inches in width. This band is broad enough to grasp the iliac crest snugly and is molded to fit firmly. The fracture site is infiltrated with a local anesthetic and the arm is gently lifted by pressure under the elbow. In this position the point of the shoulder is hoisted upward and the deformity is corrected. At this level a platform or ledge is applied to the prepared body portion so that the arm is held at the desired level. When this is in place two holes are cut in the belt on the opposite side close to the top, front and back. Through these a fabric strap is inserted. The strap passes over the shoulder on a pad directly over the inner third of the clavicle and is tightened in this position. When the strap is tightened it shoves the inner third of the clavicle down and pulls the outer third of the clavicle up because of its grip through the plaster platform on the elbow and shoulder. The advantages of this method are that a good reduction can be obtained; the immobilization is relatively comfortable; and the wrist and fingers are free, preventing stiffness. The disadvantage is that it is a somewhat cumbersome appliance and it is difficult to fit ordinary clothes over it without some little inconvenience.

The fixation is left in place for four to six weeks. Sometimes it is necessary to adjust the tension a little if the plaster slips on the iliac crest. This is easily done by inserting another layer of felt under the elbow or tightening the shoulder strap.

Recumbency. In young women and in fractures without comminution or disfiguring deformity, a good result can be obtained by simple recumbency. The patient is kept in bed with a small sandbag between the shoulders, which allows the point of the shoulder to settle downward and backward. It is important to remember that if one embarks on this program a full three weeks of recumbency is necessary and the rules must be followed strictly. Difficulty arises in keeping the patient in bed for this length of time and retaining the initial satisfactory reduction. The tendency is to allow these patients up too soon, which results in recurrence of some deformity.

Operative Fixation. All simple fractures of the clavicle may be treated by closed reduction. Those cases with considerable comminution or delay in fixation should be treated by operation and internal fixation. There are several methods available, depending upon extent of the comminution and the surgeon's preference and experience.

Medullary Wiring. This is a good method of treating fractures of the clavicle, but one should have some experience in the use of wires. The principle is to reduce the fragments as outlined previously and to transfix the fracture with a stout Kirschner wire. The wire is fixed in the cortex at either end rather than lying loose in the medullary cavity (Fig. 13–41). Only those who are expert in the technique can do it under local anesthetic blindly or with the aid of x-ray. Considerable experience is necessary to use it in this way. It is preferable to do an open reduction under the usual operating room conditions and to expose the fracture properly. A suitable Kirschner wire is inserted through the outer fragment so that it comes out the skin laterally. The fragments are then accurately reduced and held by the assistant with a clamp. The surgeon then drills the wire back across the fracture line until it is fixed in the medial fragment. The wire may be left protruding through the skin to be removed at a later date or it may be cut flush with the bone so that it does not need to be removed. The advantages of this method are that it provides secure fixation and accurate reduction and avoids immobilization of the rest of the extremity. The disadvantages are that it is an operative procedure and considerable skill is necessary to do it properly (Fig. 13–42).

Tied Wire Fixation. The alternative and sometimes preferable method is to expose the fracture site, reduce the fragments accurately and then fix them by a No. 20- or 22-gauge wire which is tied snugly (Fig. 13–43). If there is any degree of comminution this is the procedure of choice because small fragments may be aligned accurately and firm fixation provided. The disadvantages are those of an open operation and a small scar. The cosmetic appearance, however, is a consideration only in the young female.

COMPLICATIONS OF FRACTURES OF THE CLAVICLE

Early Complications. In very severe injuries, usually patients whose clavicle has been broken by direct contact violence, there may be damage of the brachial plexus and subclavian vessels. The neurovascular bundle streams out of the thoracic outlet under the clavicle on top of the first rib. At this point

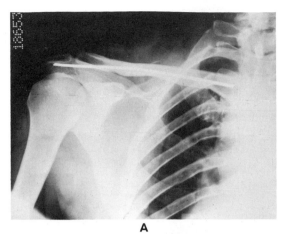

A

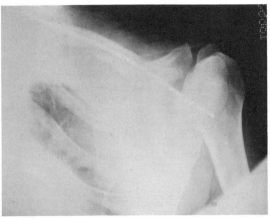

B

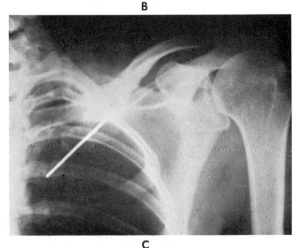

C

Figure 13–41 Single wire used in fracture of the clavicle. *A,* and *B,* In position. *C,* Wire has wandered because the end was not turned or a threaded wire used.

as it goes under the clavicle it is protected by a strong cylindrical medial bar of the clavicle so that considerable trauma is necessary to damage the plexus and break the clavicle at the same time. Sometimes direct violence, in breaking the clavicle, also fractures ribs so

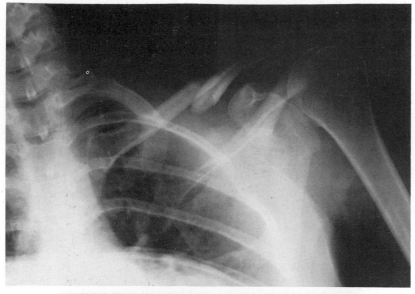

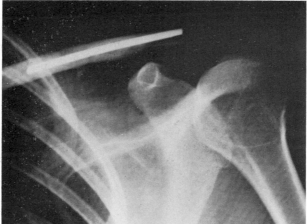

Figure 13–42 Open reduction and threaded wire fixations of the clavicle.

that pneumothorax or hemothorax is an added complication. When the force is severe enough to break the clavicle and damage the plexus, injury to subclavian vessels is common. This combination is a grave injury to the extremity.

Pathology of Combined Bone and Vessel Injury. The force comes from above or from the front and above to strike the clavicle. If it is applied from above and posteriorly, the brunt is taken on the scapula and the thick padding of posterior scapular muscles. This is a more common injury because workmen or others seeing the potential injury from a falling object run away, and it is the posterior aspect that is exposed. The clavicular injury is different. The bone breaks

the force, but as the force continues the subclavian vessels are torn as they arch over the first rib, which is used as a fulcrum (Fig. 13–44). The nerve damage, however, is at a higher site. As the force is applied the acromiomastoid division is increased so that the nerves are stretched along their length with the fulcrum of maximum tension then being the transverse process of the cervical vertebrae. The roots are torn above the clavicle or may be avulsed from their attachment to the cord.

TREATMENT. The most serious component is the vascular damage, and this should be attended to first, leaving the fracture and nerve injury until later. In many of these the vessel injury comes under control with con-

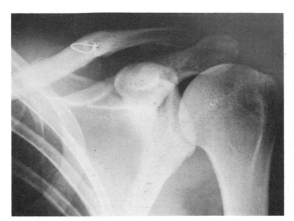

Figure 13-43 Comminuted fracture of the clavicle treated by open reduction and tied wire fixation.

servative measures, including complete bedrest, sedatives, strapping the arm at the side and the usual antishock treatment. The general condition, as indicated by pulse, blood pressure and general shock symptoms, and the swelling are indications of the progress or control of the bleeding. The pulse is often lost, but sufficient collateral circulation is usually established to nourish the extremity. Indications for exploration of the vessels are progressive swelling and shock which occur early. The first part of the subclavian artery is exposed and ligated. If the patient's condition allows, the fracture is fixed with a tied wire suture at the same time.

The nerve damage is left for consideration until later for several reasons. Since the site of nerve damage is usually much higher, the neck needs to be explored. This is not possible at the time of injury because of the patient's condition. Meticulous dissection is necessary for nerve freeing or suturing, and the extensive hematoma makes this difficult in the early stages. When the acute reaction has subsided it is possible also to obtain a more accurate impression of the specific roots involved and so plan exploration more minutely. For these reasons exploration is better left for three or four weeks. The technique has been described in the chapter on nerve injuries.

Late Complications. These are more common and include malunion and pressure from excessive callus.

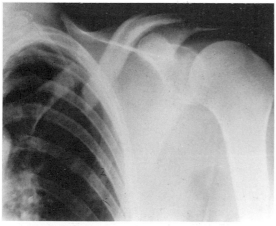

A

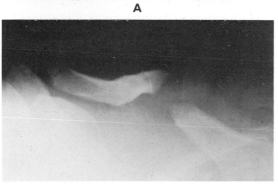

B

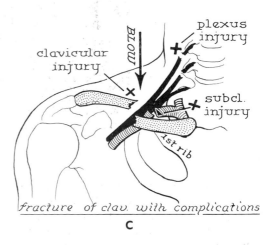

C

Figure 13-44 Fracture of the clavicle. *A* and *B*, Fractures of medial third of clavicle. *C*, Mechanism of neurovascular complications.

MALUNION OF THE CLAVICLE. Many fractures of the clavicle unite with a little alteration of normal alignment and some shortening (Fig. 13–45). This results from the point of the shoulder falling forward, buckling the fracture line. The disability is a cosmetic one only. There is rarely significant interference with function. If it is recognized early it may be adjusted by manipulation of the fracture fragments. Later, osteotomy is performed if the deformity warrants. When this is done the fracture should be supported with a bone graft similar to that described in the treatment of nonunion. Exuberant callus is common but rarely of sufficient severity that removal is necessary. Shortly after solidification of the fracture most of the excess callus gradually disappears, and some months later it is common to have very little remain of a once obvious knob.

NONUNION OF THE CLAVICLE. Nonunion of the clavicle for a long time has been regarded as a rare complication, possibly because of the greater frequency of this fracture in young people. As more of these injuries have been encountered in the older age group, the incidence of nonunion has increased. Secure immobilization apart from open reduction is difficult to obtain in the clavicle. Accurate assessment of union is also difficult. These two factors contribute to the increase of this complication (Fig. 13–46).

Technique of Bone Grafting of Clavicle. The fracture site is approached through a transverse incision parallel with the clavicle on the

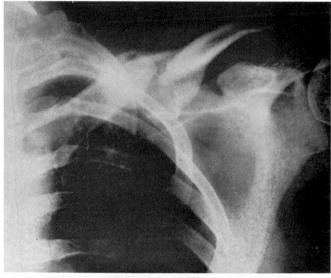

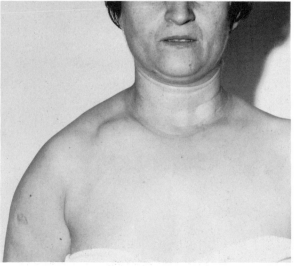

Figure 13–45 Malunion of the clavicle with excess callus formation.

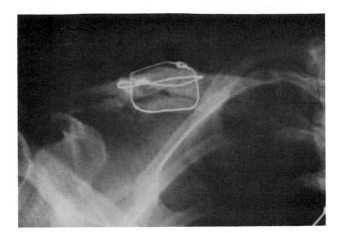

Figure 13-46 Nonunion of the clavicle treated by iliac graft and wire fixation.

superior surface. The fragments are exposed by subperiosteal dissection and aligned satisfactorily. The abnormal position usually encountered is downward and forward slipping of the outer fragment. This is corrected by levering this piece backward and lifting it up. The fragments are wedged into position and held by bone-holding forceps. Debridement and alignment of the fragments are done carefully to avoid damage to the subclavian vessels lying directly below. In compound injuries, gunshot wounds for example, the scar must be separated very carefully. It is not unusual for callus on the inferior aspect to become adherent to the adjacent soft tissue, and it is possible to tear the subclavian vessels on elevating or freeing the fracture fragments. After suitable alignment is obtained a graft is removed from the iliac crest, which the author prefers to fix to the fragments with a tied wire suture. The graft is applied along the posterior or posteroinferior surface and, as the knob is tightened, the fragments are accurately lined, with the graft becoming snugly ap-

plied along the prepared ends. Placing the graft away from the subcutaneous surface avoids exuberant callus. The technique of insertion of the wire suture is carried out carefully. Holes are dilled through the fragments and the graft so that the single loop holds both. Use of a perforated Kirschner wire facilitates this act. A single square knot is sufficient. The first portion of the knot is held with a needle driver while the second part is applied and drawn taut. As the knot is tightened the graft becomes snug and acts as a splint, contributing to the fixation of the fracture site. The arm is fixed in an iliac forearm type of plaster or body swathe. Fixation is continued until the fracture is solid, usually eight to 12 weeks.

Complete Defects in the Clavicle. Compound injuries, gunshot wounds in particular, may leave segments of the clavicle missing. In some instances this does not constitute significant impairment since the scar tissue forms a degree of support (Fig. 13–47). In others an excessive degree of mobility is contributed, requiring bridging of the gap.

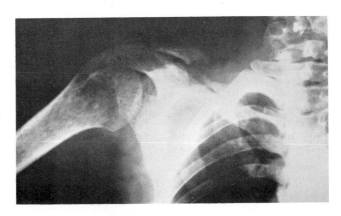

Figure 13-47 Traumatic defect of clavicle left untreated. No excessive instability in an elderly patient.

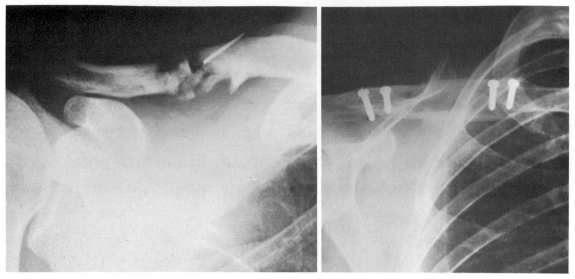

Figure 13–48 Complete defect of the clavicle treated by dual tibial grafts and screw fixation.

The lesion occurs most often in the middle third of the clavicle with a gap of ½ inch or more between the ends (Fig. 13–48). The pseudoarthrosis which remains may cause little disability, but usually weakness and instability necessitate reconstruction.

Technique. Dual iliac grafts are satisfactory and are placed to bridge the defect applied in onlay fashion at each end (Fig. 13–48). The ends are secured with tied wire sutures and immobilization is in an iliac arm plaster. Fixation is necessary for at least 16 weeks. Tibial cortical grafts with screw fixation may also be used and form a satisfactory alternative.

Fractures of the Outer End of the Clavicle

Fractures of the outer end of the clavicle are seen next in frequency to those of the midshaft zone. They usually result from direct violence and comprise a group of several specific types. A common deformity is a splintering of the lateral tip of extension of the fracture, often into the acromioclavicular joint (Fig. 13–49). Very little displacement of the fragment occurs and there is no instability of the acromioclavicular zone. A further type of greater importance is a transverse fracture, which really simulates acromioclavicular dislocation (Fig. 13–50). In some instances considerable instability results in this type of fracture.

Treatment. When there is minimal displacement all that is necessary is to support the arm in a sling for two to four weeks. When the fracture line is of the transverse type, simulating suspensory ligament impairment, the fracture should be stabilized by wire fixation to avoid recurrence insta-

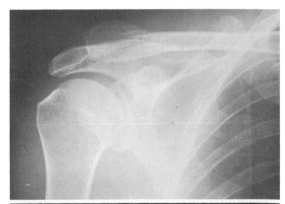

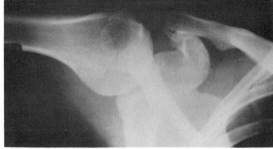

Figure 13–49 Fractures of outer end of clavicle. Simple comminution without displacement.

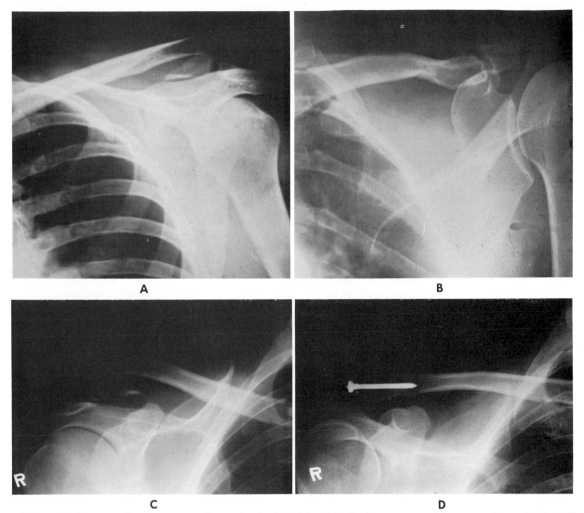

Figure 13–50 *A* and *B*, Fractures of outer end of clavicle with displacement requiring operative reduction. *C*, Displacement before reduction. *D*, After reduction and screw fixation.

bility. In some instances a small separated fragment which involves the acromioclavicular joint and which is well lateral to the suspensory ligament area may be excised, correcting the deformity and preventing any further acromioclavicular complications.

Fractures of the Sternal End of the Clavicle

These fractures are uncommon and result from direct force supplied at an angle from the lateral side causing splintering of the sternal end. It may be recalled that the sternal end is a thick strong cylindrical tube so that considerable trauma is necessary to break the clavicle at this point. It is more

common to encounter severe crush or "stave-in" injuries in which the adjacent portion of the sternal notch, sternum and rib elements are depressed rather than the inner end of the clavicle breaking. These constitute serious injuries. Fractures result in minimal deformity because of the splinting effect of the costoclavicular ligament below and the fascial suspension of the sternomastoid above and in front. These two forces tend to control the deformity.

Treatment. When there is significant deformity such as displacement of the splinters they are replaced by gentle pressure, with the patient under a general anesthetic. Adhesive or Elastoplast dressing is sufficient fixation. If any pieces are grossly displaced they should be excised.

Dislocations of the Acromioclavicular Joint

Dislocation of the acromioclavicular joint is a not uncommon injury, particularly in athletes. Three separate grades may be identified: acromioclavicular subluxation, acromioclavicular dislocation, and acromioclavicular dislocation with rupture of suspensory ligaments.

Acromioclavicular Subluxation. In this injury the outer end of the clavicle wrenches free of its capsular attachments and comes to ride slightly above the acromion. After a fall a sudden pain is experienced, followed by a swelling in the joint area and limitation of motion. Tenderness may be localized at the acromioclavicular joint, and there is increased mobility both superoinferiorly and anteroposteriorly which can be verified by x-ray. However, the displacement is not to a degree equal to the thickness of the clavicle, which separates this group from the succeeding type of dislocation. The clavicle has a springy action when pressed with the examining finger, but this is not excessive (Fig. 13–51).

TREATMENT. Such injuries may be treated conservatively by use of a soft tissue type of dressing which applies pressure over the lateral end of the clavicle and under the elbow, towing the elbow up and pressing the medial aspect. This may be supplied by adhesive strapping or by one of the commercial devices that is a fabric strap type of sling.

Acromioclavicular Dislocation. The more severe degree of acromioclavicular injury is one in which there has been sufficient disruption of the joint to allow the clavicle to be displaced in a superior fashion to approximately its own thickness, indicating that the retaining capsular structures have been ruptured. X-ray examination shows the lateral end of the clavicle to be clearly popping up above the acromion.

These injuries are identified by the deformity, the pain at the acromioclavicular site, and the bouncing looseness of the lateral end of the clavicle in a superoinferior fashion. A further element is some slight anteroposterior instability of the clavicle, but this is not extensive.

TREATMENT. Most of these injuries are best treated by some form of wire fixation. In this fashion secure immobilization is provided.

Technique. A light general anesthetic is preferable but a local can be used if desired. The patient is placed in the supine position, and two wires are threaded through the acromion, across the joint into the clavicle. The wires are inserted in criss-cross fashion (Fig. 13–52). The first wire starts a little toward the posterior surface of the acromion at a point where a good purchase in the bone may be obtained. The clavicle is held in a reduced position by the assistant and the wire is drilled into the cortex. The first wire usually just holds the dislocation and may catch only a quarter of the clavicle. This is used as the fixing wire. Second and third wires are then inserted more accurately and extend a little farther along the clavicle. They are carried along for 1½ to 2 inches. Care must be taken in guiding them. They are inserted from below upward rather than from above downward to avoid the great vessels. It is never necessary to insert the wires so far along the clavicle that the vessels might be damaged. The first wire is removed, leaving the second and third wires in place in the clavicle. If threaded wires are used, they may be left just under the skin. If ordinary Kirschner wires are used, they should be left outside the skin and the ends bent at a right angle or fixed with a small cross-bar such as is used on external fixation

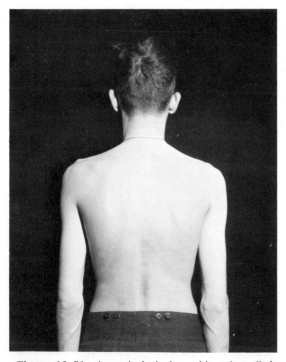

Figure 13–51 Acromioclavicular subluxation. Only conservative treatment is required.

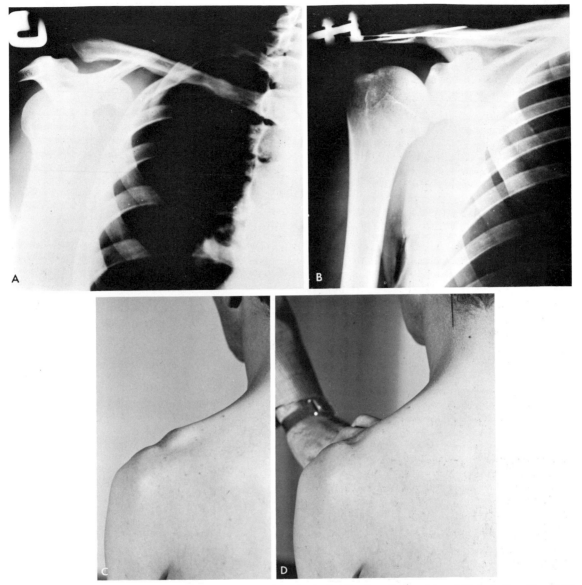

Figure 13–52 Acromioclavicular dislocation treated by dual wire fixation. Before (*A* and *C*) and after (*B* and *D*) reduction and fixation.

apparatus for jaws. Four weeks is usually sufficient fixation time. Just as in intramedullary wiring for fractures of the clavicle, fixation of the end of the wire to prevent wandering is most important if a threaded wire is not used.

Complete Acromioclavicular Dislocation. A more severe degree of this injury may be recognized in which there is a frank dislocation of the lateral end of the clavicle with partial or complete rupture of the suspensory ligaments. This is recognized by the greater deformity and the dropping down of the shoulder (Figure 13–51). More impor-

tantly, considerable anteroposterior instability can be demonstrated in these injuries by grasping the acromion and clavicle and exerting alternate anterior and posterior pressure. When the suspensory ligaments are torn, not only is there an upward displacement of the clavicle but there is a downward and forward displacement of the acromion, carrying the upper limb with it.

Frequently the x-rays show some calcification along the upper aspect of the coracoid which is due to trauma involving the suspensory ligaments avulsing periosteum.

TREATMENT. More precise treatment is

essential in these injuries and some form of internal fixation is required.

Two methods have been advanced which are effective in providing improved fixation. One is the method of Bosworth, which is a lag screw fixation from the clavicle to the coracoid, and the other is suggested by Aldredge and consists of tied wire fixation of the clavicle and coracoid.

Technique. A superior incision is used starting behind the acromioclavicular joint and extending over the clavicle to the coracoid. The acromioclavicular joint is explored and any debris is removed and the acromioclavicular capsule repaired. If it is feasible the conoid and trapezoid ligaments are identified and sutures inserted which are tied after either the screw or the wire has been inserted. Using the Bosworth screw, a $3/16$ inch hole is drilled from the clavicle into the base of the coracoid; a lag screw is inserted and tightened until the clavicle is at the level of the acromion, and then the sutures of the suspensory ligament are fixed.

In using the tied wire suture the loop is inserted around the clavicle and under the coracoid, with two loops being inserted and then tightened with a pair of wire tiers, thereby effectively reducing the acromioclavicular dislocation.

In all instances the Bosworth screw needs to be removed some eight weeks after insertion to avoid fracture of the clavicle. Frequent examples of fracture have been seen when the screw has been retained because of the rotatory stress which abduction and circumduction place on the clavicle. In most instances the tied wire fixation is removed also because of its limiting effect on the clavicular rotation, although this may not always be essential (Fig. 13–53).

When there has been disruption of the suspensory ligaments, the author prefers to replace the ligament by a new fascial ligament extending from the coracoid to the clavicle and to the spine of the scapula. The method is applicable in acute injuries in which there has been rupture and is also effective in chronic or recurrent acromioclavicular dislocation. This method is described in the next section.

Chronic or Recurrent Acromioclavicular Dislocation.

Most injuries of this type heal well with the methods which have been outlined. When the suspensory ligaments do not heal or the dislocation persists because of inadequate treatment, considerable disability

may result (Fig. 13–54). When these ligaments are torn, the strut effect of the clavicle is lost so that the point of the shoulder drops downward and inward. After a time both local and radiating discomfort may develop. Local pain and limitation of movement arise from the distortion of the acromioclavicular joint. Radiating symptoms develop from pressure traction of the neurovascular bundle beneath the coracoid. For these reasons it is desirable to reconstruct the ligaments and restore the suspensory effect (Fig. 13–55).

CORACOBRACHIALIS TENDON FIXATION. An ingenious and effective procedure has been introduced by Vargas in which the principle is to restore the coracoclavicular strut by utilizing the fascial covering of the coracobrachialis or the short head of the biceps. Other techniques are those of Neviaser and the author.

Vargas Technique. The acromioclavicular region is approached through an anterior longitudinal incision extending from the top of the clavicle distally over the coracoid and along the inner margin of the biceps for 6 inches (Fig. 13–56). The subjacent clavicle and the coracoid process are exposed. The coracobrachialis and the short head of the biceps are identified; these muscles are traced distally and a band of fascia separated from the anterior surface. The band of fascia is about 1 inch wide and is cut as far distally as good fascial tissue is available. This strip is then reflected proximally, preserving its attachment to the coracoid. A hole is then drilled through the clavicle just above the coracoid and in the area of the conoid and trapezoid ligaments. The prepared strip is then split in two and half is threaded through the clavicle. The acromioclavicular dislocation is reduced and, as it is held in this position by the assistant, the two strips are tied together, restoring the ligament. Usually the fascial fixation is supported by insertion of two Kirschner wires through the acromion into the clavicle such as is carried out in fresh dislocations. This technique allows freedom of movement of the arm and hand during the period of immobilization (Fig. 13–57). Fixation is carried out for six weeks (Fig. 13–58). The one disadvantage of the technique is that sometimes the strip of fascia which is obtained from the anterior surface of the biceps is short or may be somewhat deficient, or difficulty is encountered in stripping it.

Neviaser Technique. An ingenious and very

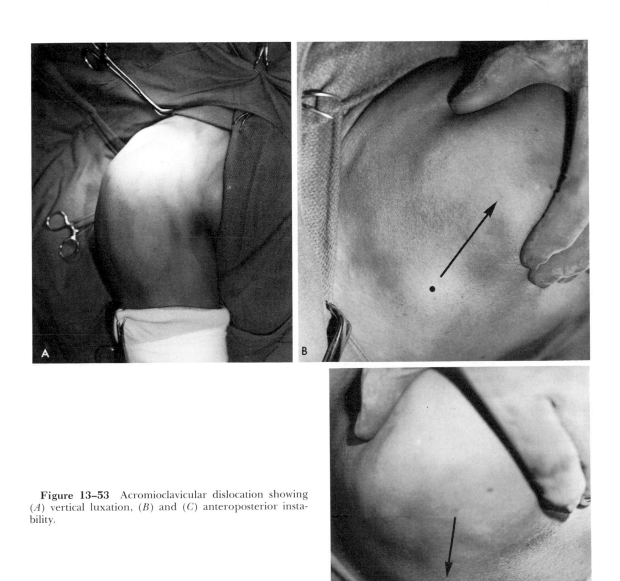

Figure 13–53 Acromioclavicular dislocation showing (*A*) vertical luxation, (*B*) and (*C*) anteroposterior instability.

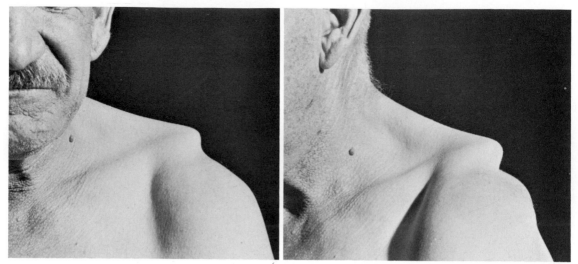

Figure 13–54 Longstanding acromioclavicular dislocation. Note downward and forward dislocation from suspensory ligament rupture.

satisfactory method of controlling acromioclavicular dislocation has been suggested by Dr. Neviaser. The principle is to use the coraco-acromial ligament, which is separated from its coracoid attachment and reflected proximally to be sutured into the clavicle under tension. As indicated in Figure 13–59, the fixation is then held in place with a Kirschner wire.

Bateman Technique. In some instances of complete dislocation with rupture of the suspensory ligaments the anterior luxation in addition to the superoinferior displacement is considerable. In these circumstances the likelihood of neurovascular compression is much greater (Fig. 13–60). For this reason the author prefers a method in which there is reconstruction of the conoid and trapezoid ligaments with a piece of fascia; in turn, the fascia, after being attached to the clavicle, is carried posteriorly to the spine of the scapula so that the alignment of the clavicle is restored by being pulled backward as well as downward.

In these injuries, particularly when acute, the degree of anterior luxation is surprising if it is assessed under anesthesia. In the method of Bosworth, or any other method which pulls the clavicle forward, this anteroposterior luxation is ignored.

A superoinferior incision is made in the usual fashion just medial to the acromioclavicular joint and extending from ½ inch above the spine of the scapula across the clavicle to the region of the coracoid. Through this incision the spine of the scapula is ex-

posed over a distance of about ½ inch mediolaterally; the coracoid process is exposed, and the scapula is denuded of soft tissue over a ½ inch region at about the point of the suspensory ligament attachment.

A piece of fascia ¾ inch in width and at least 6 inches in length is removed from the opposite thigh. A knot is tied in the piece of

(Text continued on page 433)

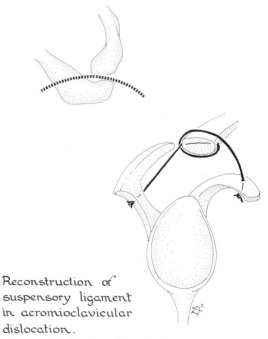

Reconstruction of suspensory ligament in acromioclavicular dislocation.

Figure 13–55 Plan of repair of suspensory ligaments with fascia and restoration of anteroposterior relationship of the clavicle in grade 3 dislocation.

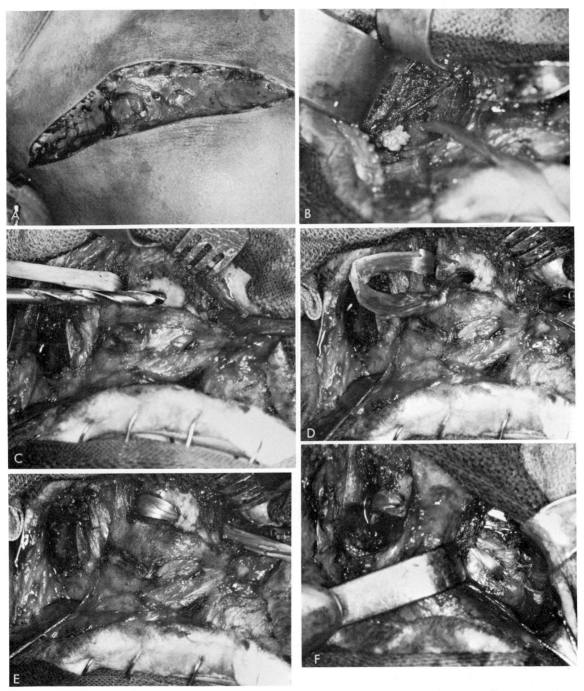

Figure 13–56 Steps in fascia reconstruction of acromioclavicular dislocation and suspensory ligament rupture. *A,* Superoanterior incision. *B,* Fascia is anchored by a knot in the spine of the scapula and pulled up over the clavicle. *C,* Preparation of hole in clavicle. *D,* Insertion of fascia through and around the clavicle from the back to the front. *E* and *F,* Fascia fixed through the coracoid anteriorly, restoring the ligament.

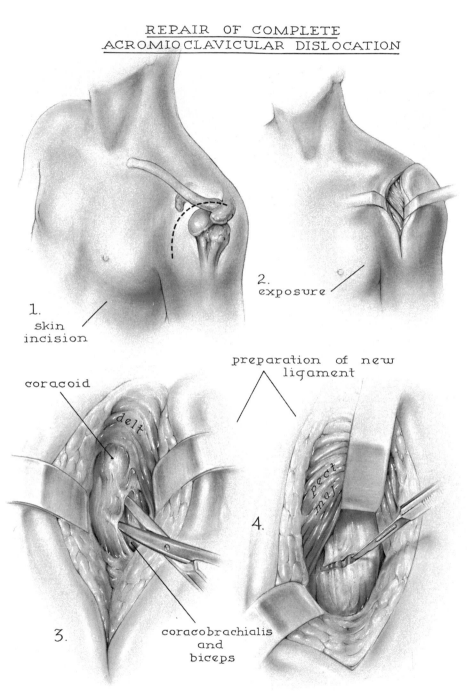

REPAIR OF COMPLETE
ACROMIOCLAVICULAR DISLOCATION

1.
skin
incision

2.
exposure

coracoid

preparation of new
ligament

delt

pect.
maj.

3.

4.

coracobrachialis
and
biceps

Figure 13–57 Technique of repair of recurred acromioclavicular dislocation (Vargas). 1, Incision. 2 and 3, Exposure of superficial aspect of coracobrachialis and short head of biceps. 4, Preparation of the new ligament from the common tendon. 5 and 6, The new ligament is reflected proximally. 7 to 11, The new ligament is anchored in the clavicle.

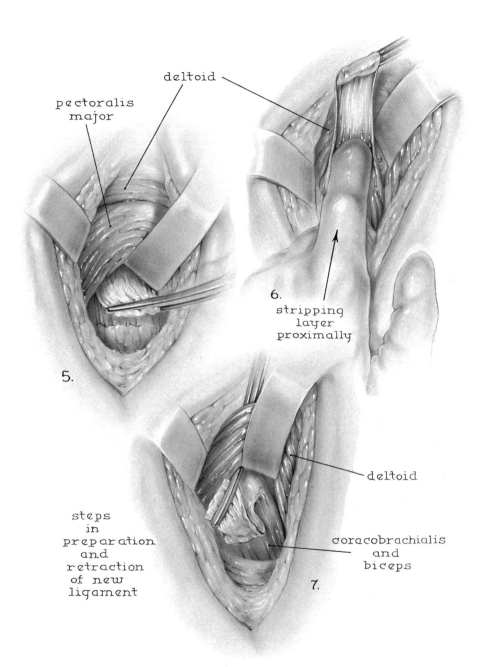

Figure 13–57 *Continued.*

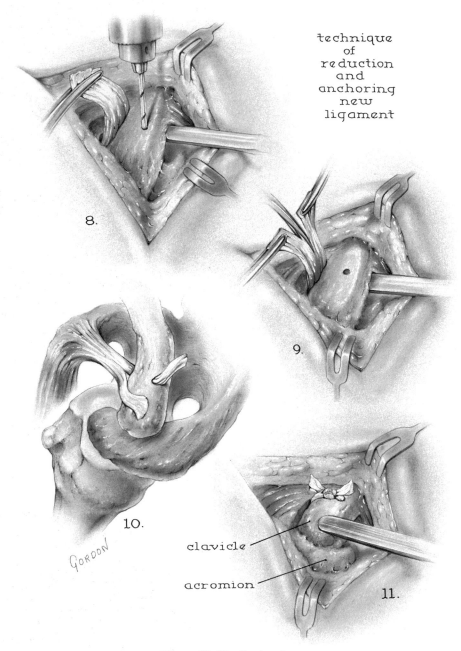

technique
of
reduction
and
anchoring
new
ligament

8.

9.

10.

GORDON

clavicle

acromion

11.

Figure 13–57 *Continued.*

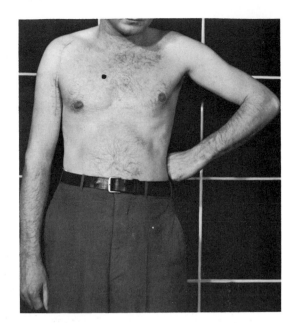

Figure 13–58 Postoperative result of Vargas procedure.

fascia and it is anchored through the spine of the scapula. The fascia is then brought beneath the muscle up over the clavicle, wrapped around the clavicle and taken through the ³/₁₆ inch hole drilled in the clavicle. The fascia is then brought downward and forward to the coracoid and anchored through a further hole in the coracoid. In this fashion the suspensory ligaments are restored, the acromioclavicular dislocation is reduced, and the anteroposterior luxation of the clavicle is corrected.

In chronic or recurrent dislocations there has often been deterioration of the joint so that it may be necessary to excise the outer half inch of the clavicle, carrying out an acromioclavicular arthroplasty in the usual fashion. It should be emphasized that simple excision of the outer end of the clavicle in this grade of acromioclavicular dislocation is not enough. As a rule, the instability from the loss of the suspensory ligament creates a deformity which is a significant impairment (Fig. 13–61); it should be repaired appropriately.

DISLOCATIONS OF THE STERNOCLAVICULAR JOINT

The medial end of the clavicle is much more securely fixed than the lateral end so

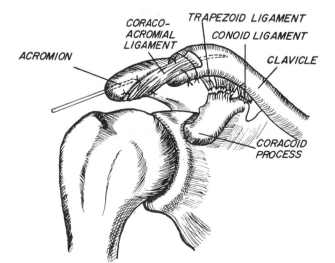

Figure 13–59 Technique devised by Dr. J. S. Neviaser.

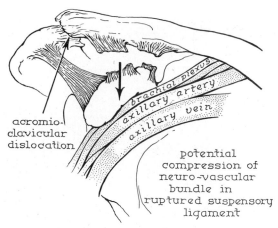

Figure 13–60 Pressure may develop on the neuro-vascular bundle from persistent suspensory ligament rupture.

that dislocation is not nearly so frequent. The mechanism of injury is a blow applied from the back and laterally so that the medial end is shoved upward and outward (Fig. 13–62). Very rarely the medial end may be pushed beneath the sternum.

TREATMENT.

Fresh Injuries. The principle of reduction is to apply sufficient leverage to lift the bulbous medial end back into the socket. A general anesthetic is necessary. The shoulder is pulled backward and pressure is exerted on the front and the top of the clavicle with the opposite hand. Usually it slips back into place with a thud. The reduction is retained by application of a clavicular cross, keeping the point of the shoulder in the extended position. A compression dressing is applied

over the medial end of the clavicle. Fixation is continued for four weeks (Fig. 13–63).

Old Injuries. Neglected and recurrent dislocations may cause no more disability than that resulting from an altered appearance. In most instances some posttraumatic sterno-clavicular arthritis develops. When symptoms warrant it, the medial end of the clavicle may be resected; if there has been no progressive joint damage, the medial end may be replaced in the socket and a fascial sling inserted to snub it into place.

Technique. A transverse incision is made 3 inches in length and centered over the acromioclavicular joint. The scar tissue and capsular debris are removed and the sternal end of the clavicle returned to the socket in the sternum. A piece of fascia $3/8$ inch in width is removed from the opposite thigh and inserted in figure-of-eight fashion through drill holes in the clavicle and sternum. Drill holes of $3/16$ inch are inserted in the sternum with care and extended obliquely from the midline toward the socket. A periosteal elevator is inserted to prevent the drill from progressing too far. A transverse hole is drilled in the medial end of the clavicle approximately $1/4$ inch from the end and about $1/4$ inch below the cortex. The fascia is inserted through the drill holes in the sternum with the loop medially and the two ends brought out through the joint and then criss-crossed and tied through the hole in the clavicle. In this fashion pressure is exerted downward and inward, snubbing the clavicle in place. Fixation in a clavicular cross is continued for a period of six weeks.

Omer Technique. Some authors have recommended that, in addition to the fascial

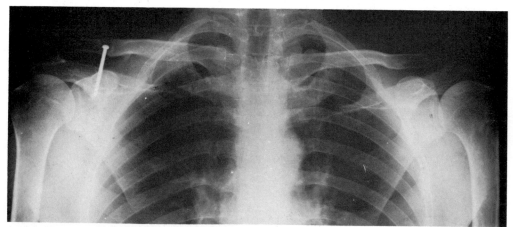

Figure 13–61 Screw fixation for acromioclavicular dislocation. Note fracture through clavicle. Screw should be removed postoperatively.

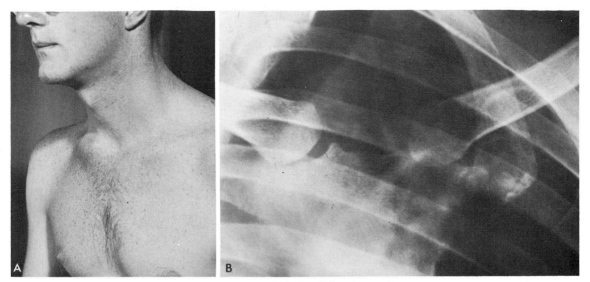

Figure 13-62 *A*, Acute sternoclavicular dislocation. *B*, X-ray appearance.

reconstruction of the ligaments, a step oste-otomy be cut in the clavicle as described by Omer. In this technique a horizontal step osteotomy is made at the clavicular attach-ment of the sternocleidomastoid muscle, and the sternomastoid is detached from the medial segment. The osteotomy reduces the stress of the long lever on the healing sterno-clavicular joint and favors the solidification of the ligamentous reconstruction. The shortening of the clavicle reduces stress on the long lever arm.

Internal Derangement of Sternoclavicu-lar Joint. Rupture of the intra-articular

disc may occur in injuries, particularly in young athletes, which are of less severity than those causing sternoclavicular disloca-tion. The disc may be wrenched free of the sternal attachment or torn so that it protudes into the joint in a fashion similar to meniscus tears in the knee. The symptoms are local pain, a catching sensation on flexion or cir-cumduction of the arm, and a clicking sensa-tion felt by applying the palm of the hand over the sternoclavicular joint. When symp-toms are persistent the joint may be explored and the fragments removed. The capsule needs to be repaired carefully and, in some

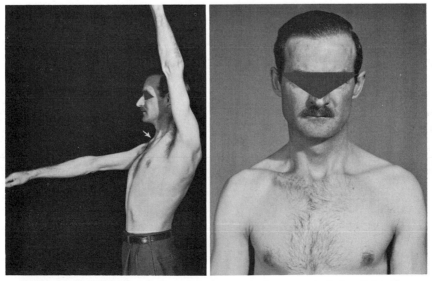

Figure 13-63 Before and after operative repair for sternoclavicular dislocation.

instances, fascial reinforcement is required because the ligament exerts a snubbing effect on the medial end of the clavicle and a degree of subluxation may ensue following its fragmentation.

FRACTURES OF THE SCAPULA

The scapula is not nearly so frequently injured as are the other two components of the shoulder girdle, the clavicle and the upper end of the humerus. The common distribution of fractures which is seen are fractures of the neck and body, fractures of the acromion, and fractures of the coracoid process.

FRACTURES OF THE NECK OF THE SCAPULA

The commonest fracture is that of the neck, which occurs as a result of falls in which the patient lands on the point of the shoulder (Fig. 13–64). The bone may give way at the base of the neck, impacting the neck into the body and leaving the glenoid intact, or the glenoid may be shattered and the fracture extend into the head and the base of the neck (Fig. 13–65). The fracture is suspected by the history of injury, local pain and tenderness and some deformity of the shoulder. When there is comminution of the neck, the point of the shoulder is flattened as a result of the medial displacement.

Treatment. In the impacted fracture, manipulation and reduction are not necessary unless shortening of the neck is sufficient to favor subluxation or interfere with abduction. These fractures are immobilized in a well fitted shoulder spica with the arm abducted in the midposition. In cases with deformity and considerable shortening of the neck, reduction should be attempted. This is accomplished by placing traction on the humerus, the principle being to bring the broken glenoid and neck back into place by tension exerted through the attachment of the shoulder capsule. The fist is placed in the axilla and used as a wedge. The point of the shoulder is levered outward over it. It may be necessary to apply a little controlled traction with the arm abducted, holding the humerus at a right angle. Fixation is carried out by application of a shoulder spica with the assistant maintaining the lateral traction. Immobilization is necessary for six to eight weeks.

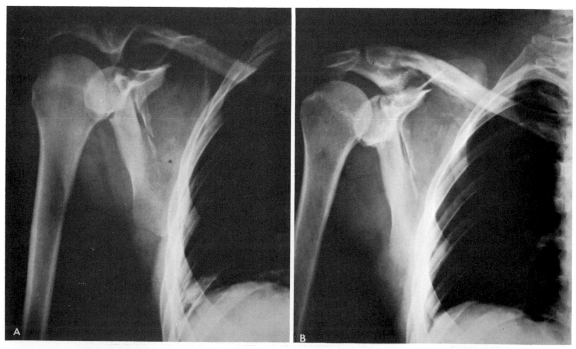

Figure 13–64   Fracture of neck of scapula. *A,* Before reduction. *B,* After reduction.

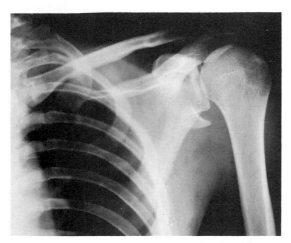

Figure 13–65 Chip fracture of the glenoid.

Comminuted fractures of the scapula are not common, but if there is gross displacement of the articular surfaces open reduction should be carried out.

TECHNIQUE.   The shoulder is approached from the posterior aspect, a longitudinal incision being made and extending from the spine distally for 4 inches. The deltoid is retracted anteriorly and laterally. The fibers of the infraspinatous are split longitudinally, exposing the posteroinferior aspect. As a rule, the fragments of the glenoid can be levered and pressed into satisfactory position. If they are unstable they may be fixed by a tied wire suture. Fixation is obtained by a shoulder spica with the arm abducted to 75 degrees. Sometimes the fragments are too small and fragile to be held adequately. Since the articular surfaces of the shoulder are not closely applied to one another and it is not a weight bearing joint, a good result with satisfactory range of motion can be expected even with considerable articular damage. The arm should be fixed in abduction to favor return of function of the abductors and rotators and to avoid inferior capsular contraction.

Restoration of Function After Fractures of the Scapula. If the shoulder has been maintained in proper position, restoration of abduction and rotation is considerably facilitated. Nonunion in these fractures is most uncommon and a period of six weeks immobilization is normally sufficient. The plaster is removed, the arm is carried in a sling, and assisted active movements are initiated and gradually increased.

FRACTURES OF THE ACROMION

The acromion serves as a protecting overhang, effectively guarding the upper angle of the humerus and rotator cuff structures. It is damaged by force applied from the back or from the back and above. Backward falls with the shoulder landing on sharp edges will produce these fractures. The usual site is at the junction of the acromion with the spine (Fig. 13–66). These fractures rarely require manipulation and heal following six weeks immobilization in a shoulder spica. A persistent epiphyseal line may be erroneously interpreted as a fracture (Fig. 13–67). The line is definitely in the acromion; there is no displacement, and often the opposite shoulder shows the same deformity. Sometimes the acromion may be sufficiently depressed that it impinges on the greater tuberosity in abduction of the arm. Under these circumstances the acromion should be gently levered upward by pressure on the elbow, using the head of the humerus as a buttress. This corrects the depression. The arm is then immobilized in an abduction plaster. It is important to immobilize the arm in full abduction in these injuries so that impingement on the coraco-acromial arch is avoided. In the neglected cases in which the acromion has formed a bent-over, beak-like obstruction, partial acromionectomy may be carried out.

FRACTURES OF THE CORACOID

The coracoid process may be avulsed by a strong muscle pull (Fig. 13–68). The attach-

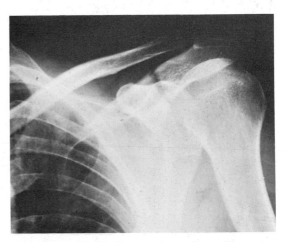

Figure 13–66 Fracture base of acromion.

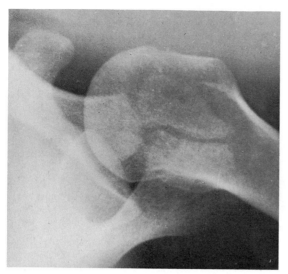

Figure 13–67 Persistent epiphyseal line of metacromion may be erroneously mistaken for a fracture. Usually the condition is bilateral.

ments of the coracobrachialis, short head of the biceps and pectoralis minor exert powerful tension so that the tip is displaced downward and medially. The resulting disability is weakness in these structures and also in the suspensory ligament. Considerable disability results from the latter. If the ligaments are involved, the injury is treated by fixation and a shoulder spica or by transfixion of the acromioclavicular joint to control subluxation. A rare complication is pressure on the neurovascular bundle, which is an added indication for open reduction and restoration of the suspensory ligaments.

Usually direct violence has fractured the coracoid. If the fracture is at the base, immobilization in a shoulder spica for six weeks is sufficient. When the damage is closer to the tip, the trauma has been applied more anteriorly so there is much greater likelihood of damage to the neurovascular bundle. The treatment of this complication dominates the situation. A splintered tip is a secondary consideration. Exploration of the nerve lesion is indicated after the posttraumatic reaction has subsided when motor and sensory systems warrant. The technique is considered in the chapter on nerve injuries.

FRACTURES OF THE CERVICAL SPINE

Many fractures of the cervical spine have serious connotations, but the gamut runs from body chips to avulsed posterior spinous processes. The serious lesions are those which are complicated by spinal cord or nerve root damage, so that the consideration of these injuries falls largely into two groups: fractures without cord implication, and fractures with cord or nerve root involvement.

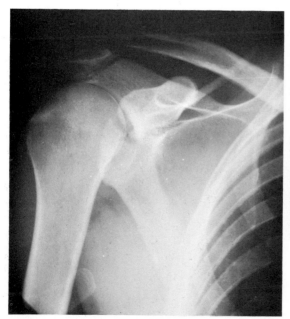

A

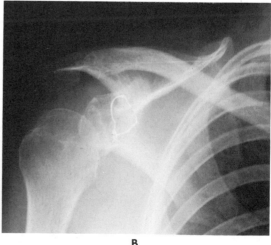

B

Figure 13–68 *A,* Fracture of coracoid. *B,* Healing following internal fixation.

FRACTURES OF THE SPINE WITHOUT NEURAL INVOLVEMENT

Fractures of the Posterior Spinous Processes. Fractures of the posterior spinous processes are avulsion injuries in that the tremendously strong ligamentum nuchae may withstand the damaging force better than the bone to which it is attached. The usual mechanism is an unguarded flexion act, or one carried out with application of excessive extension force first. The clay shoveler's fracture is a good example of the unguarded application of force. This injury results from an unexpected forward jerk for which there has been inadequate preparation. The workman in lifting a load of clay and throwing it sideways or backward over his shoulder expects the load to have left the spade and, hence, his burden to be lightened. Unexpectedly the load clings to the shovel so that as he brings it backward in preparation for the next scoop, there is a forceful unexpected dragging application that jerks the head forward and, if sufficiently severe, pulls loose one of the lower spinous processes.

The commonest site is the posterior spinous process of C.7. There are several reasons for this (Fig. 13–69). At the lower point of the cervical spine relative fixation occurs in that there is less motion here than in the midcervical area. The long and heavy

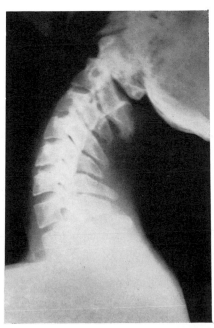

Figure 13–69 Avulsion of spinous process of C.7 in flexion-extension injury.

ligamentum nuchae is firmly attached to the tip of this process but is much less firmly attached to the other posterior tips. The relative immobility of this spine, the strong attachment and the elongated lever combine to pull the tip off at this point more frequently than elsewhere.

TREATMENT. Sometimes this injury is accepted as a simple sprain and it is not until x-ray studies show the avulsed tip that the true damage becomes apparent. Initially a soft cervical collar is applied to ameliorate the acute discomfort because it is quite a painful injury. A high percentage of these patients continue to have discomfort if the tip is not excised. Often it is a relatively small fragment.

When the fracture is closer to the base or even extends to the lamina, a much broader contact is possible and immobilization for a period of six or eight weeks is often followed by good healing. With the smaller fragments excision and repair of the ligament has become the method of choice.

Chip Fractures of Vertebral Bodies. Two distinct types may be recognized under this heading. The commonest is separation of a small bony spur or osteophyte in a spine that is already the seat of degenerative changes (Fig. 13–70). Spur formation is commonest at the C.5 and C.6 area near the middle of the cervical spine excursion. Flexion and compression forces tend to be focused more at this level than elsewhere in the spine.

An incomplete compression or flexion type injury may dislodge a small bony spur.

TREATMENT. This lesion should be treated as a cervical sprain with adequate immobilization for at least six weeks until the acute symptoms have subsided. Sometimes the fragment will unite satisfactorily, but often it remains apparently separated. The significance of identifying the fragment really is that it serves as an indication that significant trauma has been applied to the area, sufficient force having been used to produce a more than purely soft tissue involvement. The spicule may appear not to unite, but this does not seem to be of significance.

Extension Injuries. Forced backward bending or extension of the cervical spine places stress on the anterior longitudinal ligament. With distraction force focused anteriorly, tearing of the ligament can occur or a small chip may be pulled from the anterior edge of the vertebral body. As a rule,

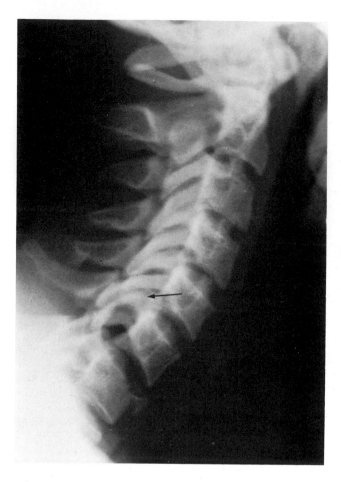

Figure 13–70 Chip fracture of posterior aspect of vertebral body C.5.

this is more painful and more significant than the osteophyte chip; more force has been involved and more damage has been done. For this to occur, significant stretching of the anterior longitudinal ligament has occurred and such a force, if increased, could favor subluxation of the facets.

X-ray examination will show the avulsed fragment, but often careful assessment delineates swelling in front of the anterior limit of the vertebral bodies, indicative of a large hematoma. Some of these lesions require cervical traction during the acute symptoms, followed by the application of a hard cervical collar or a plaster collar. The discomfort and the incapacity resulting from these injuries is usually more extensive than from the chipped osteophyte. A period of eight to 12 weeks immobilization is often necessary for subsidence of the discomfort.

Vertebral Body Fractures. Fractures below the atlas and axis without dislocation are of the flexion-compression type (Fig. 13–71). In the absence of cord involvement or any suggestion of dislocation or subluxation, a period of halter traction of 48 to 72 hours followed by the application of a Minerva jacket will usually be sufficient. The Minerva jacket is worn for 12 to 16 weeks and a firm cervical collar for an additional two months.

The management of the fractures which are complicated by dislocation or cord damage is a much more complex problem and is considered in the next section.

Fractures of Laminae Pedicles and Articular Processes. As a rule, fractures of the process are sometimes seen complicating a dislocation. Rarely, a linear crack may be identified without significant displacement, and such a fracture is handled in the same way as a compression fracture of the vertebral body. A period of preliminary chin traction may be necessary to relieve the muscle spasm, but often this is not necessary and a Minerva jacket may be applied directly. These fractures heal in about 12 weeks, but a cervical collar should be used for a further two months. The more complicated aspect of these fractures occurring with dislocation is discussed later.

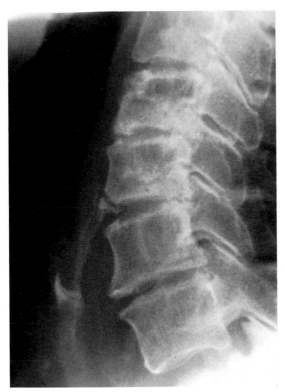

Figure 13–71 Lip fracture of vertebral body. Clear-cut edges identify this as a recent change.

Fractures of the Atlas. The atlas is subject to two separate types of injury, one a compression type of injury from falls on the head, and the other a hyperextension type of compression which implicates the posterior arch (Fig. 13–72). Either of these injuries may be accompanied by extensive cord damage and considerable dislocation of fragments, but this is not common.

Usually fractures of the atlas are not extensively displaced and may be treated satisfactorily by closed methods. A preliminary period of light traction may be necessary to steady the head, but prolonged application is unnecessary. As soon as the patient is comfortable, a Minerva jacket should be applied and worn for a period of 12 weeks.

Fractures of the Axis. The odontoid process is the vulnerable zone of the axis, but fractures can also occur through the lateral masses (Fig. 13–73).

TREATMENT. Fractures of the odontoid without cord involvement are treated by preliminary cervical traction; sometimes skeletal traction is preferable to halter traction in these lesions. The traction is continued until satisfactory position of the displaced odontoid has been obtained. When it is in

good position and the postinjury reaction has subsided, a Minerva jacket is applied and left in place for 16 weeks. At this point x-rays should be taken to determine the likelihood of union. If there is some question, immobilization should be continued for a further two months. After removal of the plaster a cervical collar is worn for an additional three months.

Some authorities advocate open reduction and internal fixation of these injuries because of the considerable instability of the axis. This should not be carried out as a primary procedure or during the early postinjury period. When difficulty is encountered in obtaining a satisfactory reduction or realignment of the odontoid is difficult, consideration should then be given to surgical therapy.

The technique employed is to leave the cervical traction in place during the exposure and carry out wire fixation of the axis and atlas with a wire loop passed underneath the posterior arch of the atlas and then tied in wrap-around fashion about the spine of the axis (Fig. 13–74). This exerts a posterior pull on the atlas, favoring accurate realignment of the odontoid process. In an early case wire fixation appears to be all that is necessary. If the case is encountered at a later period, say some six to eight weeks

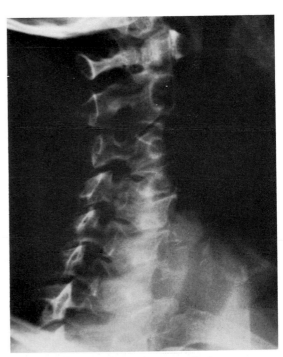

Figure 13–72 Fracture of atlas.

A

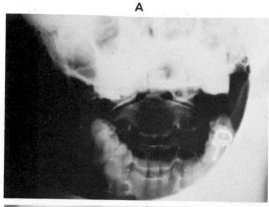

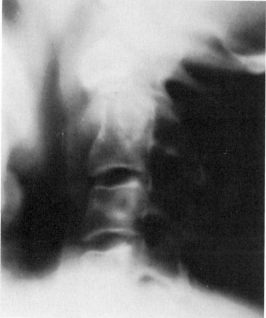

B

Figure 13–73 *A* and *B*, Fractures of odontoid process.

after injury, then the addition of some means of stabilizing the atlas to the axis is desirable. An iliac bone graft may be inserted between the posterior arch of the atlas and the axis with the wire loop so applied that it wedges the bone block in place, favoring snug fixation.

Fractures of the Lateral Mass of the Axis. When this occurs without dislocation it is usually a forced extension type of injury, or extension plus some compression force from above has been involved so that dual forces apply. The atlas may be damaged at the same time.

As a rule, there is not much displacement (unless there is accompanying cord damage) and open reduction or manipulation is not required.

TREATMENT. These injuries are treated by a preliminary period of light traction followed by application of a Minerva jacket for 12 to 16 weeks. A firm cervical collar is worn for a further two months.

Atlantoaxial Dislocations. Several different types of dislocation are encountered between the occiput and the atlas and the axis. These are discussed under the heading of Dislocations of the Cervical Spine.

FRACTURES OF THE CERVICAL SPINE WITH CORD IMPLICATIONS

A cardinal consideration in the management of all neck injuries is the prevention of cord or nerve root damage. No matter where the injury has occurred, the neck should be immobilized with the head and neck in the midposition, and unwarranted movement in all directions should be prevented. The management of these cases requires skill and experience, and often the team approach with the cooperation of orthopedist and neurosurgeon provides the best therapy for the patient.

Many patients do not survive such injuries more than a matter of hours. Following transportation to a hospital, the initial step should be the insertion of head tongs for skeletal traction and control of the deformity. This procedure can be carried out without menacing the patient's general condition with the use of only a few cubic centimeters of a local anesthetic. The type of skeletal apparatus that is used depends largely on the surgeon's preference. There are many advocates of the Crutchfield tongs because of the security of fixation and maneuverability obtained. Another good type of tong is that designed by K. G. McKenzie, which has the virtues of extreme simplicity of insertion and reliability of fixation. The McKenzie tongs

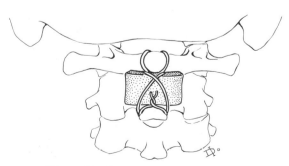

Figure 13–74 Atlanto-axial arthrodesis.

are inserted at a point about an inch above and behind the ear where a small area may be shaved, 2 cc of 2 per cent Novocain injected, a small puncture made in the skin, and the tongs applied with one or two gentle taps of a hammer while the opposite side is held with a weighted resistance. Initially seven to 10 pounds of traction is applied, pending the decision on further management of the problem.

Opinions have long differed as to the necessity for operation in these cases. For a very extensive presentation of the technical considerations, the reader is referred to Crenshaw's Campbell's Operative Orthopaedics, 4th edition, from which many of the following observations have been drawn.

The principles that are followed are dictated predominantly by the extent of neural involvement. Special consideration must also be given to dislocations in which there has been no neural involvement but which are not easily reduced.

Contradictions to Operative Treatment. Surgical treatment is not indicated in the following circumstances: (1) steady improvement of paralysis during the first 24 hours, (2) a negative manometric test, despite malalignment of the vertebrae, and (3) when complete paralysis has been immediate and has lasted more than 24 hours. Although these criteria have strong advocates, they require in-depth assessment. One can never rely implicitly on the history obtained that paralysis was complete; some authorities believe that many more of these patients should be explored.

Indications for Operative Treatment. Operation is performed: (1) when the paralysis is incomplete initially and shows some increase over the first 24 hours; (2) when there is a positive manometric test, regardless of partial or complete paralysis; and (3) when there is no improvement of the paralysis over a period of 24 hours even though it was initially incomplete and despite realignment of the dislocation.

Considerable judgment is required in deciding the time of surgical intervention. These patients are critically injured and in extensive shock and do not stand the operative procedure well.

The patient with a fracture-dislocation and transient or no cord signs whose fracture is not appropriately reduced within four or five days in spite of the use of skeletal traction requires open reduction of the dislocation, but laminectomy or cord decompression is not usually necessary.

FRACTURE DISLOCATIONS OF THE CERVICAL SPINE

In the early case the application of skeletal traction restores good alignment in a high percentage of patients (Fig. 13–75). When this is accompanied by a diminishing neurological deficit, operative intervention is not necessary. If the reduction of the deformity does not improve an incomplete paralysis,

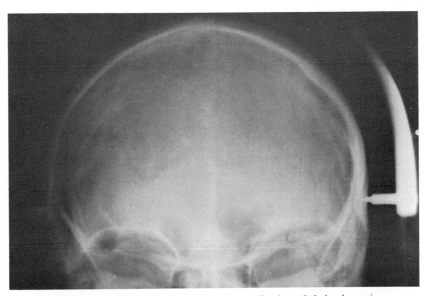

Figure 13–75 Skull prong insertion for application of skeletal traction.

then surgical intervention with decompression is required.

W. A. Rogers, pioneer in the management of cervical spine injuries, has been an advocate of the operative management of these lesions. He found that incomplete reduction by skeletal traction was likely to be followed by deformity and luxation at a later date and possibly further cord injury. When there is any doubt regarding stability, exploration and stabilization should be carried out. The operation is done with the skeletal traction in place. The patient continues with the traction for eight to ten weeks, at the end of which time a Minerva jacket may be applied for a further three months. These patients should be approached from the posterior aspect so that the dislocation may be properly realigned and cord decompression carried out if necessary. The anterior approach to the vertebral bodies in these injuries is unsatisfactory (Fig. 13–76).

DISLOCATIONS OF THE CERVICAL SPINE

Not all dislocations are accompanied by cord damage but it occurs in a high percentage.

Dislocation of the Atlas. Spontaneous dislocation of the atlas has been encountered frequently in rheumatoid arthritics and occasionally in patients with severe nasopharyngeal infection. The mechanism of dislocation is that the transverse ligament of the atlas becomes slack as a result of stretch of its attachment to the atlas such as may occur in the extreme osteoporosis of rheumatoid arthritis or in the case of hyperemic decalcification associated with extensive local infection.

TREATMENT. Sedation and gentle extension followed by halter traction usually produce satisfactory reduction. Often these patients are extremely frail and fragile and have respiratory complications, so a heavy Minerva jacket of plaster is undesirable. A preferable arrangement is a type of thoracic brace with a Fiberglass or Plexiglass chin and suboccipital extension.

Dislocation of the Atlas Without Fracture of the Odontoid. When this is the result of injury, extensive cord damage almost always occurs and often the lesion is fatal. If the odontoid does not crack across its base and the atlas shifts forward, it must crush the spine between it and the odontoid. If the

patient survives, skeletal traction is applied, followed by plaster fixation for three months. Considerable instability may result from this injury and require atlantoaxial stabilization. However, cases have been reported in which traction and skilled manipulation have reduced a complete atlas dislocation.

Dislocation of the Cervical Spine. Severe flexion force with mingled rotatory compression may produce a unilateral dislocation, so that the apophyseal facets overlap and lock on one or sometimes both sides.

T. R. Beatson has called attention to the difficulties in identifying subluxation, unilateral dislocation and bilateral dislocation in routine x-ray investigation. Experimental and clinical study was made of the significance of the degree of displacement of one vertebral body on the other as seen on the routine lateral views as a possible guide to the extent of facet involvement. By reproducing various degrees of dislocation experimentally it was found that a unilateral dislocation could be anticipated if the amount of displacement was less than half of the vertebral body's anteroposterior depth. Bilateral facet dislocation should be suspected when the displacement is greater than half the anteroposterior dimension.

UNILATERAL DISLOCATION. The usual configuration is a sliding forward of the lower facet of the upper vertebra on the superior facet of the lower body. Cord or nerve root signs may accompany these lesions.

Treatment. Skeletal traction with head tongs is instituted, with 15 to 20 pounds being applied gradually. X-ray examination is carried out every hour or so to assess the response to the pull. It may be necessary to double the amount of weight, which can be done quite safely if the tongs have been properly introduced. Most dislocations can be reduced over a period of six to eight hours with increases in weight.

When closed methods fail after a reasonable trial (three to four days) and the patient's general condition warrants, open reduction should be carried out with the cervical traction in place (Fig. 13–77).

BILATERAL DISLOCATIONS. Many bilateral dislocations have extensive cord damage and require open reduction, sometimes with laminectomy (Fig. 13–78). Some form of fixation should then be introduced. In the simple dislocation, wire fixation to the spinous processes is adequate. When there is considerable instability or extensive laminec-

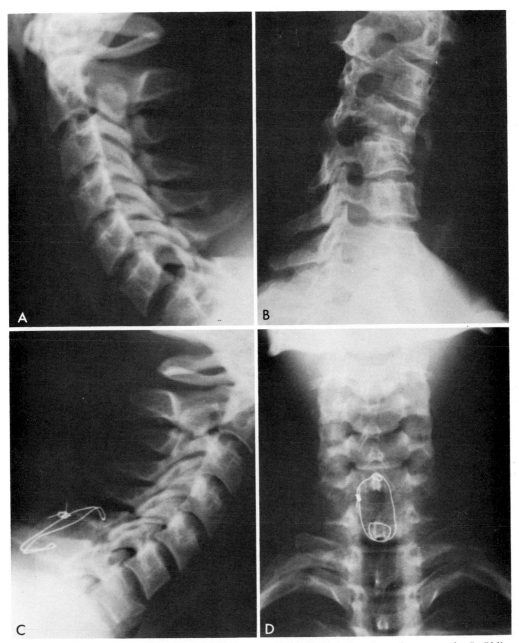

Figure 13–76   Fracture dislocation of cervical spine. *A,* Routine lateral view shows fracture only. *B,* Oblique view shows dislocation. *C* and *D,* Views following operative reduction and wire fixation.

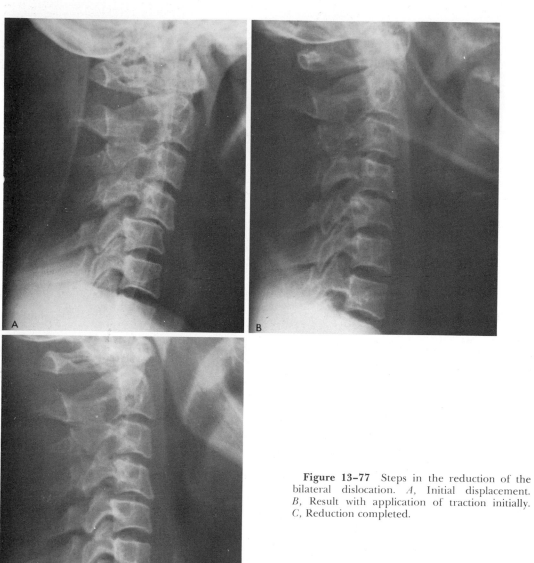

Figure 13–77 Steps in the reduction of the bilateral dislocation. *A*, Initial displacement. *B*, Result with application of traction initially. *C*, Reduction completed.

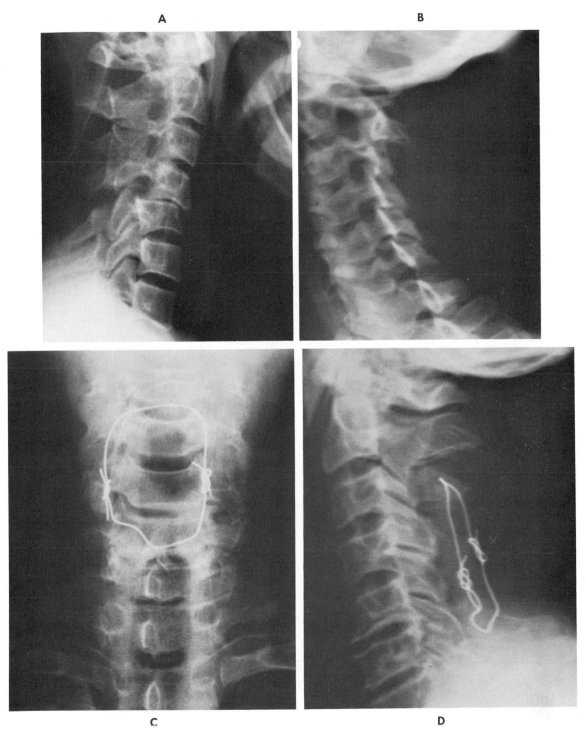

Figure 13–78 Dislocation of cervical spine before (*A* and *B*) and after (*C* and *D*) reduction and fixation.

tomy has been required, it is preferable to add a bone graft after the method of Robinson and Southwick.

Following reduction, the skeletal traction is left in place for four to six weeks, followed by the application of a Minerva jacket or special neck and shoulder brace for a further three months.

REFERENCES

Adams, J. C.: Recurrent dislocation of the shoulder. J. Bone Joint Surg. *30B*:26, 1948.

Aitken, A. P.: Fractures of the proximal humeral epiphysis. Surg. Clin. N. Amer. *43*:1573–1580, 1963.

Aufranc, O. E., et al.: Unilateral rotary subluxation of C-3 on C-4. J.A.M.A. *185*:1031–1035, 1963.

Aufranc, O. E., et al.: Bilateral shoulder fracture-dislocations. J.A.M.A. *195*:1140–1143, 1966.

Aufranc, O. E., et al.: Comminuted fracture dislocation of the proximal humerus. J.A.M.A. *195*:770–773, 1966.

Bailey, R. W.: Acute and recurrent dislocation of the shoulder. J. Bone Joint Surg. *49A*:767–773, 1967.

Baker, D. M., et al.: Fracture dislocation of the shoulder – report of 3 unusual cases with rotator cuff avulsion. J. Trauma *5*:659–664, 1965.

Beatson, T. R.: Fractures and dislocations of the cervical spine. J. Bone Joint Surg. (Brit.) *45B*:21–35, 1963.

Bell, H. M.: Posterior fracture-dislocation of the shoulder – a method of closed reduction: A case report. J. Bone Joint Surg. *47A*:1521–1524, 1965.

Blazina, M. E., and Saltzman, J. S.: Recurrent anterior subluxation of the shoulder in athletes. Proceedings American Academy of Orthopedic Surgeons, January, 1969. J. Bone Joint Surg. *51A*: 1969.

Bloom, M. H., et al.: Diagnosis of posterior dislocation of the shoulder with use of Velpeau axillary and angle-up roentgenographic views. J. Bone Joint Surg. *49A*:943–949, 1967.

Boyd, H. B., et al.: Recurrent dislocation of the shoulder: The staple capsulorrhaphy. J. Bone Joint Surg. *47A*:1514–1520, 1965.

Bruckner, H.: Evaluation of 216 primary and 50 habitual shoulder joint luxations. Mschr. Unfallheilk. *69*:324–327, 1966.

Bryan, R. S., Dimichele, J. D., Ford, G. L., and Gary, G. R.: Anterior recurrent dislocation of the shoulder. Report of a series of Augustine variation of Magnuson-Stack repair. Clin. Orthop. *63*:177–180, 1969.

Cave, E. F.: Immediate fracture management. Surg. Clin. N. Amer. *46*:771–788, 1966.

Chakrabarty, R. P.: A new surgical approach for recurrent dislocation of the shoulder. J. Indian Med. Ass. *47*:542–544, 1966.

Ciugudean, C.: A new procedure for treatment of acromioclavicular luxation. Rev. Chir. Orthop. *52*:485–486, 1966.

Crenshaw, A. H. (ed.): Campbell's Operative Orthopaedics. 4th ed. St. Louis, The C. V. Mosby Co., 1965.

Dameron, T. G., and Reibel, D. B.: Fractures involving the proximal humeral epiphyseal plate. J. Bone Joint Surg. *51A*:289–297, 1969.

Danis, A.: New technic for the treatment of recurrent dislocation of the shoulder. Acta Orthop. Belg. *32*:729–742, 1966.

Dewar, F. P., et al.: Fracture dislocation of the shoulder.

Report of a case. J. Bone Joint Surg. *49B*:540–543, 1967.

Dimon, J. H., 3rd.: Posterior dislocation and posterior fracture dislocation of the shoulder: A report of 25 cases. Southern Med. J. *60*:661–666, 1967.

Dubousset, J.: Posterior dislocation of the shoulder. Rev. Chir. Orthop. *53*:65–85, 1967.

Fahey, J. J., et al.: Fractures and dislocations in children. Postgrad. Med. *36*:39–54, 1964.

Figiel, S. J., et al.: Posterior dislocation of the shoulder. Radiology *87*:737–740, 1966.

Fontaine, R., et al.: Arterial complications in shoulder dislocations and their sequelae. Apropos of 6 personal cases. Ann. Chir. *20*:1048–1056, 1966.

Gal, A.: Severe cervical spine injuries. J. Trauma *5*:379–385, 1965.

Geneste, R.: Recurring dislocations of the shoulder treated by Bankart's operation. Rev. Chir. Orthop. *52*:665–666, 1966.

Gilchrist, D. K.: A stockinette-Velpeau for immobilization of the shoulder-girdle. J. Bone Joint Surg. *49A*:750–751, 1967.

Jacobs, B., et al.: Acromio-clavicular joint injury. An end result study. J. Bone Joint Surg. *48A*:475–486, 1966.

Lam, S. J.: Irreducible anterior dislocation of the shoulder. J. Bone Joint Surg. *48B*:132–133, 1966.

Mauck, R. H., et al.: Bilateral posterior shoulder dislocation; an orthopedic case report. Virginia Med. Monthly *93*:452–454, 1966.

McLaughlin, H. L., et al.: Recurrent anterior dislocation of the shoulder. 11. A comparative study. J. Trauma *7*:191–201, 1967.

Murphy, B. D.: "Cotton forker's injury" fracture of the upper dorsal spinous processes. Texas J. Med. *60*:520, 1964.

Neer, C. S.: Prosthetic replacement of the humeral head: Indications and operative technique. Surg. Clin. N. Amer. *43*:1581–1597, 1963.

Neviaser, J. S.: Posterior dislocations of the shoulder: Diagnosis and treatment. Surg. Clin. N. Amer. *43*:1623–1630, 1963.

Oster, A.: Recurrent anterior dislocation of the shoulder treated by the Eden-Hybinette operation. Follow-up on 78 cases. Acta Orthop. Scand. *40*:43–52, 1969.

Patterson, W. R.: Inferior dislocation of the distal end of the clavicle. A case report. J. Bone Joint Surg. *49A*:1184–1186, 1967.

Perry, B. F.: An improved clavicle pin. Amer. J. Surg. *112*:142–144, 1966.

Rapp, G. F.: Posterior dislocation of the shoulder. J. Indiana Med. Ass. *60*:923–924, 1967.

Riesel, H.: A contribution of the bilateral shoulder luxation. Mschr. Unfallheilk. *69*:327–329, 1966.

Rook, F. W., et al.: The treatment of acromioclavicular dislocation by use of a lag screw. Southern Med. J. *60*:371–377, 1967.

Scott, K. J., Jr.: Treatment of recurrent posterior dislocations of the shoulder by glenoplasty. Report of 3 cases. J. Bone Joint Surg. *49A*:571–576, 1967.

Sherk, H. H., and Nicholson, J. T.: Rotatory atlanto-axial dislocation associated with ossibulum terminale and mongolism. J. Bone Joint Surg. *51A*:957–964, 1969.

Teshima, S., et al.: Our surgical technique for acromio-clavicular dislocation. Arch. Jap. Chir. *35*:407–513, 1966.

Trillat, A., et al.: Recurrent luxation of the shoulder and glenoid labrum lesions. Rev. Chir. Orthop. *51*:525–544, 1965.

Tsuchiya, H.: Bristow-McMurray's operation for recurrent anterior dislocation of the shoulder joint. Orthop. Surg. (Tokyo) *17*:711, 1966.

Tveter, K. J., et al.: Posterior luxation of the shoulder joint. T. Norsk. Laegeforen. *86*:847–850, 1966.

Wagner, A.: Traumatic luxation of cervical vertebrae in children. Wiad. Lek. *18*:865–867, 1965.

Warrick, C. K.: Posterior dislocation of the shoulder joint. Brit. J. Radiol. *38*:758–761, 1965.

Weitzman, G.: Treatment of acute acromio-clavicular joint dislocation by a modified Bosworth method. Report on 24 cases. J. Bone Joint Surg. *49A*:1167–1178, 1967.

Welply, W. R.: Fractures and dislocations of the cervical spine — early treatment. Manitoba Med. Rev. *46*:175–181, 1966.

Willoughby, D. V.: Acromio-clavicular separations. A simple, effective method of conservative treatment. Med. Serv. J. Canada *21*:339–347, 1965.

Wilson, F. C., Jr., et al.: Results of operative treatment of acute dislocations of the acromio-clavicular joint. J. Trauma 7:202–209, 1967.

Chapter XIV

NERVE INJURIES

The main nerves of the upper limb stream through the neck and shoulder on their way from the spinal cord to the hand. In this way the zones of the neck and the shoulder are securely joined anatomically and physiologically; it follows that clinically and therapeutically the two zones then share much in common. Disorder in one area implicates the other whether it be injury or disease, so that neural and related neurological disorders in particular cannot possibly be considered comprehensively without attention to both zones (Fig. 14–1).

INVESTIGATION OF PLEXUS INJURIES

MECHANISM OF INJURY

Attention is directed toward careful assessment of the way in which injury has occurred. The manner of application of force and the type of trauma profoundly influence the type of injury and, therefore, the treatment and prognosis. The damaging force may be a heavy blow from a bump on the shoulder; a projectile fall from a vehicle, spreading the acromiomastoid dimension; severe traction on the distal portion of the

limb as when the arm is caught in a machine belt; or the blow of a hockey or lacrosse stick across the front of the supraclavicular zone. For many years practitioners of karate have been familiar with the vulnerability of the plexus above the clavicle and have taken advantage of the disposition of these nerves to attack the area with a sharp incisive blow with the side of the hand in chopping fashion midway between the root of the neck and point of the shoulder above the clavicle (Fig. 14–1).

EXAMINATION

When nerve injury is suspected, the whole area must be carefully assessed (Fig. 14–2). If there is a wound of any kind, its relation to underlying soft parts must be visualized since this often gives an indication of which structures might be involved. In dealing with supraclavicular lesions, palpation of the plexus can be carried out by gently tilting the head and neck to the opposite side and feeling the plexus as it streams across the posterior triangle. Massive avulsions of the plexus from the spinal cord, a serious but fortunately infrequent lesion, can often be diagnosed by feeling the curled-up, avulsed roots lying just above the clavicle. Similarly,

450

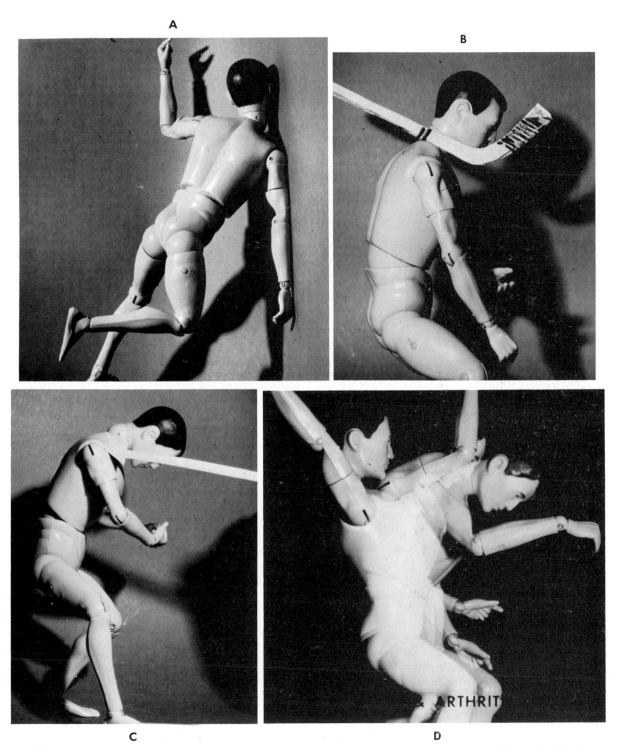

Figure 14–1 *A*, Mechanism of nerve injury in projectile falls. *B*, Shoulder angle blows. *C*, Frontal force. *D*, Twisting trauma.

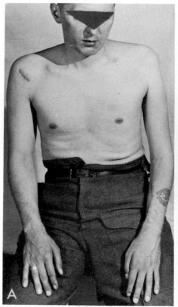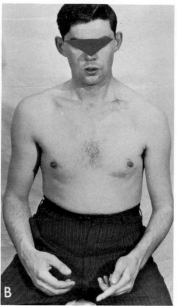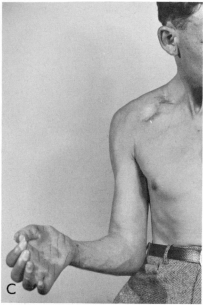

Figure 14–2 Plexus injuries from external wounds. *A*, C.5, C.6 paralysis. Note deltoid atrophy. *B*, C.7 paralysis. Note triceps and forearm extensor atrophy. *C*, C.8, T.1 paralysis. Note extensive hand changes.

gentle tapping of the roots as they are put on the stretch may evoke a tingling response in the periphery, indicating the possibility of physical continuity.

Motor System. Considerable information can be obtained from simple clinical muscle testing. There are a few key muscles which provide a general impression of the level of the injury, all of which can be tested quickly. Abduction of the shoulder is chiefly dependent on the deltoid and, hence, the upper roots of the plexus. Flexion of the elbow depends upon continuity of C.5 and C.6, whereas extension of the elbow is activated by C.7. Action of the interossei and thenar group in the hand is dependent on C.8 and T.1.

These cardinal movements give a quick indication of the level of the lesion. Motor assessment usually acts as a guide to the areas of likely alteration in sensation.

Sensory Examination. In assessing a plexus injury, sensation should be carefully tested in the area at the back of the neck and over the shoulder as well as in the arm, the forearm and the hand. In serious avulsion lesions, altered sensation due to the involvement of the posterior branches may be picked up by some change in the appreciation of light touch and pinprick in the paraspinal zone of the same side. Loss of sensation over the lateral aspect of the shoulder im-

plicates the posterior cord and accessory nerve, whereas changes in the forearm and hand will clearly implicate the medial and lateral cord. True anesthesia about the neck and shoulder or proximal arm zones is uncommon, but it occurs frequently in the more distal portion of the limb and it is an indication of serious damage.

Electrical Investigation. Special examination of motor and sensory systems is an important and essential part of the investigation of these injuries.

SIMPLE GALVANIC AND FARADIC ASSESSMENT. A good indication of the severity of the motor involvement can be obtained from assessing the response of muscles to application of direct and indirect currents. The test can be done simply, and often more complicated investigation is not necessary. It has long been established that when the nerve supply to a muscle has been cut, the muscle loses its response to indirect (faradic) current but retains its reaction to a direct (galvanic) current. When a muscle is paralyzed clinically but still responds to the faradic current, the nerve supply is in physical continuity and the muscle should recover. When response to faradism is lost, however, more serious damage has occurred and recovery will likely occur only by regeneration. Under these circumstances surgical exploration for possible repair of the nerve is usually necessary. Faradic and galvanic responses are sometimes difficult to obtain immediately after injury, but, this situation alters in a matter of days. In longstanding lesions, however, absence of all electrical response indicates replacement of muscle fibers by fibrofatty tissue, so that recovery should not be expected.

ELECTROMYOGRAPHIC EXAMINATION. The most accurate method of assessing muscle damage is by means of the electromyogram (Fig. 14–3). The examination is effected by inserting small unipolar electrodes directly into the muscle to be evaluated and by observing the magnified pattern on the cathode ray oscilloscope. The electrical patterns of normal and denervated muscles are so characteristic that even minute changes can be identified. Normal muscle produces a broad deflection similar to the electrocardiograph pattern and is easily recognized on the cathode ray screen. These deflections are referred to as motor unit action potentials (M.U.A.P.). Denervated muscle, on the other hand, emits small continuous deflections which are not under voluntary control and are called fibrillation action potentials. When fibrillation is present and persistent, it is indicative of denervation and serious damage. As a muscle recovers after injury, the earliest sign of reinnervation is a pattern of new or nascent motor action potentials. These deflections are intermediate in form between fibrillation and normal M.U.A.P. and gradually assume a more normal outline. As in the case with assessment by direct and indirect currents, when no action potential of any type can be recorded from the muscle it has been replaced by fatty or fibrous tissue (Fig. 14–3).

The minute changes in muscle can be measured and recorded. A photographic record is obtained of these, as with an electrocardiograph. The examiner has a further advantage in being able to discern certain properties from the audible accompaniment of the electromyogram. Typical motor unit action potentials have a staccato quality that is clearly discernible when the patient is asked to bring a given muscle into action. This contrasts strongly with the fibrillation action potentials not under voluntary control which have little audible intensity.

Technique of Examination. The electromyograph is pictured in Figure 14–4. The patient sits on a stool or chair in front of the machine in a relaxed position, and the skin over the zone to be assessed is prepared with iodine. A small needle electrode is inserted directly into the muscle to be tested. The individual muscle can be picked out by moving the extremity and by asking the patient to make

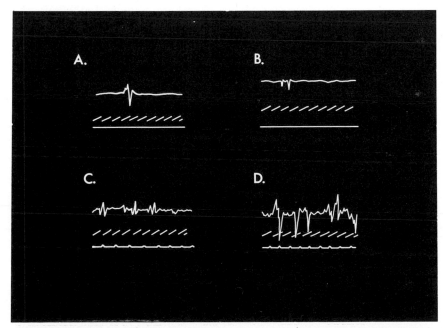

Figure 14–3 Electromyographic tracings. *A,* Normal motor unit action potentials. *B,* Fibrillation action potentials. *C,* Nascent units. *D,* Normal interference pattern.

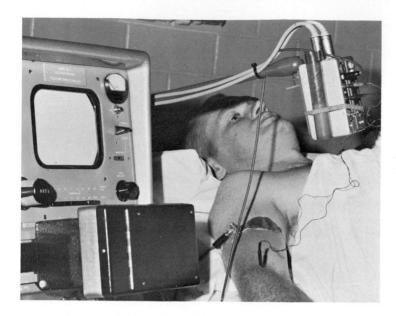

Figure 14–4 Electromyograph. Cathode screen, camera recording, multiple electrodes.

whatever motions are feasible to assist in the identification. After the needle has been inserted, the surface electrode is applied some distance from the needle electrode.

Nerve Conduction Times. Assessment of the conduction time in a suspected nerve may also be carried out by the electromyograph. Conduction time is compared with the normal nerve on the opposite side and the deficiency is recorded.

Assessment of Sensation. Clinical testing of light touch and pinprick is carried out routinely, but in addition there are more precise methods. These tests are of value in demarcating total or complete anesthesia in contrast to hyperesthesia because the principle on which they are based depends upon the presence or absence of sweating. When a peripheral nerve is cut, the autonomic supply to the area of autonomous sensory innervation is lost, and sweating in the denervated zone disappears. In medial cord injuries, for example, profound loss of sweating by the fingers occurs if the lesion is complete. In using Richter's dermometer, a small electrode with a battery source of current is applied to the dry nonsweating area and a much greater resistance to the passage in the current is encountered than when the electrode slides over the sweating zone, which provides a superior skin contact to the electrode.

Assessment by the use of a dye which changes color on application to the sweating area as compared to the nonsweating zone will outline the sympathetic loss accurately.

CERVICAL PLEXUS INJURIES

Branches of the upper spinal nerves C.1 to C.4 ramify at the side and upper front of the neck (Fig. 14–5). They do not constitute a plexus in the true sense of the word, but the intermingling and association is such that they may be considered as a separate unit as opposed to the constituents of the brachial plexus, which arises lower down. The branches are nearly all sensory and, as such, have a quite superficial distribution. They consist of the lesser occipital, great auricular, cutaneous colli and supraclavicular nerves. Injuries to these nerves are not frequent but they are encountered in a variety of circumstances so that their entity should be clearly understood.

Sources of Injury. Direct trauma is the only damaging force, in contrast to brachial plexus lesions in which forces of traction, pressure and even radiation also operate. Lacerations accidentally or directly applied may involve branches of the cervical plexus. A more common source is accidental involvement in a surgical procedure in this region, such as exploration and dissections, particularly for malignant disease, exposure of the posterior triangle, operations on the clavicle or procedures designed to remove tissue such as lymph glands for biopsy.

Signs and Symptoms. Because of their sensory function and superficial position, unpleasant pain in the distribution of the individual damaged nerves is the persistent complaint. Sensitive trigger areas caused by

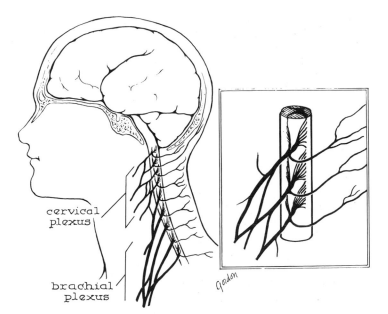

Figure 14–5 Origin of cervical and brachial plexus.

the pressure of neuromata develop. Alterations in sensation of touch can frequently be detected, but zones of true anesthesia are rare. Subjective numbness in addition to directly altered sensation is also apparent.

The posterior branches of these upper roots supply a zone of skin near the midline posteriorly and innervate the erector spinae and adjacent muscles. Direct injury to these elements is almost never seen, but they have considerable importance anatomically. These posterior branches, being a part of the common segmental nerves from the cord, are implicated in intradural, extradural and foraminal lesions of the spinal cord at these levels. Their real importance lies in the fact that electromyographic changes can often be detected in these muscles, thus implicat-

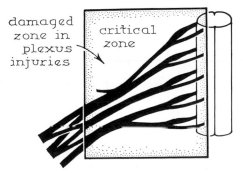

Figure 14–6 Main distribution of branches of the cervical plexus.

ing the cord or common nerve roots at this level as opposed to more peripheral lesions (Fig. 14–6).

Treatment. The branches are of sufficient size to be repaired surgically. The result is worth the effort because the best way to treat a bare nerve ending is to place it properly in another nerve. Excision of the neuromata and end-to-end suture materially decrease the unpleasant pain and diminish the sensory loss.

SUPRACLAVICULAR PLEXUS INJURIES

Lesions of the plexus above the clavicle are the most serious of all injuries to the shoulder region. Not only is the shoulder involved, but the whole extremity may be paralyzed. Many of these are irreparable, and amputation is more often necessary for these than for any other shoulder injury.

Etiology and Pathology. Traction force applied to the shoulder neck angle is the commonest cause of supraclavicular plexus trauma in industrial and civilian accident cases. No two injuries are exactly alike. A study of the functional anatomy of the plexus and an analysis of the ways in which force strikes the region aids understanding of the various lesions.

FUNCTIONAL ANATOMY. The factors which contribute to the injury pattern from a structural standpoint are: (1) the nature of nerve substance, (2) the intimate protecting surroundings, like the fascial sleeve, (3) the disposition of these parts in the region, and (4) the effect of more distant structures.

Nerves are soft semielastic structures not comparable to tubes or rigid elements. So much attention has been focused on adjacent protecting parts that the influence of the nerve structure itself on the type of injury has been neglected. The zone of the plexus most affected is from the spinal cord to the level of trunk formation. Over this zone the direction of nerve bundles changes three times (Figs. 14–6, 14–7). Fibers arise from front and back of the spinal cord in the transverse plane and then unite to form a spinal root. They intermingle and then divide again in a different fashion and in a different plane, forming the three cords. It is over this zone that most of the damage is encountered. The principles of force application cannot be applied too exactly because of this intermingling of fibers which amounts almost to a weaving or network-like course. Nerve substance is of jelly-like consistency so that it may also be molded like putty. It is possible, therefore, to dent or sever the filling of a tube without cutting the outside covering (Fig. 14–8). The covering, like that of a wiener casing, may not crack, yet the filling may be seriously crushed. These properties of weaving distribution and soft consistency allow a most distorted separation or tearing of cylinders at various levels and to various degrees (Fig. 14–9). Added to this is the innate elasticity of

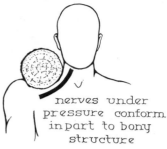

Figure 14–8 Innate elasticity of nerve substance allows some molding under stress.

the fibers so that, after being cut, they recoil and lie in disorder (Fig. 14–9). More recoil is possible than might be suspected because, upon occasion, the roots are found in a tangled heap just above the clavicle after severance from the spinal cord.

The surroundings of the critical zone from spinal cord to nerve cord level exert profound control. The important ones are the fascial sleeve (Fig. 14–10), the bony foramina, the transverse processes and the scalene muscles. As the nerve roots stream from the cord into the foramina, they enter a fascial sheath or sleeve derived from the prevertebral fascia. This is anchored to the transverse processes and surrounds the roots and then the trunks. It continues downward and distally, enveloping the vessels at the level of the clavicle. It is reinforced in this zone by subclavian and clavipectoral fascia extending to the coracoid region where it is diverted as the plexus flares into its infraclavicular branches. This sheath guards the soft nerve trunks and resists longitudinal stretch particularly. The nerve roots in leaving the spine pass through a gutter formed by the intervertebral foramen medially and continued laterally by the anterior surface of the transverse processes. They pass from above downward across this bony projection, closely related, and then angle a little anteriorly. Beyond this they are related to soft structures only until thorax and clavicle are reached. Chiefly the scalene muscles cushion the course.

The plexus streams diagonally across the shoulder neck angle, taking the shortest course, while neck and shoulder form a right-angled scaffolding. In blows from above, the innate elasticity allows nerve trunks to stretch a little, sinking into the soft tissue padding conforming to the rigid support.

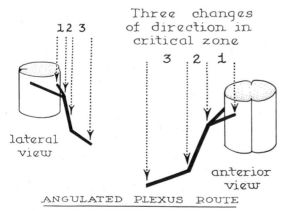

Figure 14–7 Multiangulated course of brachial plexus. (1) The roots start from the cord almost at a right angle. (2) Roots pass down and forward over transverse process. (3) Roots turned laterally and downward toward the clavicle.

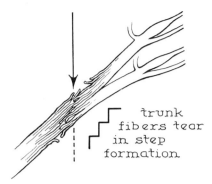

Figure 14–9 Components of the plexus roots tend to rip in step-like fashion.

More distant parts have an effect on the critical zone also. The cords are stretched between two relatively fixed points, the spinal cord at one end and the embedded distal branches at the other. More tension is exerted by the proximal anchorage than the distal. The distal anchorage is movable as a unit, however, and is capable of producing a rotatory stress focused at the roots when the arm is flailed about (Fig. 14–11, *C*). Similarly, the arm may be clamped and the spine flexed, reversing the action. These properties of two-point anchorage and then mobility of the anchoring element make possible a tremendous variation of stress application.

Force Mechanism. From the description of the numerous anatomical elements that come into play, it is obvious that a myriad of stress patterns may operate. No two closed plexus injuries are the same, but some

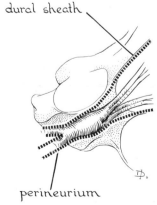

Figure 14–10 Fascial sleeve from the dura continues as perineurium of the plexus nerve trunks.

rough grouping by force application is helpful. In this study it is an analysis of the clinical picture rather than the appearance at operation which is most informative. There are three common ways in which these injuries are sustained: blows from above, falls on the neck and shoulder, and traction on the arm, either rotatory or direct pull.

FORCE FROM ABOVE. Force striking the shoulder from above is a common cause of brachial paralysis (Fig. 14–11, *A*). In industry particularly, falling objects, timbers, trees, masonry, rocks or cables may drop on a workman's shoulder. If the blow is anticipated, the posterior aspect bears the brunt as the patient in attempting to escape from the danger exposes his back. If the falling object is not seen, it drops more squarely on the point; only rarely is it applied from the front. The lateral part of the superior aspect bears the brunt so that the cords are stretched downward with tension applied directly to the root area (Fig. 14–11, *A*). Force from the back tends to shove the shoulder point forward; the nerves are tightened and stretched but no hard fulcrum or obstruction is encountered. The force coming from above tends to pull roots out from the cord rather than to stretch them, or it tears them as they go through the foramina. These are the most serious lesions because, if the tear occurs high up in the foramina or from the cord, repair is impossible.

FALLS ON THE NECK AND SHOULDER. Hurtling downward and sideways so that the head and shoulders are the landing points is also a common mechanism in these injuries. In such a fall the acromiomastoid dimension is violently increased (Fig. 14–11, *B*). Powerful stretch is transmitted to the nerve elements across the neck shoulder angle. In this maneuver it is the mobility and position of the head and cervical spine rather than the arm that exert most influence. The shoulder girdle bears the brunt of the distal point stress and this cannot shift backward or forward enough to affect the nerves. Arm influence is so much farther away from the critical zone that it must be less influential than that of the neck.

Whatever may be the minute controlling forces, the important result is whether the stretch is to the front or to the back. If it is to the front, damage is close to roots and cord. If it is to the back, the transverse processes insert as a fulcrum so that maximum stretching and tearing lies farther

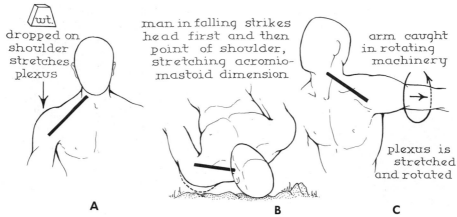

Figure 14–11 *A* to *C*, Common force applications producing brachial plexus damage.

laterally. The importance of this is that sometimes more can be done to repair the damage if there is a good proximal segment. If the force is powerful enough, one would expect to find either fairly complete avulsion from the cord or damage at or distal to the transverse processes. In the author's experience, this is the situation commonly encountered at operation.

TRACTION ON THE ARM. The third common injury mechanism is pull applied to some more distal part of the extremity so that severe traction is focused at the neck shoulder angle (Fig. 14–11, *C*). Examples of this type of injury are arms being pulled into machinery or hands caught in revolving belts so that the whole extremity is flailed about like a windmill. As might be expected, these injuries are not quite so severe as the two preceding groups. Strain is applied over a longer zone so that a broader area is affected. A stretching and tearing of nerve occurs, with fibers giving way at different levels. No fulcrum is inserted to cut fibers sharply. Extensive intraneural hemorrhage occurs, followed by fibrosis. These patients often end up having the distal part, forearm, or hand amputated because of the severe damage to the hand. They continue to complain of the burning electric shock-like pain that seared them at the moment of their injury. This pain is due to the traction nerve damage and is not the ordinary phantom limb sensation that follows amputations.

When a rotatory element is prominent in the injury mechanism, the direction in which the extremity is flailed controls which roots are predominantly affected. If it is counterclockwise, the lower parts are stretched most;

a clockwise flail affects the upper roots most (Fig. 14–11, *C*).

No matter what the intricate pattern of injury may be, the picture at operation is similar in all serious plexus injuries. The roots may be completely avulsed and then are found as a tangled heap just above the clavicle. The fascial sheaths are empty, but usually even in these cases some remnant of sleeve will still be found. Scalenes may be torn, and sometimes the phrenic nerve is gone also.

In incomplete lesions sheaths are thickened and fibrotic, nerve fibers are stretched and torn, intraneural vessels are torn, and much bleeding scar tissue infiltrates among the bundles. The longer after injury that operation is done, the more rubbery hard does the scar tissue become. At four to six weeks it is easy to dissect and separate nerve bundles. At six to 12 months dissection is much more difficult because of the strangulating scar.

Diagnosis of Supraclavicular Injuries. Diagnosis of brachial plexus injuries involves more than simple recognition of the paralysis. The lesion must be classed as to severity, site and level.

DIAGNOSIS OF THE TYPE OF LESION. In classifying nerve injuries, the routine which is most widely followed is that introduced by H. J. Seddon, in which the term neurotmesis is used to describe complete motor and sensory paralysis due to rupture of nerve fibers; axonotmesis indicates complete motor and sensory paralysis with interruption of axons but without serious anatomical disturbance; and neurapraxia is the term used to define a transient lesion which has largely motor signs and minimal sensory loss. In this last entity there is no anatomical damage, and recovery should occur quickly without surgical intervention. In the first group, surgery is necessary; in the second group, surgery is sometimes needed. If examination shows a minimal sensory deficit and good response to the indirect or faradic current, the lesion is likely a transient one and the trunks are in continuity. Profound anesthesia with absent faradic response indicates serious nerve damage, and any recovery will occur only by regeneration. Beyond these two broad groups, an indication of severity is difficult and the latter picture may be due to irreparable cord avulsion, rupture of the roots, severe stretching and intraneural scarring, or a partial rupture and associated stretching. Operative exploration is the only way of further differentiating this group.

DIAGNOSIS OF THE LEVEL OF THE LESION. The level of the plexus damage is determined by careful assessment of the muscles involved and an accurate knowledge of the local neural anatomy. At this point some consideration should be afforded normal anatomical variations and the anomalies that may be encountered. The normal anatomical distribution of fibers to the muscles must be kept in mind, but there is considerable variation in the respective contributions to individual muscles. The make-up of the plexus also varies and a pre- or postfixed plexus may be encountered (see Chapter IX). In the upward shift or prefixed type, the major contribution to the plexus involves segments C.5, C.6, C.7 and C.8. Such muscles as the deltoid and spinati may receive no contribution from C.6, all the fibers coming from C.4 and C.5, whereas the coracobrachialis is supplied by C.7 alone, and there is a major contribution from T.1 to the plexus.

Considerable confusion on the part of students is encountered in the appreciation of cord versus nerve root versus peripheral nerve lesions, and in differentiating plexus from nerve root or peripheral nerve injury. If a lesion is in the spinal cord, no sensory loss is encountered in either ventral or dorsal areas. Spinal nerves divide shortly after they are grouped together into dorsal and ventral divisions. The posterior division supplies segmental trunk muscles and the skin over an area of the back medial to the acromion. Therefore, if there is involvement close to the primary division, in addition to the usual signs and symptoms there is anesthesia over the posterior aspect of the trunk. If the lesion

lies farther distally, this division must escape damage. The sympathetic supply is carried in the peripheral nerves and not in the roots or primary division, so a lesion medial to the plexus, for example, from a prolapsed disc, does not cause the alteration in sweating which is so characteristic of peripheral nerve damage (Fig. 14–12).

Upper Roots. Roots C.5 and C.6, and sometimes C.7 to a varying degree, are the most frequently injured. The reason for this is that these upper nerves bear the brunt of downward traction force and encounter the stress first. The force is dissipated as the more distal roots are affected and the leverage is decreased. Damage of the upper roots in the common form results in paralysis of the deltoid, supra- and infraspinatus and biceps. In the very high lesions there is also involvement of the diaphragm, rhomboids, and serratus anterior. The area of sensory loss follows C.5 and C.6 distribution over the neck shoulder zone (Fig. 14–2, *A*).

Involvement of C.7. When in addition to the above muscles there is added paralysis of latissimus dorsi, pectoralis major, serratus, coracobrachialis and brachialis and weak-

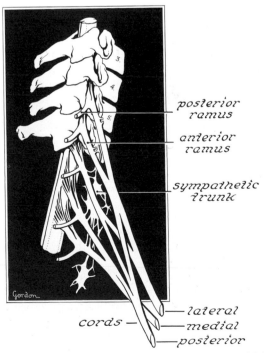

Figure 14–12 Diagrams showing point at which sympathetic fibers join peripheral nerves. This point is outside the foramen, therefore, sympathetic fibers are not involved because of disc or foraminal pressure.

ness of triceps, involvement of C.7 has occurred (Fig. 14–2, *B*).

Involvement of Lower Roots. C.8 and T.1 are involved when there is paralysis of the flexors of the wrist and small muscles of the hand. In addition disturbance of T.1 frequently produces a Horner's syndrome (Figs. 14–2, *C* and 14–13).

Complete Plexus Lesions. All the roots may be avulsed high in the neck close to the cord. This produces a typical picture: the injured arm hangs at the side as a useless flail extremity (Fig. 14–14). The only way that it can be moved is by shrugging the shoulder with the trapezius or lifting the hand with the opposite uninjured one. Palpation of the supraclavicular area frequently identifies a nodular rubbery swelling lying just above the clavicle, representing the curled-up retracted nerve roots.

Treatment of Supraclavicular Plexus Injuries. The treatment of brachial plexus paralysis is a long and tedious process. The paralyzed muscles should be splinted in the position of relaxation and electrical stimulation applied until regeneration has occurred. There has been considerable controversy regarding the advisability of surgical intervention. The author is strongly of the opinion that more of these cases should be explored early. If there is clear-cut evidence that the lesion is in continuity, and therefore that the

neurapraxia is transient, only the conservative program is necessary. If, on the other hand, investigation indicates complete interruption of some roots, exploration should be carried out. There are many arguments in favor of such a program. Despite careful clinical and electromyographic studies, it is not possible to tell whether the root has been divided completely, partially avulsed with intraneural scarring, or stretched over a distance of inches with resulting intraneural fibrosis. Nerves regenerate slowly, and it has been established both experimentally and clinically that the degree of motor recovery depends upon the preservation of the myoneural end plate mechanism. Much can be done by electrical stimulation to preserve muscles while axon regeneration is awaited, but in plexus injuries, 18 to 24 months' treatment may be necessary before the question of possible recovery is settled. Therefore, it is preferable to explore early rather than carry on treatment for a lengthy period only to have clinical verification of a complete neurotmesis.

From the standpoint of prognosis, as well as rehabilitation, an accurate concept of the extent of damage is most essential. If the lesion is irreparable, reconstruction is needed, and the earlier this program can be instituted, the better the result. Sometimes amputation is the solution and the earlier

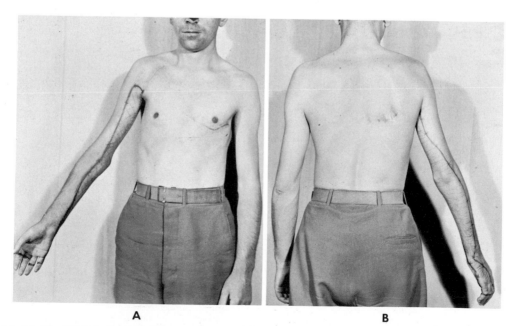

A   **B**

Figure 14–13 Clinical picture of damaged roots C.7 and C.8. Distribution of sensory loss in common plexus lesions. *A*, C.5–C.6 roots. *B*, C.7–C.8–T.1 roots.

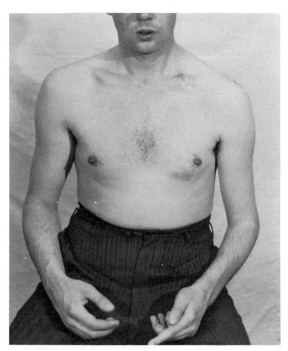

Figure 14–14 Typical supraclavicular plexus injury. Note forearm paralysis.

this is done, the better it is from the standpoint of rehabilitation. The program of muscle re-education, utilizing the unparalyzed remainder, must be started early for maximum results. Nerve lesions differ from other injuries because there is a profound effect on other structures not directly damaged. Joints become stiff, and ligaments become contracted; it is most discouraging to have innervation eventually occur but to find the joints so stiff that they cannot be moved. Everything possible should be done to speed reinnervation and preserve the functional elements.

As far as the lesion itself is concerned, often much more can be accomplished at operation than is anticipated beforehand. Partial lesions may be sutured or strangulating scar excised. An understanding of the mechanism of injury demonstrates how variable may be the level and type of the damage. No one can predict the results of force applied to the nerve tissue because of the inherent elasticity. The author has encountered traction lesions at operation which took the form of complete division of isolated nerve roots. These could be resected and repaired in the usual fashion. The site of damage can never be so accurately predicted that the case may be labeled as hopeless and

abandoned. The length of the transverse process and the point of application of stress to it as a fulcrum changes the point at which the nerve root may give way. In one instance this may be high up in the intervertebral foramen, in another, with longer transverse processes, the cut may be well out in the posterior triangle (Fig. 14–15). These lesions are so serious that the patient should be given all possible help.

GENERAL CONSIDERATIONS. Pain is a distressing symptom in many of these injuries and sometimes not much can be done. It would seem that the most severe causalgic symptoms follow extensive stretching rather than complete avulsion. Stretching and tearing produces widespread hemorrhage and fibrosis. Removal of as much scar as possible and separation and freeing of the nerve bundles always decreases, although it may not completely abolish, the pain. All surgeons dealing with nerve injuries have noted the change in the appearance of the hand immediately after operation even when the nerve is completely divided. Some vasomotor factor is stimulated, affecting the nutrition in the damaged area. This is strikingly apparent after operation on plexus lesions.

There has been more reluctance to operate on patients with these problems than those with more peripheral lesions. The deterrents have been the possibility of damage to adjacent vital structures and the possibility of vascular or other complications. Because exploration can be accomplished without any such harmful sequelae, this should not be a consideration. Since many of these cases are medicolegal problems, the prognosis has a most important bearing on financial settlement for the patient as well

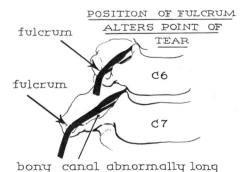

Figure 14–15 Influence of transverse process length on the level of root ruptures.

as on his present and future disability. This is a further reason for exploration, in addition to the need for accurate assessment of the damage to plan the treatment program.

CONSERVATIVE TREATMENT. *Splinting of Paralyzed Muscle.* Injuries of C.5 and C.6 result in loss of power in the shoulder abductors. These are antigravity muscles and become stretched easily. Constant stretching damages muscle fibers and delays recovery. This is prevented by using a light cantilever abduction splint which rests the arm at a right angle with the elbow in gentle flexion (Fig. 14–16).

Preventing Joint Stiffness. The extremity must be taken out of the splint at least twice daily and the joints put through a normal range of motion. If the arm is allowed to stay at the side, adduction and internal rotation contractures develop easily. This is guarded against by proper massage and passive movement. When the hand is involved, it is desirable to splint the fingers in the position of relaxation, but a removable splint should be used to prevent joint stiffness (Fig. 14–17).

Electrical Stimulation. When the nerve supply to a muscle is cut, there is profound disturbance to the muscle fiber and the motor end plate mechanism. The muscle fiber shrinks progressively and may never regain its normal size. The longer the muscle is denervated, the more extensive becomes the atrophy. Closely associated with atrophy of the muscle fibers is damage to the myoneural or end plate mechanism. This is the area of contact or the stimulating point of the muscle fiber. The mechanism degenerates when the nerve has been cut and may never recover. The formation of new muscle end plates is slow and most difficult; a long process of specialization is needed, and some authorities have doubted that it can be accomplished. Atrophy of muscle fibers affects the plate mechanism adversely also. The only method at our command to counteract these changes is electrical stimulation of the muscle. As soon as paralysis occurs and the

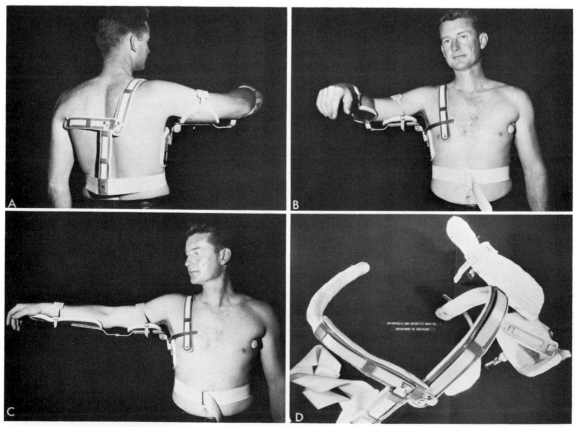

Figure 14–16 Cantilever abduction brace for abductor paralysis.

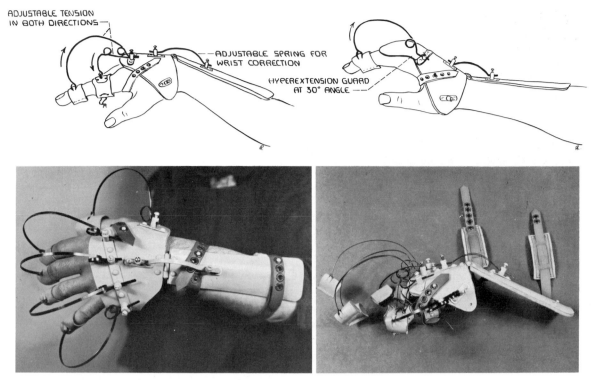

Figure 14–17 Universal splint for hand deformity is particularly useful in nerve injuries.

immediate reaction to injury has subsided, electrical stimulation should be started and continued until reinnervation appears. Stimulation is started by the physiotherapist and, if possible, should be done three or four times daily, depending upon the response. Fifteen to 20 contractions of each muscle are done. If the injury is a lesion in continuity (neurapraxia), indirect or faradic current can be used. In most cases direct stimulation of the muscle is needed and this is best accomplished with a direct or galvanic current. Preference for certain currents has been advocated and has some experimental support. However, it is agreed that it is of greater importance to have some form of electrical stimulation done rather than wait for a special current from a special apparatus.

So often these lesions need stimulation for so many months that continued attention from the physiotherapist becomes a problem from a financial and accommodation aspect. It is possible to teach these patients to carry on their own electrical stimulation, using a small apparatus such as that designed by the author. This is a very simple machine with a battery as a source of direct current. The current is controlled by a series of resistances so that it is quite harmless. The controls are all on one side on a treatment panel, which allows them to be operated by the unparalyzed hand, and they are easily adjusted. The current is applied through skin electrodes which are fixed in holders conforming to the pattern of the lesion so that individual electrode holders can be used. The practiced physiotherapist adjusts and applies the machine, marks the points of stimulation for application of the electrodes and teaches the patient to use it himself. The patient reports every four to six weeks for check-ups and follow-up study. The battery lasts for six to eight months and the patient rarely wears one out; it is a standard battery that is easily replaced. The machine is small and compact and is easily carried about (Fig. 14–18).

Re-education of the Muscle. More than recovery of voluntary contraction is necessary. The muscle must be taught to function properly in the various patterns of movement for purposeful action. So often the pattern of composite movement has not been relearned after voluntary power has returned in the individual muscle. Rehabilitation includes the restoration of function of the part

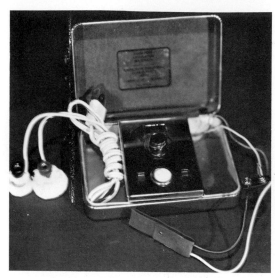

Figure 14–18   Miniature stimulator.

as a whole, not merely individual movements. If the hunching habit of the shoulder persists after deltoid power has returned, the proper pattern has not been restored and the extremity is still disabled. The patient must be taught again to properly fix his scapula as the "new" deltoid is used.

OPERATIVE TREATMENT.   Operation is carried out in these patients when clinical and electrical investigation indicates structural interruption of one or more roots. Some observers have recommended this as early as 10 to 14 days after injury, but it has been the author's preference to wait a period of four to six weeks. Such an interval allows repeated examination, and sometimes more definite outline of the lesion is obtained. During such an interval tissue reaction to the bruising and hemorrhage of injury subsides and adhesions have not become too firm to interfere with dissection.

Technique of Plexus Exploration.   The operation is done under a general anesthetic, preferably with intratracheal intubation. The neck and side of the head are shaved on the injured side and the whole upper extremity is prepared as well. The classic supine position on the operating table has been altered to a sitting posture (Fig. 14–19). The patient is placed in the sitting position with the head rotated away from the injured side. In this way the point of the shoulder drops and remains dependent, increasing the length of nerve trunks which can be explored above the clavicle. The operating field is lifted to directly in front of the surgeon and remains

comfortably accessible during the long and sometimes tedious dissection. An almost vertical incision is used, extending from the midpoint of the lateral border of the sternomastoid to the middle third of the clavicle. It may terminate at the inner third to reach the lower roots, or veer toward the outer third when exploration of the fifth and sixth roots is most important (Fig. 14–20). The external jugular vein is ligated and the sternomastoid muscle is retracted. The omohyoid is exposed and divided; the suprascapular and transverse cervical vessels are ligated. The brachial plexus is then obvious, streaming out between the scalenes. The dependent position of the shoulder places the structures of the posterior triangle on a gentle stretch, facilitating dissection and identification in layers. Through the vertical incision access to the front and back of the roots is afforded. Once the upper root is identified, the structures may be "wiped" forward and medially, allowing dissection from the posterior aspect (Fig. 14–21). Frequently this is a help since scar tissue may not have penetrated to this layer and the roots may be more easily identified.

Following the identification of the upper roots and trunks, from the side as it were, dissection is continued along the anterior and posterior aspect, following the roots distally into the interval between the two scalenes. The scalenus anterior may then be "wiped" or retracted medially and the rest

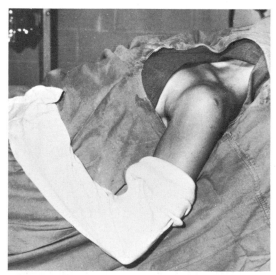

Figure 14–19   Position and draping for supra-clavicular plexus exploration.

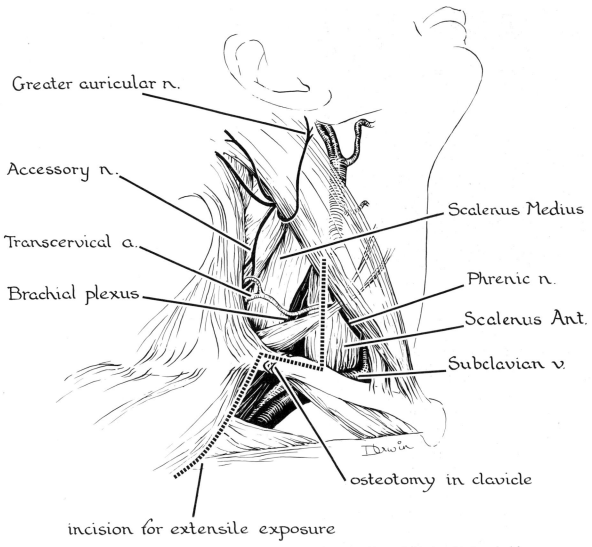

Greater auricular n.

Accessory n.

Transcervical a.

Brachial plexus

Scalenus Medius

Phrenic n.

Scalenus Ant.

Subclavian v.

osteotomy in clavicle

incision for extensile exposure

Figure 14–20 Surgical anatomy of brachial plexus exposure. Above, behind and below clavicle.

of the roots identified in serial fashion. Once the correct plane of the trunks has been obtained, dissection toward the medial side is greatly facilitated even in densely scarred areas. The plexus may be followed distally and freed well under the clavicle. The dependent position of the shoulder tends to pull the clavicle out of the way and allows the trunks to be explored well beneath the clavicle. At the same time the trunks remain closer to the surface instead of dropping posteriorly, as is the case with the body in the horizontal position when a sandbag behind the scapula pushes the whole girdle anteriorly, obstructing the base of the posterior triangle.

When further exposure is necessary, the incision described is extended in a Z-fashion with the transverse limb along the middle third of the clavicle and the distal arm extending from the lateral third of the clavicle. The clavicle is divided just lateral to the midpoint and retracted by steel wires placed through drill holes which are inserted before the bone is divided. These wires serve as retractors and as a quick method of fixation at closure.

Bridging the Gaps in the Plexus Above the Clavicle. In many instances a sizeable gap remains to be bridged after following the above procedures. Extra length is obtained by extension of the incision in Z-fashion

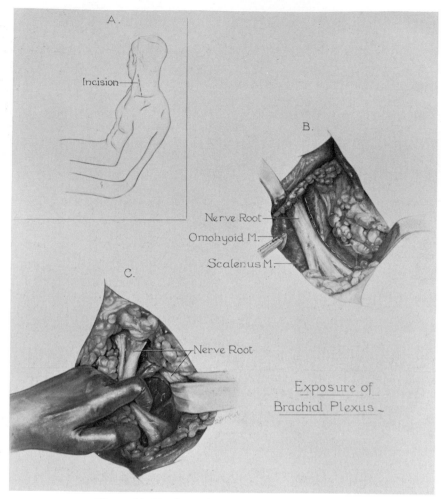

Figure 14–21 Supraclavicular plexus exploration.

distally to below the clavicle close to the junction of the outer and middle thirds. To the incision below the clavicle, the fibers of the deltoid are separated longitudinally just lateral to the deltopectoral groove to protect the extension of the veins in this area through to the subclavian vein. At a point just medial to the coracoid, digital dissection will identify the neurovascular bundle. The attachment of the pectoralis minor to the coracoid is severed, and the fibers of the pectoralis major are retracted strongly or a portion of these fibers are cut obliquely.

It is then possible to mobilize the nerve trunks below the coracoid and they can be pulled up above the clavicle a moderate distance. Some extra length is obtained by this maneuver, but usually it is not enough to bridge the gap.

At this point it will be found that extra length is gained for the nerve trunks by shortening the clavicle, pulling the pieces on top of each other by means of the retracting wire sutures. A piece of the center of the clavicle amounting to 3/4 to 1 inch is then resected and the ends of the clavicle are wired together securely. In fixing the clavicle it is shortened; it will be found that extra length can be gained by further pulling the distal segment of the nerve upward. Three-quarters of an inch to 1¼ inches may be gained by this maneuver, and usually suture can then be carried out without tension. By first wiring the clavicle together and then completing the suture, a firm splint is obtained which takes the tension off the suture line and prevents its being torn apart by movement of the shoulder girdle (Fig. 14–22).

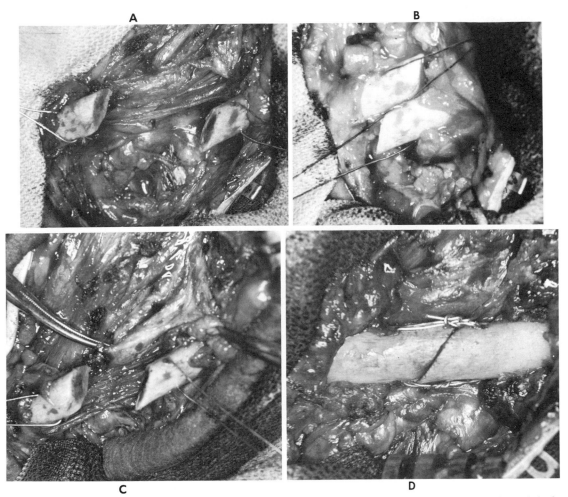

Figure 14-22 Steps in obtaining extra nerve length to bridge gaps in repair of supraclavicular plexus injuries. *A*, Osteotomy of clavicle. *B*, Overlap of clavicular ends possible with moderate traction indicating amount of clavicle that may be resected. *C*, Resection of approximately one inch of clavicle shortens the supraclavicular gap appreciably. *D*, Completed osteotomy with shortening of clavicle. The retracting wires serve as a means of fixation.

Postoperatively the arm and shoulder are mobilized in a body spica with the point of the shoulder elevated slightly.

INJURIES BEHIND THE CLAVICLE

Fracture of the inner third of the clavicle from excessive force often involves the plexus at this point. Serious vascular injuries nearly always occur also. Under these circumstances the vascular damage dominates the picture (Fig. 14-23).

Two types of injury are to be identified: (1) the traction injury in which excessive force pulls the artery and vein over the first rib as a fulcrum and at the same time seriously stretches the adjacent neural structures; and (2) a second, less severe injury which results from force sufficient to break the clavicle but not penetrate strongly beyond it so that there is a contusion type of injury to the neural elements but the subclavian vessels are usually not torn.

Treatment. When there is evidence of progressive vascular damage, immediate exploration of the subclavian vessels is required. The vascular damage is dealt with and, if the patient's condition permits, appropriate nerve repair is also carried out at the same time. Should his condition be critical, however, the vascular damage alone is controlled and the plexus is explored again after recovery from this primary and emergency surgery.

In less severe injuries, even though definite plexus contusion has occurred, it

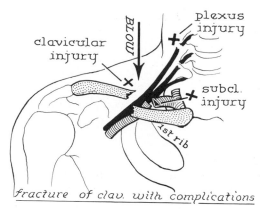

Figure 14-23 Fracture of the clavicle, showing mechanism of neurovascular complications.

may not be necessary to explore the nerves. The decision to do this depends upon the electromyographic findings; if they indicate significant denervation of any group of muscles, this constitutes strong evidence for surgical exploration.

Frequently this type of injury is followed by symptoms of late compression of the neural elements due to scar formation or exuberant callus. Under these circumstances a portion of the clavicle can be excised and the ends reunited effectively, decompressing the neurovascular bundle.

INFRACLAVICULAR PLEXUS INJURIES

Etiology. The elements of the brachial plexus are frequently involved by several mechanisms applied in the area below the clavicle. Thus we can recognize (1) direct trauma, (2) indirect trauma, and (3) complications of fractures and dislocations.

DIRECT TRAUMA. Falls on the armpit may seriously damage nerves and vessels in the axilla. Workmen, for example, in falling from a height may impale the axilla on a sharp edge in their descent, either crushing or cutting some of the axillary contents (Fig. 14-24). Similarly tumbles through windows or glass doors are a not uncommon source of direct laceration of the plexus in the axilla.

INDIRECT TRAUMA. In industry a not infrequently seen serious injury results from the arm's being caught in heavy belting of a machine. The force is often enough to break the humerus at the point of the belt application, and the continued pull is applied to the

soft tissues in such a way that tears of the nerves occur at a higher point in the arm. Damage to the nerves resulting from this mechanism often extends to the area of the axilla.

DISLOCATIONS OF ACROMIOCLAVICULAR AND GLENOHUMERAL JOINT. Forceful dislocation of the shoulder may stretch the posterior cord, axillary and circumflex elements. For some time this mechanism was thought to cause the nerve damage by pressure of the head of the humerus on the cords. As one assesses this mechanism experimentally in cadavers, it appears to be a stretch lesion resulting from abduction and rotation of the humerus, with the head of the humerus acting as a fulcrum, increasing the stretch action as the arm is abducted and externally rotated and extended.

Complete acromioclavicular dislocations with rupture of the suspensory ligament can also implicate the neurovascular bundle (Fig. 14-25). As a rule, this is a late development resulting from failure to reconstruct the suspensory ligaments. A gradual increase in forward and downward displacement of the shoulder girdle results from loss of continuity of the conoid and trapezoid ligaments. Traction on the neurovascular bundle develops intermittently but gradually becomes more continuous. Symptoms of radiating pain and

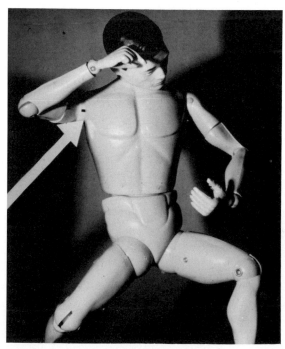

Figure 14-24 Axilla injuries.

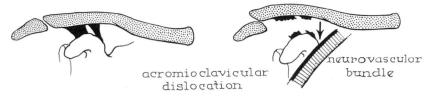

acromioclavicular
dislocation

neurovascular
bundle

Figure 14-25 Neurovascular bundle injury in acromioclavicular dislocation and suspensory ligament rupture.

weakness in the hand develop. Repair of the suspensory ligament by re-establishing the stability of the shoulder girdle relieves the pressure on the neurovascular bundle, and it is not necessary to do a separate exploration of these structures.

DAMAGE TO INDIVIDUAL CORDS OF THE PLEXUS

Lateral Cord of the Plexus. This cord and its branches are infrequently involved. Damage to the outer cord produces paralysis of the muscles supplied by the musculocutaneous nerve, lateral anterior thoracic nerve and a portion of the median nerve (Fig. 14-26). There is motor loss involving the biceps, the coracobrachialis, the brachialis and the pectoralis major. Clinically weakness of flexion at the elbow is the most prominent sign. The sensory deficit is in the distribution of the lateral cutaneous nerve of the forearm along the lateral surface of the forearm.

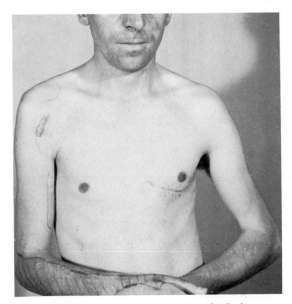

Figure 14-26 Lesion of lateral cord of plexus.

Medial Cord. Injuries of the medial cord produce signs and symptoms mainly involving the hand. There is paralysis of the muscles supplied by ulnar and median nerves. The sensory loss involves the area supplied by the medial cutaneous nerve of the arm and forearm as well as median and ulnar nerves, including the palmar surface of the hand and fingers and the medial border of the forearm and arm (Figs. 14-27 and 14-29).

Lesions of the Posterior Cord. The posterior cord is in a more vulnerable position than either of the other cords, possibly because in lying posteriorly it is more susceptible to cutting trauma from the back in falls or wounds. When the posterior cord is injured, there is paralysis of the muscle supplied by the axillary, radial, thoracodorsal and subscapular nerves. This means paralysis of the deltoid, teres, latissimus dorsi, subscapularis, brachioradialis, and extensors of the elbow, wrist and fingers. Sensation is lost over the dorsal surface of the forearm and the hand (Figs. 14-28 and 14-29).

Treatment of Infraclavicular Lesions. The same principles apply to the management of these lesions as have been outlined for injuries that occur above the clavicle. All the conservative and supportive measures are the same as those applied to the paralyzed muscles. Wounds and lacerations of the axilla tend to be below the supply of the deltoid and shoulder group so that, from the standpoint of splinting, it is chiefly the hand that needs attention. Contractures are prevented by proper physiotherapy and adequate splinting. A splint of the Universal type, such as is illustrated in Figure 14-17, is the most satisfactory.

OPERATIVE TECHNIQUE. The indications for exploration of this area are the same as for injuries above the clavicle. When signs of a complete lesion are present on electrical investigation and clinical examination, operation is required. The arm is placed in abducted and externally rotated position on

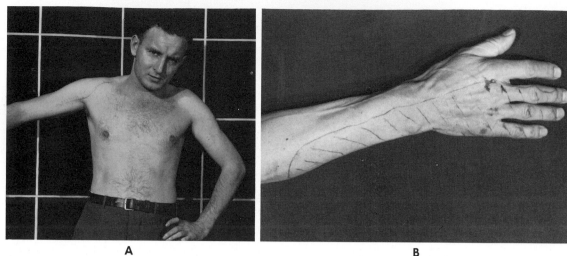

Figure 14–27   *A* and *B*, Medial cord lesion, and indication of area of hand involvement.

the table. The area is exposed by an incision extending from the clavicle across the anterior fold of the axilla down the medial surface of the arm. The incision is deepened by blunt dissection through the axillary fascia, and the neurovascular bundle is exposed without difficulty. In high lesions it may be necessary to detach the medial origin of the deltoid from the clavicle. If possible, the cords are identified above the lesion and traced to the scar area. Dissection is then continued below the site of injury and through the disordered zone of scar. The technique of nerve repair may be mentioned briefly. The result of repairing injured nerves is critically dependent upon the accuracy with which the suture is performed. It is facilitated by using proper instruments which cut and trim the nerve ends accurately. A neurotome

such as that designed by Tarlov is most useful. The nerve should be handled by rubber covered forceps to prevent more damage; the finest of suture material should be used. The author prefers No. 6-0 fine mersilene or ophthalmic silk on a swaged needle and supports the suture line with an autogenous plasma clot. Use of the plasma allows fewer sutures to be inserted and, hence, less foreign body irritation from the stitches. The contraction of the clot splints the suture line, favoring regeneration of axons across the gap.

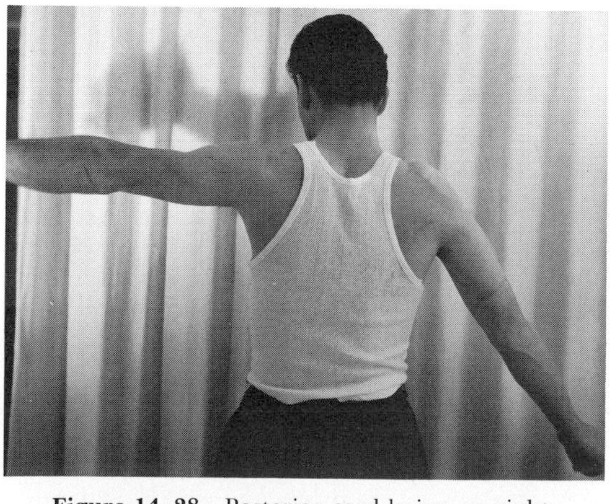

COMMON INFRACLAVICULAR BRANCH INJURIES

AXILLARY NERVE INJURIES

The axillary nerve lies in a vulnerable position in the shoulder and is frequently injured. The damage arises most often as a complication of dislocations and fractures of the upper end of the humerus (Fig. 14–30).

Mechanism of Injury. The nerve branches from the posterior cord and leaves the main trunk on the upper border of the subscapularis, accompanied by the posterior circumflex vessels, and passes through the quadrilateral space to the posterior border of the deltoid. It lies directly below the joint capsule and then winds around the surgical neck of the humerus on the undersurface of the deltoid. In the axilla it may be easily compressed against the head of the humerus or neck of the scapula. It is invariably accom-

Figure 14–28   Posterior cord lesion on right.

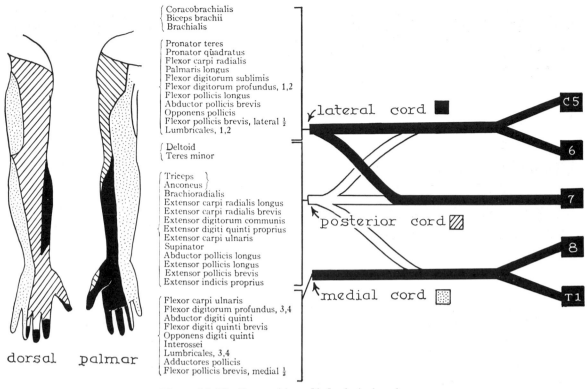

Coracobrachialis
Biceps brachii
Brachialis

Pronator teres
Pronator quadratus
Flexor carpi radialis
Palmaris longus
Flexor digitorum sublimis
Flexor digitorum profundus, 1,2
Flexor pollicis longus
Abductor pollicis brevis
Opponens pollicis
Flexor pollicis brevis, lateral ½
Lumbricales, 1,2

Deltoid
Teres minor

Triceps
Anconeus
Brachioradialis
Extensor carpi radialis longus
Extensor carpi radialis brevis
Extensor digitorum communis
Extensor digiti quinti proprius
Extensor carpi ulnaris
Supinator
Abductor pollicis longus
Extensor pollicis longus
Extensor pollicis brevis
Extensor indicis proprius

Flexor carpi ulnaris
Flexor digitorum profundus, 3,4
Abductor digiti quinti
Flexor digiti quinti brevis
Opponens digiti quinti
Interossei
Lumbricales, 3,4
Adductores pollicis
Flexor pollicis brevis, medial ½

lateral cord

posterior cord

medial cord

C5
6
7
8
T1

dorsal   palmar

Figure 14–29 Composition of infraclavicular plexus.

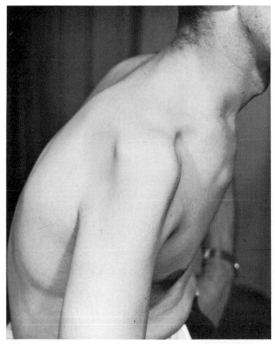

Figure 14–30 Deltoid paralysis from axillary nerve injury.

panied by a large plexus of vessels. In dislocations of the shoulder, as the head slips out from the inferior aspect of the capsule, the nerve is in a vulnerable position and may be stretched. In blows on the posterior aspect of the shoulder or in backward falls, the nerve may be compressed against the neck of the scapula (Fig. 14–31).

Signs and Symptoms. Damage to the axillary nerve results in paralysis of the deltoid and an area of decreased appreciation to light touch and pinprick about the size of a 50 cent piece over the lateral aspect of the shoulder. Atrophy of the deltoid is obvious and results in an angular prominence of the shoulder joint. The shoulder also drops a little, leaving the acromion and coracoid prominent.

Treatment. The deltoid is splinted in the relaxed position with a cantilever splint, and electrical stimulation is applied. Nearly all injuries of the axillary nerve are mild stretches in continuity so that recovery is the rule. When the nerve has been divided by stabs or gunshot wounds, or when no recovery is apparent either electrically or clinically over

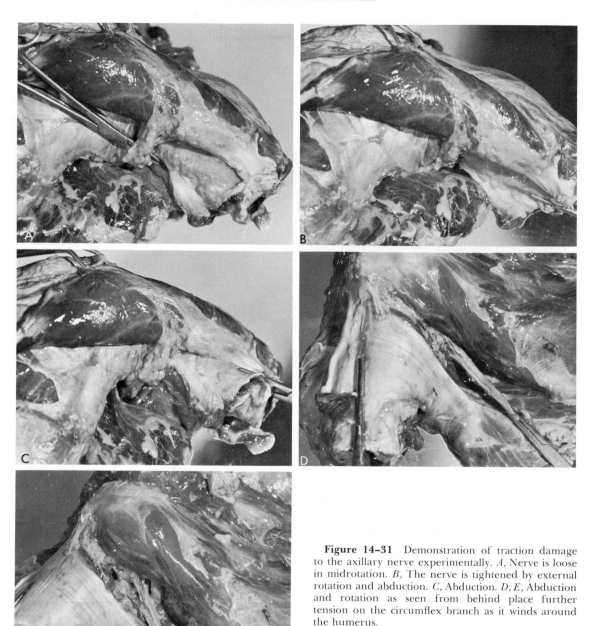

Figure 14–31 Demonstration of traction damage to the axillary nerve experimentally. *A,* Nerve is loose in midrotation. *B,* The nerve is tightened by external rotation and abduction. *C,* Abduction. *D, E,* Abduction and rotation as seen from behind place further tension on the circumflex branch as it winds around the humerus.

a period of four to six months, the nerve should be explored and repaired.

OPERATIVE TECHNIQUE. The nerve is approached through a right-angle incision over the posterior aspect of the axilla. It is identified as it comes through the quadrilateral space and turns toward the deltoid. In repairing the nerve, extra length may be obtained by mobilizing it into the axilla and beneath the deltoid.

IRREPARABLE PARALYSIS OF THE DELTOID

Most deltoid paralyses are eventually overcome, but this is not always so. In young people particularly, the deltoid deficit can be overcome fairly satisfactorily by training the auxiliary muscles. By instruction and practice it is possible to abduct the arm without the deltoid when the rotator cuff and biceps are intact; if this is accomplished, there is no need for reconstruction (Fig. 14–32). The serious deltoid defect usually arises from plexus injuries and is associated with damage to the supra- and infraspinati also. Under these circumstances there are no auxiliary muscles to help replace the loss and serious disability results. Traction injuries of roots C.5 and C.6 are the commonest source of irreparable paralysis. Several operations have been devised, but replacement of abduction power remains a difficult problem. The most satisfactory procedures have been the tendon transfer, as devised by Mayer, or an arthrodesis of the shoulder. Arthrodesis stabilizes the joint and produces some power of abduction. When paralysis is extensive, with involvement of the serratus anterior, biceps and pectorals as well as the deltoid, girdle movement is seriously hampered. Arthrodesis under these conditions does not produce so satisfactory a result as we are used to expecting in the nonparalytic lesions for which it is usually done. It leaves a rigid, poorly powered shoulder.

The author has approached this problem by utilizing the trapezius and the acromion as a method of restoring abduction. Often the trapezius is the only useful muscle in the area which escapes completely. Even after an arthrodesis, the burden falls largely on this muscle, so that any measure to improve

its mechanical advantage is of value. The leverage of this muscle is improved by transferring its lateral attachment to the humerus, fixing it as far down the shaft as possible. To be effective the muscle must be firmly anchored in the new position. These considerations have been met by including the acromion and part of the spine of the scapula in the transfer, leaving the muscle attachment intact. In this way the acromion and spine provide a means of solid fixation to the humerus. By rotating the acromion and spine slightly, extra length in the transplanted tendon is gained. This technique allows transfer of a large mass of the trapezius, producing a strong sling suspending the upper end of the humerus and preventing subluxation. The author has used this technique in extensive, irreparable lesions and found it the most satisfactory procedure (Fig. 14–33).

Technique. With the patient in the prone position, the shoulder is approached through a T-shaped incision. The transverse limb extends from the base of the spine of the scapula posteriorly around the point of the shoulder, terminating just above the coracoid process (Fig. 14–33). The vertical limb is centered over the lateral surface of the upper end of the humerus, extending 2½ to 3 inches distally from the transverse cut. These flaps are then mobilized freely to expose the spine of the scapula, the lateral 1½ inches of clavicle, the acromion and the deltoid. The atrophic deltoid is split, exposing the joint. Dissection then continues underneath the acromion from the lateral

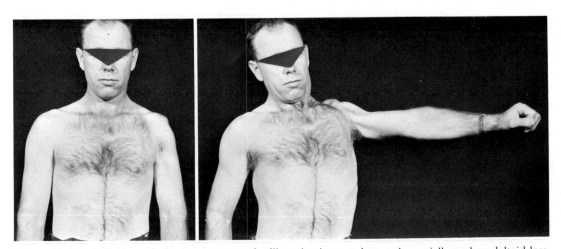

Figure 14–32 Deltoid paralysis. Accessory muscles like spinati can, at best, only partially replace deltoid loss.

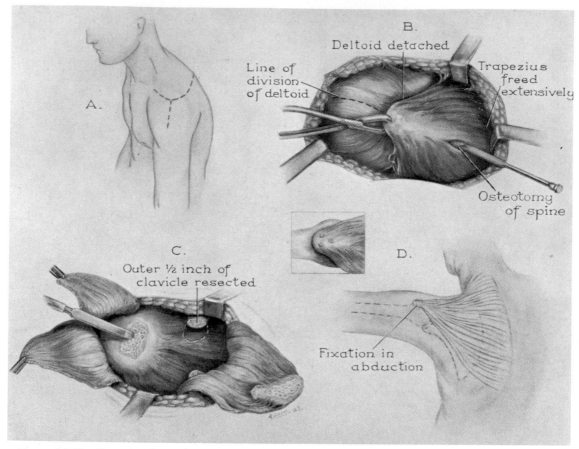

Figure 14–33 Operation for permanent paralysis of abductors of the shoulder. *A*, Incision. *B*, Osteotomy of spine. *C*, Immobilization and pulling of acromion laterally to the head of the humerus. *D*, Fixation to the humerus.

aspect, freeing the undersurface of the acromion and the spine of the scapula. A small area of the spine of the scapula is exposed well toward the medial end of the incision. A small section only is exposed so as to preserve the attachment of as many of the fibers of the trapezius as possible. The spine is cut at its base using a periosteal elevator as a guide from the lateral side. The cut extends obliquely downward and laterally. This frees a broad cuff of trapezius still attached to the spine and the acromion. The superficial surface and adjacent areas of the separated portion are mobilized freely. This provides a broad mass of muscle to be pulled laterally as a hood over the upper end of the humerus. The outer ¾ inch of the clavicle is excised, avoiding damage to the suspensory ligaments. The undersurfaces of the acromion and the spine are prepared for fixation to the humerus by roughening the cortex. The arm is abducted to a right angle and a corresponding area is prepared on the upper lateral aspect of the humerus. The acromion is fixed to the humerus as far distally as possible; firm traction is applied, stretching the trapezius cuff. Two or three screws are used to fix the transferred acromion.

Postoperatively the arm is immobilized in a shoulder spica in 90 degrees abduction. This fixation is continued until the transplant has united firmly with the humerus, which occurs in eight to ten weeks, depending on the fixation. At four to six weeks after operation the patient is instructed to practice shrugging his shoulder while it is still encased in plaster. Two weeks later the upper half of the plaster is removed and active exercise is begun. When union is solid, the arm is placed in an abduction splint in which the arm is gradually lowered to the side. During this period physiotherapy is continued, with emphasis on a lifting shrugging action to train the trapezius in its new role. There are several points in the tech-

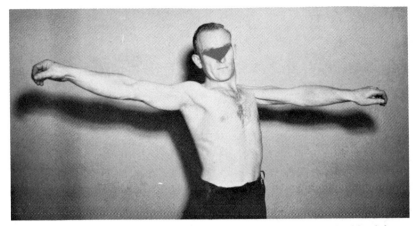

Figure 14–34 Result of trapezius transfer to the acromion in a case of irreparable abductor paralysis.

nique to which special attention should be paid. Sufficient bone is removed at the site of the osteotomy of the spine so that it does not reunite or form new bone, thereby bridging the gap. In fixing the acromion to the humerus, the humerus is kept in slight internal rotation (Fig. 14–34).

QUADRILATERAL SPACE SYNDROME

The author has encountered a group of cases showing a new or somewhat different grouping of paralysis after injury to the posterior axillary region. These patients have paralysis of the deltoid and triceps muscles, usually complete, producing a very disabling combination. Attention is called to this group because heretofore they have been somewhat loosely labeled as plexus paralysis and some aspects of the syndrome have been overlooked.

Signs and Symptoms. Following damage to the posterior aspect of the scapular or axillary area, either due to a blow or a fall backward, weakness of the shoulder and elbow is noted. Examination shows the obvious deltoid paralysis, but the association of the triceps may be overlooked since gravity simulates triceps action so well. More careful questioning may indicate that the posterior axillary area has borne the brunt of a blow. Indentation of the area from the sharp edge of a falling object, such as a tree branch or a corner of a scantling, may be responsible; or the patient may have fallen backward, landing on a protrusion such as a stick, brick, stone, sharp concrete or steel edge (Fig. 14–35).

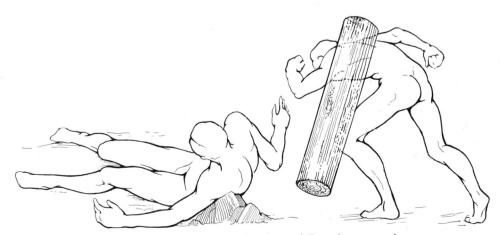

Figure 14–35 Mechanism of injury in quadrilateral space syndrome.

Mechanism of Injury and Pathology. The author has explored several such cases and the maximum disturbance may be demonstrated in the posterior infraglenoid region. The axillary nerve and the branches to the triceps are crushed against the postero-inferior glenohumeral surfaces. The branches to the triceps separate from the parent radial trunk and lie more closely related to the axillary nerve at this point, so that they may be compressed along with the axillary nerve, and the radial nerve escapes (Fig. 14–36). There are many small veins in the area and a well formed plexus almost surrounds the nerves, so that a large hematoma forms quickly from bruising trauma. Evidence of the extensive bleeding is found weeks later in the broad staining of the tissues. The boundaries of the quadrilateral space form a natural barrier, localizing the extravasation. The extensive yet localized hematoma favors scar formation, and at operation the nerves are found enmeshed in many rubbery adhesions. Definite neuroma formation may be demonstrated, amounting almost to division of the nerve. In the abducted position the nerves are particularly close to the bony surface and may be easily compressed.

Treatment. As a rule recovery occurs if a conservative program is followed. This includes proper splinting and electrical stimulation. If evidence of regeneration is not apparent within three months, the area

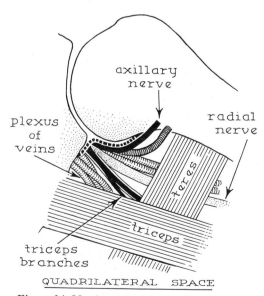

Figure 14–36 Anatomy of quadrilateral space.

should be explored and the nerves released from the strangulating scar (Fig. 14–37). The old argument that bruised nerves recover with or without treatment is not good enough in light of our present knowledge of damage to the myoneural end plate mechanism. Freeing the nerves from scar, or doing anything that will speed regeneration and improved axone conduction diminishes the damage to the muscle. Sometimes the axillary nerve in particular is stuck to the inferior aspect of the glenoid at the neck of the scapula, and sharp dissection is necessary to free it. On palpation the nerve is firm and hard and has obviously been tightly crushed.

TECHNIQUE OF EXPLORATION OF QUADRILATERAL SPACE. The quadrilateral space is approached from the back. The patient is placed on his face with the injured arm at right angles. The space is approached through a right-angle incision centered near the posterior border of the deltoid (Fig. 14–37, *B*). The deltoid is retracted laterally and the teres major superiorly. When this has been done, the nerves in the quadrilateral space may be identified as they stream through and may be followed to their respective destinations. Sharp dissection is frequently necessary to separate the branches from the scar. The nerves are carefully freed over their whole length and all adherent scar is excised. After operation electrical stimulation is continued until voluntary power has returned. In all the cases that have been explored, some recovery has occurred (Fig. 14–38). The deltoid has failed to recover in one case.

Deltoid and triceps paralysis without implication of the rest of the muscles supplied by the radial nerve is the characteristic feature. If the injury is recognized as being the result of direct damage in the quadrilateral space zone rather than an indefinite stretch lesion of the brachial plexus higher up, more rational therapy is possible.

BIRTH INJURIES OF BRACHIAL PLEXUS

The brachial plexus above the clavicle may be damaged during a difficult delivery. Forcible spreading apart of the neck and shoulder by manipulation or abnormal presentation stretches the nerve roots and even the most skillful attention is not always able

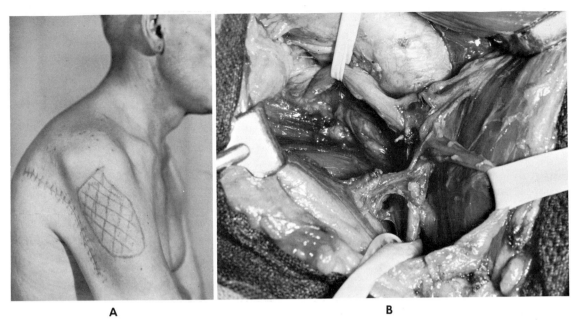

A   B

Figure 14-37 Quadrilateral space syndrome. *A,* Deltoid and triceps atrophy with zone of sensory loss. *B,* Appearance at operation. The deltoid is at the right; axillary nerve is at left above. Thickening and adhesions are seen about the circumflex and triceps branches. The radial nerve is the structure retracted and passing inferiorly.

to prevent the complication. Fracture of the humerus or clavicle may be associated, but the nerve damage is most important.

Clinical Picture. In severe trauma the limp, useless arm is striking. It hangs at the side, partly flexed at the elbow, internally rotated and with the hand turned palm outward. This is the common picture following damage to the upper roots and is labeled Erb's palsy. Less severe forms occur; sometimes only the suprascapular nerve is dam-

aged. The inferior roots C.7, C.8 and T.1 are injured when the arm gets caught above the head, and force then falls on the axilla, stretching the roots. There is little shoulder involvement in such injuries, the major defect appearing in the forearm and hand. Klumpke's name is attached to this type of paralysis. A plea is made to abandon these names as applied to these injuries because, at best, they are an indefinite classification and not scientifically descriptive. Adequate treatment

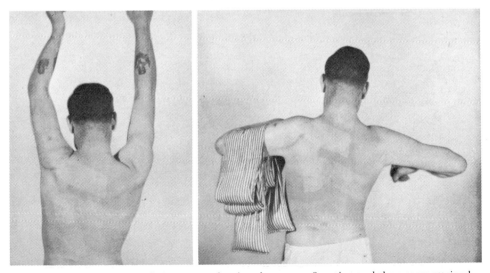

Figure 14-38 Recovery after surgery, showing the range of motion and the power attained.

rests on accurate recognition of the muscles involved, and this is not conveyed by a proper name.

All gradations from transient weakness to profound paralysis are encountered. The less extensive injuries may not be recognized for some weeks, at which point they are largely recovered.

Early Treatment. The principles of treatment are similar to those outlined for other plexus injuries and include proper splinting, electrical stimulation and, occasionally, operative reconstruction. A light splint is applied with the arm abducted, externally rotated, and the elbow at 90 degrees. Splinting is continued until voluntary power starts. Electrical stimulation is desirable but difficult in these cases. The children are frightened and the muscles are so small that accurate application is tedious. In extensive lesions electromyographic studies should be done, but again this is difficult. When no improvement occurs in a matter of months, surgical exploration should be considered. Possibly more of the refractive cases should be operated upon. The time to do this is early, at one year rather than at four years, by which time the myoneural mechanism may have degenerated irretrievably.

Treatment of Residual Deformity. Residual deformity occurs in many of these injuries. The common defect is fixed internal rotation of the shoulder. Even when there is extensive motor recovery, persistent internal rotation is difficult to prevent. Conservative measures such as passive stretching, muscle exercises and education are continued until the age of four or five years. The deformity should not be allowed to continue longer than this because more distal portions of the extremity become involved. Bone growth is altered and deformities become fixed (Fig. 14–39). The internal rotation at the shoulder favors flexion at the elbow, and lack of extension develops. The decreased range of extension becomes fixed when the relationship of olecranon to olecranon fossa does not develop normally. Release of the shoulder internal rotation diminishes these deformities.

The procedure of choice to correct adduction and internal rotation contracture is the Sever operation. The principle of this operation is to cut the shortened internal rotators, remove any obstruction from coracoid and acromion, and rotate the arm into external rotation.

TECHNIQUE. The shoulder is approached through an anteromedial incision extending from the acromion distally to beyond the pectoralis major tendon. The coracoid process is identified and severed near its tip, releasing the tension of the pectoralis minor, the short head of biceps and the coracobrachialis. The subscapularis tendon is identified, elevated and cut longitudinally across its fibers. The arm is then rotated externally. The tip or lateral edge of acromion may need to be resected to free the head completely. When the latissimus dorsi and teres muscles interfere with abduction, they may be severed through a separate incision posteriorly as suggested by Steindler. Postoperatively the arm is fixed in a shoulder spica in the corrected position for two weeks. The arm portion is then bivalved and active exercises

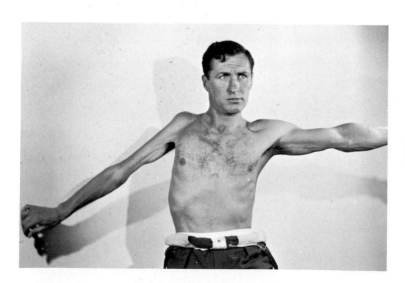

Figure 14–39 Erb's palsy of long standing. Note internal rotation deformity and adductor contracture.

started. Fixation is removed at the end of three weeks.

Treatment of Bone Deformities. In the early stages soft tissue contractures are the deforming elements. Later, bone and joint become a fixed part of the deformity and need treatment. Torsion of the shaft of the humerus is the common finding, but subluxation of the head with torsion is also encountered. Frequently abnormalities of the head of the humerus and the glenoid cavity develop.

OSTEOTOMY FOR INTERNAL ROTATION. Fixed internal rotation hampers shoulder, elbow and hand movement profoundly. The deformity may go unnoticed until an attempt is made to raise the hand to the face, at which time it becomes obvious. When the elbow is flexed, the internal rotation at the shoulder brings the hand to chest level only, and further upward movement is impossible. Patients compensate by bending the neck forward as far as possible to reach the hand. Eating, washing, combing the hair and similar actions are all profoundly hampered. Soft tissue release is not enough at this stage, and a rotation osteotomy of the humeral shaft is necessary.

TECHNIQUE. The operation is best performed just before puberty, when bone growth is not interrupted and the amount of correction needed may be accurately assessed. Some have advocated performing the osteotomy at a level 2 inches below the joint. The author has preferred to do it just below the midpoint of the shaft to obtain complete correction. The shaft is exposed through a longitudinal incision posterolaterally. The humerus is divided transversely. The distal segment is rotated externally through nearly 90 degrees until the forearm is in the lateral body line. The fragments are fixed by plate or intramedullary nail, depending upon the individual operator's preference. The arm is immobilized in a shoulder spica in the corrected position and at about 70 degrees abduction. Fixation is retained until the osteotomy is solidly united, usually 10 to 12 weeks.

Torsion and Joint Deformity. In addition to the torsion of the shafts, the contracture and deformity may be so severe that subluxation of the head of the humerus occurs. Various relationships of head to glenoid are encountered, but it tends to ride posteriorly. Longstanding, neglected cases are the commonest source of this complication.

The posterior subluxation results from the extreme internal rotation and cannot be controlled unless osteotomy is done. The routine advocated by Putti and Scagletti is done in two stages. A preliminary operation releases the soft tissue barrier after the method of Sever, and the head of humerus is returned to the glenoid by whatever maneuver is then necessary. The arm is fixed in the corrected position for two weeks and then the osteotomy is done. This is essential because if the arm were allowed to return to the side, the extreme torsion would reproduce the luxation.

REFERENCES

Bateman, J. E.: Trauma to Nerves in Limbs. Philadelphia, W. B. Saunders Company, 1962.

Cloward, R. B.: New method of diagnosis and treatment of cervical disc disease. *In* Clinical Neurosurgery. Vol. 8. Baltimore, The Williams & Wilkins Co., 1962.

Drake, C. G.: Diagnosis and treatment of lesions of the brachial plexus and adjacent structures. Clin. Neurosurg. *11*:110–127, 1964.

Dutoit, G. T., et al.: Transposition of latissimus dorsi for paralysis of triceps brachii. Report of a case. J. Bone Joint Surg. *49A*:135–137, 1967.

Frykholm, L.: Cervical nerve root compression resulting from disc degeneration and root sleeve fibrosis. Acta Chir. Scand. *160* (Suppl.), 1951.

Harris, H. H., et al.: Nerve grafting to restore function of the trapezius muscle after radical neck dissection. A preliminary report. Ann. Otol. *74*:880–886, 1965.

Howard, F. M., et al.: Injuries to the clavicle with neurovascular complications. A study of 14 cases. J. Bone Joint Surg. *47A*:1335–1346, 1965.

Lain, T. M.: The military brace syndrome. A report of 16 cases of Erb's palsy occurring in military cadets. J. Bone Joint Surg. *51A*:557–560, 1969.

Leffert, R. D., et al.: Infra-clavicular brachial plexus injuries. J. Bone Joint Surg. *47B*:9–22, 1965.

Merle D'Aubigne, R.: Nerve injuries in fractures and dislocations of the shoulder. Surg. Clin. N. Amer. *43*:1685–1689, 1963.

Miller, D. B., and Boswick, J. A.: Lesions of the brachial plexus associated with fractures of the clavicle. Clin. Orthop. *64*:144–149, 1969.

Saha, A. K.: Surgery of the paralysed and flail shoulder. Acta Orthop. Scand. Suppl. *97*:5–90, 1967.

SYSTEMIC DISORDERS OF THE SHOULDER AND THE NECK

Chapter XV

NEUROLOGICAL AND DYSTROPHIC DISORDERS

Neurological disturbances arising from the neck and shoulder are common and significant. The shoulder itself is more frequently involved in neurological disorders than is generally appreciated. Generalized disease may first come to light in this region, or the process can be largely a local one. The hand and the arm, being used for intricate tasks, may first reflect weakness or unsteadiness from disease in the neck or the root of the limb. Disorders such as the muscle atrophies should always be kept in mind in investigating persistent shoulder disability. The group as a whole includes: (1) cervical root syndromes; (2) cervical tumors; (3) dystrophic diseases about the shoulder; and (4) neurovascular syndromes.

CERVICAL ROOT SYNDROMES

A number of neck disorders evoke signs and symptoms that may be brought together as a typical root syndrome. The term identifies changes at a level starting in the spinal cord to the spinal roots through the intervertebral foramina and to the point of plexus formation above the clavicle in the posterior triangle of the neck (Fig. 15–1). Beyond this point a mingling of the roots occurs in forming the plexus so that irritation from this level distally evokes a pattern of mingled segments and the individual root orientation is altered. Thus, it is important to appreciate the anatomy of segment or root distribution as opposed to peripheral nerve or trunk distribution. The prominent examples of root lesion embrace cervical cord tumors and cervical disc or foraminal lesions.

TUMORS OF THE CERVICAL CORD

In 1887 the first recorded operation in America for a tumor of the cervical cord was carried out on a patient who had been complaining of pain in the posterior scapular area for three years. Cervical cord tumors are not common but are mentioned here because of their seriousness and the dramatically successful surgical treatment that can be offered.

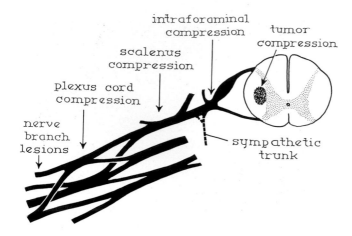

Figure 15–1 Sites of pathology evoking neural type radiating pain.

The signs and symptoms are usually clear-cut, but it is important to be aware of these in investigating shoulder-neck pain. When profound motor and sensory changes are encountered in addition to persistent pain without a history of injury, the possibility of a space-taking lesion should be kept in mind. In all other diseases of this group, the neurological findings are not nearly so definite as they are in the case of cord tumor. Pain starts in a gradual fashion but continues in the shoulder and neck, to be followed later by a sharper radiating discomfort. Characteristically the patient complains of difficulty in finding a comfortable position and the pain may persist at night with a boring, aching quality.

Pathology. Tumors of the cervical cord may be classified as intradural, extradural or foraminal according to the position which they occupy (Fig. 15–2). Tumors developing directly in cord substance are more likely to be malignant, whereas the more usual lesion arises in relation to the dura and is a slow growing, more likely benign entity. The extradural lesion, implicating an individual nerve root, produces the most typical cervical root syndromes (Fig. 15–3).

Signs and Symptoms. Root irritation develops from tumor formation; later, signs and symptoms of cord compression appear. In this way disturbances develop in the lower motor neuron such as atrophy, paralysis and decreased tendon reflexes at the level of the compressed segment. Mixed with this there is upper motor neuron irritation resulting from cord compression, but this affects the fibers below the level of pressure application so that spasticity and increased reflexes are encountered in the lower limbs. Pain and hypesthesia are present because of irritation of the posterior spinal root. Alteration in appreciation of pinprick can be outlined following the segmental distribution. The localization of these lesions may be considered best under the headings of upper, mid and lower cervical regions.

UPPER CERVICAL REGION. The distribution of pain involves the base of the head and neck and later reaches the posterior aspect of the shoulder. Movement of the neck aggravates the discomfort. There is weakness and atrophy of the cervical muscles, such as the trapezius, and diaphragm function may be impaired as a result of phrenic involvement.

MIDCERVICAL REGION. Included in this area are the segments from C.4 to C.7. A lesion at the level of the fifth cervical root produces paralysis of rhomboids, deltoid, supraspinatus, biceps and brachial radialis. The remaining muscles of the upper limb show some spasticity also, as does the lower limb. At C.5 the biceps reflex is decreased or absent, while the triceps reflex remains intact

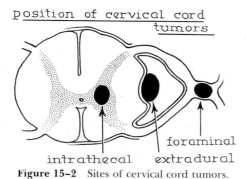

Figure 15–2 Sites of cervical cord tumors.

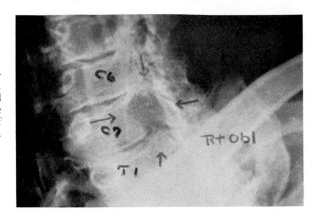

Figure 15–3 Neurofibroma of cervical root. Erosion of the intervertebral foramen may be seen. Patient gave four months' history of shoulder and right arm pain and later difficulty in writing. The lesion has eroded the vertebral body and pedicle of the seventh cervical vertebra. (Courtesy Dr. C. P. McCormack.)

at C.6; with involvement of the seventh root the triceps is implicated.

LOWER CERVICAL REGION. Segments C.8 and T.1 are involved, causing paralysis of the small muscles of the hand and weakness of wrist movement. There may be involvement of the sympathetic supply to the eye, resulting in a constricted pupil and enophthalmia (Horner's syndrome). Tendon reflexes are not significantly implicated, but some spasticity of the trunk and lower limb develops.

One of the striking types of cervical tumor is the neurofibroma arising from an individual spinal nerve. A common location for these is a lower nerve root and the intervertebral foramen. They arise from the connective tissue between fibers or bundles of fibers, forming a localized, slow-growing, fibrous lesion. The tumor gradually erodes the foramen, producing a striking x-ray picture (Fig. 15–3). Shoulder and radiating pain is the common symptom; discrete neurological signs of the nerve root develop later.

Diagnosis. In all cases suspected of a space-taking lesion, cervical myelography should be carried out. The myelogram will present important information that will aid in localization as well as give some indication of the possible type of neoplasm that may be encountered. Other special tests include cerebrospinal fluid assessment. X-ray examination of the chest, complete laboratory blood studies and sometimes a scout series of the entire skeleton should be done.

Surgical Treatment. Once a space-taking lesion has been identified it should be removed surgically by posterior approach.

EXTRUDED INTERVERTEBRAL DISCS

Irritation of cervical nerve roots due to abnormalities related to the interbody structures has now been recognized as a frequent occurrence. An understanding of this disorder and its interbody mechanics has clarified the etiology of these disturbances considerably. The syndrome has been likened to a lumbar disc lesion, but recent study has defined somewhat different pathological states.

Etiology and Pathology. The interbody elements in the mobile cervical and lumbar segments of the spine are susceptible to wear and tear changes starting as early as the third decade. The changes involve anulus, nucleus and cartilaginous plates. Fissure formation in the anulus occurs in the cervical region but less frequently than in the lumbar, so that frank herniations of the nucleus are much less common. The forces of vertebral compression are also less than in the lumbar zone so that squeezing of the nucleus through the anulus is not so frequent. The nucleus undergoes degeneration, shrinking and dehydration in the aging process, losing elasticity and resilience just as occurs in the lumbar region, but the forces imposed on it are not so disturbing. It is in the third element of this interbody system, the cartilaginous plate and its edges, that greatest deformation occurs. A series of accessory joints on the lateral edges of the vertebral bodies from C.2 to T.1 has been identified and minutely described by Luschka (Fig. 15–4). These lie anteromedial to the nerve root and posteromedial to the vertebral artery and

Luschka joints

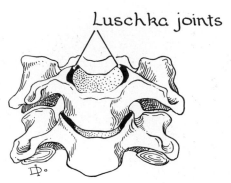

Figure 15-4   Joints of Luschka.

veins. Spur-like small lips on the upper surfaces of C.3 to T.1 form these accessory facets which articulate with cartilage-covered islands and corresponding beveled areas at the lower margin of the vertebral body (Fig. 15-5). A capsule and synovial tissue have been identified, completing these small joints. The consensus by experienced observers such as Compere is that these areas are important in the degenerative mechanics of the interbody system. The wear and tear changes related to the vertebral body edges implicate these articulations. In addition,

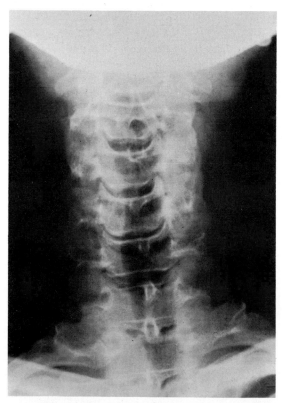

Figure 15-5   Spur formation at Luschka.

stress of motion, particularly gliding motion, is reflected in deterioration of these joints. Their proximity to nerve and vessel has been postulated as a significant irritant in the degenerative or posttraumatic reaction (Fig. 15-6).

Signs and Symptoms.   The typical case is encountered in the middle decades, 30 to 50. The patient complains of stiffness in the neck and pain in the shoulder, followed by pain in the arm and forearm, ending in the fingers. The pain follows two or three distinctive patterns which help to identify these lesions. Commonly the thumb and index finger are involved. The pain has distinctive qualities and distribution; the neck, shoulder and upper arm are involved first by a constant, steady, vaguely localized ache. Shortly there is added a sharp, radiating element with an electric shocklike quality. This becomes a pins-and-needles sensation in the fingers confined to discrete zones. Pain into the base of the thumb or into the index finger and thumb is frequent, which is in distinction to involvement of the whole hand or the middle fingers particularly, as occurs in vascular or neurovascular disorders. Pain develops intermittently and may be followed or replaced entirely by a feeling of numbness in the fingers. It is aggravated by neck movement, sudden changes in position, stepping down a step suddenly, or coughing and sneezing. The pain in the neck and shoulders may be severe enough to awaken the patient at night, and relief is obtained only by changing the position. It is deeply situated and nagging. As a rule, in localizing the lesion, involvement of the thumb and index finger indicates irritation of the sixth nerve root at the fifth space, which is the commonest site; when the middle fingers are involved, it is the seventh nerve root at the sixth space. This is the general rule, but variations due to cervical abnormalities and so-called pre- and postfixed plexuses must be kept in mind (Fig. 15-7).

The mechanism of pain production in disc lesions has been extensively investigated. Frykholm suggests that it is the stimulation of the ventral part of the cervical nerve root that produces the shoulder pain, whereas peripheral discomfort arises from irritation of the dorsal root; possibly the sclerotome interpretation as outlined by Inman and Saunders explains both types of pain (see Chapter III and Fig. 15-8). The supply to deep structures, bones and joints, does not

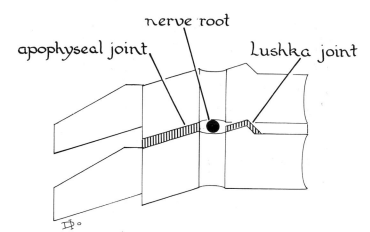

apophyseal joint

nerve root

Lushka joint

Figure 15–6 Articular relations of the nerve root.

quite correspond to the segmental cutaneous supply, so that root irritation is manifested by deep pain from one area (in this case, shoulder) and cutaneous pain in the superficial zone (in this case, thumb and fingers). As might be expected, the disc lesions of cervical and lumbar regions are not exactly alike. Greater mobility and less static compression operate in the cervical zone, which is one reason for fewer cervical extrusions.

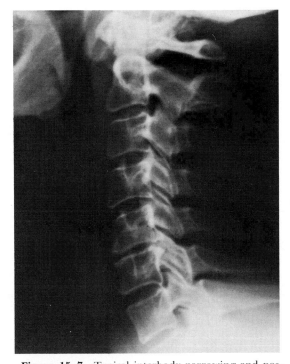

Figure 15–7 Typical interbody narrowing and posterior marginal spur formation producing cervical root syndrome.

NEUROLOGICAL DISTURBANCES

Some authors, notably Cloward, have called attention to the possibility of two separate pain system entities in cervical intervertebral disc disease. It has been suggested that in cervical spine injuries of the extension flexion variety, the pain at the root of the neck with extension to the scapular and interscapular area is on a "discogenic" basis. Cloward emphasizes that the sensory nerve which supplies the intervertebral disc, the sinuvertebral nerve (Fig. 15–8A), extends from the periphery of the anulus to the posterior nerve root (Fig. 15–8A). Then it extends through the spinal cord and out the anterior root and motor nerve to the respective muscles. These observations are based on an extensive experience with the use of the discogram in investigating intervertebral disc pathology. These complaints are prominent in traumatic disc lesions but often subside, being replaced by a soft tissue type of irritation.

The persistent radiating pain of nerve root irritation has been referred to as the "neurogenic" pain as opposed to the discogenic element. In cases of more gradual onset, progressive degenerative changes and osteoarthritic development, it is the neurogenic element which is more likely to dominate the clinical picture.

The neck is held stiffly, and in acute lesions all neck muscles may be in spasm. Movement to the side of the pain increases root compression and reproduces the radiating symptoms; tilting the head away decreases the discomfort. Paraspinal tenderness on pressure at the level of the lesion is present;

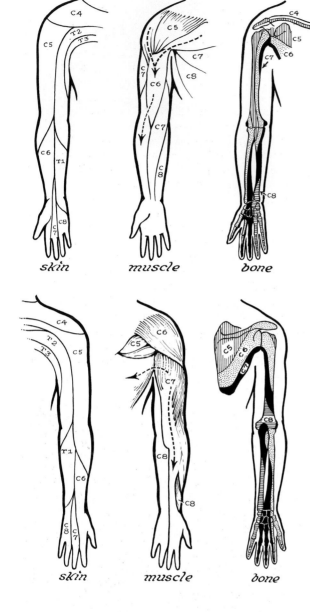

Figure 15–8 Comparison of segmental innervation of superficial and deep structures.

Figure 15–8A Location of sinuvertebral nerve.

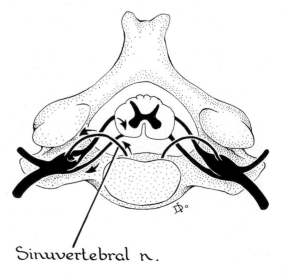

Sinuvertebral n.

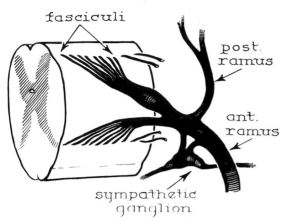

Figure 15–9 Sympathetic contribution reaches a spinal nerve beyond the zone of disc influence.

Spurling has shown that percussion of the posterior spinous process reproduces the radiating discomfort. Signs of weakness and atrophy are not prominent. In C.5 and C.6 lesions (sixth root) the biceps and deltoid are involved; in C.6 and C.7 (seventh root) the triceps is weak. Involvement of small muscles of the hand can occur but is much less common and indicates a lesion of the eighth cervical root. Alteration in appreciation of light touch and pinprick to some degree can usually be shown. It follows the pattern of the cutaneous supply; in case of C.6, the base of the thumb and the lateral border of the forearm are involved. In C.7, the thumb and index finger and sometimes the middle finger are involved.

It is sometimes difficult to outline sensory change and it rarely amounts to anesthesia. If there are signs of profound motor and sensory loss, plus loss of sweating, the lesion is beyond the level of disc and nerve root and must be looked for distally along the peripheral nerve. Difficulty arises in differentiating disc lesions from peripheral nerve injuries. One of the most reliable signs is the loss of sweating, which does not occur in disc involvement but is common in peripheral injuries. The accompanying diagram illustrates this point (Fig. 15–9). The subjective sensory disturbances follow similar distribution, that is, to the lateral border of the arm and to the thumb. If the hypesthesia is along the inside and to the ulnar area, the lesion is likely beyond root level, although rarely the eighth cervical root may be involved by disc protrusion. Root compression by discs below the C.6 and C.7 interspace is

rare, which helps to separate these cases from disorders arising from cervical disc protrusions. Tilting the head to the side of the pain increases discomfort in disc disease, whereas tilting the head and chin away from the pain side aggravates scalene disorders.

Diagnosis

REFLEXES. A very significant sign is alteration of the biceps and triceps reflex. In lesions of the sixth root at the fifth space, the biceps jerk is altered; in lesions of the seventh root at the sixth space, the triceps reflex is commonly implicated. Occasionally both may be involved.

X-RAY CHANGES. In the lateral view there is a loss of the normal cervical curvature for one or two segments; above and below the disturbed level the spine is straight and stiff (Fig. 15–10). Narrowing of the intervertebral space is present and often there is lipping of the bony margins (Figs. 15–11 and 15–12). Oblique views should always be done to show foraminal changes well (Fig. 15–13).

SPECIAL INVESTIGATIONS. Contrast studies, spinal fluid analysis and electromyo-

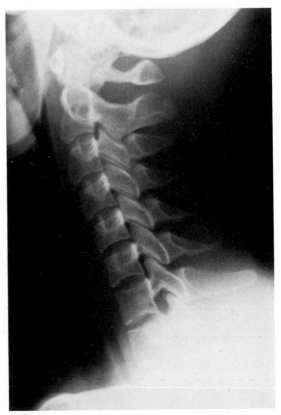

Figure 15–10 Straight cervical spine in acute nerve root irritation.

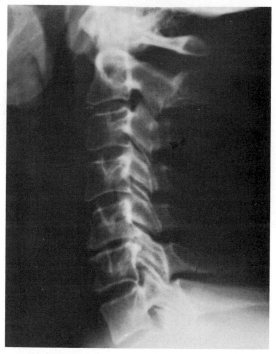

Figure 15–11 Narrowed interbody space with posterior osteophytes producing nerve root syndrome.

graphic studies are the basis of the special investigations to identify nerve root syndromes. Not every case suspected of having nerve root pressure requires any or all of

these special tests, however. Routine x-rays often clearly show the level involved; oblique views, in particular, display the foramina with osteophyte impingement. In conjunction with the clinical findings, plain x-rays may be enough to indicate the level involved. Contrast studies are often helpful, particularly in identifying the level of the greatest impingement when several zones appear narrowed. In cases with profound motor and sensory change, myelography should always be done to rule out a space-taking rather than a degenerative lesion (Fig. 15–14).

DISCOGRAPHY. Discography has a place in those instances in which it is difficult to identify the level involved, and in particular to indicate the zone which requires operative stabilization. Discography is carried out under local anesthesia, a long needle being inserted under x-ray visualization directly into the disc and a small amount of dye being inserted (Fig. 15–15).

Cloward Technique. The procedure may be done in the x-ray department or, if desired, in an operating room with adequate x-ray facilities. The patient is given a mild sedative and placed in the supine position. The right half of the neck is prepared. A superficial skin wheal is made with 2 per cent Novocain without adrenalin. The C.5–C.6

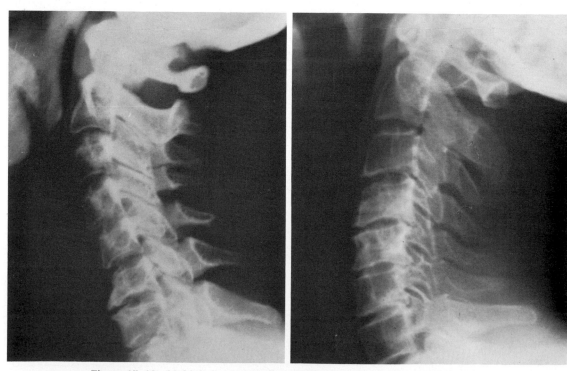

Figure 15–12 Multiple level osteophyte formation causing nerve root pressure.

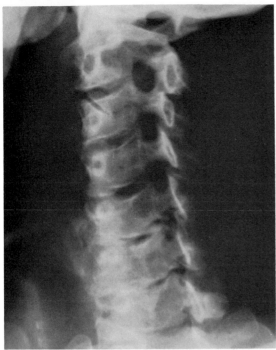

Figure 15-13 Foraminal osteophytes at C.5 and C.6 causing "neurogenic" pain are clearly shown in oblique view.

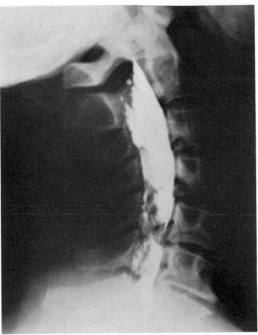

Figure 15-14 Cervical myelogram shows positive pressure on the nerve root at C.5 and C.6 involving the sixth root.

space is approached initially, but this lies directly behind the coracoid cartilage. The principle of the approach is to displace the trachea and esophagus medially and the carotid sheath with its contents laterally. This is accomplished by shoving the structures across the midline with the middle and index fingers, keeping pressure laterally on the carotid artery, which can be identified by its pulsation. Deep pressure in this interval identifies the ridges of the anterior margins of the vertebral bodies and the disc in between. This pressure is maintained and a No. 20 two-inch needle is inserted into the disc at an angle of 45 degrees. The disc space is identified by gentle probing until a sense of giving resistance is encountered in the anulus as compared to the hard firmness of the vertebral body. The needle is inserted into the anulus 1 to 2 mm. Through this needle a smaller bore No. 25 needle 1/2 inch longer is inserted and the contrast media, usually Hypaque, is injected. Normally 0.1 to 0.2 cc is all that is used, but if there is an abnormality such as rupture or separation of the anulus, as much as 0.5 cc may be needed. No more than 0.5 cc should ever be injected.

Considerable attention is given to the patient's reaction during the procedure and

to the distribution of the pain of which he complains.

The procedure should be carried out with care, with proper preparation of the skin, adequate control of the patient, and caution taken not to move the needle indiscriminately in identifying the disc space. Com-

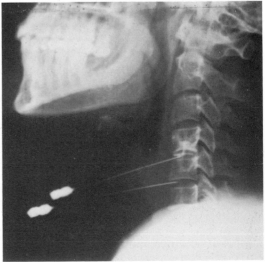

Figure 15-15 A discogram technique. Dye may be seen in the 4–5 interbody space and a needle in place prior to injection for the 5–6 space.

plications reported from discography include pain, infection and spinal cord damage. Those who have used this procedure extensively have emphasized the necessity for proper precautions and for practicing the procedure on cadavers before using it clinically.

Treatment. Cervical root syndromes resulting from disc disease respond well to conservative treatment, and these measures should be used before resorting to surgery.

CONSERVATIVE TREATMENT. Properly applied cervical traction eases the nerve root compression. In acute lesions this is rapidly effective, but in chronic states or so-called hard discs, relief is more difficult to attain. When there is extensive root fibrosis, traction is ineffective and may even aggravate the pain. The latter condition is much more apt to arise in spines involved with extensive spondylosis. The traction program may be started in the physiotherapy department, with the physiotherapist adjusting the weight according to patient tolerance. The usual application is about 20 pounds for 15 to 20 minutes. Home traction is encouraged and the patient is instructed in using his own apparatus. The patient must be taught the importance of applying the pull at the proper angle (Fig. 15–16). If too much extension is exerted, the pain may be aggravated rather than decreased. In some instances pneumatic traction is useful because the patient can adjust the pull to the precise level of relief. Intermittent traction is sometimes needed; such an apparatus consists of a small lever alternator attached to a motor that is introduced into the traction system, contributing an element of jerking pull that may be useful in longer standing lesions in which it is essential to persist with conservative means because the patient is unfit for operative treatment.

The discomfort may reach the proportions that hospitalization is required so that traction can be applied continuously and accompanied by proper sedation. Particularly in patients who appear as poor operative risks, the cervical traction may need to be continued for a matter of weeks. When the patient becomes ambulatory a light cervical collar of Plexiglas should be used; if the nerve root irritation has subsided, some stabilization during sleep is best obtained with a felt collar (Fig. 15–17).

MEDICATION. A program of medication is essential along with the traction. Light

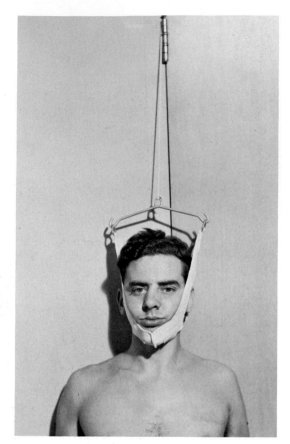

Figure 15–16 Simple application of cervical traction for home use.

sedatives, muscle relaxants and anti-inflammatory drugs enhance the effects of the physical measures. Physiotherapy and other physical modalities also help. Deep heat and massage to promote muscle relaxation, Novocain for trigger areas in the suspensory muscles and ultrasound radiation for deeper penetration all have a place. During the acute stage of pain some patients may obtain better relaxation with the use of ice.

SURGICAL TREATMENT. Those patients not responding well to comprehensive programs can be materially helped by surgical measures. The primary lesion may be dealt with by direct approach, including discotomy and anterior interbody fusion. Occasionally a large extrusion without extensive longstanding interbody change may be better handled by posterior laminectomy and discotomy.

In some instances, particularly extension flexion injuries with root irritation, the involvement of the paraspinal muscles and the scalenes in particular is prominent. Con-

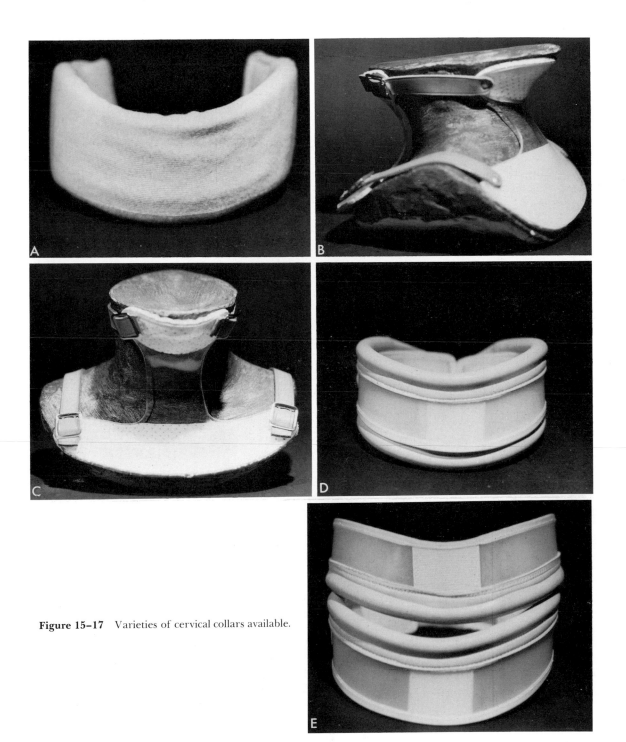

Figure 15–17   Varieties of cervical collars available.

siderable relief of both local and radiating discomfort may be obtained by simple scalenotomy.

Scalenotomy. A short 1½ inch incision is made a thumb's breadth above the clavicle and parallel to it. The deep fascia and platysma are separated along the line of the incision, and the posterior border of the sternomastoid is retracted. At this point superficial cervical vessels may be encountered and will need to be ligated (Fig. 15–18). Similarly the external jugular vein may cross the area and so will need to be clamped and ligated; as a rule, it may be retracted toward the midline. An essential step in this procedure is continued dissection just lateral to the posterior border of the mastoid muscle to identify the upper roots of the brachial plexus. Experience has shown that many anomalies exist in the configuration of the scalene muscles, and some of these implicate the upper roots of the plexus. It can happen that the plexus is buried entirely in the

scalenus anticus, so that if this muscle is cut somewhat blindly, serious damage to the brachial plexus results. For this reason the author recommends that the upper roots of C.5 and C.6 be identified and retracted posteriorly to allow precise identification of the scalenus anticus apart from any plexus involvement. After this has been done it is possible to lift the scalenus anticus and wipe the phrenic nerve from its anterior surface, retracting it medially. Digital dissection is continued toward the medial aspect of the wound, gradually identifying the medial border of the scalenus anticus. From the side and at the back, as it were, the posterior aspect of the scalenus anticus is identified and a Luer clamp inserted posteriorly, elevating the muscle. The muscle then may be cut under direct vision. The seventh cervical root is then apparent posteriorly, and if fibers of the scalenus medius also appear taut, these also can be dissected and cut. Care should be taken in all dissecting maneuvers

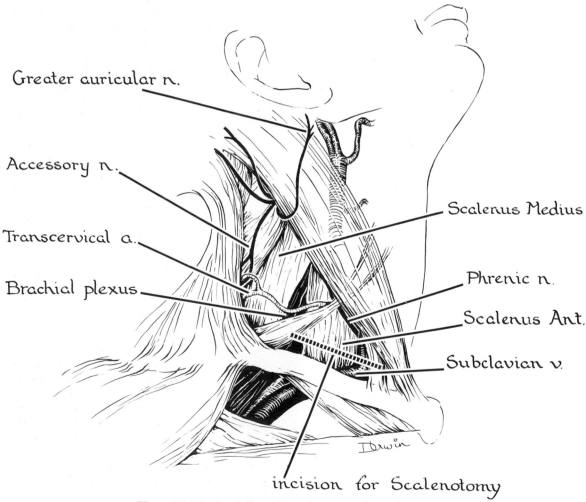

Figure 15–18 Surgical anatomy of approach for scalenotomy.

toward the medial aspect of the scalenus to avoid damage to the carotid sheath and its contents.

Discotomy, Anterior Interbody Fusion, Posterior Laminectomy. When symptoms are not relieved by a reasonable period of conservative treatment, there are surgical measures of proved benefit. In many instances the preferable approach is to the anterior portion of the spine if the lesion is in the region of C.4 to C.7. In this procedure it is possible to remove the disc material quite completely, and if there is a posterior herniation it is often possible to draw this forward by gently curetting the interspace.

Following discotomy some form of interbody arthrodesis should be carried out. The method described by Cloward in 1958 has been modified by many contributors. The principle is to insert a graft in dowel fashion between the contiguous bodies in such a way that it will be locked in place. Unless proper precaution is taken in doing this, the graft may subsequently slip out, causing pressure on the esophagus and trachea. In the author's hands the use of a baled graft which is locked into position with the help of strong cervical traction by the anesthetist has met most of the requirements successfully.

The anterior aspect of the spine is approached by an oblique 4 inch incision along the anterior border of the sternocleidomastoid muscle at the level of C.4 to C.7 (Fig. 15–19, *1*). (If the surgeon prefers, a transverse incision may be used, but the oblique one affords better exposure should abnormalities of blood supply or other obstructions be encountered.) Dissection continues through the platysma separating the interval between the upper border of the thyroid, trachea and medial border of the sternomastoid muscle (Fig. 15–19, *2*). In keeping toward the midline the small strap muscles then come into view and are incised or dissected and reflected medially. At this point the superior thyroid-vein may course across the wound and need to be ligated. Sometimes the pyramidal lobe of the thyroid gland extends proximally or there may be exuberant thyroid tissue from one pole extending to the wound area. As a rule, these structures can be retracted, but occasionally a superior pole of the gland needs to be resected (Fig. 15–19, *3*).

Traction medially will pull trachea and esophagus from the midline, and by digital palpation the anterior aspect of the vertebral bodies can be identified (Fig. 15–19, *4*). As a rule, there is sufficient spur formation that the column is easily felt; often the spur formation is a good guide to the desired level for discotomy.

One assistant retracts the trachea and esophagus with a pair of right-angle retractors medially, and the other assistant retracts the neurovascular bundle under the edge of the sternomastoid muscle laterally. The pretracheal fascia is incised and the spine comes into view covered by a thin layer of prevertebral muscles and prevertebral fascia.

At this point the precise level is checked by radiological visualization, using a hypodermic needle inserted in one space as a marker. Depending upon the equipment and the operator's routine practice, the level is identified using plain films or the fluoroscope.

When the appropriate level or levels have been identified with certainty, the anulus is incised and the nuclear material curetted.

A longitudinal trough about $5/16$ of an inch wide is then cut in the vertebral bodies extending two thirds of the way through on both sides of the contiguous plates (Fig. 15–19, *5*). This produces a trough $5/8$ to $3/4$ of an inch in length. With a curved curet the undersurfaces of the cortex and medullary cavity are cleaned, but the anterior cortex is left in place to serve as a locking ledge for the graft.

The assistant cuts a postage-stamp size graft from the iliac crest incorporating the lateral cortex and the cancellous bone as far as the medial cortex but not through it (Fig. 15–19, *6*). The graft is then cut appropriately so that it may be wedged into the prepared trough. The author prefers to cut a T-shaped graft and use the root of the T as a handle to insert the bailed ends under the cortex with the assistant putting firm traction on the cervical spine. The excess of the T is then excised.

A felt collar dressing is applied immediately after operation and within 48 hours this is changed to a light Plexiglass collar. Depending upon the number of disc spaces treated, the degree of stability, the size of the patient, and so forth, immobilization in bed is continued for three to four weeks; then the patient is allowed up, but must wear the cervical collar for a further six to eight weeks (Fig. 15–20).

Posterior Laminectomy. In the majority of patients the anterior approach is the method

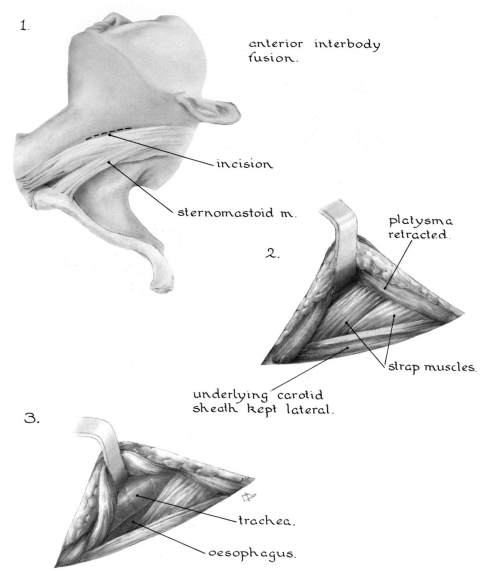

1.

anterior interbody
fusion.

incision

sternomastoid m.

2.

platysma
retracted.

strap muscles.

underlying carotid
sheath kept lateral.

3.

trachea.

oesophagus.

Figure 15–19   Technique for anterior interbody fusion. 1, Incision may be slightly oblique or transverse. 2, Superficial dissection. 3, Deep dissection.

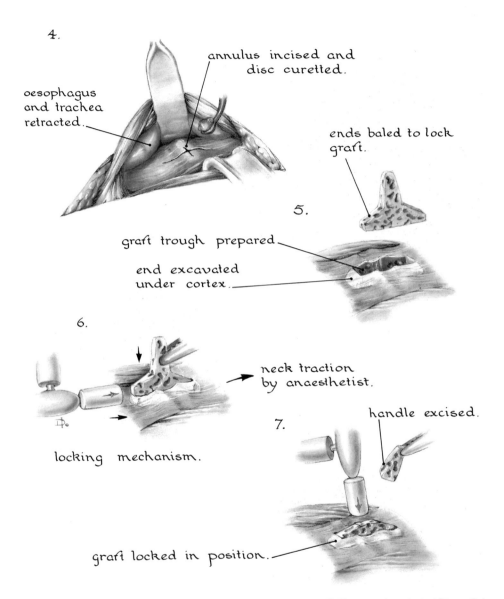

Figure 15–19 *Continued.* 4, Midline structures firmly retracted medially, exposing the midline of the vertebral column. 5, Longitudinal trough is cut in the two vertebral bodies with the cortex at the ends of the trough undercut to allow locking of a baled graft into place. 6 and 7, Locked graft in place with traction released.

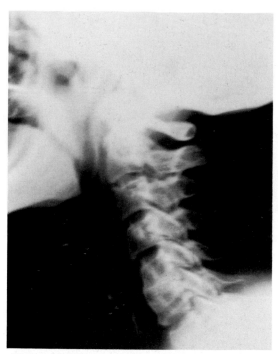

Figure 15–20 Appearance following anterior interbody fusion.

of choice, particularly when only one or two spaces may be involved. When multiple areas may be implicated and there may be some question of a space-taking lesion, posterior laminectomy is preferable. It is carried out in the usual fashion, with resection of the contiguous portions of laminae and direct exposure of the cord (Fig. 15–21).

In some instances when one is dealing with a single level lesion in which the herniation appears to be well lateral and posterior, the approach may be made through the area of the apophyseal joint after the method suggested by Frykholm. In this procedure the bone just medial to the articular area is ground away and finally resected in the floor of the facet. When a portion of this bone on the medial side is removed along with the ligamentum flavum, the lateral border of the spinal cord and nerve root origin with the axilla can be exposed and dealt with appropriately.

NEUROVASCULAR SYNDROMES OF THE NECK AND SHOULDER

The funneling together of nerves and great vessels at the junction of neck and arm has laid the foundation for a large group of disorders with distinctive symptoms and signs. Neck, shoulder and arm discomfort characterize these states. The quality, distribution and course of the pain differ considerably from that encountered in the cervical root syndromes. The clavicle lies in the middle of this area, acting somewhat like the constriction of an hourglass so that three zones of irritation may be identified: one above the clavicle, one behind the clavicle, and one below the clavicle. The differences between vascular and neural pain were pointed out previously and these should be reviewed for a complete understanding of these syndromes (see Chapter IX).

MYELOPATHY DUE TO SPONDYLOSIS

In many instances the effects of degenerative changes comprise a generalized spondylosis, and more than one level of spine may be implicated. Not infrequently the changes at one level reach the point where a much more extensive neurological deficit develops (Fig. 15–22).

Clinical Picture. As a rule, there is a history of nerve root pain of long standing before symptoms develop indicative of extension of the pathological process. In the beginning these symptoms usually include a sense of weakness and clumsiness in the hands, dysesthesia of the fingers and then some weakness in the lower limbs. Added to these findings later will be atrophy of the muscles of the hand and shoulder and spastic weakness in the legs. Tendon reflexes in the upper limb are usually increased.

The sensory changes tend to follow the previous nerve root involvement but increase from the zone of autonomous supply to implicate more extensive areas in the hand. In the later stages some involvement of the posterior columns with altered postural sensibility in both limbs may occur.

Vertebral vascular ischemia may be a complication of severe cervical spondylosis and cervical myelopathy. Under these conditions arteriosclerosis and intimal plaque formation contribute an element of ischemia to the vertebral vascular system which may be accentuated further by pressure on the vertebral artery by osteophyte formation (Fig. 15–22, *A*). To the usual neurological deficit of the myelopathy there are added severe intermittent attacks of vertigo due to the ischemia. In many instances arteriograms will demonstrate significant intimal changes

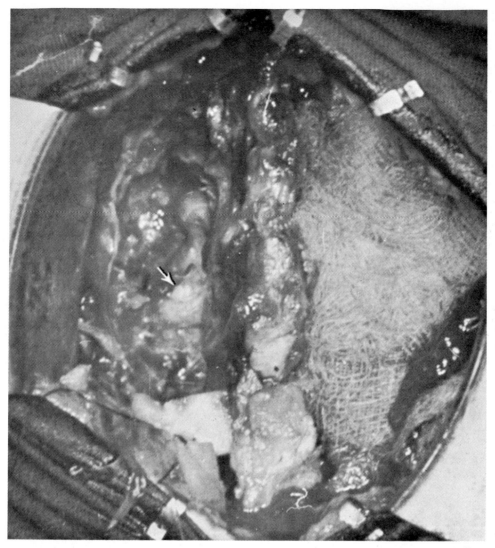

Figure 15–21   Posterior laminectomy and discotomy. Nerve root C.7 is arched over a large soft disc extrusion. (Courtesy Dr. C. P. McCormack.)

of the vascular tree in addition to the spondylosis (Fig. 15–23).

Treatment.   As a rule, the patient has had a comprehensive program of conservative measures for the predominant root irritation stage of the disease, and the development of cord signs is a progression from this state. In some instances a more acute process may develop which is suggestive of a space-taking lesion; sometimes even myelographic findings simulate this disorder also, so that it is difficult to be certain of the precise lesion with which one is dealing. When there are obvious cord signs and the condition of the patient will permit, posterior laminectomy to decompress the cord should be carried out.

In the usual fashion the posterior spinous processes, laminae and articular facets of the cervical spine are exposed from C.3 to C.7. The laminae and spinous process at the level of most extensive involvement are then completely removed (Fig. 15–22, *B*). Inspection of the cord is carried out and further laminectomy is performed as appears necessary and is guided by any apparent compression of the cord. When excessive decompression is necessary, stabilization is desirable. This may be carried out relatively simply by taking a piece of the fibula and splitting it longitudinally, wiring the two halves in place to posterior spines above and below the resected area.

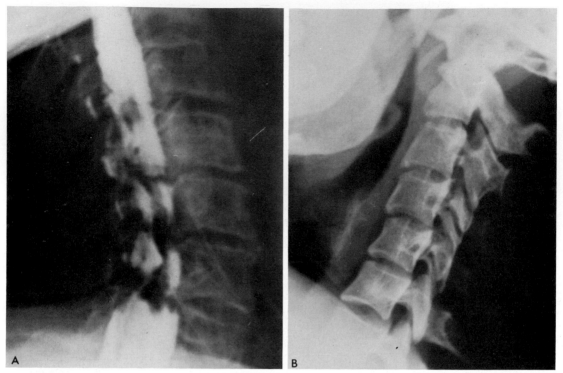

Figure 15–22 *A*, Cervical myelopathy indicated in the myelogram; *B*, following posterior laminectomy.

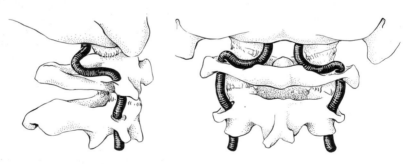

Vertebral artery - head A.P.

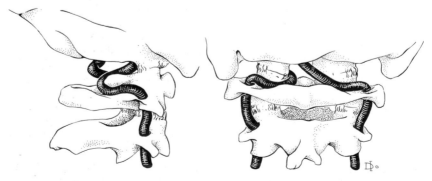

Vertebral artery - head rotated

Figure 15–22A Anatomical and physiological aspects of the vertebral artery.

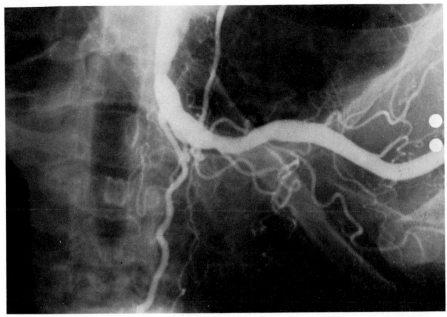

Figure 15–23   Arteriogram showing carotid constriction and arteriorsclerotic narrowing compromising the baso-vertebral system. Such changes contribute to vertebrobasilar ischemia in cervical spondylosis and myelopathy.

Postoperatively the head and neck are supported in an appropriate cervical splint which may be a soft felt collar to start with, progressing to a firm Plexiglas collar when ambulation is allowed at the end of three to four weeks.

When the lesion is at a higher level, C.2, C.3 or C.4, it would appear that the posterior approach is superior, with laminectomy and stabilization being carried out at the same time.

CERVICAL RIB, SCALENE DISTURBANCES AND ABNORMALITIES OF THE FIRST RIB

These disturbances have been considered in detail in Chapter XIV, Nerve Injuries.

Lesions Related to a Normal First Rib

Spontaneous or Fatigue Fracture of the First Rib. Sudden pain in the shoulder with radiating symptoms following strenuous unaccustomed activity may be due to fracture of the first rib (Fig. 15–24). The predisposing forces are the groove on the first rib and the scalene muscle attachment. Strong muscle pull, with the scalenus attached posteriorly and the subclavius anteriorly, is a suggested cause. Indirect violence has been postulated because it is most difficult to damage the first rib by external force without injuring the clavicle. Follow-up x-rays show a typical healing process, so apparently it is a fatigue or stress-like type of fracture that occurs.

TREATMENT.   Limitation of movement until the discomfort has subsided is indicated. In many patients the findings are incidental, although the painful episode can be recalled; frequently it has resulted from carrying heavy loads such as bags of coal or canoes.

High Riding First Rib. Variation in the shoulder slope and the shape of the thoracic cage is frequently seen. Improper posture and congenital deformities of the cervical spine can contribute to the abnormal position of the first rib. Normally the axis is downward and forward, and when this plane is altered so that the anterior end is tipped up, the rib becomes more horizontal and, consequently, abnormal stress may be applied to the neurovascular bundle which loops over it; for example, cervical scoliosis resulting from congenital hemivertebra alters the first rib, disturbing the thoracic inlet. The rib on the convex side of the curve will be higher, with possible resultant traction on the neurovascular bundle. Shoulder and radiating symptoms often develop but may not be apparent until middle life because of early body adaptation. Symptoms may appear after debilitating illness or injury.

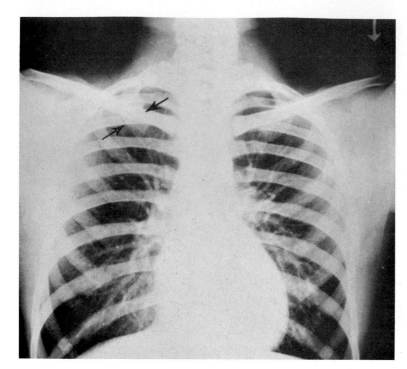

Figure 15–24 Stress fracture of the first rib.

TREATMENT. Conservative treatment is usually sufficient; occasionally scalenotomy or resection of the first rib is required.

NEUROLOGICAL DISORDERS ABOUT THE SHOULDER

The shoulder is involved in neurological disorders more frequently than is generally appreciated. Generalized disease may first come to light in this region, or the process may be largely a local one. The hand and the arm, because they are used for intricate tasks, may first reflect weakness or unsteadiness as a result of disease at the root of the limb. Disorders such as the muscle atrophies should always be kept in mind in investigating persistent shoulder disability. The group as a whole is considered under (1) myopathies, (2) neuroarthropathies, and (3) poliomyelitis. Many of the lesions are quite uncommon, but extensive research, particularly biochemical, is shedding new light on the incidence and the etiology.

MUSCULAR DYSTROPHIES

The muscular dystrophies are a group of disorders characterized by progressive de generation of muscle, which develops apart from any active nervous system disease. Shoulder involvement is not uncommon, and it is particularly important to differentiate these lesions from nerve injuries about the shoulder. The characteristic finding is muscle wasting unaccompanied by any sensory change. The common deformity is atrophy of muscle, but rarely hypertrophy or pseudohypertrophy is the presenting sign. Different types are recognized according to the distribution of the atrophy and certain other properties.

Etiology and Pathology. A strong hereditary tendency is noted in these diseases. The pattern of transmission has been worked out in some instances; the pseudohypertrophic form, for example, appears as a sex-linked character transmitted by healthy females to males only. The origin of the hereditary fault has not been elucidated. Generalized metabolic and muscular metabolic abnormalities have been suggested. Pathologically the process is a degeneration of muscle fibers, which are gradually replaced with fibrous tissue. The degeneration is patchy, with areas of fibrosis alternating with apparently normal muscle fibers. Fibrous tissue is later infiltrated with fat, which in large amounts gives the pseudohypertrophic appearance.

Clinical Features. These disorders tend to begin early in childhood or adolescence, which sets them apart from diseases such as progressive muscular atrophy and myasthenia gravis. Painless atrophy of muscle in a symmetrical distribution is the feature. There are no sensory changes. Vague aching and weakness in lifting the arm followed by obvious wasting is characteristic. There may be other similar cases in the family, or a history of hereditary incidence may be obtained. No true relation of injury or infection has been established, although in industrial cases the patient nearly always relates the onset to some traumatic incident.

Facioscapulohumeral Muscular Dystrophy

There are separate types of dystrophy, but in the shoulder area that most frequently encountered is the facioscapulohumeral dystrophy of Landouzy. As a rule, weakness of the facial muscles ushers in this disorder, producing a characteristic loss of expression or a mask-like appearance. This abnormality is rarely noted by the patient, and the first symptoms to become apparent have to do with the shoulder. Weakness is noted, which progresses and is accompanied by wasting. The wasting process involves the flat muscles about the shoulder particularly, such as deltoid, trapezius, pectoralis and latissimus. The long muscles, such as biceps and triceps, are relatively little involved. As the disease progresses there may be involvement of the trunk and lower extremities. In common with most of the muscular disorders, the disease begins at an early age. The earlier it begins, the poorer the prognosis. It does not always progress and remissions are common, during which the atrophy changes very little (Fig. 15–25).

Treatment. No specific curative therapy has as yet been advanced. Physiotherapy for prevention of joint contractures and exercises to maintain and improve the power of the involved muscles is all that can be done. In some cases electrical stimulation has been applied, and it may have a beneficial effect. The most satisfactory method is to have the patient fitted with his own stimulator and to teach him to use it himself. He learns to stimulate the deltoid, pectorals, and so forth, as routinely as he cleans his teeth. Since the course is unpredictable, continued use of the uninvolved joints and muscles is important. Advantage should be taken of any remissions to improve general body health. Patients may go for years without significant change. If the disease becomes progressive, the involvement of respiratory, trunk and swallowing muscles may prove fatal.

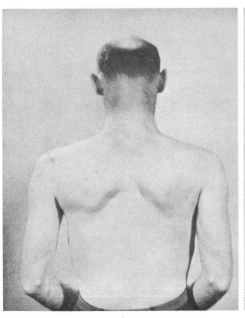 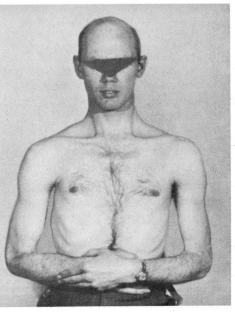

A   B

Figure 15–25 Fascioscapulohumeral dystrophy. *A,* Atrophy of flat muscles of shoulder girdle. *B,* Lack of facial expression and pectoral atrophy.

Pseudohypertrophic Muscular Dystrophy

Apparent enlargement of muscles may occur as another form of muscle substance disorder. This is a generalized process which, as a rule, starts in the lower extremities almost simultaneously with shoulder involvement.

Clinical Features. In the shoulder area certain muscles become enlarged, noticeably the deltoid, spinati and triceps. Occasionally the biceps and the serratus anterior are involved. They become prominent, producing a bulky or chunky contour. On palpation, the muscles are firmer than normal, but they are not so strong. The calves and glutei of the legs are involved, and weakness of this group produces a lordotic stance and waddling gait. The disease is characterized by the absence of sensory abnormalities or central nervous system signs. There are no mental abnormalities. Pseudohypertrophic muscular dystrophy usually begins between the ages of 10 and 15 years and follows through the stage of enlargement to one of atrophy and gradual progressive weakness of the involved muscles. In contrast to progressive muscular atrophy, the small muscles of the hand and feet characteristically escape.

Treatment. The pseudohypertrophic form of muscular dystrophy is progressive, although when it starts in early adult life the progress may be very slow. Muscle exercises are initiated to improve the power of the intact groups. Joint contractures are controlled, but gradual involvement of more muscles, particularly the muscles of respiration and swallowing, occurs. Death usually is a result of the pneumonia which develops following respiratory paralysis.

MYOTONIC DYSTROPHIES

These are a group of muscular diseases less frequently seen than the previous dystropies; they are characterized by an abnormality in the contraction pattern of the muscle. The usual finding is an inability to relax after contraction, so that the individual action is prolonged as relaxation is resisted. Associated with this is a varying degree of weakness and progressive atrophy. A strong tendency to familial distribution is recognized, but the cause of these disorders has not been established. Various types are recognized and are classed according to the character of the contractile action and the age incidence.

Dystrophia Myotonica or Myotonia Atrophica

This is an inherited disorder frequently afflicting several members of a family. It is a rare disease and may be recognized first in childhood. Muscles about the shoulder, the sternomastoids, and facial muscles gradually become atrophic. Later the forearm, the hands and the quadriceps are involved. The initial symptoms are weakness and loss of control in certain movements, such as lifting the arm or turning the head. In addition to the atrophy and weakness, the muscles have an uncontrolled or involuntary persistence of any movement which is initiated. The initial contracture is slow and is followed by stiffness or sustained contracture; for example, in grasping, flexion of the fingers persists and the patient has trouble relaxing the grip. Tapping a muscle may initiate a contraction which is carried on if resistance is applied. There are other defects such as gonadotrophy which frequently accompany this disorder, separating it from similar disturbances. The muscles most frequently involved are the sternomastoids, and atrophy is severe in these. It may proceed to a point where lifting the head from the pillow is difficult or entirely impossible. When it develops in childhood, it frequently progresses till puberty and then remains stationary.

Treatment. The patient should continue his usual activities as long as possible. Undue fatigue and overexposure to temperature extremes should be avoided.

Congenital Myotonia

A similar form starting as a congenital disorder is also recognized. Atrophy and the abnormalities of muscle contraction are not quite so obvious.

Treatment. Research is throwing much new light on these disorders. Quinine reduces the myotonia and is administered orally. The effectiveness of quinine is ascribed to its curarizing action at the myoneural zone. The myotonia is also abolished by cortisone, as indicated by McEachern, but the increased contractility returns when the hormone is stopped. Further work is needed to elucidate the effectiveness of cortisone. In addition to proper drug therapy, attention is also directed toward preventing contractures, particularly adduction contracture of the shoulder. Proper physiotherapy, including adequate exercises for uninvolved groups, is prescribed.

Periodic Paralysis

One of the most dramatic diseases of this group is that labeled "periodic paralysis." Sudden attacks of profound muscle weakness progressing to flaccidity involve shoulder girdle and arm or pelvic girdle and leg. The attacks are recurrent and occur chiefly in young females, although males suffer also. Biochemical research has revealed a striking abnormality in the blood potassium level during attacks and this is the basis of effective therapy.

Etiology and Pathology. Substantial evidence has accumulated indicating that this disease is closely related to changes in the blood potassium level. During attacks the serum potassium drops from 18 to 22 mg per cent to as low as 5 mg per cent. It would appear that mucles drain the serum calcium supply abnormally under certain conditions. Administrations of adrenocortical extract, glucose or epinephrine may produce attacks. Symptoms are dramatically relieved by giving potassium. There are most significant implications in this modality as related to muscle activity in general: In patients with periodic paralysis, attacks may be produced by giving insulin and glucose. The muscle weakness and fatigue of diabetic coma are related to the hypopotassemia and are relieved by administration of potassium. This brings up the possibility of relatively minor muscle disturbances, which are very common, having some relation to the same mechanism.

Clinical Features. The present symptoms are sudden loss of voluntary power in symmetrical groups of muscles in the proximal part of the extremity. The process may start in the shoulder, with loss of power in the deltoid, biceps and triceps. It rarely involves more distal groups or small muscles. There are no sensory changes. The paralysis is a true loss of voluntary power and may last four to five days, then disappear as suddenly as it came. Between attacks the muscles seem quite normal. It is not a psychic or hysterical disorder. Tendon reflexes are lost and electrical responses are altered. Attacks may be associated with menstruation and follow a menstrual period closely. They may cease suddenly and not recur for many months. The tendency is to grow out of the attacks, but they may increase in frequency, resulting in considerable muscle weakness and muscle atrophy. The frequent involvement of several members of a family is characteristic.

Thyroidal and Menopausal Dystrophy

Attention is directed to two new disorders of this neuromuscular group that have recently been recognized. These are thyroidal and menopausal muscular dystrophy. Although they are predominantly generalized disease, the shoulder region is implicated and it becomes important to be aware of them in investigation of shoulder problems. Further significance lies in the biochemical investigation associated with these lesions and their response to divergent therapy. In one instance the thyroid balance is faulty, in the other there is a relation to cortisone action.

Menopausal Muscular Dystrophy. Increased muscle weakness, usually starting in the pelvic girdle but implicating the shoulder too, has been described and is associated with the menopause. Women of the menopausal age are most frequently afflicted, but the condition is described in men also. The profound weakness is relieved by cortisone, as reported by McEachern, and preliminary observations suggest treatment by administration of 100 mg daily for a period of several weeks. Careful supervision is mandatory during this period.

Thyroidal Neuromuscular Disorder. Generalized muscular disturbance in which the shoulder and upper extremity participate has been reported recently by McEachern as being associated with thyroid disturbances. Weakness and abnormal fatigability occur along with hyperthyroidism. The muscle disturbance may follow many patterns and the exact relationship is not quite clear. In one instance it is similar to a periodic paralysis and in another it is a chronic process resembling progressive muscular atrophy. For the present discussion it is important to keep the possibility of thyroid dysfunction in mind in investigating obscure muscular disorders. Correction of the primary lesion is usually effective.

Myasthenia Gravis

Myasthenia gravis is a disease of adult life characterized by a profound fatigability and increasing weakness of skeletal muscles. The neck and shoulder are implicated in the process, although the initial signs appear in the muscles of face and mouth, progressing later to the limbs.

Etiology and Pathology. Many intriguing observations have been recorded relating this disorder to abnormality of the thymus gland. The general properties are most suggestive of an endocrine or metabolic disease. Autopsy findings and those of surgical exploration are conflicting. Tumor formation or hyperplasia is recorded in 50 per cent of autopsies, whereas at operation the percentage is 10 or less. Nerve and muscle show almost no change, so it is presumed that the abnormality lies at the myoneural junction. The clinical condition has been compared to chronic curare poisoning, but the precise mechanism is not yet clear.

Clinical Features. This disorder contrasts with many of those previously discussed because it rarely begins before puberty and usually is not obvious until much later. Weakness begins in the eye and facial muscles, producing the typical ptosis and blank expression. Neck muscles are involved next, leading to a forward tilt of the head and stooped shoulders from the loss of power. This extends to the rest of the skeletal muscles. Symptoms are worse toward the end of the day. Difficulty in chewing and swallowing is prominent. Oddly enough, wasting and atrophy of the muscles are not prominent in contrast to the extreme changes seen in progressive muscular atrophy.

Treatment. This is a chronic disease punctuated by remissions. Thymectomy has been recommended, and the consensus is that it is beneficial. Not all patients are helped, however, and the improvement may be very slow. During exacerbations, rest and proper bed care are essential to prevent undue fatigue and respiratory complications in particular.

Progressive Muscular Atrophy (Amyotrophic Lateral Sclerosis)

The first symptom of this generalized disease may appear as weakness in movement of the shoulder. The disturbance most frequently starts in the upper extremity in early middle life and is characterized by a progressive wasting and paralysis. A relationship to activity has been suggested in that the disease sometimes appears to start in the muscle groups most actively used by the patient in his occupation.

Etiology. In contrast to the previous disorders which were due to disturbance in muscle substance, progressive muscle atrophy is primarily a disease of nerve tissue. There is a patchy degeneration of the anterior horn cells, resulting in peripheral nerve degeneration. Trauma has no proved relationship.

Clinical Features. This disorder has been called chronic "poliomyelitis," which serves to indicate the adult incidence, the slow progress and the predominant lower motor neuron quality. It differs a great deal from poliomyelitis because it is a progressive malady and a disturbance of later life. Symptoms appear first as weakness and clumsiness in certain muscle groups. The muscles about the shoulder, such as deltoid and supra- and infraspinatus, are often first involved. A little later the lattissimus, triceps and pectorals are implicated. This results in progressive weakness and insidious atrophy. Movements such as lifting, holding and reaching become progressively less dependable and are avoided as much as possible.

Although shoulder involvement is prominent (Fig. 15–26), the disease may start in other muscles, or other groups may be involved at the same time. The small muscles of the hand, the interossei in particular, are frequently involved; examination may show atrophy and fibrillation of the tongue. If the disease is suspected, careful inspection usually shows that several muscle areas are affected. No matter where the wasting starts, there are signs of pyramidal irritation in the lower limbs. Sensation is not involved and no definite pattern of wasting and weakness corresponding to nerve distribution is followed. The presence of wasting in other areas, plus lower limb involvement, serves to differentiate this lesion from other shoulder disturbances. Fibrillation or twitching of the muscles is characteristic. This may not be obvious but can be illustrated by gentle tapping of the muscle, which will induce quivering.

Initially the disease may be confused with spinal cord tumor, but the minimal sensory disturbance distinguishes it and there are no spinal fluid abnormalities. Bilateral wasting of the small muscles of the hand may result from cervical rib pressure, but this is differentiated by the characteristic peripheral

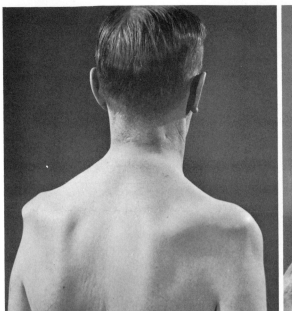 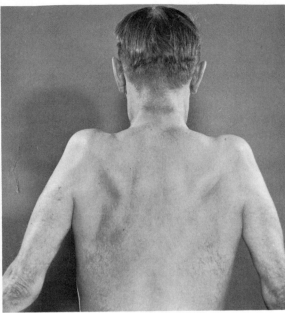

Figure 15–26 Amyotrophic lateral sclerosis.

nerve pattern of paralysis and anesthesia. X-ray clarifies the disturbance. Muscular dystrophies occur at a much earlier age and are not likely to be confused. The only similar disturbance is myotonia atrophica; the increased tone or aftercontraction tension is characteristic. Syringomyelia often starts as atrophy in the upper limbs and increased tone in the lower limbs, but it has a characteristic and prominent sensory disturbance. Peripheral nerve injuries differ from amyotrophic lateral sclerosis because of the distribution of the paralysis and the anesthesia, which follows individual nerve distribution.

Treatment. At present there is no specific effective remedy for the disease. The results of the wasting and muscle weakness are treated. Physiotherapy is used to prevent contractures and to enhance the effectiveness of uninvolved groups. In the upper limbs, self-help devices are an aid. These are discussed under poliomyelitis management. The progressive and generalized nature of the disease makes reconstruction inadvisable.

NEUROARTHROPATHIES OF THE SHOULDER

Despite the tremendous advances in the eradication of syphilis and the greatly improved methods of neurological investigation, neurotrophic joints are still encountered. Shoulder complaints may be the first indication of diseases such as syringomyelia or syphilis. Both these disorders may progress sufficiently to obliterate normal joint sensation so that subluxation and instability of the shoulder are presenting symptoms. We tend to think of neurotrophic joints as occurring much more commonly in the lower extremity because of their weight-bearing. The shoulder is an exception to this because of the high incidence of syringomyelia in the cervicothoracic region. Syringomyelia is particularly characteristic of this group (Fig. 15–27). Posterior column disease, such as occurs in subacute combined degeneration, diabetes and transverse myelitis, can produce similar changes but is rare. The term Charcot's joint has come to be applied to this abnormality when the fundamental pathology is any of the above primary causes. The condition is a widespread and progressive degeneration of the insensitive articular structures. Trauma may precipitate the condition, and the true nature may become apparent after a relatively minor incident.

Etiology and Pathology. In each of these primary disturbances the effects on the joint are the same. The changes develop because of profound loss of sensation in articular and periarticular structures. The normal response for protection of the joint is lost so that it is constantly carried beyond the normal range or fails to respond with a normal reparative process to minor injury. The lack of response gradually produces instability. The increased

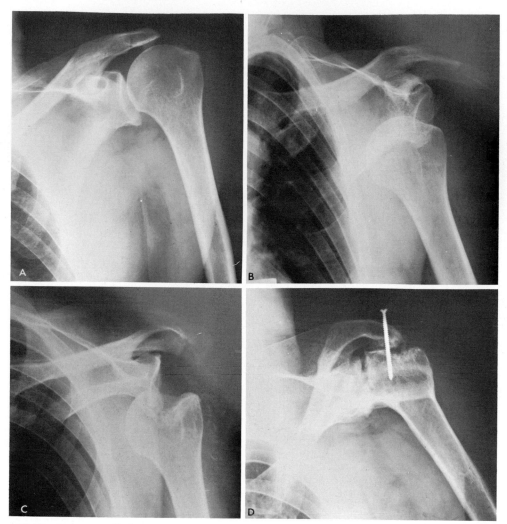

Figure 15–27 Syringomyelia involving the shoulder. *A*, Apparently normal shoulder. *B*, Six months later. *C*, Dislocation with joint destruction. *D*, Following arthrodesis.

laxity is then further aggravated and in a more severe fashion by more and more acute trauma. The range of insult even to minor trauma is increased. The vicious cycle of injury, instability and more profound injury continues until the insensitive joint is grossly disorganized. When such a joint is exposed at operation, gross destruction of articular cartilage is apparent. There are pitting and erosion of subchondral bone, deep depressions, detached loose fragments, marginal hypertrophy and large spurs. The joint capsule is stretched and the articulation is grossly unstable.

Clinical Features. When the shoulder is involved, a similar picture is presented whether the underlying disease is syringomyelia, syphilis or subacute combined degeneration. The distinguishing features of the primary disease are apart from the joint. The neurotrophic joint is recognized at once by the gross laxity and wide instability unaccompanied by pain. The disorganization is way beyond and out of proportion to the complaints. Examination shows laxity of the shoulder in all directions. In some instances it is obviously subluxed, with the head hanging below the glenoid (Fig. 15–28). Mostly the head is dislocated anteriorly. The muscles about the shoulder contract normally, but disuse atrophy makes them thinner than usual. As the joint is examined passively, the ligamentous, capsular and muscular laxity is apparent, allowing the instability. Coarse crepitus, catching sensations and moderate effusion are also apparent. Pain is strikingly absent. As the shoulder is moved passively, any protective pain that occurs arises from the accessory joints such as the acromioclavicular or sternoclavicular. The x-ray shows a characteristic picture, with extensive joint destruction, irregularities and incongruities in the articular surfaces, lipping of joint margins and separated, devitalized fragments.

Signs and Symptoms. Syringomyelia is a disorder of the spinal cord characterized by the development of cystic areas replacing normal spinal cord substance. Cavities develop in the posterior horn of gray matter and appear as elongated spaces. As these expand and dilate, the anterior horns of gray matter are compressed, producing some motor disturbances also. The position of the primary pathology in the posterior horn of gray matter results in distinctive disturbances in sensation. The appreciation of light touch is retained, but the sensitivity to pain, heat and cold is grossly disturbed. The combination of retaining touch and losing thermal appreciation is labeled dissociated anesthesia and usually begins on the medial aspect of the forearm, extending to the chest and pos-

terior shoulder areas. Sometimes it is chiefly the posterior shoulder area that is involved. The patient notices the dulled temperature sense in the hands when washing or from burning the fingers with a cigarette without feeling pain.

Examination shows characteristic local and neurological signs. The shoulder is lax and unstable. There is gross limitation of movement and weakness of all shoulder muscles. Areas of dissociated anesthesia over the posterior shoulder and scapular zone may be outlined. The small muscles of the hands are frequently involved, and this weakness and atrophy spread to the forearm flexors and later to the arm. In the lower limb there may be signs of moderate pyramidal tract compression, resulting in increased tone and hyperactive reflexes, but the disturbance is not nearly so profound as in the upper extremity.

Treatment. When the shoulder is involved, the lesion is a progressive and disabling one. Instability and laxity of the joint lead to subluxation and partial dislocation,

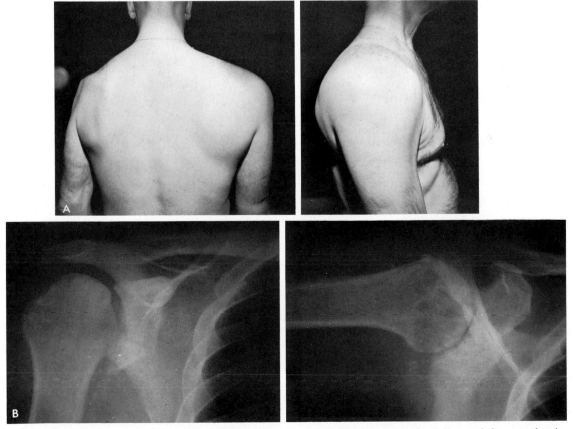

Figure 15–28 Neurotrophic shoulder. *A*, Clinical picture; note swelling on right side. *B*, X-ray of changes, showing gross joint destruction.

interfering with all upper extremity movements. As this increases, pressure occurs on the axillary vessels and brachial plexus. This aggravates any motor and sensory disturbance already present in the hand and may continue. For these reasons, arthrodesis of the shoulder is advised. In some cases when systemic conditions contraindicate extensive surgery, a protective apparatus around the shoulder or a sling may be worn. For all who wish to continue using the extremity, arthrodesis is the procedure of choice.

TECHNIQUE OF ARTHRODESIS IN NEUROTROPHIC JOINTS. These joints are difficult to fuse, and all possible aids must be called upon to obtain a successful result. Arthrodesis can be carried out by methods previously described, but some combination of intra-articulation fusion by bone grafts and internal fixation should be used. The disintegration of the joint surfaces and the deep incongruities make accurate apposition difficult. Surfaces must be excised until healthy layers of bone are exposed and an accurate approximation is possible. When this has been done, rigid internal fixation should be used and the arm immobilized in plaster postoperatively. Plaster fixation is usually necessary for six months (Fig. 15–27, *D*).

TREATMENT OF UNDERLYING DISEASE. The disease in the spinal cord should be treated also, and in this connection x-ray therapy has been the most successful. When the intraspinal process becomes acute or fulminating so that swelling and expansion seriously interfere with lower limb function, it may be necessary to do a decompression laminectomy.

Syphilitic Arthropathy

Shoulder involvement is not nearly so frequent in syphilis as in syringomyelia because of the location of the underlying cause. The lower extremities suffer more in syphilis because of the constant trauma of weight-bearing. When the shoulder is involved, a typical neurotrophic joint occurs similar to that described under syringomyelia (Fig. 15–28). Signs and symptoms develop after moderately severe trauma, such as that sufficient to produce a fracture. The fracture may fail to heal as expected, and the neurotrophic complication develops. A fracture of the anatomical or surgical neck may progress to nonunion, at which time investigation discloses the true nature of the disturbance.

Treatment.

SHOULDER. If the complication is a nonunion without significant joint disturbance imposed, it should be grafted in the usual fashion, followed by prolonged immobilization and intensive systemic therapy. If a joint lesion has become well established, with disintegration of the head, arthrodesis should be carried out as outlined in Chapter VII.

SYSTEMIC THERAPY. Concentrated antisyphilitic treatment should precede definitive shoulder surgery. Follow-up after operation should be most careful.

Subacute Combined Degeneration, Diabetes and Transverse Myelitis

Shoulder involvement is rarely seen in these disorders; the lower extremities are usually the seat of any neurotrophic arthropathy that develops. The treatment of the primary condition overshadows local therapy because of the widespread effects of the disease.

POLIOMYELITIS

Poliomyelitis is an acute viral infection with worldwide epidemiology. It is caused by a RNA virus of the picorna group pathogenic for man and primates. Three distinct types of virus have been identified antigenically. The accepted course of infection is by oral ingestion, with extension to lymphatic channels and the bloodstream from the G.I. tract, following which the central nervous system may be invaded.

Immunity results from development of serum antibodies for all three types of virus. The incubation period varies from three to 35 days, with six to 20 days being the commonest period.

Four distinct forms of the disease have been identified clinically: (1) inapparent infection, (2) minor illness, (3) nonparalytic poliomyelitis, and (4) paralytic poliomyelitis. It is the latter group with which we are principally concerned.

The development of Salk vaccine has marked a major achievement in control of the disease. Parenteral administration of formalin-inactivated strains grown in monkey kidney tissues successfully produces active immunization. After two years, however, booster doses are necessary to maintain immunity. In some instances, oral administration of attenuated strains has been used successfully. Monovalent oral (Sabin) vaccines produce high levels of neutralizing antibodies and are now the recommended method. Administration of type (2) is followed in eight weeks by type (1) and then by type (3) after a further six weeks. A polyvalent vaccine is given to adults in two doses, eight weeks apart.

SHOULDER INVOLVEMENT IN POLIOMYELITIS

This acute infective disease is usually suspected from the constitutional and meningeal signs and later verified by the lower motor neuron paralysis. It can happen that the general symptoms are overlooked and that flaccid paralysis is the first abnormality to be recognized. When the distribution of the effects of the virus is focused on the upper extremity, the shoulder area is frequently involved. Weakness and paralysis of the abductors of the shoulder may be the first alarming symptoms of the disease.

Etiology and Pathology. Poliomyelitis is caused by a group of filtrable viruses probably transmitted by droplet infection to nasopharyngeal mucous membranes and, thence, to the gastrointestinal tract. It probably reaches the central nervous system by absorption from the alimentary canal. An inflammatory reaction is initiated, with hyperemia and edema of the spinal cord. The nutrition of the anterior horn cells is impaired, and if sufficiently severe, necrosis of the horn cells results. There is a spotty distribution so that localized complete paralysis is rare but widespread partial paralysis is common. When the anterior horn cells die, the peripheral nerves degenerate and permanent paralysis results. The horn cells may be subjected to transient pressure only and later recovered. Muscle recovery follows regeneration of the axons if the muscles have been properly protected. The most recent investigations indicate that there are at least three poliomyelitis viruses.

Clinical Features. The initial symptoms are headache, fever, malaise, sore throat, gastrointestinal upsets and irritability. Examination shows stiffness of the neck, fever of 102 to 104° F, and an increased spinal fluid count. These general symptoms may not be recognized, and the patient awakens one morning to find some parts paralyzed. In the upper extremity the shoulder and hand groups are the most often involved. The deltoid is the shoulder muscle most frequently affected, and it may be involved on both sides. The whole upper extremity may be paralyzed, including all the shoulder muscles. Poliomyelitis is differentiated from other neuromuscular disorders by the acute process, the young age group affected, the seasonal incidence, the absence of sensory involvement, the rapid predominant motor involvement and the initial meningeal disturbances. ·

Treatment. In underdeveloped countries where epidemics still occur the principles of treatment include relief of pain, control of deformity, development of uninvolved muscles and appropriate operative reconstruction for residual defects.

DURING ACUTE STAGE. Management of the shoulder involvement is closely related to the disturbance in the rest of the extremity and is based upon the assumption that extensive recovery may occur even when the initial paralysis is severe. During the onset of the disease, general supporting measures and good nursing are all that can be done. Muscle tenderness is treated by moist heat, and when the inflammation has subsided sufficiently, splints are applied to control deformity and prevent contracture. The shoulder is supported in a position of relaxation compatible with the relief of pain. An effort is made to have it abducted as close to a right angle as possible. This is accomplished by degrees, lifting the arm on pillows and allowing it to rest in abduction. The position is altered several times daily, changing rotation. Shortly, pillows are replaced by light splints. When the patient can sit up, a platform is arranged in front to support the arm at shoulder level. When he is ambulatory, light comfortable splints are applied to maintain the arm in a position of function with the shoulder abducted and flexed. Bilateral involvement is common, necessitating abduction splints on both sides. This is best accomplished by using a single central yoke, which is applied over the head with a platform attached at each side.

DURING CHRONIC STAGE. Once the acute reaction has subsided and muscle tenderness in particular has disappeared, more concentrated therapy can be tolerated. The length of the acute period varies considerably; it may be a matter of weeks or several months. Tenderness is not always confined to the paralyzed muscle in the shoulder. The axillary region seems to remain sensitive longest.

In the shoulder the problem is to prevent adduction contracture while paralyzed abductors are recovering. If the patient is bedridden, the position is shifted several times daily. Gentle passive stretching is initiated and continued once the sitting position is reached. If the paralysis is extensive, special attention is needed to prevent the cuff from freezing, limiting rotation. Suspensory slings are a great help during this stage. They may be attached to the bed or applied to a wheel chair. Two leather loops are suspended by springs from a metal rod. The rod is ⅜ inch in diameter and about 5 feet long. It is bent at a right angle so that about 2 feet extends forward over the top of the chair when it is fixed to the back. After the patient is seated in the chair, the springs are adjusted so that the arm is held away from the body in 80 to 90 degrees abduction. Stand feeders and other similar stationary supports are used in combination with the suspensory slings. These self-help devices are a tremendous aid in extensive paralyses.

Besides therapy to prevent contractures, treatment must be given both paralyzed and unparalyzed muscles. Electrical stimulation is started to aid muscles and also to assist in relearning movement patterns. Accessory muscles such as biceps, triceps and spinati, if less involved, are educated to take over the deltoid action. Assisted active movements are started and gradually increased.

MANAGEMENT OF RESIDUAL DEFORMITIES. After some months a point is reached at which improvement stops. This may be six or 26 months, but it is then assumed that indefinite treatment will produce little useful improvement. The problem then is to make the best of what has occurred. When the shoulder is but a small part of an extensive lesion involving upper and lower extremities, mechanical aids are relied upon. Such vital acts as eating, shaving and washing are aided by the suspension sling and stationary feeder. The trapezius frequently escapes, so it may be used in a hunching motion to help raise and lower the shoulder. If the forearm rests on a support, such movement then may be developed to get the hand to the face. Tendon transfer or arthrodesis is not recommended in extensive lesions of the rest of the extremity. More commonly the residual defect is loss of abduction at the shoulder,

with paralysis of deltoid and spinati. The treatment of this defect depends upon the effectiveness of adjacent accessory muscles.

Biceps and Triceps Intact. When the muscles have escaped or have recovered well, a concentrated effort is made to improve their action to compensate for the deltoid loss. Specific exercises are given and trick movements are encouraged, such as swinging the arm into flexion and then abduction to learn a new action pattern. When this is disappointing, the contribution of these muscles to abduction can be increased by shifting their proximal attachments to the acromion. The anatomical and physiological basis of this operation is referred to in Chapters II and III.

Biceps and Triceps Transfer. This operation works best when accessory muscles such as the spinati, latissimus and serratus are functioning well. The technique followed is that recommended by Ober.

Technique. The long tendons are exposed through separate incisions at the front and back. Anteriorly the coracoid process is exposed and the short head of the biceps is detached. The top of the coracoid is severed with tendon to facilitate attachment to acromion. The tendon is pulled laterally and free of the pectoralis to be attached under tension to the acromion. Tied wire sutures are used as fixation. The long head of the triceps is exposed posteriorly and freed. With a small flake of bone it is detached from the scapula and pulled forward. It is fixed to the edge of the acromion in similar fashion. The arm is immobilized in an abduction splint for four weeks. During a further two weeks, the arm is lowered gradually.

Reconstruction for Extensive Paralysis. The real problem is the patient with paralysis of the accessory muscles as well as the deltoid. Often the only muscle which remains intact is the trapezius. All power of abduction is lost under these circumstances and serious disability results. The rest of the extremity may not be afflicted, so the patient is left with a good forearm and hand which cannot be used because of the shoulder weakness. When this is so, there are two procedures that help considerably. The first is some form of trapezius transfer, such as that suggested by Mayer. The author has modified this technique and found it most helpful in these problems. When there is extensive paralysis so that the scapula is not well powered, the result of arthrodesis is disappointing and trapezius transfer is preferable. The technique of this operation was outlined under reconstruction for brachial plexus paralysis earlier in this chapter.

Arthrodesis of the Shoulder in Polio. In some instances stabilization of the shoulder by arthrodesis is preferable to tendon transfer. This operation is only considered in the more extensive lesions. It must always be kept in mind that the result of arthrodesis in the paralyzed shoulder is not nearly so good as we are accustomed to expect in other conditions for which the operation is performed. When the accessory muscles are paralyzed, the girdle is not well controlled. A further consideration is that arthrodesis may be done at a wider angle in children because they accommodate and accustom themselves much better than an adult to the sticking out of the scapula behind and on rotation. This accounts for the superior results in children. Arthrodesis may be performed by any of the methods previously described (Fig. 8–84).

REFERENCES

Auquier, L., et al.: Neuralgic amyotrophy of the upper limb (Parsonage-Turner syndrome) and cervicobrachial neuralgia. Rev. Rheum. 32:516–521, 1965.

Chyatte, S. B., et al.: Early muscular dystrophy: Differential patterns of weakness in duchenne, limb-girdle and facioscapulohumeral types. Arch. Phys. Med. 47:499–503, 1966.

Cloward, R. B.: The anterior approach for ruptured cervical disks. J. Neurosurg. 15:602–617, 1958.

Cloward, R. B.: Cervical discography. Ann. Surg. 150:1052–1053, 1959.

Frykholm, R.: Cervical nerve root compression resulting from disc degeneration and root sleeve fibrosis. Acta Chir. Scand. Suppl. 60, 1951.

Mayer, L.: Tendons, ganglia, muscles and fascia: In Dean Lewis Practice of Surgery. Hagerstown, Md., W. F. Prior Co., Inc., 1947.

McEachern, D.: Disease and Disorders of Muscle Function. In The Musculoskeletal System. New York, The Macmillan Co., 1952, p. 94.

Ober, F. R.: Operation to relieve paralysis of deltoid muscle. J.A.M.A. 99:2182, 1932.

Poulet, J., et al.: Syringomyelic arthropathy. (Apropos of a case with arthrographic examinations.) Presse Med. 76:981–982, 1968.

Roger, J., et al.: Familial and recurring form of amyotrophic paralysis of the scapular girdle. Rev. Neurol. (Paris) 112:557–559, 1965.

Spurling, R. G., and Scoville, W. B.: Lateral rupture of the cervical intervertebral discs: A common cause of shoulder and arm pain. Surg. Gynec. Obstet. 78:350, 1944.

Stamatoiu, I., et al.: Late scapuloperoneal form of progressive muscular dystrophy. Neurologia (Bucur.) 10:21–27, 1965.

Verger, P., et al.: Infantile pseudomyopathic neurogenic amyotrophy. Two new cases. Pediatrie 21:585–593, 1966.

Walbom-Jorgenson, S.: Neuropathy of the shoulder joint primarily diagnosed as sarcoma. Clin. Radiol. 17:365–367, 1966.

Chapter XVI

ARTHRITIS AND RELATED SYSTEMIC DISEASES

Possibly nowhere in medicine is there offered a more fruitful field for a combined effort of the specialities than in the treatment of arthritis. Pioneer work has been done by the American Rheumatological Association in developing a working classification of the diseases of this field, which is reproduced below. From this broad group, prominent examples that affect the shoulder and neck region have been selected for description and study.

ARA NOMENCLATURE AND CLASSIFICATION OF ARTHRITIS AND RHEUMATISM

Polyarthritis of Unknown Etiology
    Rheumatoid arthritis
    Juvenile rheumatoid arthritis
    Ankylosing spondylitis
    Psoriatic arthritis
    Reiter's syndrome
    Others
"Connective Tissue" Disorders
    Systemic lupus erythematosus

    Polyarteritis nodosa
    Scleroderma (progressive systemic sclerosis)
    Polymyositis and dermatomyositis
    Others
Rheumatic Fever
Degenerative Joint Disease
(Osteoarthritis, Osteoarthrosis)
    Primary
    Secondary

RHEUMATOID ARTHRITIS AS IT AFFECTS THE SHOULDER AND NECK

Rheumatoid arthritis is a polyarthritis of unknown etiology. It has been distinguished from rheumatic fever chiefly by the chronicity of joint involvement.

In rheumatic fever, in distinction to rheumatoid arthritis, the patient is acutely ill, with pyrexia and multiple, usually large, joints involved in an acute inflammatory process. Frequently there is also some clinical evidence of cardiac involvement. Joint in-

514

volvement of an evanescent nature characterizes rheumatic fever, but should the changes persist, the state then may emerge into a true rheumatoid arthritis.

Shoulder Involvement. Rheumatoid arthritis in the shoulder is not uncommon as part of a polyarthritis but it is rare as an isolated lesion (Fig. 16–1). In assessing the possibility of a lesion being of rheumatoid character, the clear difference between this state and totally unrelated disorders such as traumatic bursitis, tendinitis, calcified tendinitis and cuff lesions can be clearly demarcated; none of these latter bear any relation to the rheumatoid lesion whatsoever. In understanding the shoulder as an articular complex, a further factor of significance is the dominance of involvement of the glenohumeral mechanism in rheumatoid arthritis; the bicipital mechanism and the subacromial bursa are almost always involved in the rheumatoid lesion, but this is not so in other disturbances implicating the glenohumeral joint.

Etiology of Rheumatoid Arthritis. No universally accepted cause of rheumatoid arthritis has been documented. Some evidence has been accumulated supporting infection as an etiological agent. The other two theories which have achieved prominence in recent years are arthritis caused by immunological processes and arthritis as an autoimmune disease manifestation. It has been possible to examine each of these theories by animal experimentation.

Experiments have been carried out in animals and a type of arthritis to which animals are sensitized has been produced by intra-articular injection with fibrin or inflammatory exudates. This indicates that possibly a secondary autoimmune response can prolong and extend the primary response to an inflammatory agent. The possible role of mycoplasmas in rheumatoid arthritis has been supported by experimental work. In several animal species, organisms of this type are a recognized cause of polyarthritis. The rheumatoid-like diseases in swine are characterized by acute onset, sometimes with periods of exacerbation and remission, with the joint tissues showing hyperemia, edema, swelling and villous hypertrophy of the synovial membrane. Microscopically there is infiltration of plasma cells and lymphocytes in the synovium.

The interest of the rheumatologist in connective tissue disorders in general has been a stimulus to the theory that rheumatoid arthritis is a primary autoimmune disease. The hypothesis advanced is that it may be one of a group of connective tissue diseases that result from an immunological reaction between abnormal lymphoid cells and host tissues. The resultant pathological reaction embraces hyperplasia of lining cells, mononuclear infiltration of the synovial tissue, deposition of fibrinoid and cartilage erosion. Plasma cells, however, which are so conspicuous in rheumatoid arthritis are not evident. A transient type of arthritis with migratory joint involvement has been produced in rats following injection of Frehan's complement which has lent credence to the contribution of this factor. Essentially, these are reactions to microbacterial products. However, the more serious lesions which result from this experimental method, such as balanitis, uveitis and spondylitis, produce a lesion more closely resembling Reiter's syndrome. The adjuvant arthritis in rats may be due to the undirected stimulus to the immunological system which, for reasons unknown, becomes directed against articular tissues; or it could result from the persistent reaction in microbacterial components.

Production of an experimental lesion completely resembling rheumatoid arthritis has not resulted from any one of these three processes, but microplasmal arthritis in swine resembles the human lesion most closely. The efforts to implicate bacteria as a cause of rheumatoid arthritis have been unsuccessful; to date, attempts to isolate a true virus from rheumatoid synovial fluid have been unsuccessful, but the inflammatory theory persists strongly.

Pathology. The tissue changes in rheumatoid arthritis start in the synovium but eventually involve all elements of the musculoskeletal system. Once the reaction is chronically established in the joint structures, profound secondary changes in muscles, bone, nerves and vessels may eventually dominate the picture.

SYNOVIUM. Ultramicroscopic studies have enlarged our knowledge of these changes. The initial one is a marked edema with the production of a mononuclear exudate consisting of lymphocytes, plasma cells and macrophages. There are areas of destruction of synovial cells with the deposition of fibrin. Extensive hyperemia with dilated venules and capillaries develops. This results in the production of a less viscous than normal synovial fluid. The distention of tissue by the inflammatory exudate initiates the pain and tenderness, as well as leading to the decrease in joint motion.

JOINT CAPSULE. Some inflammatory reaction is present initially, with lymphoid and plasma cell infiltration extending from the synovium (Fig. 16–1). Later the capsule becomes fibrotic and thickened. Similar changes extend also to the para-articular ligaments and tendons and the immediately subarticular bone marrow space. In the same fashion as the synovium, the ligaments and tendons which merge with the outer portion of the joint capsule become infiltrated with inflammatory cells, with lymphocytes and plasma cells predominating. The extension from capsule to subarticular marrow space may be through defects in articular cartilage and subchondral bone plate associated with panus formation, or through vascular channels normally connecting with the synovium. The inflammatory reaction initiates increased vascularity, which contributes significantly to the bony atrophy in the area. The striking discrepancy in this process is its failure to invade the fatty elements. At operation a ravaged rheumatoid joint will show that the synovium has been destroyed but the infrapatellar fat pad has remained immune. These changes have been interpreted as a passive or a secondary reaction resulting from extension from the synovium, rather than a primary process taking place within the capsule itself.

In the shoulder the capsular thickening is particularly significant because it implicates the dependent inferior folds, gluing them together, and grossly interferes with motion, abduction and flexion. This pathological change, which is so strongly reinforced by gravity, has been a major obstacle to successful arthroplasty of the shoulder.

MUSCLES, TENDONS AND BURSAE. Changes in the tendon sheath and muscle attachment are similar to the synovial reaction. In the shoulder the subacromial bursa is extensively implicated in more than half the patients. Involvement of muscles arises from the multiple tendon attachments about the joint. Extension of this process implicates nerve endings, and it is probable that this is the dominant factor initiating the deforming muscular spasm.

After joint reaction has become chronic, further change involves the muscles, largely as a result of inactivity. Atrophy of muscle fibers occurs and collections of cells appear between fibers and about vessels and nerves. In some instances this inflammatory infiltration is quite extensive, initiating what has been described as a "myostatic change." When this occurs, more severe muscle signs appear in the form of weakness and tenderness; even electromyographic changes, including fibrillation, can be identified. Enzyme estimations are also abnormal.

CARTILAGE AND BONE CHANGES. Destruction of articular cartilage occurs, with a fibrous panus formation extending over the damaged areas (Fig. 16–2). Recent observations have shown that the death of the cartil-

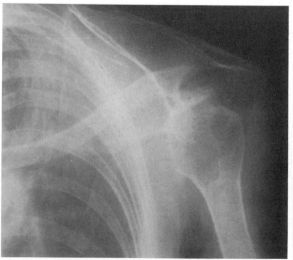
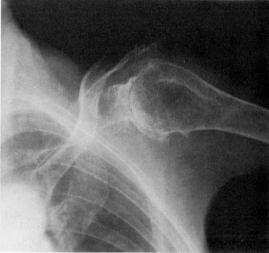

Figure 16–1 Rheumatoid arthritis of the shoulder. Note narrowed joint space, erosion at capsular reflection and extreme osteoporosis.

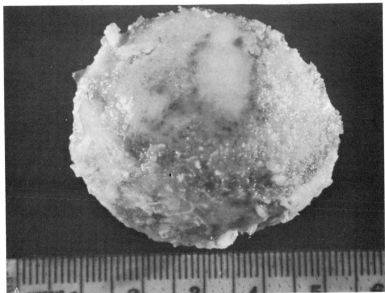

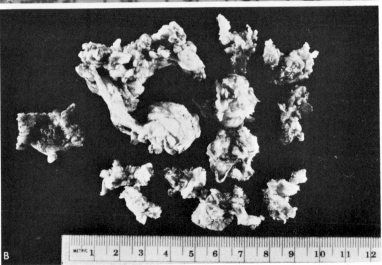

Figure 16-2 Cartilage and bone changes in rheumatoid arthritis. *A*, Humeral head; *B*, joint debris.

age cells probably precedes the panus formation. Previously it was felt that the panus formation invading the cartilage caused the death of the chondrocytes, but this would appear not to be so. In some fashion this is related to failure of replacement of the matrix polysaccharide. Portions of subchondral bone plate may also become necrotic in zones adjacent to the panus formation.

In the later stages of the disease, organization of the inflammatory reaction enhances replacement by fibrous tissue, leading to marked thickening of the joint capsule. Fibrous and bony ankylosis results from the organization of the fibrinous synovial exu-dates. If there has been extensive involvement of subchondral bone, the organization may consolidate adjacent bony surfaces, leading to ankylosis.

VASCULAR LESIONS. Vasculitis is common in rheumatoid arthritis, and severe associated skin changes may appear, including purpura, incipient gangrene and profound peripheral erythema. A high titer of rheumatoid factor and peripheral neuroarthropathy are frequent accompaniments of profound vascular changes. In some instances biopsies have shown cellular infiltration of the small arteries, and the more extensive vascular alterations favor incipient necrosis of the area.

RHEUMATOID NODULES. These consist of masses of connective tissue distributed in para-articular fashion. Sokoloff has suggested that these nodules began as areas of necrosis around small arteries. They are commonest as subcutaneous deposits related to major joints but may appear in almost any part of the limb. Similar granulomas have been identified involving heart, lung, aorta and kidney. Lesions similar to the granulomas may also be found in tendons and, when present, form a weak zone which is a frequent site of rupture of the tendon.

Clinical Picture. Rheumatoid arthritis presents a characteristic picture; women are involved three times as often as men, with onset commonly occurring between 30 and 45 years of age. Shoulder disturbance is often part of a multiple upper limb involvement. The patient complains principally of aching pain, stiffness, night pain and restricted abduction and rotation. Both upper limbs are usually involved if this zone is implicated at all, with the master arm presenting the more extensive involvement.

Signs and Symptoms

GENERAL. Other joints, particularly the interphalangeal joints of the same sides, are swollen and stiff, presenting the characteristic fusiform appearance. Subcutaneous nodules may be identified over bony prominences in para-articular distribution. The slowly progressive change in the small joints of hands and feet is followed by typical deformity.

LOCAL. In the usually thinly upholstered patient, the involvement of the shoulder is obvious from the generalized swelling. The fullness implicates the glenohumeral joint and spreads to the subacromial zone. Tenderness is present over the whole joint. Movement is restricted in all directions, abduction and rotation being particularly impeded. Shoulder movement is possible only by a girdle action, producing obvious scapular rotation.

As the disease progresses, swelling continues and luxation of the head in the glenoid occurs. The joint grates as movement is attempted and pain is considerably increased. In longstanding cases, partial subluxation is frequent.

Laboratory Findings. Rheumatoid factor is present in 70 to 80 per cent of patients. The sedimentation rate is elevated, and a chronic hypochromic anemia is common during the active stage of the disease. Synovial fluid shows characteristic changes, including cloudiness, a deeper yellow or greenish tinge, decreased viscosity and increased white cell count.

Pathological Signs. Soft tissue swelling due to effusion is an early finding, followed by osteoporosis as the cardinal change. The glenoid and head of the humerus are markedly osteoporotic, the joint space is decreased, and the head of the humerus appears to be riding at a higher level than normal.

At the point of synovial reflection from cortical surfaces there is a tendency for bony erosion to form. In the case of the shoulder this is particularly prominent along the inferior aspect. It would appear that unprotected intra-articular bone does not stand the chronic pressure (which is increased in the joint as a result of the synovial hyperplasia) nearly so well as the part covered by cartilage.

In later stages subluxation is favored, accompanied by incongruity of articular surfaces. The joint space is almost totally obliterated. Subluxation probably results from the mechanical factors, principally increase of the intra-articular pressure and dependency of the head of the humerus as related to the glenoid. The changes in the shoulder suggest that anatomical mechanical factors significantly influence the deformities, possibly as much as the disease itself.

Treatment

LOCAL TREATMENT. The principles are to splint the area involved, treat the disease systemically and then restore joint function with physiotherapy and surgery if necessary. The program is best carried out under direction of a rheumatologist, who continues supervision of the systemic program should surgery become necessary.

So often shoulder involvement is but a minor part of widespread systemic disease that other areas, particularly the knees and the hands, receive maximum attention. In the acute phase bedrest with the shoulder suspended at intervals in springs and slings is recommended, followed by use of a light cantilever type brace to prevent severe adduction contractures.

Once the acute reaction has subsided, physiotherapy, including actively assisted motion, is started. The program includes conductive heat, massage, pulley exercises and whirlpool therapy.

SYSTEMIC TREATMENT. The rheumatologist is best equipped to handle all the conservative program. Since this disease so often follows a long and chronic course, a clear understanding is essential of what can be done at various stages to encourage the patient and to help him to maintain complete confidence in the doctor. The principles of rest, relief of pain with salicylates, balanced diet, planned exercises and control of deformities are the accepted general measures. In addition to this, anti-inflammatory drugs are now used consistently. Considerable variation in the patient's response, along with the differences in the stages of the disease, govern which drug or combination of drugs is likely to be the most effective.

Gold Therapy. In most clinics gold therapy has continued to be used and, in some instances, has proved the most effective measure. The drugs commonly applied are gold thioglucose (S-Solganal) and gold thiomalate (Myochrysine). These are given in small doses of approximately 10 mg to assess the patient's reaction, followed by 25 to 50 mg at weekly intervals for a period of months. The continuation of this program depends entirely upon the patient's response. If a favorable response is obtained, the use of 50 mg once a month may be continued for several years. Many contributions have been made to the literature delineating the toxic effects of gold therapy, which include severe dermatitis, hematological disorders and kidney lesions.

Antimalarial Drugs. In some instances chloroquinine and related drugs have been advised. The high incidence of side effects, particularly ophthalmological disturbances, has limited the use of this therapy.

Corticosteroids. In 1949 Hench and his colleagues introduced the use of corticosteroids. They are extremely effective in suppressing the symptoms due to joint inflammation and generalized fatigue. However, there has been no evidence that they effectively suppress the specific disease process. Candidates for steroid therapy are those patients with severe unremitting disease who, in spite of an adequate period on a conservative program, have continued to have fever and anemia, with weight loss, effusion and progressive deformities. The usual plan is to administer sufficient drugs to control the symptoms and then gradually withdraw the medication. The starting dose is small; for example, prednisone in a dose of 3 to 4 mg three times a day is initiated, with a further program depending upon the patient's response. In some instances intra-articular injection of corticosteroids has been recommended, but experience has indicated that this must be controlled very carefully. In the shoulder, in particular, repeated intra-articular injections are to be avoided. Numerous examples of neurotrophic joints with extensive destruction of the articular elements have been recorded. This constitutes a serious complication and one which is almost impossible to eradicate.

Phenylbutazone. This has proved an effective anti-inflammatory drug. It has a special value in many orthopedic conditions apart from rheumatoid arthritis, but in some rheumatoses it is the drug of choice. The initial program is provision of 100 to 300 mg per day for a period of some weeks and, depending upon the response, reduction of the amount to 100 mg a day. Toxic reactions may be frequent with this drug, including edema due to sodium retention, irritation of gastric ulcers and agranulocytosis. For this reason the drug must be administered with caution and continual observation maintained.

Indomethacin. Indomethacin is an indol derivative which, on initial clinical trials, indicated significant clinical response. In some clinics this is the drug of choice, the dosage being a 25-mg capsule daily at bedtime, followed by the addition of a second capsule a week later and a third capsule at the end of the third week to make a daily dose of 75 mg. Use of the drug in this progressive fashion is essential because many patients evidence poor tolerance.

Cytotoxic Agents. In patients with rapidly advancing disease who have failed to respond to the usual forms of treatment, cytotoxic agents such as nitrogen mustard have been applied experimentally. Satisfactory results have not been obtained, so that at the present time nitrogen mustard and all similar drugs have been reserved for the more extreme cases. Similarly, intra-articular injection of these substances has not proved satisfactory.

SURGICAL TREATMENT. Surgical attention to the shoulder nearly always is but a part of an ongoing program of supervision lasting over a period of years. It sometimes happens that the clinical course is such that the shoulder symptoms become dominant, particularly those resulting from subluxation of the head of the humerus. Under these circumstances replacement arthroplasty is advisable (Fig. 16–3). In all these cases it is extremely important to proceed with the cooperation of the rheumatologist since the surgical treatment is but one episode of an extensive

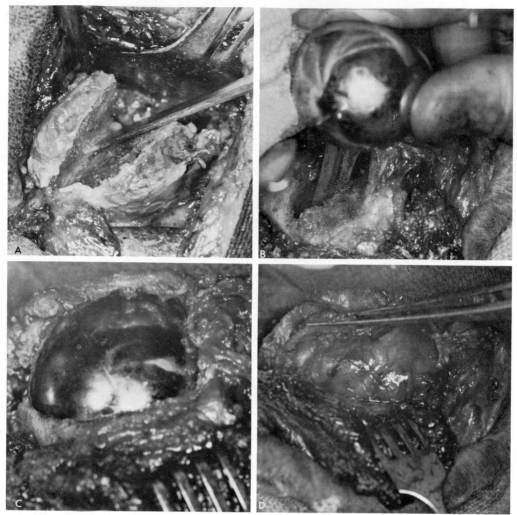

Figure 16–3 Arthroplasty for rheumatoid arthritis. *A,* Excision of head; *B,* preparation and insertion of prosthesis; *C,* prosthesis in place; *D,* closure of capsule over prosthesis.

program. These patients always require meticulous systemic control, and the medical management frequently is much more difficult than the surgical therapy.

Operative Technique. The patient is placed in the sitting shoulder position and the usual superoanterior incision is made, extending from just behind the acromioclavicular joint over the top of the shoulder parallel to the fibers of the deltoid for approximately 5 inches. The incision is deepened between the deltoid fibers (Fig. 16–3, *A*), the coracoacromial ligament is incised and an acromioclavicular arthroplasty is performed. This procedure is carried out routinely to provide adequate exposure and also to make use of its contribution to pain-free increased girdle action.

The capsule of the shoulder joint is incised medial to the long head of the biceps, extending down through the subscapularis. In this fashion the joint is opened and it may be adequately debrided. The head of the humerus is then elevated by the assistant through the aperture in the capsule and the toilette of the head is carried out. In most instances resection of the head and replacement with a prosthesis such as the Neer or other type is required (Fig. 16–3, *B, C* and *D*).

When shoulder reconstruction has been inordinately delayed, destruction of the capsule is sometimes extensive. Under these circumstances an effort should be made to repair it as well as possible, using fascia lata or some form of synthetic suture.

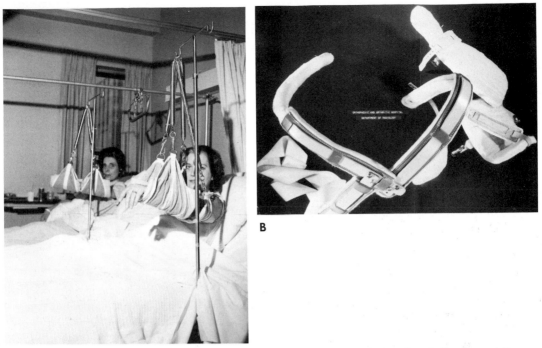

Figure 16-4 Postoperative arthroplasty routine. *A*, Springs and slings suspension. *B*, Cantilever splint.

The arm is placed in suspension for a period of 48 hours and then transferred to the springs and slings apparatus (Fig. 16-4, *A*). As the wound heals and some motion is obtained, the cantilever splint is added (Fig. 16-4, *B*).

The significant complication of all these procedures is the reforming of capsular adhesions on the anterior aspect of the joint. Gravity is a constant menace, favoring gluing together of the infra-articular structures. For this reason the author has persisted in using

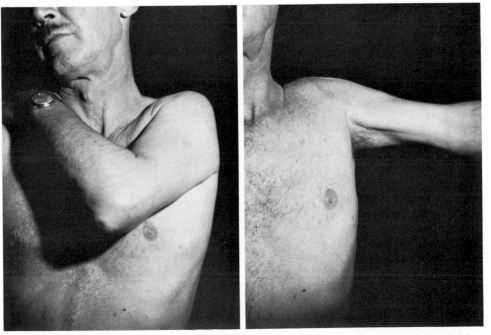

Figure 16-5 Postoperative result four months following arthroplasty for rheumatoid arthritis.

the cantilever splint for some months following surgery in an effort to minimize the periarticular fibrosis.

Extensive recovery of motion is difficult to obtain, but it may be anticipated that with careful physiotherapy the patient will at least get the arm up to a right angle (Fig. 16–5). The salient feature is that nearly always the pain is markedly diminished and the joint reaction subsides extensively. When the capsule is properly repaired the element of neurovascular pressure from subluxation of the head also is removed.

OSTEOARTHRITIS OF THE SHOULDER

Osteoarthritis has been considered in detail in Chapter VIII. A somewhat different type of prosthetic arthroplasty using the cortical contact type of prosthesis can be carried out (Fig. 16–6). The technique is presented here again since, if it is desired, the rheumatoid shoulder may be treated in the same fashion (Fig. 16–7).

ACUTE INFECTIOUS ARTHRITIS OF THE SHOULDER

The shoulder is not often involved in acute arthritis but it can occur. The widespread and effective use of antibiotics has controlled infection following compound fractures and osteomyelitis of the upper end of the humerus, which were the usual sources of articular involvement. Contamination after penetrating wounds and compound fractures remains a source of this lesion. In some instances repeated steroid injections favor a low-grade contamination, with changes which eventually look almost like a neurotrophic shoulder.

Signs and Symptoms. The diagnosis is usually obvious, with exquisite pain localized unhesitatingly to the shoulder area. The pain persists on any action, and there is increasing limitation of movement because of muscle spasm and acute soreness.

On examination the whole shoulder contour is disturbed by a generalized enlargement. Tenderness is present all over, but the superoanterior aspect is the most sensitive. The muscles are stiffly contracted, holding the shoulder and arm close to the side of the body. The signs and symptoms of an acute systemic process such as fever, leukocytosis

and increased sedimentation rate are also present. The x-rays show a narrowing of the joint space and osteoporosis of the humerus and glenoid.

Treatment

ASPIRATION. The joint should be aspirated and as much exudate as possible removed. Penicillin or an appropriate antibiotic, depending upon the susceptibility of the organism, is injected into the joint. Repeated aspiration and antibiotic injection may be necessary. Systemic antibiotic therapy is also continued. The shoulder is immobilized in a sling or light abduction plaster with the upper half removed. Immobilization is continued until the acute phase has subsided and then active motion is gradually restarted.

DRAINAGE. It is rare that the process is so rapid and fulminating that it is not controlled by repeated aspiration and antibiotics. When this happens, however, the joint must be drained. An incision is made over the superoanterior and posterior aspects. Through-and-through Penrose drains are inserted and may be removed as soon as the discharge has stopped. In some instances it is possible to set up a continuous drainage of antibiotics, with the irritation continuing for several days. If the exudate is particularly sticky, the effectiveness of the antibiotic will be enhanced by the use of a detergent.

GOUT OF THE SHOULDER

Gout has long been recognized as a metabolic disease involving many joints. Symptoms related to the shoulder are uncommon as a single entity but may be recognized as part of the generalized process. In nearly all instances involvement of the shoulder is a late manifestation occurring in patients who have extremely severe disease.

Pathology. No joint is exempt from the involvement of metabolic arthritis, but those of the lower extremity are much more commonly involved. The characteristic finding is a deposit of urates in the periarticular structures and cartilage adjacent to the epiphyseal area. The deposits produce local necrosis, which is followed by a foreign body reaction and proliferation of fibrous tissue (Fig. 16–8).

The crystals have been identified as monosodium urate monohydrate, and a characteristic tophaceous nodule consists of a multicentric deposit of urate crystals and

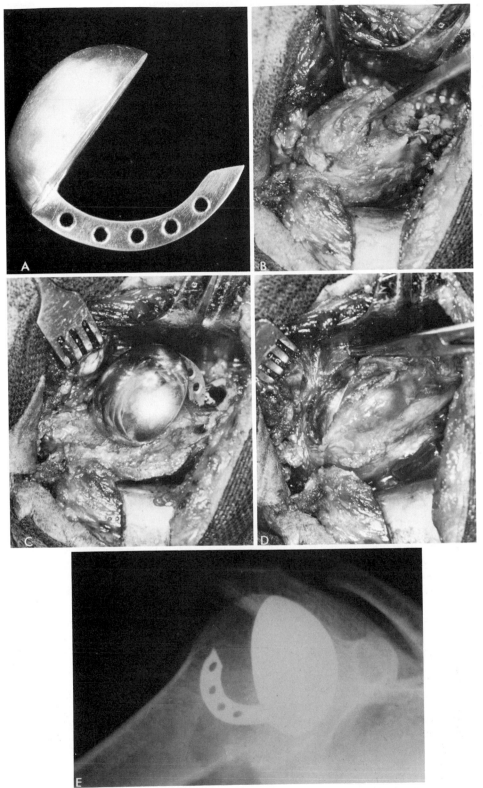

Figure 16–6 Alternative technique for shoulder arthroplasty. *A*, Vitallium plate cortical contact prosthesis. *B*, Preparation of head for resection with an osteotome. *C*, Prosthesis being inserted. *D*, Closure of capsule, *E*, Postoperative x-ray appearance.

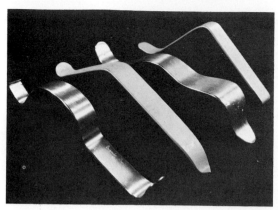

Figure 16–7 Set of special shoulder retractors which is of considerable help in all shoulder surgery.

intercrystalline matrix together with inflammatory reaction and foreign body granuloma. The process produces cartilaginous degeneration and considerable synovial irritation. Ultimately destruction of subchondral bone and proliferation of the adjacent zone develops as a result of the panus infiltration, producing a characteristic appearance. The laboratory findings of an increase in blood uric acid are diagnostic.

Treatment. The primary need is for treatment of the systemic condition. The most effective remedies are colchicine 0.5 or 0.65 mg every one or two hours until the pain is relieved or until diarrhea, nausea or vomiting occurs. Intravenous colchicine in 1 to 3 mg doses is effective and minimizes the intestinal irritation. Phenylbutazone is extremely effective but must be used with high initial doses of 400 to 600 mg followed by doses of 100 mg four times daily. A diet of milk, fruit juice, eggs and cereals and high fluid intake is also required.

If the shoulder is acutely involved it should be splinted by a light abduction splint until the acute attack has subsided; this should be followed by a program of active and assisted active motion. The shoulder is so rarely involved that surgical attention is not often required; should articular changes be extensive, arthroplasty may be required.

PSEUDOGOUT OR ARTICULAR CHONDROCALCINOSIS

In 1958 the Czechoslovakian authors Zitman and Sitchek first identified a condition of chondrocalcinosis polyarticularis which they differentiated from other metabolic arthritides such as gout. Subsequently the term pseudogout was applied to what is a gout-like syndrome in which there is a deposition of calcium thyrophosphate dehydrate (C.T.P.D.) crystals in the joint.

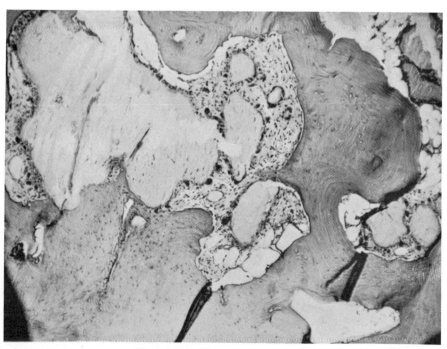

Figure 16–8 Gout of the shoulder.

Pathology. Deposits of crystals in fibro-cartilaginous structures are encountered, with the knee being involved in about 90 per cent of all cases. Microscopically the deposits are composed of microcrystalline aggregates of C.T.P.D. Synovial biopsy shows inflammatory and reparative changes consistent with the clinical state of the joint at the time of the biopsy. The precise mechanism of the crystal precipitation in the cartilage has not been identified. Presumably an acute attack results from the rupture of a preformed deposit into the adjacent large tissue area of the synovial cavity. Crystals have been identified initially in all fluids obtained from acutely inflamed joints in these patients.

The shoulder may be involved, but only rarely. It presents a picture of acute irritation very similar to that of calcified tendinitis. However, there are a frank effusion and generalized joint tenderness. The diagnostic criteria for pseudogout include the demonstration of the crystals obtained by biopsy, typical calcifications on the x-rays and an acute synovitis.

Treatment. Specific treatment has not been identified for this condition, but relief has been obtained by aspiration of the joint followed by injection of corticosteroids. In some instances phenylbutazone also appears to be of benefit. Caution should be observed, however, in carrying out repeated intra-articular injections.

SCLERODERMA

Progressive systemic sclerosis or scleroderma is a disease whose main histopathological feature is hyperplasia of collagen. The primary change involves the skin, but the changes in this zone subsequently give rise to contractures which lead to extensive limitation of joint movement. The upper extremities are involved much more frequently than the rest of the body, and the shoulder is implicated correspondingly.

Pathology. The onset is insidious, usually occurring in the fourth to fifth decade; it involves females much more often than males. Microscopically there is extensive hyperplasia of collagen with a diffuse distribution. In many instances vascular changes precede the cutaneous involvement. The skin is puffy and swollen initially, and this is followed by thickening and induration. Later the skin and subcutaneous tissues become tight and stretched; they are firmly bound to the underlying structures, thereby grossly restricting activity.

Clinical Course. The course of the disease is variable, but the majority of the cases follow an extremely chronic process. There frequently is prodromal appearance of changes in the hand and fingers, similar to Raynaud's disease. The skin is puffy and edematous; subsequently it becomes pigmented and indurated, with atrophy and fibrosis. Skin and muscle contracture follows, and subsequently the joints of the upper limb are involved. There is restriction of joint motion, diminution of joint space, loss of articular cartilage and, eventually, extensive articular destruction. In 30 per cent of the patients signs of cutaneous sclerosis occur after the phase of spastic phenomena; in approximately 25 per cent, the first changes implicate the joints directly.

Treatment. No completely satisfactory method of treatment of this progressive systemic disturbance has been delineated. Some promising new drugs such as ethylenediamine dihydroxide, ethacrynic acid and potassium para-aminol benzoin (Potaba) have been used. In the case of the shoulder, physiotherapeutic measures maintain mobility for a period, but eventually the skin contracture is such that motion is lost and no physical methods appear to prevent the progressive changes.

SYSTEMIC LUPUS ERYTHEMATOSUS

A connective tissue disorder predominant in women of the child-bearing age, which runs a varied and sometimes very chronic debilitating course, has become known as systemic lupus erythematosus.

Pathology. The changes are confined to connective tissue and include a variety of lesions, including verrucous endocarditis, segmental thickening of the basement membrane of the glomerular tuft of the kidney, periarteric fibrosis in the spine and the presence of hematoxylin bodies in heart, kidney, lymph nodes, spleen and synovial membranes. At some stage, in almost all cases, the somewhat characteristic cutaneous erythematous lesions develop. The most frequent sites are the face, the neck, the upper chest and the back. In 75 per cent of patients there is involvement of the kidneys with a focal glomerulonephritis.

Clinical Features. In approximately 90 per cent of patients there is some joint involvement that begins in the small joints of the upper extremity, but the shoulder may be implicated fairly rapidly. Characteristically there is a polyarthritis, but without evidence of acute irritation. The symmetrical changes resemble those of rheumatoid arthritis extensively. Fever, fatigue, generalized weakness and weight loss are systemic signs ushering in the disease. The shoulder involvement is usually a part of generalized involvement of the upper limb.

Treatment. No specific agent to combat this condition has been identified. The most widely used medications are steroids and salicylates. The local treatment consists of splinting the joints during the acute stages, followed by a program of active and assisted active motion in the chronic stage. Surgical therapy of the joints is not applicable except in longstanding cases of maximal severity.

POLYMYOSITIS

A disease related to the group of collagen disturbances has been identified with increasing frequency during recent years. It consists of muscle weakness and implicates the trunk muscles particularly, but the shoulder region is occasionally involved. Acute pain and soreness referable to the muscles is often present, with weakness progressing to the point where the patient may not be able to use the limbs in controlled fashion.

The characteristic findings can be identified electromyographically; consistent changes include fibrillation on voluntary effort and low amplitude, short duration, polyphasic potentials. Enzyme studies show gross abnormalities also. Biopsy of the muscles shows cellular infiltration among muscle fibers comprised of plasma cells and lymphocytes and some follicle formation. Subsequently considerable atrophy appears in the muscle fibers.

The condition is to be separated from steroid and metabolic myopathies. In the former, signs of hypercortisonism are present, and the electromyographic studies do not show the same profound changes.

Treatment. When the lesion has been identified by electromyographic and muscle studies, prednisone 15 mg daily is started. Painful areas are splinted and physiotherapy initiated. Steroid therapy is carefully controlled to prevent hypercortisonism; it may need to be continued three to four months.

RHEUMATOID ARTHRITIS OF THE CERVICAL SPINE

Approximately 60 per cent of patients with rheumatoid arthritis have some involvement of the neck. The changes are often extensive and include apophyseal joint changes, vertebral subluxation, atlantoaxial subluxation, osteoporosis, ankylosis, disc narrowing, vertebral and plate erosion, odontoid erosion and erosion of spinous processes.

Apophyseal Joint Changes. The surfaces of the apophyseal joints become irregular and eroded. Marked changes are frequent at C.2 and C.3. The joint space is thinned, and the cortex is osteoporotic. These alterations predispose to a serial subluxation of the whole spine.

Atlantoaxial Subluxation. Roughly one quarter of the patients will show atlantoaxial subluxation. This change has been defined as a distance greater than 3 mm radiologically between the anterior margin of the odontoid and the posterior margin of the atlas.

Neurological signs are not always present, and a considerable degree of displacement can develop without these occurring. Cregan has contributed pioneering work in the treatment of cervical subluxation. When persistent neurological signs develop, atlantoaxial cervical stabilization is necessary. Cregan has indicated the difficulties that arise from extensive disease in this area, leading to fragmentation of atlas and extensive instability. A method of stabilization of the occiput to the spine as devised by him is reproduced here (Fig. 16–9).

Subluxation in Lower Cervical Spine. Although the atlantoaxial and atlanto-occipital zones are the critical ones, luxation at C.3–C.4 and C.4–C.5 occurs alone or in conjunction with the disease at a higher level. Treatment for this lesion is the same, with protection by a collar and cervical traction with tongs or a halo followed by surgical stabilization. Operation from the posterior aspect appears to be the most satisfactory approach. Often these people require tracheostomies and approach from the front is difficult. In addition, stabilization of the area

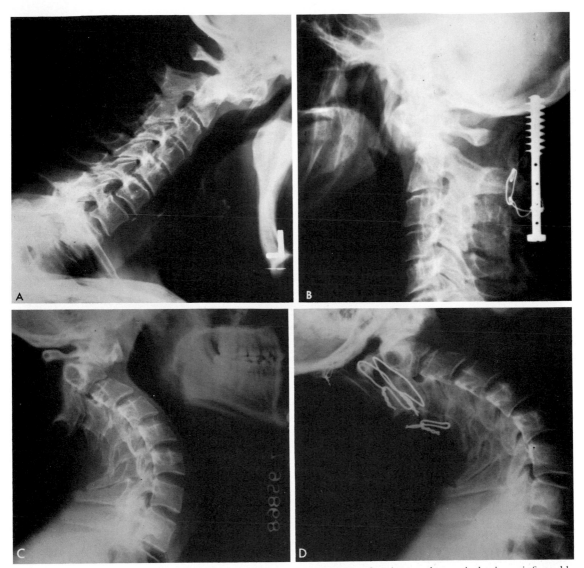

Figure 16-9 *A* and *B*, Before and after operation for screw fixation of occiput to the cervical spine reinforced by autogenous bone grafting. (Courtesy Dr. J. C. Cregan.) *C* and *D*, Alternative method of occipital cervical stabilization.

with some form of internal fixation may be more complicated if the anterior approach is used.

Osteoporosis. At least 20 per cent of patients with rheumatoid arthritis with cervical change show considerable osteoporosis. A prevalence of involvement of the upper segment or cervical spine occurs and contributes to the likelihood of subluxation.

Interbody Changes. Narrowing of all disc spaces occurs in a large percentage of patients. Erosion of the end plate often accompanies this and is more frequent at the lower levels.

Spinous Processes. When interbody narrowing is marked and there is considerable osteoporosis, posterior spinous processes may impinge and erosion subsequently occurs.

Treatment. During the acute stages, in addition to routine systemic therapy, splinting with a light Plexiglas collar molded to fit the individual patient is required. When incipient subluxation occurs, halter traction is used. When neurological signs appear, halo or ice tong traction followed by stabilization is necessary. In some patients without neurological signs surgical stabilization is still required.

ANKYLOSING SPONDYLITIS

Ankylosing spondylitis has many distinctive features which suggest its classification as a separate disease from rheumatoid arthritis.

The characteristics which tend to distinguish this entity are a predominance in young men, ligamentous calcification of the spinal column, increased incidence of recurrent iritis, and aortitis resulting in aortic insufficiency. A pattern of dominant inheritance and absence of rheumatoid factor and rheumatoid nodules is also evident (Fig. 16–10).

Most patients with ankylosing spondylitis have a different and better prognosis than those with rheumatoid arthritis. The response to drugs is similar. One of the most important contrasting features is the pattern of joint involvement. The sacroiliac joints are always involved in ankylosing spondylitis. A further common distribution is to the symphysis pubis, manubrium sternae, acromioclavicular, costovertebral and dorsolumbar spine, C.1, C.2 and C.3 of the cervical spine, and occasionally C.4–C.7 (Fig. 16–11). In both conditions the shoulder may be involved, although this is more frequently

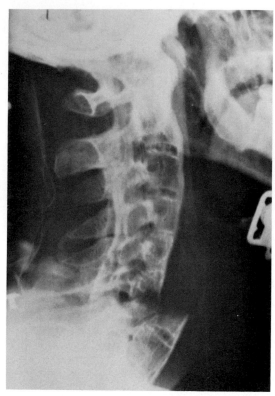

Figure 16–11 Fracture dislocation of the cervical spine in ankylosing spondylitis. Extreme degrees of dislocation because of the rigidity of the fragments may be encountered.

seen in rheumatoid arthritis than ankylosing spondylitis.

Ankylosing spondylitis is usually considered to be a process which starts in the sacroiliac joints and spreads upward in the spine; hence, the theory that an ascending infection of general origin is responsible. A further important difference is the development of syndesmophytes, particularly in the dorsolumbar region, which may sometimes occur before sacroiliac arthritis. Although differences in the manifestation of the two diseases in the cervical spine can be identified, they are usually not the basis of the diagnosis. There will be evidence of the dominant disease to a greater degree elsewhere. The tendency to subluxation is more apparent in rheumatoid arthritis than in ankylosing spondylitis. The changes in the lower part of the spine differ considerably with the extensive syndesmophyte formation, a distinct contrast to the changes found in rheumatoid arthritis.

Considerable differences in the incidence between the two sexes with these diseases has been identified. Rheumatoid arthritis in-

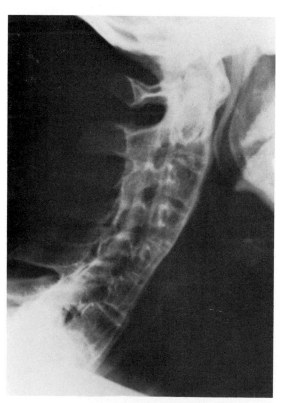

Figure 16–10 Ankylosing spondylitis.

volves two or three women for every man, whereas the ratio of ankylosing spondylitis is closer to ten men for each woman.

A frank hereditary influence occurs in ankylosing spondylitis and is present to a much greater degree than is the case with rheumatoid arthritis. There is rarely involvement of the shoulder joint along with the cervical spine in ankylosing spondylitis. In general, if there is no involvement of the peripheral joints early in the disease, these are not likely to complicate the ankylosing lesion.

Surgical Treatment. In some instances progressive deformity of the cervical spine reaches a point at which it is difficult for the patient to see far enough ahead of himself to stand or walk comfortably. In many instances this is the result of progressive flexion contracture at the hips, and considerable improvement may be obtained by surgery (Fig. 16–11).

In other cases the cervical spine deformity may progress to the point where osteotomy would be extremely helpful. Attempts have been made to do this, but difficulties are encountered in giving these patients an intubation anesthetic and in performing a tracheostomy.

A significant contribution in this field has been made by E. H. Simmons in the form of carrying out osteotomy of the cervical spine under a local anesthetic. He has recently devised a most ingenious method of cervical laminectomy under local anesthesia which is applicable to this area. The problems of general anesthesia, tracheostomy and intubation in these patients are formidable, so that the use of a local marks a significant advance when it may be applied.

The principle is to use light sedation, place the patient in the sitting position and approach the posterior spinous elements under local anesthesia. The site applicable for correction of anterior kyphosis is at the cervicothoracic junction.

A total laminectomy, including the posterior spinous process of C.7, is carried out, with extension carried well laterally to the articular elements. When this zone has been adequately freed, gentle posterior pressure is made on the forehead to bring the neck from the flexed position to one of greater extension. Usually this is accomplished with an audible snap. The head is then fixed in this position with the aid of the halo apparatus and the position is maintained until fusion has taken place in the corrected alignment.

REFERENCES

Benedek, T. G., et al.: Ankylosing spondylitis with ulcerative colitis and amyloidosis. Report of a case and review of the literature. Amer. J. Med. *40*:431–439, 1966.

Bland, J. H., et al.: Rheumatoid arthritis of cervical spine. Arch. Intern. Med. (Chicago) *112*:892–898, 1963.

Bleck, E. E.: Arthritis of the C1–C2 and C2–C3 intervertebral facets. G.P. *33*:94–95, 1966.

Bose, K. S.: Osteotomy of the cervical spine. J. Indian Med. Ass. *42*:576–578, 1964.

Brichard, M.: Arthroplasty of the shoulder by vitallium prosthesis. Acta Orthop. Belg. *31*:817–820, 1965.

Calabro, J. J., et al.: Management of ankylosing spondylitis. Amer. J. Occup. Ther. *19*:255–258, 1965.

Carter, J. B., et al.: Myasthenia gravis and rheumatoid spondylitis. Co-existence in 3 cases. J.A.M.A. *194*:913–914, 1965.

Claessens, H., et al.: Arthritis and arthrosis of the scapulo-humeral joint. J. Belg. Med. Phys. Rhum. *20*:73–82, 1965.

Conlon, P. W., et al.: Rheumatoid arthritis of the cervical spine. An analysis of 333 cases. Ann. Rheum. Dis. *25*:120–126, 1966.

Cregan, J. C.: Internal fixation of the unstable cervical spine. Ann. Rheum. Dis. *25*:242–252, 1966.

David-Chausse, J., et al.: Ankylosing spondylitis beginning in childhood. Rhumatologie *18*:198–210, 1966.

DePalma, A. F.: Arthrodesis of the shoulder joint. Surg. Clin. N. Amer. *43*:1599–1607, 1963.

Durrigl, T.: History of ankylosing spondylitis. Lijecn. Vjes. *87*:789–793, 1965.

Francois, R. J.: Microradiographic study of the intervertebral bridges in ankylosing spondylitis and in the normal sacrum. Ann. Rheum. Dis. *24*:481–489, 1965.

Gleason, I. O., et al.: Atlanto-axial dislocation with odontoid separation in rheumatoid disease. Clin. Orthop. *42*:121–129, 1965.

Grantham, S. A., Dick, H. M., Thompson, R. C., and Stinchfield, F. E.: Occipitocervical arthrodesis. Indications, technic and result. Clin. Orthop. *65*:118–129, 1969.

Hart, F. D.: Lessons learnt in a 20 year study of ankylosing spondylitis. Proc. Roy. Soc. Med. *59*:456–458, 1966.

Hench, P. S.: Discussion. Proceedings of the American Rheumatic Association Annual Meeting. Rheumat. Dis. *13*:352, 1954.

Kanefield, D. G., Mullins, B. P., Freehafer, A. A., Furey, J. G., Horenstein, S., and Chamberlin, W. B.: Destructive lesions of the spine in rheumatoid ankylosing spondylitis. J. Bone Joint Surg. *51A*:1369–1375, 1969.

Kinsella, T. D., et al.: Ankylosing spondylitis; a late re-evaluation of 92 cases. Canad. Med. Ass. *95*:1–9, 1966.

McGill, I. G.: An unusual neurological syndrome associated with ankylosing spondylitis. Guy Hosp. Rep. *115*:33–36, 1966.

Merle D'Aubigne, R., et al.: Technic of arthrodesis of the shoulder by a posterior approach. Rev. Chir. Orthop. *52*:155–161, 1966.

Mukerjee, S. K.: Synovial chondromatosis in shoulder joint. Proc. Roy. Soc. Med. *61*:665–667, 1968.

Newman, P., and Sweetman, R.: Occipito-cervical fusion. An operative technic and its indications. J. Bone Joint Surg. *51B*:423–431, 1969.

Ott, V. R., et al.: Differentiation of ankylosing spinal disease. Arch. Phys. Ther. (Leipzig) *17*:141–148, 1965.

Robinson, H. S.: Rheumatoid arthritis — atlanto-axial subluxation and its clinical presentation. Canad. Med. Ass. J. *94*:470–477, 1966.

Rometti, M.: Radio-clinical aspects of cervical curvature disharmonies. Rhumatologie *18*:27–30, 1966.

Rosenberg, M. A., et al.: Fracture dislocation of the cervical spine with rheumatoid spondylitis: Case report and review of literature. J. Canad. Ass. Radiol. *16*:241–243, 1965.

Schulutko, L. I.: Some problems of treatment of Bech-terew-Strümpell-Marie rheumatoid arthritis. Beitr. Orthop. Trauma *12*:412–415, 1965.

Serre, H., et al.: Atlanto-axial dislocation in rheumatoid arthritis. Rheumatism *22*:53–58, 1966.

Sharp, J.: The differential diagnosis of ankylosing spon-dylitis. Proc. Roy. Soc. Med. *59*:453–455, 1966.

Simmons, E. H.: Personal communication, 1969.

Sokoloff, L.: The pathology of rheumatoid arthritis and allied disorders. *In* Hollander, J. L. (ed.): Arthritis and Allied Conditions, A Textbook of Rheumatology. 7th ed., Philadelphia, Lea & Febiger, 1966.

Sokolowski, A.: Our observations on the relationship between the clinical picture and patient's age in ankylosing spondylitis. Rhumatologia (Warsz.) *3*: 103–109, 1965.

Verhaeghe, A., et al.: The shoulder in rheumatoid arthritis. Rhumatologie *20*:189–200, 1968.

Verjans, H.: The indications for arthrodesis of the shoulder. J. Belg. Med. Phys. Rhum. *20*:28–33. 1965.

Williams, K. A.: Ankylosing spondylitis. Brit. J. Clin. Pract. *19*:647–654, 1965.

Section

VI

TUMORS OF THE SHOULDER AND THE NECK

CHAPTER XVII

TUMORS OF THE SHOULDER AND NECK

The neck and shoulder constitute a significant site for the development of tumors. The tissue components themselves comprise elements with frequent neoplastic complication. The chest and the breast, notorious sites of primary malignant disease, are intimately connected, so that the region is susceptible to common metastatic involvement. The peculiar propensity of thyroid tumors for bone is also a menace.

Associated areas not commonly thought of as integral parts of the shoulder, like the axilla, the upper spine and the root of the neck, also contain structures which, when implicated by tumor processes, commonly involve shoulder or neck. Proximity to important viscera in the chest, the mediastinum and the neck implicates the shoulder area in symptoms from these when it is not itself involved. The cervical spine harbors tissue which, with neoplastic change, can produce symptoms pervading the whole region, and yet there may be little evidence of distortion of this area on the surface. In the first case on record of the successful removal of a spinal cord tumor, the patient had complained of pain in the shoulder for three years. The mobility of the shoulder, in itself, is a function which generates discomfort, focusing attention on the moving part, and yet the true nidus may lie at some distance.

Significant neoplastic changes may primarily implicate the soft tissues or bony elements. Any abnormal swelling or persistent pain without swelling in a child is an indication of possible neoplastic change. Palpation quickly separates soft tissue swelling from lesions of hard consistency or deep structure origin. Soft tumors are located chiefly above the clavicle and at the back of the axilla. Bone tumors producing symptoms in this region involve the spine, humerus, scapula or clavicle and, occasionally, the first rib; these usually represent a serious complication. Many advances have been made in interpreting skeletal pathology, and superior methods of diagnosis are continually being established. Improvement in radiological and pathological interpretations of bone neoplastic change has led to the identification of new entities as well as better understanding of the old. The methods of treating these lesions have also improved. Surgical techniques have not altered greatly, but the use-

533

fulness of radiation has increased, and some forms of drug therapy now show new promise for control of certain tumors.

INVESTIGATION AND DIAGNOSIS OF SUSPECTED TUMORS

Thorough and complete investigation is mandatory in examining a suspected bone neoplasm. This involves not only accurate clinical assessment and consideration of the region implicated, but also meticulous radiological investigation and laboratory studies. In all instances, if at all possible, the final diagnosis must rest upon accurate tissue examination. Although putting together the results of all these investigations is essential, much information is to be gained from each facet, and no one procedure should be omitted in the hope of skipping quickly to an answer by the use of another. The modern armamentarium for tumor treatment is developing so many tools that an in-depth assessment of any lesion in any given category or precise group must be carried out.

SPECIAL POINTS IN THE HISTORY

As a generalization, the more serious lesions of bone malignancy are encountered in the early years and in the second decade in particular. The upper end of the humerus is the third most common site of primary malignant bone tumor. In the history of these lesions pain is the cardinal symptom and is usually the first symptom to call the attention of the patient to the area. The usual mode of onset is a nagging discomfort in the general shoulder-neck region which may be difficult to define. This soon changes, with the pain assuming a more constant occurrence and persistent boring quality. The patient cannot get comfortable. No position alters the pain; sleep is interfered with, and sedation gradually has only a transitory affect. In a patient under 30 without a history of significant trauma, who complains of a persistent discomfort in the shoulder area, the possibility of serious bone or joint involvement must be kept uppermost. The pain may not be severe. The one characteristic that should arouse suspicion is the persistence, since nearly all painful disorders of the shoulder respond to rest or to change in position with a decrease in discomfort. Continuation of the pain should make one look farther and more carefully.

A history of injury is associated in so many cases, and often the patient is certain that his trouble arose from this incident. Our present knowledge suggests that injury does not cause bone tumors; trauma, however, often calls attention to an area already the seat of disease, and from then on the patient is aware of the process. Any pertinent incident should be carefully documented, since medicolegal controversy frequently develops following injury.

Limitation of movement is the next most frequent symptom. This may be active or passive, but in the early stages it is almost always active and results largely from the production of pain on motion. Later, passive movement, too, is hampered and, finally, the patient develops a characteristic picture. The face is thin and drawn from months of pain; the expression is anxious; the shoulder is kept rigidly still, supported close to the side by the good arm; the posture is stooped; and any jar is exquisitely painful. Fracture may occur following an unusually trivial trauma and may be the first indication of more serious disease, particularly of cystic lesions in the upper end of the humerus.

SPECIAL POINTS IN EXAMINATION

Careful and complete physical examination is essential and includes a general examination as well as the suspected local area. There should be routine examination of neck, chest, breasts, abdomen, pelvis and prostate. In patients past middle life particular care is exercised in this routine to disclose primary tumors. Secondary tumors in the shoulder region can be the first sign of serious malignant disease of viscera. A pathological fracture of the neck of the humerus, for example, may be the first indication of widespread disease.

Swelling. Abnormal masses are detected by inspection and palpation. Unusual contour may be obvious, but often overlying soft tissues mask the lesion. The clavicle, the upper end of the humerus and the scapular region are palpated for unusual swelling. The outline, consistency and relation to skin and deep structures of any mass are assessed. Invasion of soft tissues is checked. A soft, freely movable lesion is not usually serious. A firm, adherent enlargement, diffuse in outline, somewhat tense, gradually increasing in size, is significant. Attention should be paid to the overlying skin. If it is soft and freely movable, the subjacent swelling does not suggest aggression. If it is thin, somewhat stretched and adherent, suspicions should be aroused. Note is made of any throbbing sensation or sense of vascularity of the swelling. The axilla and supraclavicular fossa should always be searched for enlarged lymph glands. Vascular abnormalities are noted, for example, venous engorgement of the arm or chest due to subclavicular or mediastinal obstruction.

X-RAY INVESTIGATION

The radiologist can help tremendously in the diagnosis and investigation of bone tumors and should be consulted early. Much of our improved knowledge of these problems has come from the efforts of these colleagues. If skilled opinion is not immediately available, x-ray films can always be mailed to a recognized center in the area. Although it is asking a great deal to expect even an expert to express an opinion on films which may not be quite the caliber and technique to which he is accustomed, he can still guide and direct the investigation in a most helpful fashion. Routine views, as outlined previously (Chapter IV), are done first. When a suspicious area is demonstrated, further special views are in order. Films are made to show greater structural detail and soft tissue shadow. A "scout" series of the rest of the skeleton is indicated, particularly in cystic lesions. Chest plates are essential to rule out possible secondary involvement of the lung or a primary chest tumor, since the shoulder lesion might then be the metastatic one.

LABORATORY INVESTIGATION

There are a few tests that are most important in this investigation, and most laboratories are sufficiently well equipped to do them. These include the determination of alkaline and acid phosphatase levels, blood calcium and phosphorus, Bence Jones protein in the urine, and urinary calcium by the Sulkowitch method.

Accepted Figures in Common Laboratory Tests of Bone Disease. The normal values for alkaline phosphatase (osteoblastic formation): adults, King-Armstrong units 5.0 to 12.5; Bodansky units, 1.5 to 5.0 per 100 cc; children, much higher, up to three times this

figure. Acid phosphatase: King-Armstrong units, 0.6 to 3.0; Bodansky units, 0.5 to 1.0 per 100 cc. Serum calcium level: adults, 10.0 to 11.5 mg per 100 cc; children, 4.0 to 6.0 per 100 cc, and higher in infants. Serum phosphorus: adults, 2.3 to 4.0 mg per 100 cc; children, 4.0 to 6.0 mg per 100 cc, and higher in infants. Urine calcium: Sulkowitch test, weak to moderate, varies with diet. (The Sulkowitch test is a quick means of determining urine calcium levels.) Bence Jones protein: negative.

Diagnostic Value of Laboratory Tests. Biochemical analysis is gradually pushing to the foreground in the study of all bone disease, and there are findings of particular significance in tumor investigation.

PHOSPHATASE LEVELS. Phosphatase is an enzyme present in many body tissues. It is elaborated in bone as an alkaline phosphatase and is intimately connected with the calcification process. During new bone or osteoblastic bone formation, an increased amount is present at the site and the excess passes into the blood. Its specific action is to break up inorganic phosphorus compounds, increasing phosphoric acid locally, which then forms calcium phosphate. Nearly all the alkaline phosphatase is derived from bone, and the blood level roughly parallels the bone level. It is, thus, a reliable evidence of osteoblastic activity. It is also used as an indication of liver function since it is normally excreted by the liver. When disease interferes with liver function, phosphatase in the blood is increased because it remains unexcreted. Another enzyme, acid phosphatase, is also significant in tumor analysis. It is formed normally in large amounts in the prostate and stays within normal limits in health and also in cases of prostatic malignancy that have not metastasized. When the tumor has gone beyond the prostate, the enzyme is detected in abnormal amounts in the blood stream.

Discussion of Phosphatase Levels. The study of the phosphatase level has come to play an important part in the diagnosis of bone lesions; in some cases it is helpful in the prognosis and assessment of reaction to treatment. An elevated alkaline phosphatase level is encountered in Paget's disease, hyperparathyroidism, metastases (osteoblastic or osteolytic), osteogenic sarcoma, carcinoma of the prostate and rickets. Normal or slightly elevated levels are encountered in giant-cell tumor, Ewing's tumor, reticulum cell sarcoma of bone, plasma cell myeloma and osteomalacia. Normal levels are encountered in senile osteoporosis, inflammatory diseases of bone, osteochondromas, osteomas, chondromas, extostoses, benign fibromas and solitary bone cysts. Serum acid phosphatase is markedly elevated in a high percentage of patients with carcinoma of the prostate with bone metastases. In primary bone tumors no disturbance in blood calcium or phosphorus should be anticipated. When the tumor is forming new bone rapidly, the alkaline phosphatase is elevated. A high acid phosphatase determination in light of our present knowledge is highly suggestive of carcinoma of the prostate. This does not mean, however, that a significant rise is always found.

Significance of Repeated Phosphatase Analysis. Repeated phosphatase determinations are significant in that they may indicate the course of the disease. A favorable process may be interpreted from a drop in acid phosphatase, whereas marked elevation usually indicates an unfavorable course. When metastases from carcinoma of the prostate show marked new bone formation, the alkaline phosphatase is also elevated. This latter is produced by the bone around the malignancy; the acid enzyme, in contrast, is derived from the malignancy itself or from the metastases to other regions and not from reaction of the bone around the metastases (Luck).

High level phosphatase determinations may show a drop after amputation, excision of the tumor or its inactivation by radiation. If a fall in the phosphatase does not occur, one may suspect the presence of secondary involvement. If the level rises after staying within relatively normal range for some time, again metastases may be suspected. Similarly a lesion which has been treated by x-ray therapy, apparently satisfactorily, will cause a drop in phosphatase; if this returns to the high level, reactivation is probable. These findings cannot be followed rigidly, but they help as a general guide.

CALCIUM AND PHOSPHORUS LEVELS. Calcium and phosphorus levels are not usually altered in primary bone tumors. Diagnostic variations occur in endocrine or metabolic bone lesions, however, and the shoulder may be involved in any of these. Recklinghausen's bone disease as a result of hyperparathyroidism is a classic example. Blood calcium is raised, phosphorus is lowered, and urinary calcium is increased. Renal osteodystrophy is the term given to bone and blood changes due to parathyroid hyperplasia; it is believed

to be stimulated by renal insufficiency. Blood calcium is low in this disease, as is also calcium urinary excretion, while the phosphorus level is high. Calcification of tissues, sometimes generalized, is encountered. Paget's disease is a profound skeletal disturbance in which decalcification and then new bone formation may occur. The shoulder, particularly the humerus, may be implicated in either or both these processes. During the osteoporotic phase, moderately increased blood calcium and lowered phosphorus may occur, but the urinary excretion is nearly always normal.

Menopausal osteoporosis is mentioned at this point because slight biochemical abnormalities are encountered. There may be a slight increase in blood calcium and decrease in blood phosphorus and an increase in urinary calcium. This is similar to Recklinghausen's disease; in this lesion, however, there is always a raised alkaline phosphatase, which is not so in the menopausal syndrome. In some malignant lesions with both osteolytic and osteoblastic formation, calcium levels are raised along with the alkaline phosphatase, but the phosphorus level remains unaltered.

PROTEIN LEVELS. Recent investigation indicates that protein is more important in some bone diseases than has previously been appreciated.

Multiple Myeloma. Profound disturbances of protein metabolism occur in multiple myeloma. These consist of the appearance of urinary Bence Jones protein, altered serum globulin content and abnormal amyloid deposits.

Menopausal Osteoporosis. Changes occur in the skeleton during the menopause which sometimes produce symptoms, chiefly in the back and pelvis. Biochemical changes occur at the same time, so the condition may be confused with some of those, such as Recklinghausen's disease. The demineralization that occurs has been attributed to deficient protein bone matrix, which leads to a general decalcification. Blood and urine levels of calcium are increased slightly and blood phosphorus is lowered. The alkaline phosphatase remains unaltered, in contrast to hyperparathyroidism and malignant bone lesions.

BIOPSY

Tumor investigation is completed by biopsy study. Before this step is taken, all the information derived from history, examination, x-ray and laboratory analysis should be collected and studied. The biopsy procedure is important and should be done by one who is prepared and equipped to carry treatment of the case to completion. Undesirable complications result from intervention made too hastily or by unqualified personnel. Tumor may be disseminated, profuse hemorrhage encountered, and wounds be difficult to close, leaving fungating masses. These complications are prevented by systematic preparation, complete co-operation of auxiliary services, and meticulous technique.

Technique. The pathologist should be at the operation to observe the gross appearance of the lesion and to guide the surgeon in removing representative tissue for study. There is a tendency to do quick sections, but in dealing with bone tissue this has serious limitations. The preparation of material for study is often not good enough for even the expert pathologist to express an accurate opinion as to whether a lesion is benign or malignant. It has not been established that serious harm occurs from doing a formal surgical removal of tissue for careful preparation and study. It is important to remove representative tissue and to prepare a meticulous tissue section from which an accurate diagnosis can be made.

Biopsy should be regarded as a major operation and must be performed under the usual rigid aseptic technique of bone procedures. An easily approachable area is chosen for section where there is no serious skin involvement. Tissues are handled gently. Representative areas, as indicated by x-rays and gross examination, of cortex, medulla and adjacent soft tissues are removed. Bleeding is controlled by electrocoagulation, Gelfoam or Surgical gauze. The wound is closed tightly in layers and should never be drained. Sutures are not removed until the wound is well healed because of the danger of fungating extension. In some instances aspiration biopsy will do, particularly when there is a question of inflammatory disease. This is also done under meticulously sterile conditions. The selected area is infiltrated with 2 per cent Novocain and a large bore needle, No. 18 to 20, is introduced after puncture of the skin. It is advanced into the tumor mass and a core of tumor tissue sucked out. If desired, a guide wire can be used and a small tube with teeth on the end guided over the wire, and a segment reamed

from the tumor. X-ray visualization can be used to localize the lesion, if necessary. In most cases involving the shoulder formal biopsy is preferable.

TUMORS OF THE SHOULDER

SOFT TISSUE TUMORS

Skin, subcutaneous tissue, lymph glands, muscles, connective tissue, nerves, vessels and some viscera produce soft tumors that need to be differentiated from one another. The areas about the shoulder in which these are commonly found are (1) above the clavicle at the front and back, and (2) in the axilla.

Supraclavicular Area

Sebaceous Cysts. The common tumor or swelling over the back of the shoulder and adjacent neck area is the sebaceous cyst, which appears as a soft, globular enlargement with a small black dot in the center, representing the blocked sebaceous duct. It is in the skin, so it moves with the skin; it is usually small, but can reach 2 to 3 inches in diameter. The outline is round or oval, not lobulated. Cheesy sebaceous material is expressed on pressure or excision. These do not cause significant disturbance unless they are secondarily infected or break down and suppurate. They may be excised under a local anesthetic. The excision should include a small piece of skin with the blocked duct.

Lipomas. Tumor-like collections of normal fat occur frequently over the posterior aspect of the shoulder, back and neck. Occasionally fat in the supraclavicular area looks like a tumor, but it is not so clearly demarcated as a true lipoma of the back or neck. Lipomas are soft, lobulated, painless and sharply demarcated. They are not fluctuant or adherent to deep structures. The lobulation is due to fibrous septa passing between the fat deposits, which aids differentiation from the sebaceous cyst. The rubbery consistency of the lipoma further separates these two lesions. The lipoma is a true tumor but has no tendency to malignant change. Symptoms result solely from local pressure. Occasionally trauma results in hemorrhage into the area, causing considerable pain. These swellings commonly are present for a long time without causing symptoms. When they become noticeable or the patient feels they have increased in size, they should be excised. Occasionally in some occupations, as in lifting weights on the shoulder, pressure is irritating, forcing excision of the tumor (Figs. 17–1 and 17–2).

Neurofibromas. Pigmented, firm nodules, usually multiple, are common in this region. Most of these are neurofibromas growing from branches of the cutaneous nerves. They arise from the connective tissue sheath of the nerves and are small and painless. They are found all over the body, sometimes as a generalized neurofibromatosis. A plexiform type is occasionally encountered. Treatment is not required unless, as occurs rarely, there is a sudden enlargement and irritation. Tumors occasionally arise from the brachial plexus either as part of a generalized neurofibromatosis or as a solitary tumor. Neurofibroma is a common lesion and occasionally becomes malignant. The treatment is resection of the tumor and sufficient nerve trunk on either side so that all tumor tissue is removed (Fig. 17–3).

Lymphatic Swellings. Lymphatic enlargement is common in this region. The inferior, deep, cervical lymph glands lie here and are frequently implicated in infections, tumors, blood and reticuloendothelial disorders. These glands drain the back of the neck and scalp, superficial pectoral region and lateral part of arm and forearm;

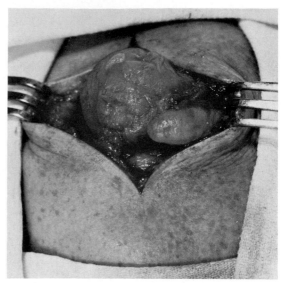

Figure 17–2   Deep lipoma of shoulder.

therefore they are involved in infective or neoplastic processes from chest, neck, back of the shoulder and back of the tongue.

In addition to local lesions, these glands are involved in generalized systemic disturbances such as leukemia, Hodgkin's disease or tuberculosis. The glands are relatively superficial, not much subcutaneous material being present. The area is examined frequently, so these glands may be the first to be noted by the patient in some of the generalized processes. The type of enlargement varies from a tangled inflammatory mass to the multiple discrete rubbery nodules of the lymphoblastomas. Simple local infection in the neck, tongue or back may still be the cause. Study of other areas discloses the irritating lesion. Because these glands are obvious and accessible, biopsies are frequently taken from them. The glands lie close to the accessory nerve and care must be taken to avoid damaging it. A cluster of glands lies around the nerve as it crosses the posterior triangle, and it is easily cut or crushed (Fig. 17–4).

Axillary Swellings

Discomfort in the shoulder arises from lesions in the axilla, which are sometimes overlooked. Lymph tissue is the common source of axillary enlargements.

Lymphatic Involvement. A tender, rounded swelling which comes up quickly

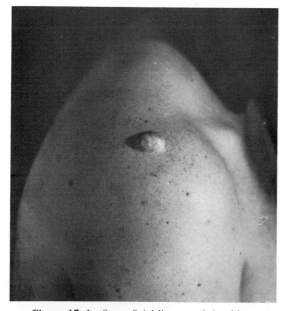

Figure 17–1   Superficial lipoma of shoulder.

A

B

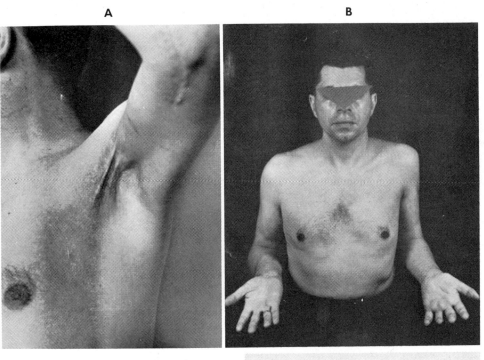

Figure 17–3 Neurosarcoma of brachial plexus. *A*, Biopsy scar. *B*, Extensive changes in hand. Note swollen fingers and thenar atrophy. *C*, Tumor removed in resection.

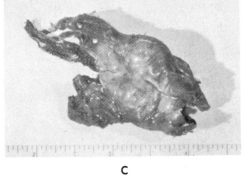

C

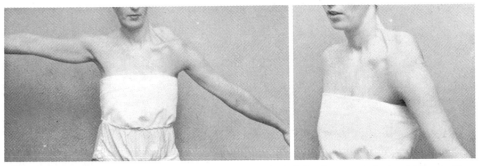

Figure 17–4 Patient with trapezius and levator scapula paralysis following cervical gland biopsy. Note extensive deformity, with altered neck contour and winging of scapula.

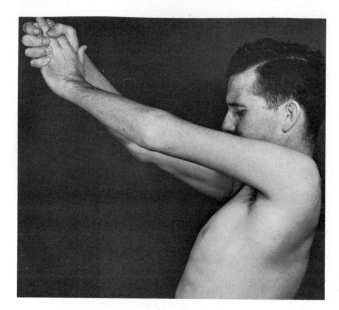

Figure 17-5 Axillary adenitis from elbow infection. Note swollen axilla.

is most probably a lymphadenitis. There are 20 to 30 glands which communicate with this region and drain the shoulder, back, front of chest, breast, upper abdomen, hand and forearm. Infection in any of these areas may produce a swelling in the armpit. These glands are susceptible also to the other causes of adenopathy outlined previously, but infection is by far the commonest cause. A hangnail, olecranon bursitis or pimple on the chest may lead to pain, soreness and limitation of shoulder movement. Infection arising in the axilla itself is common since hair follicles become inflamed by repeated use of irritating antihidrotics. Recurrent infection may be so well established that massive excision and replacement by skin grafting is needed. Calcification is occasionally seen in these glands (Fig. 17-6).

BONE TUMORS

Every practitioner should be on guard when a young patient, particularly between 10 and 25 years of age, complains of continuous, dull, aching shoulder pain followed by limitation of movement and local tenderness since this may be the early indication of a bone tumor. Swelling or even thickening is a late sign, and if recognition is delayed until this appears, the case may be hopeless. The symptoms are so often related to some accident or traumatic incident that everyone needs to be on guard (Fig. 17-7). Sometimes

the initial x-ray fails to show the lesion, so that all cases of persistent pain should be re-examined in a month's time, rather than labeling the patient as psychoneurotic.

TUMORS OF THE UPPER END OF THE HUMERUS

The upper end of the humerus is the third most frequent site of the body for the development of neoplastic change. In addition, it is a not infrequent site for metabolic disturbance, infections, parasitic disorders

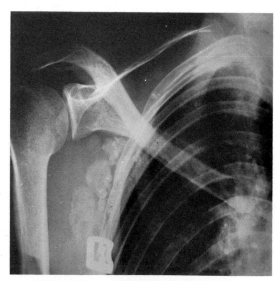

Figure 17-6 Calcification of axillary glands.

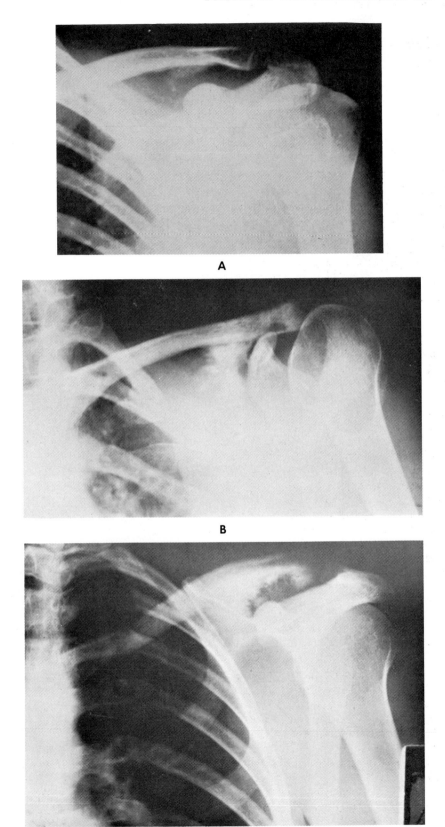

Figure 17–7 *A*, Blow on the shoulder blamed for persistent pain. *B*, Two months later. *C*, Advanced osteogenic sarcoma.

and other systemic disturbances. Changes suggestive of neoplasm and neoplastic-like disorders most commonly take the form of a circumscribed area of rarefaction which then may have certain specific qualities and changes characteristic of many lesions. The following tumors have been identified in the upper end of the humerus: (1) giant-cell tumor, (2) benign chondroblastoma, (3) aneurysmal bone cyst, (4) solitary bone cyst, (5) fibrous dysplasia, nonossifying fibroma, (6) benign osteoblastoma, (7) solitary enchondroma, (8) osteogenic sarcoma, (9) chondrosarcoma, (10) Ewing's tumor, (11) myeloma, (12) reticulum cell sarcoma, and (13) secondary bone tumors. These lesions may be confused with entities such as Paget's disease, osteomyelitis, lipoid granulomata and some chronic inflammatory states.

Solitary Bone Cyst of Humerus

The upper end of the humerus is the commonest site of the lesion known as solitary bone cyst. A translucent or cystic expansile area of bone is seen lying juxta-epiphyseal, but always diaphyseal in site. It is definitely demarcated and occasionally trabeculated. It is of clinical importance that the second commonest pathological fracture encountered in the upper end of the humerus is due to the solitary bone cyst.

Clinical Features. There is no complete agreement on the origin of the solitary cyst. The occurrence of a fracture from a relatively trivial trauma is a frequent first symptom. Pain occurs but is intermittent and not severe. There is gradual expansion, leaving a thin cortex which is easily fractured. Repeated fractures lead to thickening of the cortex and sometimes obliteration of the cyst. The cysts begin on the diaphyseal side of the epiphyseal plate, which is a cardinal observation in differentiating them from giant-cell tumors, which arise on the epiphyseal side (Fig. 17–8).

Pathology. The x-ray appearance and the clinical course follow a fairly constant pattern. Considerable variation in the pathological pattern is encountered, however. Grossly there is a well defined cavity which sometimes contains fluid, sometimes blood and sometimes a fibrofatty mixture. A definite lining membrane may be identified occasionally, or the edge of the cystic area may blend so completely with bone that no margin can be made out. Often it is difficult to obtain a good biopsy specimen by curetting the cavity. The lining membrane has a fibrous stroma and is avascular, with a few giant cells enmeshed in the stroma.

Diagnosis. As a rule, this lesion is easily diagnosed from its characteristic site and x-ray appearance. The only difficulty which arises in the diagnosis is in differentiating it from fibrous dysplasia or giant-cell tumor. The giant-cell tumor generally occurs at the end of the bone on the epiphyseal side. Fibrous dysplasia is encountered in the older age group; trabeculation of the cyst is usual, and the lesions occur in other bones too. There are no abnormal laboratory findings in solitary cyst, calcium, phosphorus and phosphatase all being within normal limits.

Treatment. Most of these cases should be treated surgically. Even when a pathological fracture has occurred, it appears preferable to expose the area and insert massive bone grafts.

TECHNIQUE. The upper end of the humerus is exposed through a muscle-splitting incision. Aseptic technique is followed throughout. The site of the cyst is recognized by a slight expansion or bubble formation in the cortex. A portion of the cortex is removed and the cyst explored. It is curetted, coagulated and swabbed first with carbolic acid and then with alcohol. Bone is removed from the iliac crest or medial aspect of the tibia. Bank bone can be utilized, if preferred, but it is not quite so good. Whatever source of bone transplant is used, the most important step is to completely pack and obliterate the cavity; the cause of many failures in the past has been inadequate obliteration. The wound is closed in layers, and the arm is immobilized in an abduction plaster spica for eight weeks.

For a time radiation therapy was suggested in the treatment of these lesions, but experience has shown that surgery is preferable. The difficult cases are those which persist to adult life, or those not treated radically enough at the primary operation. All these cases should be x-rayed again at six-, 12-, and 18-month intervals after operation. Recurring cases sometimes require radical block resection of the diseased bone and massive grafts to repair the defect. Most patients do well; deformity and disability are not serious problems.

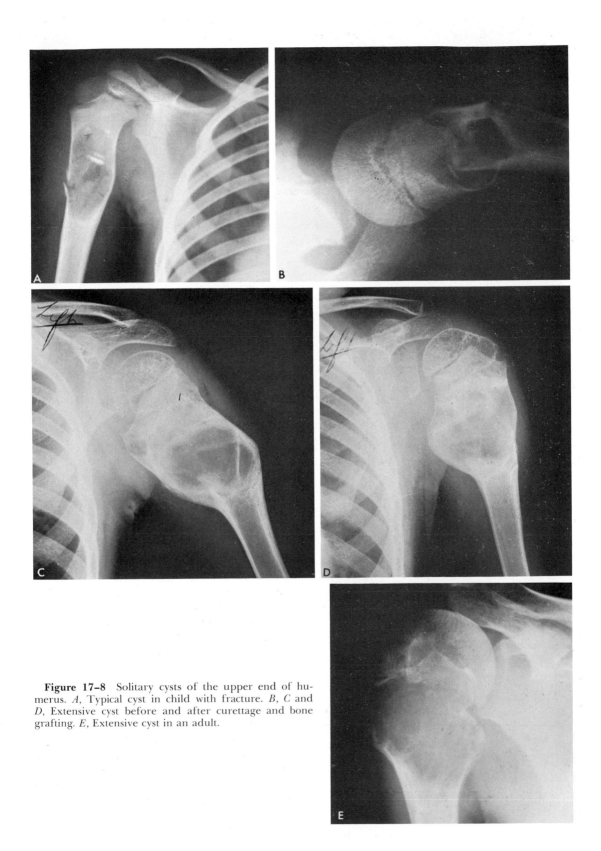

Figure 17–8 Solitary cysts of the upper end of humerus. *A*, Typical cyst in child with fracture. *B, C* and *D*, Extensive cyst before and after curettage and bone grafting. *E*, Extensive cyst in an adult.

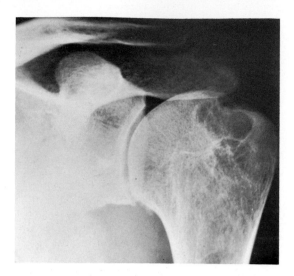

Figure 17–9   Giant cell tumor.

Giant Cell Tumor

This is a primary, benign bone tumor which occurs at the ends of long bones. The upper end of the humerus is not a common site, but neither is it rare.

Clinical Features.   Swelling is usually the first sign and is followed by disturbance in joint function. Tenderness is present on palpation. In the x-ray it appears as a well localized, cystic process on the epiphyseal side of the upper end of the humerus. Frequently the tumor is eccentrically situated, so that it appears as a blister or bubble-like development with trabeculation and, later, shows more uniform expansile properties (Fig. 17–9).

Pathology.   This tumor is usually benign, but improved laboratory methods and more careful study have permitted recognition of a more aggressive or telangiectatic form. Grossly an expanded portion of the cortex is recognized, but there is no extension into the soft tissues or adherence to soft tissues. As the tumor grows there is a tendency to transverse expansion rather than longitudinal progression. When cut into, the tumor has a characteristic currant-jelly appearance. Extending through the jelly-like area are fibrous strands and enmeshed spicules of bone. Microscopically it consists of a mass of multinucleated giant cells enmeshed in a vascular stroma.

Treatment.   If the tumor is accessible, surgical excision and obliteration of the cavity is the preferred treatment. If it is not accessible, radiation may be used. Several factors determine the prognosis. The earlier the tumor is diagnosed and treated, the better the outlook. In general, the prognosis is good, but just as in any of these conditions, follow-up x-ray studies should be done at six months and a year. Some observers have classified these tumors according to microscopic appearance.

Benign Chondroblastoma of Humerus

A lesion somewhat linked to giant-cell tumor has been identified; it is characteristically located in the upper end of the humerus. Codman originally called attention to this lesion and it sometimes is referred to as Codman's tumor. The tumor occurs in young patients and presents a vacuolated cystic appearance localized to the epiphysis. Recurrence of the tumor after the age of 25 is extremely uncommon. Attention is called to the area because of persistent pain, often an aching sensation, continuing at night in spite of resting of the extremities. In some instances slight swelling is apparent, and frequently there is persistent local tenderness. Radiologically the tumor appears cystic, with bubble-like striations and a patchy calcification. Grossly it appears as a grayish yellow mass with irregular zones of calcification and hemorrhage scattered through it. Microscopically giant cells, areas of calcification and zones of fibrous tissue replacing hemorrhagic fields are found.

The treatment recommended is complete

excision and replacement by bone grafts, either cancellous or cortical, supported by cancellous bone. Radiation has some effect on this tumor, but it is less effective than resection and replacement with bone. The ultimate prognosis is good.

Aneurysmal Bone Cyst

A somewhat rare, benign tumor occasionally affects the upper end of the humerus and has been described by Jaffe (1950) as having striking radiographic features. The term aneurysmal is used to indicate the "blow-out"-like distension of the cortex, leaving a thin shell. Characteristically it has an eccentric situation, tending to involve cortex on one side only. These patients almost always have well localized pain to the shoulder region, sometimes becoming extremely acute, with associated restriction of shoulder motion in all directions. Identification of the lesion can be made with reasonable certainty by x-ray examination (Fig. 17–10), but formal biopsy should be carried

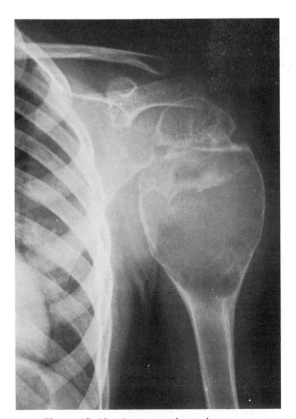

Figure 17–10   Aneurysmal type bone cyst.

out. The treatment of these lesions is surgical, with curettage of the cystic area and packing of the cavity with autogenous bone.

Fibrous Dysplasia

Fibrous dysplasia produces translucent cystic areas in long bones and not uncommonly involves the upper end of the humerus. It is a disease of adolescence or early adult life. The shoulder lesion may be single or part of a more general skeletal involvement. The clinical course is quite similar to that of solitary bone cysts, but these patients are older and it is not uncommon to have a fracture through the cortex as the first significant symptom of the disease.

Pathology. On gross examination the translucent bony areas are represented by a thin, trabeculated cortex filled with a grayish white fibrous tissue in which there are islands of calcification. The lesion occupies a segment of the bone and, in the x-ray, ends at right angles to the cortex and does not have a tapering or pointing extremity suggestive of progression (Fig. 17–11). Microscopically the cystic areas are composed of fibrous tissue, with a stroma showing varying areas of vascularity. Giant cells are encountered and osteoblast clusters are seen occasionally.

Treatment. Recurrence or progression of this lesion is not so common as in the case of solitary cysts. Conservative methods are satisfactory; the arm is immobilized in plaster for fractures, and excision or bone grafting is rarely needed. Often considerable decrease in the translucency is apparent after a fracture has healed.

Generalized Osteitis Fibrosa Cystica

Hyperparathyroidism may produce generalized skeletal cyst formation. An adenoma of the parathyroids alters phosphorus and calcium metabolism profoundly, so that there is increased calcium loss in the urine. This leads to decalcification and areas of cyst formation in which the upper end of the humerus may be involved in common with other bones.

Pathology. This is a metabolic bone disease and the laboratory findings are the key to diagnosis. Increased parathormone depresses the blood phosphorus level, causing increased excretion in the urine. The combined calcium and phosphorus level tends to

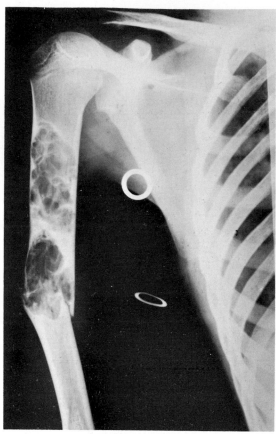

Figure 17–11 Fibrous dysplasia.

lated. The increased phosphorus blood level depresses calcium, and tetany may develop.

Nonossifying Fibroma or Fibrocortical Defect

A cystic-appearing, small lesion implicating the ends of long bones, which develops out of the fibrous tissue in the periosteum, has occasionally been identified in the upper end of the humerus (Fig. 17–13). If one is encountered there, it is common to find lesions in other bones, particularly the lower end of the femur or the upper end of the tibia. Many of the lesions do not require treatment. When there are symptoms and local signs, surgical excision can be carried out. In some instances the lesion is much more extensive, taking on a multiple cystic appearance; under these circumstances it is referred to as nonossifying fibroma. In contrast to the fibrous cortical defect, the larger size of this lesion makes it necessary to carry out excision more frequently; occasionally pathological fractures have been reported.

Osteoid Osteoma

In 1935 Jaffe proposed the concept of osteoid osteoma as a clinical pathological

remain constant, so that increased calcium appears in blood to compensate for phosphorus loss. The calcium is drained from the bones, resulting in a general decalcification and increased calcium in the urine.

The local cystic change is similar to fibrous dysplasia, but there are more osteoblasts apparent. The cystic area tends to merge with decalcified bone and is not so well demarcated (Fig. 17–12). The cyst is in decalcified bone, but in fibrous dysplasia the rest of the bone is usually quite normal. There is hyperplasia and increased activity of osteoclasts. The parathyroid pathology varies; a single adenoma or diffuse hyperplasia of all the glands may be encountered. The systemic features and profound biochemical changes govern prognosis and disability more than the local bone or gland abnormalities.

Treatment. When the diagnosis is established, the parathyroid region should be explored and dealt with as indicated by the local findings. Following excision of a tumor, the blood chemistry must be carefully regu-

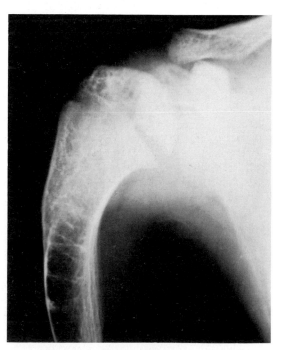

Figure 17–12 Osteitis fibrosa cystica.

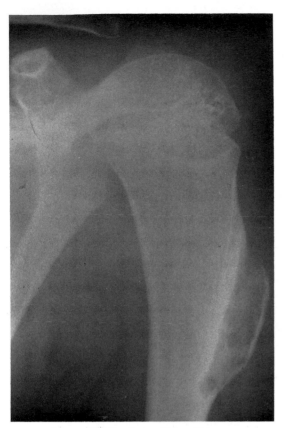

Figure 17–13 Nonossifying fibroma.

entity related to a small but painful bone lesion occurring primarily in an age group of 10 to 25 years. A clinical characteristic is the presence of symptoms of some years' standing, frequently before the lesion has been identified. In the case of the shoulder, persisting aching pain can be expected in the upper part of the arm, or implicating the shoulder joint, with some restriction of motion. The principal clinical findings include an exquisite point of local tenderness, usually related to the lateral cortex of the humerus. In many instances there is extensive muscle atrophy as a result of the restriction of motion because of the persistent pain. A significant clinical finding is relief of the pain from administration of aspirin.

The x-ray appearance is typical, demonstrating a small sequestrum-like density surrounded by a clear halo-like zone, beyond which bone is normal. The recommended and most successful treatment is complete excision of the lesion. At operation it appears as a round, hemorrhagic granular pit, deep in the cortex or at the junction of the medullary cavity and cortex. Normally it is no larger than a ten cent piece. The lesion has a characteristic microscopic appearance, presenting a rounded zone of closely packed new trabeculae and osteoid tissue. Calcification of trabeculae proceeds irregularly as the lesion ages. The overlying cortex reacts in a typical fashion, producing a layered condensation of essentially normal bone.

Benign Osteoblastoma

A separate tumor entity has been identified which, histologically, resembles a conventional osteoid osteoma with the exception that there are a greater number of osteoblasts and they are larger in size. The lesion itself is considerably larger than the ordinary osteoid osteoma, which has given rise to an alternate title of giant osteoid osteoma.

It is a vascular osteoid, forming benign tumor characterized by a large number of osteoblasts. It is rarely encountered in the upper end of the humerus. As a rule, it is a relatively small tumor, but may show a considerable degree of translucency, with bulging of the shaft. Alternate areas are radiopaque because of the heavy calcification of the osteoid. The principal reason for separating it from the osteoid osteoma is its size and quite different radiological appearance; yet, histologically, many of its elements resemble the osteoid osteoma. The proper treatment is complete surgical excision and replacement by appropriate bone grafts.

Osteochondroma of Humerus

The commonest benign tumor of bone is the osteochondroma or osteocartilaginous exostosis. It occurs frequently on the upper end of the humerus, usually on the medial side just below the head. The majority of these tumors develop in the first three decades, producing pain and limitation of motion as the early symptoms. The typical lesion has a stalk one to two inches long with a bulbous tip capped with cartilage. This projects upward at an angle above 60 degrees with the shaft (Fig. 17–14). The lesion may develop on the lateral aspect, in which case it more often projects at a right angle. The base is broad and bends with the shaft. The growth may extend to the point where it impinges on the glenoid, but more commonly the limitation of movement is from entanglement under the soft tissues. The tumor starts on the metaphyseal side of the

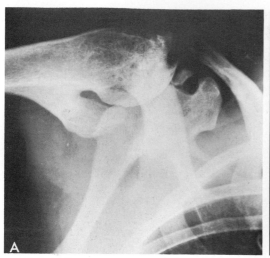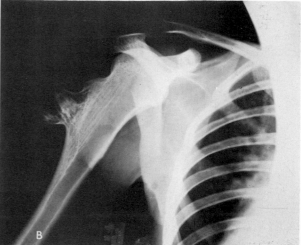

Figure 17–14 Typical osteochondroma; *A,* medial aspect; *B,* lateral aspect.

epiphyseal plate; the tip is covered with cartilage and growth continues at the top, usually until puberty.

Treatment. Surgical excision is the treatment of choice. Those lesions on the medial side may best be approached from the posteromedial aspect. Excision should include the periosteal layer and cartilaginous cap, cutting the base flush with the shaft. These lesions may rarely become malignant. Any osteocartilaginous tumor which starts to grow rapidly should be widely excised.

Solitary Enchondroma

The upper end of the humerus may be the seat of a solitary enchondroma. Occasionally this lesion resembles solitary cyst or fibrous dysplasia in that it has a cystic appearance (Fig. 17–15). Next to the small bones of the hands and the feet, the humerus is a not uncommon site. Instead of a cystic appearance, the impression of a solid deposit is more common, with patchy, calcified flecks scattered throughout. This is a benign lesion, often coming to light because of an easily produced fracture. Pain with some limitation of movement may occur in the absence of fracture. The metaphysis is the characteristic site. The diagnosis is made on surgical exploration. Sometimes whole segments of the shaft are replaced by bluish white cartilage. Microscopically the cartilage has a typical benign appearance; the cells are uniform in size, with a single small, or occasionally double, nucleus.

Treatment. Excision is the method of choice, with curettage of the area and re-

placement with cancellous bone. Radical resection is not so essential as in giant-cell lesions, nor is recurrence nearly so frequent. Occasionally a chondroma undergoes malignant change, usually evidenced clinically by persistent pain after previous therapy. Radical resection is indicated. Radiation therapy has not been effective in treatment of cartilaginous lesions.

Osteogenic Sarcoma

Osteogenic sarcoma occurs in the upper end of the humerus, next in frequency to the lower end of the femur and the upper end of the tibia. It is the commonest primary malignant tumor about the shoulder.

Clinical Features. The tumor is commonest between the ages of 10 and 25 years. The cardinal symptom is persistent pain that is unrelieved by rest and the usual simple remedies. Local tenderness is the earliest reliable sign. The appearance of swelling varies with the make-up of the tumor, but it is a late sign. The whole shoulder is swollen, tense and tender; superficial veins are dilated. The hands and fingers are swollen from the persistent, cramped position in which the arm is held at the side of the body and from local venous obstruction.

The x-ray appearance is commonly a mixture of cystic formation and new bone growth. In some the latter appearance is so dominant that it is difficult to separate the lesion from pure cyst. In others the new bone formation is predominant (Fig. 17–16, *B*). A cardinal indication of aggression is perforation of the cortex and extension into

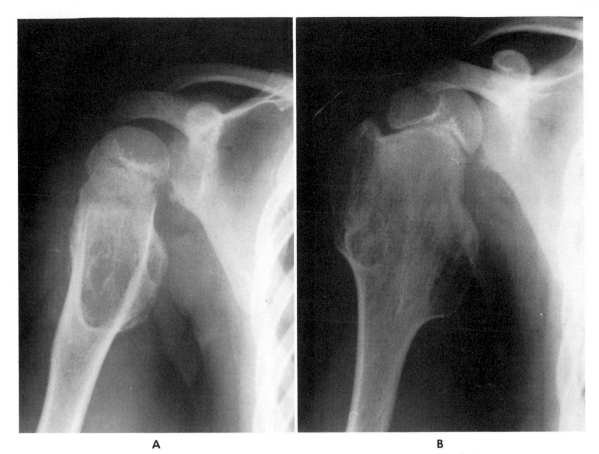

Figure 17–15 *A* and *B*, Enchondroma of humerus.

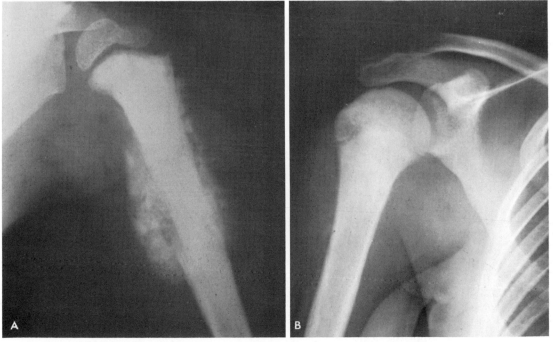

Figure 17–16 Osteogenic sarcoma. *A*, In a child; *B*, adult sclerosing form.

the soft tissues. At this point pathological fracture is common. Emphasis has long been placed on the "sun ray" appearance of bone spicules growing at right angle to the cortex (Fig. 17–16, *A*). Authorities such as Lichtenstein indicate that this appearance is not diagnostic. It may be seen in metastatic lesions, in some neurogenic tumors and even in Ewing's tumor. It is emphasized that osteogenic sarcoma, by its very nature, must be anticipated in a variety of appearances, so that biopsy is essential for the diagnosis. The telltale features are the progressive melting away process, which does not stay within the bounds of the shaft of the bone. Gradually, a soft tissue shadow develops which is most suggestive of the malignant properties.

This tumor is differentiated from giant-cell tumor by its aggressive, extensile appearance, the raised blood phosphatase and the soft tissue shadow. Malignant giant-cell lesion is hard to separate clinically and radiologically from the lytic form of sarcoma, but the treatment is so similar that this does not matter. On cursory investigation a solitary cyst is similar, but the lack of expansile progression, blood changes and the benign clinical course are distinguishing. The blood phosphatase is elevated in osteogenic sarcoma and falls when disarticulation is done, and, if found at a high level again, is suggestive of recurrence or a secondary tumor.

Pathology. The normal architecture of the medulla and the cortex is completely obliterated, being replaced by cystic hemorrhagic areas that alternate with soft, new bone formation. The osteogenic property may dominate, producing a hard, sclerotic mass extending through the shaft into soft tissues, or soft elements may dominate, extending along the medullary cavity and into the shaft.

The microscopic appearance varies from a highly cellular neoplastic form to a predominantly osteogenic type, with much new atypical bone and cartilage and a minimum of stroma. Intramedullary sections tend to be more cellular, with large osteogenic cells, with little stroma and many large atypical cells, spindle cells or tumor giant cells.

Treatment. The only treatment that offers a glimmer of hope is early, radical surgery. The prognosis is very poor. A five-year survival rate, as presented by Lichtenstein, and Budd and MacDonald, is between 5 and 15 per cent. The lungs are involved so early, particularly in shoulder lesions, that most of these patients do not survive longer

than two years after operation. When an early, single metastasis is encountered in the lung, consultation with a thoracic surgeon regarding possible lobectomy or pneumonectomy is indicated. Disarticulation of the shoulder would appear to offer as much as forequarter amputation in these lesions. If there is extensive soft tissue invasion, forequarter amputation is the procedure of choice. Even in apparently aggressive tumors, operation is advisable. Patients are most appreciative of the comfort and the relief of pain that result from removal of the tumor.

TECHNIQUE OF DISARTICULATION OF SHOULDER. A tourniquet can be used, but most surgeons prefer to work without it. A stout, rubber band is applied and held in place by heavy pins.

The incision begins at the front, over the clavicle, lateral to the coracoid. It is carried outward and downward, following the anterior axillary fold, and crosses the axilla. The posterior limb swings down in racquet fashion, across the posterior deltoid, curving forward to meet the anterior limb (Fig. 17–17).

Dissection. Dissection proceeds from the front, with the branches of the thoraco-acromial arch being clamped and tied and also the cephalic vein. The deltoid is divided across its insertion, opening the shoulder joint. The long head of the biceps, the subscapularis, the pectoralis major, the latissimus dorsi and the teres major are divided close to their bone attachments. The capsule is cut across, dividing the supraspinatus, the infraspinatus and the teres minor muscles. The axillary artery and vein are identified by palpation. These are ligated separately, if possible, and doubly with heavy chromic catgut or silk. The nerve trunks are pulled down

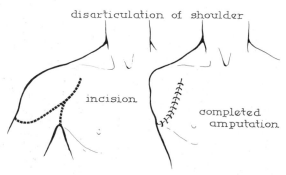

Figure 17–17 Incision for disarticulation of shoulder.

gently and cut and allowed to retract, avoiding strong traction. The other vessels are ligated. If a tourniquet has been used, it is released at this point. The subscapularis and triceps are cut across and the upper extremity falls free. Muscles may be replaced in various ways to fill the resulting dead space. The pectoralis major, the latissimus dorsi, and the cuff remnants are tacked to the glenoid. The deltoid edges may be folded over into this space also. The wound is closed in layers. A Penrose drain is inserted and is removed in 48 hours. A pressure dressing is applied and the bandage carried across and around the chest (Fig. 17–18).

FOREQUARTER AMPUTATION. This operation is needed for malignant disease when there is any suggestion of spread that will involve the joint or go beyond the confines of the upper end of the humerus. It is a major procedure. Proper preparation, including adequate blood for transfusions, is essential. The operation may be done either from the front or the back, depending upon the operator's preference. Some feel that the major vessels may be exposed and ligated with greater ease from the back.

From the Front. The incision extends laterally along the upper border of the clavicle and dips down, following the anterior axillary fold (Fig. 17–19). After the vessels have been ligated, the incision is completed posteriorly and upward, meeting the anterior limb.

Dissection. The clavicle is disarticulated at the sternum or cut across at the junction of the inner and middle thirds. The muscles and ligaments attached to the clavicle are severed close to the bone. The pectoralis minor is then divided and the extremity allowed to rotate and drop backward and outward. This exposes the axillary contents. The axillary artery and vein are identified and separated by careful dissection. The vessels are then doubly ligated with silk or heavy chromic catgut. The nerve trunks are severed while under definite tension and then allowed to retract. The incision is continued to the back; the trapezius and the transversus coli are cut; and the suprascapular and transverse cervical arteries are tied. The muscles attached to the medial border of the scapula are then cut close to the bone and the serratus magnus and latissimus dorsi are cut, freeing the extremity. The wound is closed in layers and a pressure dressing applied. Sutures are removed when the wound is healed, about the twelfth or fourteenth day following operation.

From the Back. This operation may also be done with the patient on his face. In this case the muscles along the medial border of the scapula are divided and the scapula is allowed to rotate with the extremity downward and forward. It is then retracted more laterally. The serratus anterior is cut and the axillary contents come into view. At this point they lie quite deep in the wound and considerable retraction is necessary to complete their identification and dissection. The vessels are ligated and the nerves cut as just described. The patient is then rotated on his side and the operation is completed from the front. (In doing the operation from the

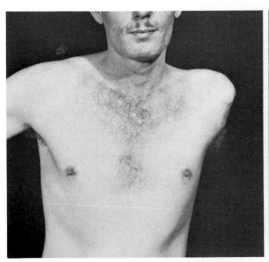 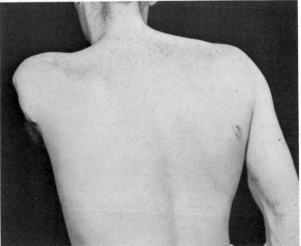

Figure 17–18 Postoperative result of disarticulation of shoulder.

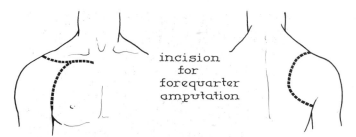

incision
for
forequarter
amputation

Figure 17-19   Incision for forequarter amputation.

back first, the major portion of the dissection is completed before the anterior segment is reached. In doing it from the front, possibly the vessels are a little more quickly identified and ligated, but the operator still needs considerable time to complete the posterior dissection.)

Chondrosarcoma

Tumors displaying malignant properties stemming primarily from cartilage elements have been placed in a separate category. They are occasionally encountered in the humerus, but the pelvis and the femur are more common sites. Compared with osteogenic sarcomas, they appear later, are much slower growing, metastasize less frequently and are much rarer. Figure 17-20 shows chondrosarcoma of the first rib.

Clinically a mass may be present for some time without producing significant discomfort. Sudden increase in size or discomfort is suggestive of aggressive change. Radiologically punctate calcification or a stippled appearance in the shaft with an indistinct or fuzzy adjacent zone of cortex is characteristic. The mass is often large, plastered on the cortex and irregularly calcified.

Histologically chondrosarcoma is separated from osteogenic sarcoma by the basic malignant element arising from cartilage rather than the primitive bone cell. Lichtenstein and others have drawn attention to this differentiation.

Treatment.   Radical local excision or disarticulation of the shoulder may be done. The survival rate is much higher than in osteogenic sarcoma. Attention is drawn to the need of careful assessment of any large cartilage tumor for malignant change. It is the impression of authoritative observers that many early malignant cartilage changes are overlooked. In view of the relatively satisfactory result that can be expected from radical surgery, such lesions should be more carefully analyzed.

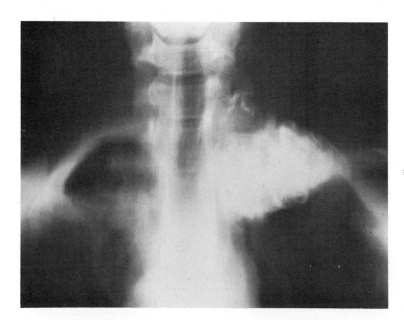

Figure 17-20   Chondrosarcoma of rib (laminogram).

Fibrosarcoma

A primary malignant fibroblastic tumor has been recognized as occurring occasionally in the upper end of the humerus. No distinguishing clinical features are apparent, and the diagnosis is made on histological section. An oval cystic lesion with suggestive cortical distribution and beginning soft tissue invasion is typical. The head, neck and upper shaft of the humerus may be involved, and radiological differentiation from malignant giant-cell tumor and osteogenic sarcoma is difficult. The treatment is the same, disarticulation of the shoulder.

Ewing's Tumor of the Humerus

The upper portion of the shaft of the humerus may be involved by Ewing's sarcoma. The humerus is involved next in frequency to the femur and the tibia. This is an insidious lesion, present for some time in the medullary cavity before symptoms direct attention to the area. Persistent, dull, aching pain, pain at night, tenderness over the upper shaft of the humerus and, later, limitation of shoulder movement are the early clinical findings. The typical x-ray shows a mottled disintegration of the shaft (Fig. 17–21). A moth-eaten appearance extends irregularly up and down the shaft and later involves the cortex in a patchy fashion. Periosteal reaction, in the form of an onion-skin effect is noted beyond the limits of the disintegration site (Fig. 17–21). This layered or onion peel-like reaction is seen so often in Ewing's tumor that it has been designated as being completely characteristic. It is most suggestive, but other lesions such as metastatic carcinoma, neuroblastoma and reticulum cell sarcoma may show the same thing. It seems best to regard it as a usual periosteal reaction to several lesions, rather than diagnostic of one.

Further clinical features recognized as characteristic of this lesion include fever, secondary anemia and leukocytosis. These are late findings and again are only suggestive rather than diagnostic. It is a disease of youth, with most cases occurring between the ages of 10 and 25 years.

The tumor is closely simulated by reticulum cell sarcoma, neuroblastoma and acute osteomyelitis. Reticulum cell sarcoma is encountered in older patients and has a diagnostic histological appearance. The blood and systemic changes are not so com-

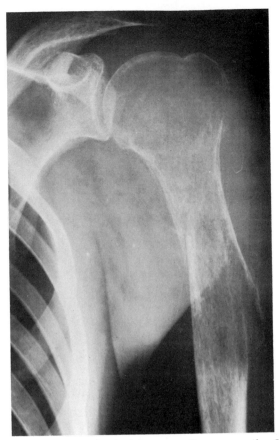

Figure 17–21 Ewing's tumor of upper end of humerus.

mon, nor does tumor tissue extend into the soft parts so extensively as in Ewing's. Much more of the bone is involved than is usually apparent from the x-ray examination (Fig. 17–22). Microscopically the tumor is made up of masses of small, round cells of characteristic uniform size and appearance and with minimum intercellular substance intervening. A characteristic arrangement in sheets or along blood vessels is described but is not uniformly encountered. The cells have poorly limited cell boundaries and nuclei are crowded together. Areas of hemorrhage and necrosis are frequent. There is no suggestion of bone formation. Metastases occur to other blood-forming regions such as ilium, ribs and vertebrae. Viscera such as lung and liver may also be involved. Laboratory findings are significant in that calcium, phosphorus and phosphatase levels are rarely altered.

Treatment. The lesion is easily confused with reticulum cell sarcoma, osteomyelitis, secondary carcinoma and neuroblastoma. Reticulum cell tumor occurs in an older

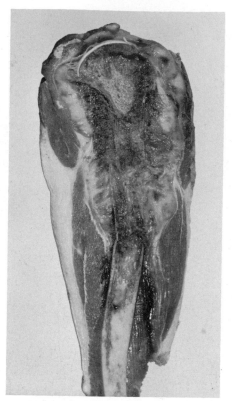

Figure 17–22 Ewing's tumor of the upper humerus. Note the extensive shaft soft tissue involvement when compared to the x-ray in Figure 17–21.

age group and has a characteristic cytological picture which comes to light when special stains are used. Osteomyelitis may be confused with Ewing's tumor when found in young children because of the frequent leukocytosis, fever and secondary anemia. Biopsy, chemotherapy and response to radiation distinguish the two. Secondary carcinoma occurs in older patients; clinical signs and the biopsy are distinguishing. Neuroblastoma is difficult to separate clinically and radiologically from Ewing's sarcoma. Both produce a similar periosteal reaction, both occur in young people, and in both the lesions may be multiple. Neuroblastoma occurs in very young patients, most under ten. It has a characteristic histological appearance, with the cells distributed in classic "rosette" fashion.

Ewing's tumor has a miserable prognosis despite early and accurate diagnosis. The treatment of choice in humeral lesions is immediate radiation followed by disarticulation of the shoulder (Fig. 17–23). The immediate result is most gratifying, but most patients succumb to multiple secondary tumors in two to three years. Palliative radiation is used in recurrences and metastases.

Multiple Myeloma of the Humerus

The humerus, in company with the rest of the skeleton, may be involved in this primary malignant disease of the bone marrow cells. In the shoulder region the clavicle is possibly more frequently involved than the upper end of the humerus. Primary symptoms of the disease are reflected from the spine and chest more often than from the long bones. The spine is a frequent site, and when the cervical vertebrae are affected, shoulder or shoulder plus radiating pain is prominent. The disease occurs after 30 years of age, and usually between 40 and 60. Occasionally the upper end of the humerus is the source of the initial complaints, but x-rays generally show that skull, spine and pelvis are also riddled. The bones have a pocked appearance, with small, sharp, punched-out zones (Fig. 17–24). Several may coalesce, forming a larger defect (Fig. 17–25). The pocking may be so diffuse that normal architecture is obliterated and only a thin, fragile shell remains. Pathological fracture is common. In roughly half the patients the urine shows Bence Jones protein. This develops as a cloudy precipitate when urine is heated to 45 to 60° C, and disappears with further heating. Increased serum calcium is frequent, but the phosphorus level is not altered correspondingly, which distinguishes this disorder from Recklinghausen's disease and renal osteopathy. The blood changes include alteration of the albumin-globulin ratio and rise in serum protein. In roughly 50 per cent of patients the globulin fraction is increased above the albumin level, accounting for the rise in the protein level. The mechanism of these blood changes appears to be associated with the breakdown of the myeloma cells, and present investigation indicates that this is a complex process. The uric acid level has also been reported raised in this disorder. Renal complications and amyloidosis are other features receiving increased attention in the investigation of this disease.

Pathology. A typical skeletal lesion appears as a small cortical elevation which cuts easily or is quite brittle. Medullary substance may have permeated the cortex, extending into soft tissue. Normal marrow is replaced by a grayish white vascular tumor

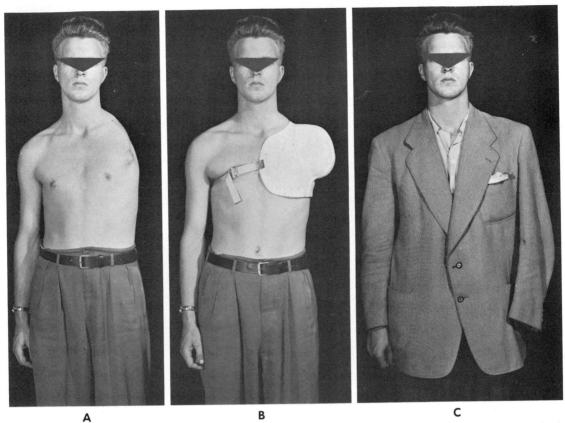

A	B	C

Figure 17–23 Forequarter amputation for Ewing's tumor. *A,* Postoperative appearance; *B,* shoulder prosthesis; *C,* improvement of appearance in wearing a coat with use of prosthesis.

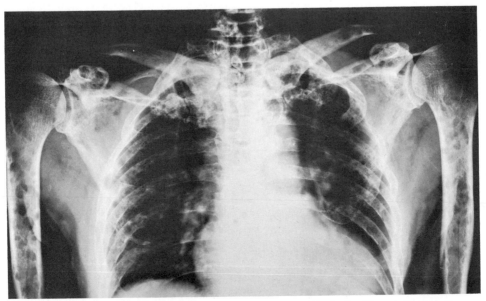

Figure 17–24 Multiple myeloma. Massive involvement of both shoulder girdle and ribs.

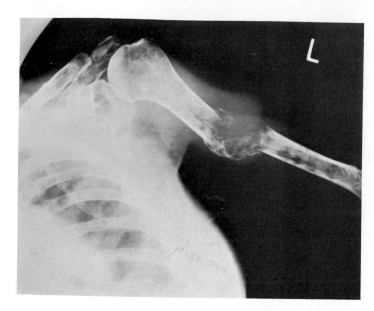

Figure 17–25 Myeloma of the humerus with coalescence of multiple foci to form a larger defect.

substance. Microscopically it is composed of sheets of cells with prominent nuclei, little cellular substance and almost no intercellular supporting network. The cell type is characteristic, being similar to a plasma cell with a large, round, stippled nucleus. The intranuclear material distribution sometimes resembles a clock face or radiates like the spokes of a wheel. In other examples the cell is much larger, with abundant cytoplasm. Lichtenstein has suggested a relationship with the blood findings between the large and small cell varieties; possibly, increased globulin is associated with the large cell type, whereas when the small cell is predominant, albumin and globulin are within normal limits. Primitive cells, myeloblasts or plasma cells may be found in the blood smear. In advanced cases plasma cells may form one third of the leukocyte blood count. Sternal puncture for examination of the marrow is recommended in all suspected cases.

Treatment and Prognosis. Multiple myeloma is a progressive, malignant disease. When it is sufficiently advanced to come into clinical focus, patients do not survive longer than two to three years, as a rule. Patients with well localized lesions last longer. No cure is available, and efforts are directed toward preventing and controlling fractures and providing relief from pain. Concentrated research is opening new avenues of therapy. Stilbamidine, as reported by Snapper, decreases the pain. Radioactivated compounds such as radioactive phosphorus are being investigated, but results are not too encouraging. To date, radiation appears as beneficial as these remedies.

Solitary Myeloma

A solitary myeloma may be encountered which follows a much more benign course. The upper end of the humerus may be the seat of a single large myeloma, but the scapula is possibly more frequently involved. The x-ray shows a somewhat sharp, punched-out lesion that is trabeculated, and without lytic involvement of the rest of the shaft, of the soft tissue or of other bones. This is a much less common tumor than multiple myeloma, but the humerus or the scapula is a common site. The cystic look, the less aggressive course and the site simulate giant-cell tumor and solitary bone cyst. Blood changes show almost none of the profound alteration associated with multiple myeloma. Many observers assume that such a lesion may later develop into multiple myeloma.

Pathology. A single tumor zone is present without cortical destruction or soft tissue invasion. The marrow is not normal and shows somewhat vacuolated zones alternating with fibrous or more vascular and cellular deposits. The cells dominating the histological picture are plasma cells, but they lack the characteristics of aggressive malignancy.

Treatment. This tumor responds to radiation, and survivals of ten years or longer have been reported. Radical section, followed by radiation, is preferred. When there is any suggestion of extension, recurrence or activation, disarticulation of the shoulder should be done provided the rest of the skeleton is not involved.

Metastatic Lesions

The upper end of the humerus is a frequent seat of secondary tumor growth extending from primary lesions elsewhere in the body. These frequently have an osteolytic or moth-eaten appearance. The characteristics of the group are the multiplicity of lesions, the frequency of pathological fracture and the occurrence in the older age group. Almost any carcinoma may metastasize to bone, but certain ones do so more frequently; thus, carcinoma of the breast, prostate, kidneys, lung and thyroid have a high incidence of skeletal involvement, and the humerus is one of the bones most frequently involved. Secondary tumors occur more often than primary tumors in this area and one must constantly be on guard for their presence. Some observers have concluded that the nearer a bone to the site of primary involvement, the more frequently is it the site of metastasis. The upper end of the humerus is close to the breast, chest and thyroid, making it a common site of secondary involvement.

Secondary tumors occur about the shoulder, and in the upper end of the humerus in particular, with surprising frequency. It can happen that a metastasis discovered here is the first indication of an established visceral malignancy (Fig. 17–26). This area is close to the lung, breast, mediastinum and neck, so tumor spread is early and rapid. Abdominal malignancies also metastasize to the shoulder and may do so without implicating the lung. Such tumor spread has been shown by Batson to occur by way of the prevertebral veins. It is possible to inject this system with opaque dye by way of the dorsal vein of the penis and demonstrate the profound venous extension to spine, pelvis, shoulder girdle and even skull without involvement of lung.

Carcinoma of the Breast. Carcinoma of the breast leads to bone involvement in roughly 5 per cent of the patients. A pathological fracture of the neck of the humerus may be the first indication of metastatic spread. The fracture is treated as usual by

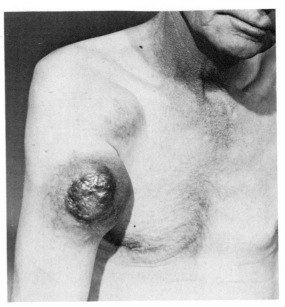

Figure 17–26 Secondary carcinoma in humerus, osteoblastic type. Primary in lung.

adequate immobilization, but x-radiation is given in addition.

Carcinoma of the Prostate. In over two thirds of prostatic malignancies there is bone involvement. Although the pelvis and spine are the most frequent sites, the humerus and scapula may also be involved (Fig. 17–27). The mechanism of such spread is presumably by the prevertebral venous network. A moth-eaten cystic appearance in the x-ray is common. Increased acid phosphatase is highly suggestive of prostatic malignant disease. The level usually falls after adequate treatment. Should a sudden rise occur again, it is suggestive of further secondary development.

Pathological fractures are treated by immobilization, but the important aspect of therapy is adequate hormone administration. Relief of pain and cessation of tumor aggression can be obtained for appreciable periods.

Carcinoma of the Lung. This tumor is one of the commonest causes of death in males. Increasing attention to and awareness of this dread tumor is needed. Skeletal metastases are common and multiple pathological fractures are frequently encountered (Fig. 17–26). The primary disease is, usually, so far advanced or proceeding so rapidly that nothing can be done apart from relieving pain. One of the most distressing tumors encountered is that occurring in the apex of the lung, where, by direct or metastatic

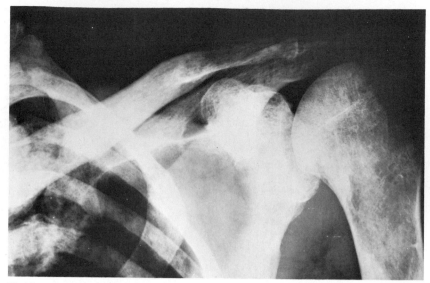

Figure 17–27   Multiple secondary deposits of carcinoma in the shoulder girdle; primary in prostate.

spread, the brachial plexus is involved. These patients, in addition to local pain, develop a typical causalgia involving the whole upper extremity. This adds a great deal to their misery, so that much sedation is essential to control the pain. A primary tumor of lung apex may produce shoulder-neck pain early in its course without metastatic involvement of the skeleton (Pancoast lesion) (Fig. 17–28).

Carcinoma of the Gastrointestinal Tract. Occasionally the shoulder is implicated from primary tumors in the abdominal cavity. Bone is involved in 3 per cent of these malignancies (Fig. 17–29). As with lung tumors, this is usually a late manifestation of the disease.

TUMORS OF THE SCAPULA

Tumors of the scapula are not encountered so often as those in the upper end of the humerus, but they occur more frequently than in the clavicle. Most of the scapular substance is in the base of the glenoid and the heavy buttresses leading from it. Tumors seem to be related to this zone more often than to the rest of the bone. As in the humerus, secondary tumors are not uncommon and arise from the same sources. Clinically tumors of the scapula tend to become apparent a little sooner than those in the humerus. There is not so much medullary cavity to hide the process, and any irregularity becomes obvious in the thin bone structure. The tumors found are similar to those described for the humerus. The common,

benign lesions are osteochondromas (Figs. 17–30 and 17–31) and giant-cell tumors (Fig. 17–32). The treatment is the same as for tumors in the humerus.

A general problem is posed in the giant-cell lesions. These commonly occur in the neck and expand to just beneath the cartilage of the glenoid cavity. Sometimes the joint surface is cracked because the egg-shell thinness of the bone withstands little trauma. These are treated by excision, curettage and obliteration with cancellous bone chips and cortical bone, if necessary. Complete resection is difficult and recurrence sometimes follows easily. When this happens, complete resection without grafting may be done, including the glenoid surface. Should there be any question of malignancy, scapulectomy, as outlined later, is the operation

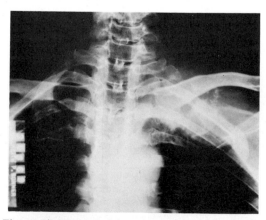

Figure 17–28   Apical lung tumor (Pancoast lesion).

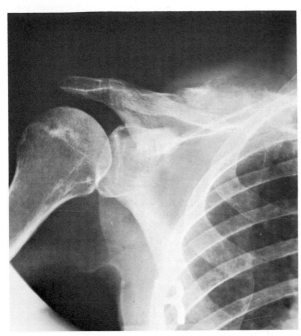

Figure 17–29 Secondary carcinoma in scapula; primary tumor was in gallbladder.

face down and the shoulder so draped that it may be moved. A curved incision is used and extends from the tip of the acromion, medially, across the spine, turning downward lateral and parallel to the vertebral border (Fig. 17–34). This allows access to all edges of the bone. The suspensory muscles along the spine are cut, then those at the vertebral border and inferior angle. The cuff muscles are incised lateral to the glenoid; the long head of the biceps is cut and clamped. The scapula is elevated and the transverse scapular vessels ligated as they extend into the suprascapular notch. The coracoid and trapezoid ligaments are cut. The scapula is rotated so that the subscapularis may be cut through. The long head of the biceps is then sutured to the clavicle and acts as a suspensory ligament, replacing, in a fashion, the conoid and trapezoid ligaments. This last step was introduced by W. E. Gallie, who emphasized the necessity of some suspensory force for the arm. If this is not provided, the extremity tends to drop limply and drag. Some support relieves this and improves the power of movement. Scapulectomy is a surgi-

of choice. Plasmacytomas are occasionally encountered in the scapula and appear in the subglenoid neck region. These are easily confused with giant-cell tumors, as the illustration shows (Fig. 17–33). Biopsy settles the issue. Treatment is the same as for giant-cell tumors. If they recur after excision and bone grafting, scapulectomy should be done.

Malignant tumors such as chondrosarcoma, Ewing's and osteogenic sarcoma are also encountered. Cartilaginous tumors seem to be more frequent than Ewing's or osteogenic lesions. Sometimes these grow to a large size. Apparently they may begin as a simple chondroma that, after some time, increase in size and assume aggressive properties. Other lesions such as those outlined for the humerus are encountered, and the pathological characteristics are similar.

Treatment. Local excision of benign lesions such as osteoma, osteoid osteoma and osteochondroma is sufficient. Benign cystic lesions such as giant-cell tumor should be resected and obliterated with bone. Malignant tumors, for example, chondrosarcoma, are satisfactorily treated by total scapulectomy. In more aggressive lesions (osteogenic and Ewing's sarcoma), forequarter amputation is recommended.

TECHNIQUE OF TOTAL SCAPULECTOMY. The operation is performed with the patient

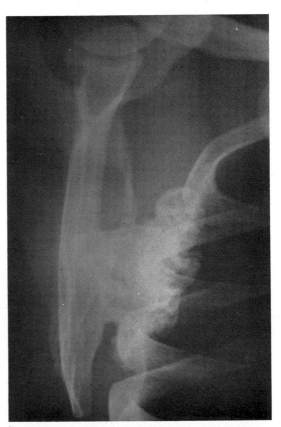

Figure 17–30 Osteochondroma of scapula.

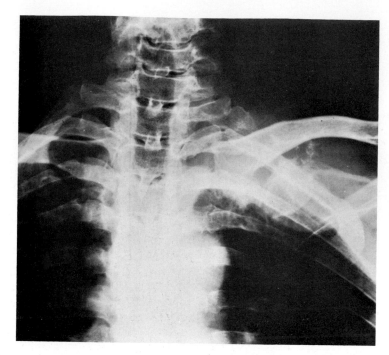

Figure 17–31 Chondroma of scapula.

cal procedure of the first magnitude, but most satisfactory results are recorded. The resulting disability is less than might be anticipated. These patients retain reasonable control and are able to lift from the side.

TUMORS OF THE CLAVICLE

The clavicle is the least common site for tumors in the bones of the shoulder. It is still susceptible to both benign and malignant neoplasms; osteomas and, occasionally, giant-cell tumors are found. Their treatment is similar to the principles outlined for such growths in the humerus and scapula. Malignancies are encountered also (Fig. 17–35). Multiple myeloma (see Fig. 17–24) has some predilection for the clavicle. Osteogenic sarcoma arises occasionally (see Figs. 17–7 and 17–36). These tumors become apparent quite early because the superficial position of the whole shaft favors attention to any irregularity or soreness. Osteogenic sarcoma poses a serious problem to therapy. Local extension rapidly involves vital structures at the lung apex or in the neck, making excision difficult. The operation of choice is forequarter amputation but, occasionally, progression is such that only local resection can be done. This may be accompanied by radiation, but the therapy is only transiently effective and recurrence is rapid. Fungating

masses add considerably to the unfortunate patient's discomfort and repeated local resection by cautery is justified.

BONE DISEASE TO BE DIFFERENTIATED FROM NEOPLASMS

In addition to tumors, the shoulder girdle is susceptible to bone diseases found else-

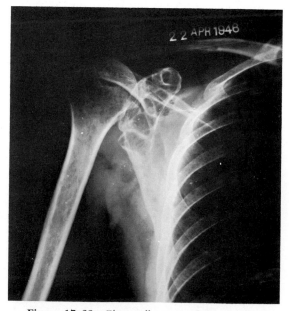

Figure 17–32 Giant cell tumor of the scapula.

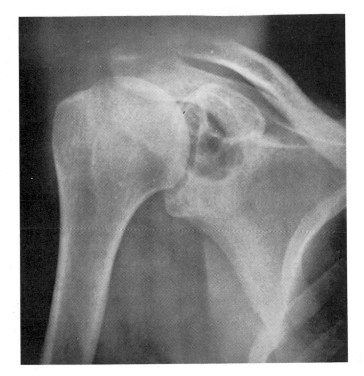

Figure 17–33 Plasmacytoma of scapula.

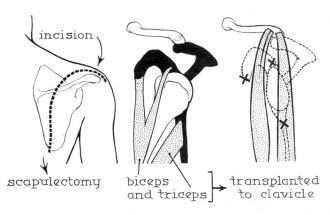

Figure 17–34 Technique of total scapulectomy.

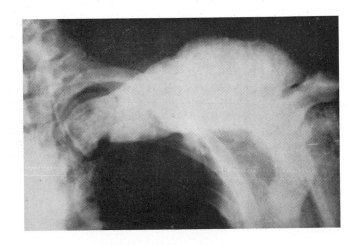

Figure 17–35 Osteogenic sarcoma of clavicle.

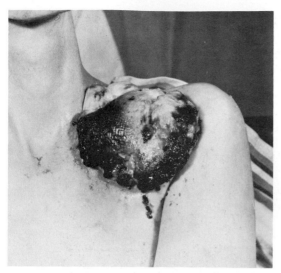

Figure 17–36 Fungating advanced osteogenic sarcoma of clavicle.

where in the body, including von Recklinghausen's disease, fibrous dysplasia, Paget's disease, osteomyelitis, syphilis and even scurvy. The mobility and constant use may focus attention on this region first in any of these generalized disorders. Many simulate tumors, particularly in x-ray films, and these have been discussed previously. Paget's disease, lipoid granulomatosis, osteomyelitis

and the very rare syphilis and scurvy merit further consideration.

Paget's Disease

The shoulder bones are implicated in this generalized constitutional disorder of later life. In this region it commonly comes to light as an osteoporotic or cystic change in the upper zone of the humerus (Fig. 17–37). As such, it may be confused with other cystic lesions like fibrous dysplasia, Recklinghausen's disease and osteogenic sarcoma. Most authorities feel that Paget's disease proceeds through several phases, so that an osteoporotic stage is encountered initially (Fig. 17–37, *A*), followed by a lithocystic phase (Fig. 17–38) and, finally, the commonly seen osteolithic stage (Fig. 17–37, *B*). It is in the early phase of osteoporosis or cyst-like change that difficulty in diagnosis arises and clinical complications are more apparent. Many cases progress through all these stages without ever producing symptoms. Nearly all patients are over 40 and males are more commonly afflicted than females. Pain, limitation of movement and some bowing or swelling of the upper part of the arm are the clinical findings when the shoulder is involved. Occasionally pathological fracture is the initial indication. The

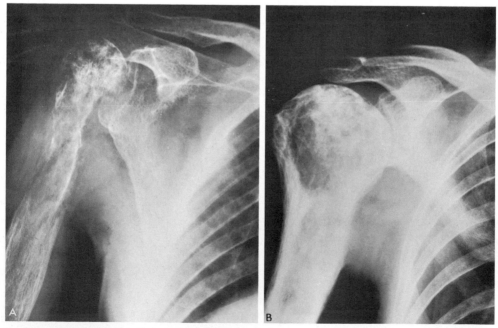

Figure 17–37 Paget's disease of the upper end of humerus. *A*, Osteoporotic or osteolytic stage; *B*, osteolithic stage.

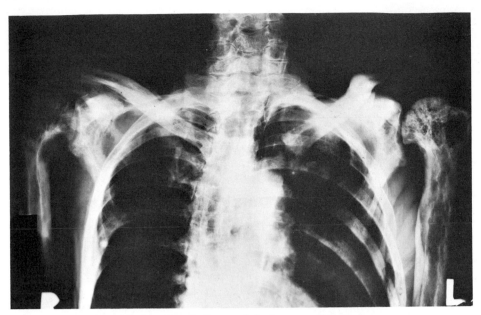

Figure 17–38 Paget's disease of the humerus, lithocystic stage.

x-rays show startling changes in the early phase of this disease.

An osteoporotic zone or segment appears in the proximal half of the humerus. This may be followed by thickening and minute cyst formation in the cortex and later by the typical hardening and gross thickening of the end stage. The process may stop anywhere along this course. In extreme cases, which have the most serious complaints, the osteoporosis is profound, amounting almost to a lytic process. The normal cortical outline disappears, and the upper portion of the shaft and head is represented by an irregularly calcified mass. Fractures are common at this stage. Investigation shows other body areas involved, but usually only one zone shows these profound changes at one time. Calcium and phosphorus in blood and urine are normal, but the serum phosphatase is elevated. Therapy is directed toward the complications of this disease since no established treatment is available for the generalized process. Fractures of the humerus are treated by reduction and immobilization in plaster. Operative fixation is usually not necessary and, in the extremely porotic lesions, is not suitable. Occasionally the osteoporosis is so marked that the fracture is months in healing; rarely they do not heal. In such cases the effect of moderate x-radiation may be assessed.

The most serious complication is malignant change, which is encountered in roughly 10 per cent of patients presenting symptoms (Fig. 17–39). The malignant process is classified as an ostegenic sarcoma and in such form is the commonest type of osteogenic sarcoma in patients over 40 years of age. It is manifested by persistent and increasing pain, radiologically aggressive lytic development and a high serum alkaline phosphatase level.

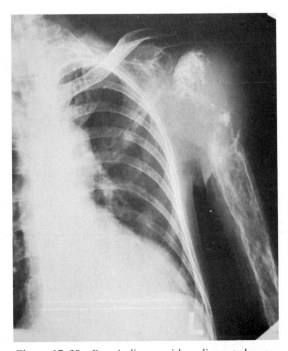

Figure 17–39 Paget's disease with malignant change.

It should be emphasized at this point, however, that such a diagnosis should be made only on microscopic section because the osteoporosis may be severe and then progress in quite benign fashion. In the shoulder region the treatment of choice is forequarter amputation. This may be supplemented by radiation.

Lipoid Granulomas

Cystic changes in scapula and humerus are encountered as manifestations of this somewhat rare group of disturbances. Letterer-Siwe disease, Hand-Schüller-Christian disease and eosinophilic granuloma are currently interpreted as different histological stages of one underlying disorder. The scapula appears to be the most frequently implicated of the shoulder bones. The basic x-ray change is a well demarcated circular defect, or several such areas coalescing in irregular fashion (Fig. 17–40). Multiplicity of lesions is the rule, with skull, vertebrae and pelvis more commonly implicated than the extremities.

In infants and in children up to two years of age the general systemic reaction is preponderant, with marked proliferation of the reticuloendothelial cells. Letterer-Siwe disease is the term applied to this phase. Later, bone changes are more prominent and the term Hand-Schüller-Christian disease may be applied. In addition to the cystic changes that are predominant in membrane bone, diabetes insipidus and exophthalmus occur. Eosinophilic granuloma is considered the late phase and has fewer bone changes and less profound systemic reaction. The early forms are easily diagnosed. Eosinophilic granuloma, however, is easily confused with other cystic changes such as fibrocystic disease, solitary bone cyst, giant-cell tumor, chondroblastoma, osteogenic sarcoma and Ewing's tumor. Biopsy determines the diagnosis. A characteristic cytological picture is present, with groups of foam cells in a granulomatous tissue. In eosinophilic granuloma, masses of eosinophils, along with the histiocytes, are diagnostic.

The treatment of these disorders is changing as our knowledge increases. An infectious process is suggested by the distribution and progress of some of these cases. The possibility of a virus lesion of bone is provocative. X-ray treatment has been the most successful measure to date. Recently the possible infectious etiology has been substantiated by R. N. Fisher, who reports successful treatment with chloromycetin of the usually fatal Letterer-Siwe disease.

Osteomyelitis

The advent of effective chemotherapy has decreased the incidence of this once dread disease. The humerus is the bone most frequently involved about the shoulder (Fig. 17–41). The metaphyseal region may be implicated in the hematogenous spread, but direct contamination from fractures and wounds is more frequent. In children the joint may be involved because a small corner lies within the capsular confines. The disease

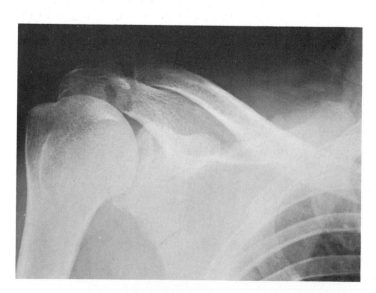

Figure 17–40 Cystic lesion of the acromion similar to eosinophilic granuloma.

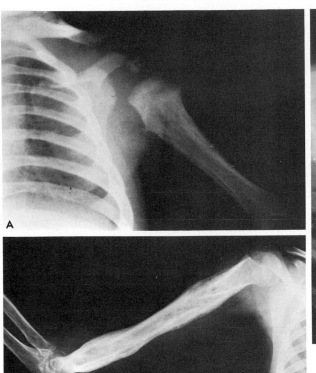

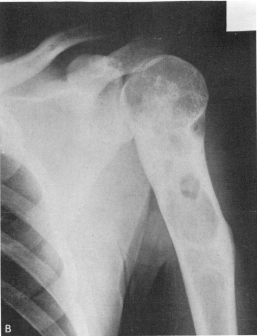

Figure 17–41 Osteomyelitis of humerus. *A*, Joint involvement in child; *B*, abscess formation with small sequestrum; *C*, extensive involvement of shaft.

may be confused with calcified tendinitis or various bone tumors, notably Ewing's. The treatment is proper chemotherapy and immobilization in plaster. In chronic cases, if sequestra are apparent, they should be removed.

Syphilis

Changes in the shoulder bones may appear in syphilis in either the congenital or acquired varieties. In the congenital variety, there are the usual cortical thickening and epiphyseal fragmentation (Fig. 17–42). Occasionally the gumma may be encountered in the humerus as a solitary lesion (Fig. 17–43).

Scurvy

Scurvy has become a rare disease, but it still is encountered occasionally. The shoulder is often involved, and striking x ray changes may be seen in the acute stage. The upper end of the humerus has a globular shadow, with the raised periosteum presenting a halo-like effect (Fig. 17–44); this appearance is diagnostic. Systemic therapy quickly controls the bone changes.

Osteochondrodystrophies

Striking bone changes result from this group of developmental disorders and the shoulder shares in these. The upper end of the humerus presents characteristic changes in achondroplasia and osteochondrodystrophy. In achondroplasia the humerus is short and thick and the head has a flattened "door-knob" shape (Fig. 17–45). Bony irregularities and exostoses close to the metaphyseal region are common. The changes rarely interfere with function to any extent because adaptation and control to counterbalance the irregularities begin at an early age. Limitation of rotation is the most significant effect.

RARE JOINT DISEASES

Two uncommon joint disorders may be mentioned which are found much more frequently in joints in the lower limb. These

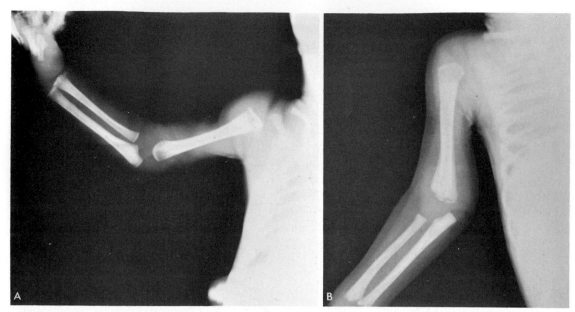

Figure 17-42 Congenital syphilis involving the shoulder. *A*, Note broadening and flattening of the head of the humerus; *B*, note cortical thickening and ragged epiphysis.

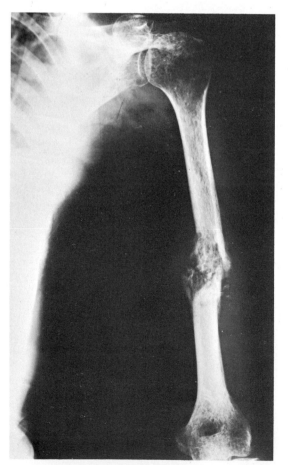

Figure 17-43 Gumma of humerus.

are osteochondromatosis and neutrotrophic changes.

Osteochondromatosis

The x-ray film is striking, showing many small halo-like bodies scattered throughout the joint (Fig. 17–46). These are cartilaginous bodies developed from the synovial lining by a process of metaplasia. Symptoms arise commonly about the third decade and consist of painful catching or locking episodes, followed by swelling and limitation of movement. The treatment is exploration and excision of the loose bodies. At operation the joint is crammed with multiple pea-sized cartilaginous bodies. Some are loose and some are embedded in synovium, while others are attached in pedunculated fashion by a synovial stalk. These latter are in the process of being pinched off to become loose within the joint. In some areas the synovial lining should be excised completely to eliminate all the potential chondromas. The joint is usually approached from the front; the deltoid fibers are separated or the anterior portion detached from the clavicle and reflected laterally.

Neurotrophic Joints

Profound joint changes occur in the shoulder from syringomyelia and syphilis (Figs.

17–47 and 15–28). These have been considered in detail in Chapter XV.

Hodgkin's Disease

In conjunction with other parts of the skeleton, the bones of the shoulder may be involved in Hodgkin's disease. Diffuse uniform sclerosis is encountered, spreading from the cortex inward. Pain and limitation of movement may accompany the generalized systemic manifestations. Somewhat similar changes are also seen in leukemia (Fig. 17–48).

TUMORS OF THE NECK

Most tumors or tumor-like lesions involving the neck implicate the soft tissues and viscera. They fall naturally into two groups, depending on their location at the front or the back. In contrast to the zone about the shoulder, there are frequent swellings implicating the front of the neck that are of non-neoplastic origin. For this reason it is extremely important to carry out meticulous

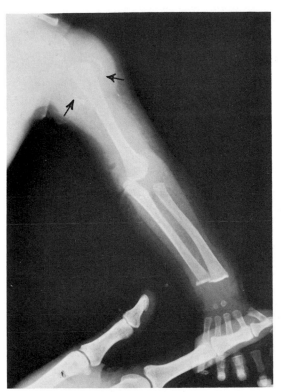

Figure 17–44   Scurvy of the shoulder.

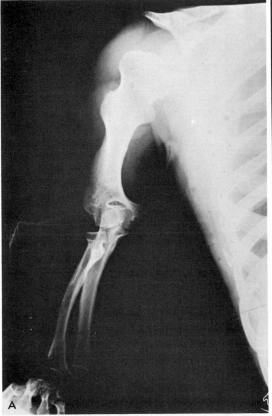

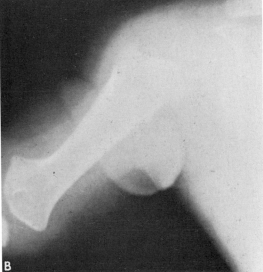

Figure 17–45   Shoulder changes in (*A*) achondroplasia; (*B*) Morquio's disease.

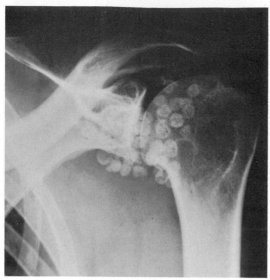

Figure 17–46 Osteochondromatosis of shoulder.

physical examination, particularly in assessing a swelling in the midline, anterior to or closely associated with this zone. In the same way inspection of the supraclavicular zone should be a routine part of a general physical examination because of the likelihood of certain systemic diseases becoming apparent in the lymph glands of this region.

ANTERIOR CERVICAL LESIONS

In the anterior triangle of the neck certain uncommon lesions may be defined.

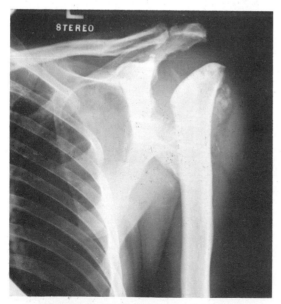

Figure 17–47 Neurotrophic shoulder.

Thyroglossal Cysts

These cysts or tumors arise from the remains of the thyroglossal duct, which extends from the base of the tongue to the isthmus of the thyroid gland. They appear in the early years of life as oval swellings in the midline. Often they consist of thyroid tissue and are firmly nodular on palpation. If soft, they are cystic with a loculated cavity, lying in the usual site just below the hyoid bone.

Dermoid Cysts

A further type of congenital cyst is identified also lying in the midline and made up of cutaneous elements in various proportions. Skin, hair follicles and sweat glands are included in these benign neoplasms. When they cause symptoms, they should be treated by surgical excision.

Branchial Cysts

A rare lesion is the laterally placed congenital cyst, which is termed a "branchial cyst." These are rounded swellings appearing below the angle of the jaw, or just at the anterior border of the sternocleidomastoid muscle. On section they contain epithelial and lymphoid elements and arise from the remnants of a branchial cyst. In some instances an opening to the surface develops as a fistula from the collection of these congenital elements. The branchial fistula arises at a higher level and, in rare instances, has an internal opening related to the base of the tongue.

Carotid Body Tumors

A tumor of the chromaffin system, developmental in nature, may appear in relation to the bifurcation of the carotid artery. It is called a potato tumor because of its loculated skin-like covering. The tumor occurs in the early decades and may be mistaken for many less significant disorders. The tumor has an important relationship to the cerebral blood pressure and this is its salient feature. Pressure on the lesion frequently produces attacks of syncope; these often have an apparently unexplained origin but are due to a tight collar, pressure from a coat or some other cervical constriction. Considerable recovery can be anticipated from surgical removal.

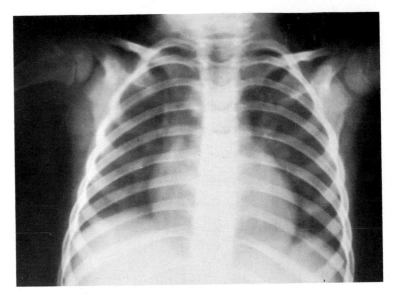

Figure 17–48 Hodgkin's disease, showing involvement of the shoulder.

Thyroid Tumors

Firm swellings at the root of the front of the neck usually implicate the thyroid gland. Neck pain is not an unusual complaint, and yet the patient may be unaware that the source is really at the front. Colloid tumor or exophthalmic lesions are easily recognized. The rare condition of woody thyroiditis produces much more acute pain and is characterized by a rapid and diffuse enlargement, along with extreme local tenderness and absence of concomitant thyroid symptoms. Carcinoma of the thyroid, although a relatively rare lesion, should be watched for. It always develops in a gland already the seat of dysfunction, and the onset of the change may be characterized by a new painful state localized to this region. The further importance of the lesion is its predilection to metastasize to bone.

TUMORS OF THE POSTERIOR ASPECT OF THE NECK

Swellings in the posterior triangle and posterior cervical region may be classified under three main headings.

Inflammatory Lesions

Many states such as infections of the tonsils, teeth and jaws may implicate the cervical lymph glands. Any of these will produce a generalized cervical adenopathy. Initially one group may be more involved than the other. Local skin inflammation and hair follicle infections also produce similar painful swellings, leading to a decrease in neck motion and considerable local pain. The characteristic of all these lesions is their rapid onset and their usually patent association with nearby inflammation.

Lymphoblastomas

The commonest initial site of involvement in leukemia and the lymphoblastomas of the lymphoid system is in the cervical lymph glands. There is little pain associated with this and almost no implication of movement in the cervical spine. In some instances it is a casual assessment of the area that identifies the swollen glands.

Secondary Carcinoma

The cervical lymph glands are important drainage mechanisms for lip, tongue, mouth, larynx, nasopharynx and esophagus. Consequently spread of a primary malignant lesion from these areas to the neck is not uncommon. Carcinoma of the stomach can also occasionally be detected in this area. Biopsy should be done of all firm, persistent swellings. Neck symptoms, apart from the truly local changes, are most infrequent.

BONE TUMORS INVOLVING THE CERVICAL SPINE

Regional demarcation of bone tumors has not been extensively developed because most contributors dwell on the delineation of a given tumor rather than interpreting its regional significance. In the case of the cervical spine, as elsewhere, we may demarcate benign, malignant and secondary bone tumors.

Benign Tumors

Many benign tumors have been identified in the cervical spine, but the commonest one is some variant of the hemangioma; other lesions have been reported, including giant-cell tumor, benign chondroblastoma, aneurysmal bone cyst, osteoid osteoma, osteoblastoma, osteochondroma and enchondroma.

Hemangioma. The hemangioma is the commonest tumor of the spine and in its general distribution frequently implicates the cervical area. Often these are small and asymptomatic, but there may be multiple lesions. Jaffe has suggested that they may represent focal varicosities rather than true hemangiomata. Radiologically they appear as an area of rarefaction, with a coarse trabecular ribbing or longitudinal striations. Pain in the area, local tenderness and, occasionally, nerve root irritation develop. A common course is collapse following a fall, after which symptoms are markedly accentuated. The tumors are more common in the thoracic and lumbar region. The outstanding characteristic is confinement to the vertebral body.

TREATMENT. This depends on the state of the lesion. If collapse has occurred, the instability produced and the distortion of the area may produce cord and radiating symptoms, requiring laminectomy. If this operation is carried out, the area should be stabilized at the same time. Radiation is effective for lesions causing local symptoms without neurological signs, or in patients suffering severe complications of injury.

Osteochondroma. A not infrequent lesion implicating the tip of a spinous process may be identified as an osteochondroma. This appears as a solitary lesion, or in company with other osteochondromata may implicate humerus and scapula. Surgical excision is recommended once this lesion has been identified. In addition to the local pain and tenderness, considerable restriction of motion results from the mechanical interference with adjacent spinous processes. A further reason for early surgical excision is

that, upon occasion, malignant changes have been reported in these lesions.

Benign Chondroblastoma. Another epiphyseal lesion that has been described in the spine is the benign chondroblastoma. It is a common tumor, also of the upper end of the humerus. It differs from the giant-cell lesions because of its cartilaginous components and areas of focal necrosis. Radiologically it may be difficult to differentiate this from osteochondroma, but the treatment is the same; the lesion should be excised completely.

Aneurysmal Bone Cyst. Aneurysmal bone cysts have been reported as involving some part of the vertebral column almost as frequently as they involve the long bones. They occur in the cervical spine, usually confined to the vertebral body, or occasionally implicating the arch and processes. Radiologically the cyst is a ballooned-out zone with soap bubble partitions initially, but when these collapse, this feature alters. However, the clear-cut translucent appearance on one side or the other is highly characteristic.

Surgical exploration and curettage with bone grafting is desirable, but where the cyst may be excised completely, this should be done. The surgeon should be prepared to encounter considerable hemorrhage; in this connection, some form of cryosurgery could be the method of choice in dealing with these lesions.

Osteoid Osteoma. These benign lesions have been reported in the cervical spine and usually involve the arch or articular processes. Persistent local pain, followed later by radiating symptoms is characteristic. Local tenderness can be identified, but because of the motion of the arch, it may be difficult to identify precisely the point from which the pain is coming. Consequently the lesion may stay hidden for some time. Any tumor in this area is extremely difficult to demonstrate in the x-rays and may be present for long periods before it is identified. When it is surgically accessible, block resection, as in the case with this lesion elsewhere, is the treatment of choice.

Solitary Bone Cyst. Although this is a common lesion in the shoulder girdle, with more than half of the cases being reported as occurring in the upper end of the humerus, solitary bone cyst has not been reported as occurring in the cervical area of the spine.

Nonossifying Fibroma. This benign lesion of bone from the fibrous elements of the cortex has occasionally been identified in the upper end of the humerus but has not been reported as occurring in the cervical spine.

Benign Osteoblastoma. An uncommon tumor with a predilection for the vertebral column has been identified; it is characterized microscopically by abundant osteoblasts, and it is vascular, osteoid and bone forming. The tumor occurs more often in the spine, including the cervical area, than elsewhere. It involves the arch and the spinous processes most frequently but can occur in the vertebral body. Radiologically the cortex is expanded and has a stippled pattern, with trabeculation. Microscopically the appearance is akin to that of an osteoid osteoma.

TREATMENT. Surgical excision should be done if feasible and followed by x-ray therapy. The latter alone may sometimes promote healing if the infected zone is surgically inaccessible.

Enchondroma. Mention is made of this lesion for completeness in considering neoplastic involvement of the cervical spine. This benign growth of cartilaginous element is the commonest tumor in the phalanges and is frequently encountered in the upper end of the humerus, but has only rarely been reported in any area in the spine.

Malignant Tumors

Primary malignant lesions are extremely rare in the cervical spine, but the area is frequently involved by secondary deposits.

Multiple Myeloma. Multiple myeloma is generalized bone marrow disease characterized by multiple and occasionally single lytic areas in the skeleton. This is a disease of older persons, and the bone deposits commonly appear in the spine, including the cervical region; it is the commonest malignant tumor identified in the cervical spine. The disease has an insidious onset, with weakness and lassitude resulting from the blood stream involvement. This is followed, later, by bone pain, neck ache and suboccipital pain due to bony involvement of the region. Vertebral body collapse occurs later in the disease, markedly increasing signs and symptoms and often precipitating cord and extensive nerve root involvement. Generalized osteoporosis can be the only early sign of bone involvement, and the condition can progress to extreme systemic prostration, with almost complete absence of the typical

punched-out areas of bone. The blood picture is best studied in sternal puncture smears of the bone marrow. A smear in which the plasma cells make up more than 3 per cent of the nucleated cells should be regarded as abnormal. Increased plasma cells of uniformly small round structure can be found in other diseases, also, such as liver disease and metastatic carcinoma. However, when the proportion reaches 10 per cent, the diagnosis of myeloma is almost certain.

Associated laboratory findings are also significant; anemia, hypercalcemia, hyperglobulinemia and renal insufficiency are common. Hypercholesterolemia with hyperglobulinemia is clearly indicative of the disease. Bence Jones protein in urine is also diagnostic of multiple myeloma. It must be recognized that hyperglobulinemia occurs in other conditions such as cirrhosis of the liver, chronic nephritis, rheumatoid arthritis, diffuse hepatitis, sarcoidosis and lymphogranuloma venereum, but when it is associated with hypercalcemia, it is highly suggestive of myeloma.

The treatment of this lesion is undergoing marked change with the advent of significant new drugs. The management of this disorder should be placed in the hands of a competent physician familiar with the new drugs that are applicable to treatment of this disease.

Management of the local lesion may demand surgical reconstruction because of involvement of the spinal cord. In some instances collapse of a single vertebral body will precipitate serious cord symptoms. Under these circumstances cervical traction is required and is followed by laminectomy and stabilization of the cervical spine. The development of new methods of chemotherapy justifies even extensive surgical measures to maintain stability of the spinal column, to prevent cord symptoms and to maintain a pain-free state as long as possible.

Osteogenic Sarcoma. Osteogenic sarcoma occurs in the upper end of the humerus (the third commonest location after lower femur and upper tibia), but has not been described as a primary lesion of the cervical spine. Similarly fibrosarcoma of the bone has been described in the upper end of the humerus but not in the cervical spine.

Chondrosarcoma. Authorities now clearly separate malignant tumors developing from cartilage elements, which maintain their characteristics but develop malignant tendencies. They occur with half the frequency of osteogenic sarcoma, the upper end of the humerus and the scapula being common sites. The tumor also has been described in the cervical spine, arising from spinous processes. In some instances it appears that these represent malignant changes in an osteochondroma. Because the cervical spine is a frequent source of injury, any accessible neoplastic lesion should be excised as soon as it has been discovered.

Ewing's Sarcoma. Ewing's tumor has been identified in the cervical spine, but its occurrence is extremely rare. It occurs in the shoulder girdle far less often than in the pelvis and all the bones of the lower limbs. The treatment of choice is radiation, but the prognosis for even a three-year survival is extremely grave.

Endosarcoma. A very rare primary tumor of bone has been identified in long bones and is mentioned because it is representative of a change in a common vertebral hemangioma, taking on malignant tendencies. It has not been described in the cervical spine.

Lymphoma. Primary tumors of lymphoid tissue are now referred to collectively as the lymphomas. Included in this group are Hodgkin's disease, lymphosarcoma and a rare lesion, giant follicle lymphoma. The cervical lymph glands represent the commonest site of early involvement of any of these lesions. Bone lesions then result from direct extension or metastatic invasion to the cervical spine.

In Hodgkin's disease 10 to 20 per cent of patients have some bone involvement during the clinical course, and as many as 50 to 60 per cent show changes in the spine at autopsy. Spinal involvement, in particular, can be an indication of the disease. Lymphosarcoma involves the skeleton to a much lesser degree than Hodgkin's, but any region of the spine may be implicated by this tumor.

The reticulum cell sarcoma is a separate malignant lymphoid tumor with distinct cell structure that shows abundant reticular fibers when stained with special silver preparations. The lesion starts in lymph glands, spreads by lymph chains and may eventually involve the skeleton. Long bones of the lower limb are most frequently involved, but the spine, including the upper thoracic and cervical regions, also may be implicated. Giant follicle lymphoma is a rare, malignant tumor that is differentiated by the large nodes and the numerous follicles with germinal centers.

Skeletal involvement can occur in the later stages, as in lymphosarcoma.

Treatment for some time depended largely upon the use of radiation, which still is effective in relieving pressure, particularly on neural elements. Chemotherapy now holds significant promise and the possibility of its use should be assessed by a physician skilled in this field.

Metastatic Lesions

A skeletal focus is frequently the presenting lesion of a malignant process involving breast, prostate, lung, kidney or thyroid gland (Figs. 17–49 and 17–50). When this is so, considerable search may be necessary to identify the primary lesion. It also frequently happens that more than one metastatic focus may be present, particularly in the spine, without giving rise to clinical symptoms and without the primary tumor being evident.

Our present form of investigation, relying as it does on x-ray studies, is grossly inadequate. Secondary deposits may be extensive and yet not at all apparent in the best of x-rays. The cervical spine, in contrast to the rest of the shoulder region, is a much more common site of metastatic deposit. Some authorities have indicated that in patients with malignant disease which terminates fatally as many as 70 per cent will show some skeletal involvement; of all the sites, the spine is the most frequently involved. It may be that if there is skeletal involvement at all, the spine will be implicated. The thoracic, first, and then the lumbar spine are the most frequent sites, but certain tumors have a predilection for the cervical spine. In addition, the cervical spine is commonly involved in any general skeletal disturbance. The changes in the x-ray that are suggestive of secondary deposits include alterations in the contour and slight body collapse; more extensive involvement is indicated by an osteolytic zone or an osteoblastic reaction.

LABORATORY FINDINGS. Cancer that is metastatic to the skeleton produces significant changes in blood chemistry. An increase in the serum calcium of 1 mg per 100 cc is important; elevation of alkaline phosphatase is also highly suggestive of skeletal metastases.

Other conditions producing hypercalcemia which must be differentiated are

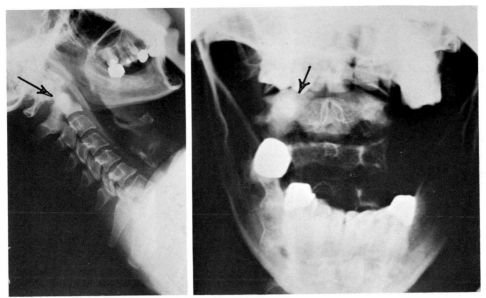

Figure 17–49 Osteoblastic tumor secondary in cervical spine; primary was in breast.

hyperthyroidism and vitamin B poisoning. Presumably it is lytic destruction of the osseous tissue at the sites of the metastases, releasing calcium into the blood stream, that is responsible for the hypercalcemia. The

significant conclusion from the laboratory studies is that a patient with any malignant disease who demonstrates a persistent elevation in serum calcium should be strongly suspected of having a skeletal metastasis. By and large it is the osteolytic rather than the osteoblastic lesions that produce the greatest degree of calcium upset. Osteoblastic lesions produce new bone at the site, rather than lysing it for blood stream absorption.

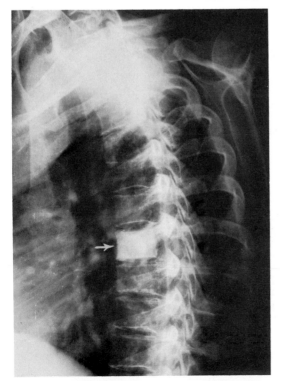

Figure 17–50 Secondary tumor in thoracic spine; primary was in prostate.

Osteolytic Metastases. To some degree the type of metastatic change encountered may be related to the primary site. When the secondary deposit is a destructive one, it appears radiologically as an area of translucency, irregularly situated, usually in the body of the vertebra. This type of change is then frequently followed by vertebral body collapse and the development of more extensive symptoms. Primary tumors commonly producing this change are hypernephroma, carcinoma of the thyroid and carcinoma of the lower bowel.

Osteoblastic Metastases. Certain primary tumors have a greater tendency to be manifested by metastases that initiate or stimulate bone growth about them, and these then appear as osteoblastic centers. Why they incite this type of reaction, rather than the lytic response, has not been determined. Carcinoma of the prostate commonly produces an osteoblastic metastasis, as does bronchogenic carcinoma. Metastases from carcinoma of the breast may be either osteo-blastic or osteolytic; sometimes both types of action are encountered in the spine (Figs. 17-51 and 17-52).

The significance of the osteoblastic lesion is that it is much less likely to be the seat of vertebral body collapse, but the osteoblastic reaction is more likely to produce symptoms localized to the area at an earlier stage than the osteolytic disturbance. The development of the new bone formation is apparently due to irritation from the tumor on the bony elements already present rather than any participation of the tumor tissue itself in the bone forming mechanism.

REFERENCES

Batson, O. V.: The vertebral vein system as a mechanism for spread of metastases. Amer. J. Roentgenol. *48*:715, 1942.

Berrett, A.: Value of angiography in the management of tumors of the head and neck. Radiology *84*:1052–1058, 1965.

Breslau, R. C.: Ganglion of the glenohumeral joint: An unusual axillary tumour. Southern Med. J. *59*: 566, 1966.

Cobey, M. D.: Hemangioma of joints. Arch. Surg. *46*: 465, 1943.

Codman, E. A.: Epiphyseal chondromatous giant-cell tumors of the upper end of the humerus. Surg. Gynec. Obstet. *52*:543, 1931.

Codman, E. A.: The Shoulder. Boston, Thomas Todd Co., 1934.

Copland, M. N.: Benign tumors of bone. Surg. Gynec. Obstet. *90*:697, 1950.

Coventry, M. B.: Differential diagnosis of malignant bone tumors. Ann. Surg. *132*:888, 1950.

Decoulx, P., et al.: Conservative scapulo-cleido-hume-rectomy for osteosarcoma of the acromion. Acta Orthop. Belg. *32*:341–354, 1966.

Du Boulay, G. H., et al.: Elusive tumours in the cervical spinal canal. Brit. J. Radiol. *37*:465–468, 1964.

Fisher, R. H.: Multiple Lesions of bone in Letterer-Siwe disease; report of a case with culture of para-colon Arizona bacilli from bone lesions and blood, followed by a response to therapy. J. Bone Joint Surg. *35*(a):445, 1953.

Geshicter, C. F., and Copland, M. N.: Tumors of Bone. 3rd Ed. Philadelphia, J. B. Lippincott Co., 1949.

Iraci, G., et al.: Intraspinal tumours of the cervical tract. A study of 68 cases. Int. Surg. *46*:154–167, 1966.

Jaffe, H. L.: Osteoid osseoma of bone. Radiology *45*:319, 1945.

Jaffe, H. L.: Aneurysmal bone cyst. Bull. Hosp. Joint Dis. *11*:3, 1950.

Jaffe, H. L.: Tumours and Tumorous Conditions of the Bones and Joints. Philadelphia, Lea & Febiger, 1958.

Jaffe, H. L., and Lichtenstein, L.: Solitary benign en-chondroma of bone. Arch. Surg. *45*:480, 1943.

Le May, M., et al.: Intervertebral disc protrusion masquerading as an intramedullary tumour. Brit. J. Radiol. *37*:463–465, 1964.

Lichtenstein, L.: Bone Tumors. St. Louis, The C. V. Mosby Co., 1960.

Luck, V.: Bone Pathology. Springfield, Ill., Charles C Thomas, 1950.

MacDonald, I., and Budd, J. W.: Osteogenic sarcoma. A modified nomenclature in view of 118 five-year cures. Surg. Gynec. Obstet. *77*:413, 1943.

Mullan, S., et al.: The use of an anterior approach to ventrally placed tumours in the foramen magnum and vertebral column. J. Neurosurg. *24*:536–543, 1966.

Nadler, S. H., et al.: A technique of interscapulothoracic amputation. Surg. Gynec. Obstet. *22*:359–364, 1966.

Ottolenghi, C. E.: Diagnosis of orthopedic lesions by aspiration biopsy. Results of 1061 punctures. J. Bone Joint Surg. *37*(a):443, 1955.

Ottolenghi, C. E., et al.: Aspiration biopsy of the cervical Spine, J. Bone Joint Surg. *46A*:715–733, 1964.

Reinhold, H.: On the rare localization of bone heman-giomas of the cervical spine. Radiol. Diag. (Berlin) *6*:355–360, 1965.

Reszel, P. A., et al.: Liposarcoma of the extremities and limb girdles. A study of 222 cases. J. Bone Joint Surg. *48A*:229–244, 1966.

Sedgwisk, C. E.: Tumours of the neck. Surg. Clin. N. Amer. *45*:553–566, 1965.

Shumrick, D. A.: A lump in the neck. GP *31*:110–117, 1965.

Snapper, I.: Treatment of multiple myeloma with stilbamidine. Clinical results and morphologic changes. J.A.M.A. *137*:513, 1948.

Snapper, I.: Metabolic bone diseases. *In* The Musculo-skeletal System. New York, The Macmillan Co., 1952, p. 139.

Stookey, B.: Compression of the spinal cord due to ventral extradural cervical chondroma. Arch. Neurol. Psychiat. *20*:275–291, 1928.

Wirbatz, W. et al.: Partial resection of the scapula in malignant hemangiopericytoma of the shoulder. Zbl. Chir. *90*:2141–2145, 1965.

Wright, J. L., et al.: An unusual chondroblastoma. J. Bone Joint Surg. *46A*:567–600, 1964.

Wronski, J., et al.: Chondrosarcoma of cervical spine causing compression of the cord. J. Neurosurg. *21*:419–421, 1964.

Zancolli, E., et al.: Interscapulo-cleidothoracic disar-ticulation. Indications and technique. Prensa Med. Argent. *52*:1122–1126, 1965.

DISABILITY EVALUATION OF THE SHOULDER AND THE NECK

Chapter XVIII

PRINCIPLES OF DISABILITY ASSESSMENT

Automobile and industrial accidents have become potent sources of upper body injuries, and many times the shoulder and neck are involved. There are automatic protective acts unconsciously assumed by the individual when the upper portion of the body is threatened with injury. In the case of the car accident, the protective act is putting the arm out in front to protect the head, neck and shoulder region as the impact is taken against the dashboard or the rear of the front seat. Such an act directs force toward the root of the limb as the forearm-elbow zone bears the brunt of the blow. In industry the shoulder-neck area is likewise an exposed zone, particularly to objects dropping from a height, and the involuntary act of the workman in attempting to escape the impact is to turn the back of his head, neck and shoulder region to the falling object. Other acts like simple stumbles, either backward or forward, involuntarily bring the upper limb into action and transmit force to the shoulder region, so that this area may exhibit more damage than the rest of the limb.

In each of these mechanisms of injury totally different components may be involved, so that a lucid understanding of the residual defects after injury requires a working knowledge of the practical anatomy and physiology of the region that has been exposed to injury processes. Some 75 per cent of litigation in courts of the United States arises out of accidents.

One of the challenges facing a surgeon treating injuries today is the practical interpretation of the end result he has obtained in treating a given case. More and more civil court judges, lawyers, industrial commissions and workmen's compensation boards are looking to the man who handled treatment of the patient to tell them in terms they can understand how much practical damage the accident has caused the patient. This seems a reasonable request, and those physicians who repeatedly treat such injuries should prepare themselves to meet these demands adequately. The surgeon may be held responsible to lawyer, judge and jury, as well as his patient, for proper assessment of the damage. Government authorities at all levels are requiring statements more and more often that assess the incapacity of the patient applying for welfare benefits, pensions, institutional care and home attention of all descriptions. The whole phase of disability and incapacity appraisal has enlarged tremendously. One natural corollary to this development is the realization that total medicine embraces the phase of rehabilitation as a further direct responsibility of the doctor. Great service is provided by the profession if it can assist in judging disability and in planning rehabilitation.

From the beginning of medicine the success of the profession has been founded on concern for the patient and the placing of his welfare above all else. There can be no more sincere motive nor surer avenue to success. The gospel of kindly interest spreads in industry as in private practice, engendering confidence and cooperation. A callous disinterested impression conveyed by an arrogant approach of disbelief in the patient's story has no place in caring for the sick and injured.

The position of the doctor is like a latch pin, because he is responsible for the patient on one side and should also be conscious of the employer's interests on the other. Industry is leading the way in providing care for the injured through both surgical reconstruction and rehabilitation, and employers are keenly conscious of the improved employee relations and increased efficiency and production that result from providing adequate medical care for the workmen. Accident prevention associations of both management and labor are cooperating to raise treatment standards to a high level.

In tackling assessment of incapacity and planning rehabilitation, a knowledge of the stages of repair and assessment of individual recuperative properties is most advantageous. The various phases of disability should be understood; the special means of investigating and controlling cases should be appreciated; and the common sources of disability of a given area should be known as well as the special peculiarities to which the region is susceptible.

STAGES OF DISABILITY

Definition. The concept of total medical care now extends from the time of injury until the resumption of productive activity. In this period several phases may be recognized, each encompassing specific responsibilities for treatment and evaluation. For practical purposes disability is defined as interference with the normal earning capacity. Four separate phases in this process can be identified, and it helps considerably to be able to define the stage in which a given patient is at the time of assessment. Often opinions are requested regarding the injured when it is possible to identify only the phase the patient has reached and to indicate in the report the further steps which must be taken to complete rehabilitation. Interpretation will be meaningful only if the doctor has a thorough knowledge of the different stages himself.

TOTAL INCAPACITY TREATMENT STAGE

This period of disability begins with the accident and continues until active treatment is discontinued. During this time the patient is treated actively, usually in a hospital; he remains in this phase until healing of his lesions has been completed. It extends to the point where ambulation is possible or he is able to start learning purposeful activities with his upper limb. The patient is completely disabled as far as work is concerned during this whole period, but the present management of injuries so often requires multiple surgical reconstructions that a planned program of active treatment must be defined from the very beginning. For example, if a man has a deltoid paralysis from a traumatic dislocation, his active treatment period will continue until the paralysis has recovered or appropriate reconstructive measures to ameliorate the residual impairment have been carried out.

TOTAL INCAPACITY REHABILITATION STAGE

Restoring the patient as nearly as possible to preinjury condition is now a recognized responsibility. Treatment, therefore, includes a rehabilitation phase during which movement, power, control and pattern movement activity are restored to a point at which the patient may reasonably resume work. As a rule, a further period of building confidence in his recovered motion is also required. Repair of a tendon or setting of a fracture or restoration of power in a paralyzed muscle is not sufficient; the workman must regain confidence and the ability to start off by himself.

In this stage structural repair is completed and functional repair progresses continually. Much of this active period is a phase of disuse resulting from the body malfunctions that follow injury, so that after physical structure has been restored, general body function must often be re-established. A period of relearning of intricate movement patterns, which were automatic before the injury but which now need careful cultivation, is essential. Proper organization and supervision during this stage helps tremendously. Group activities, a planned routine and proper instruction are best given at a rehabilitation center, if this is feasible. At the end of this stage the patient may be said to have gone as far as possible where active treatment is concerned; the point has been reached where further improvement and efficiency can be expected only from continued practice, and this is accomplished most advantageously on the job.

TEMPORARY PARTIAL DISABILITY

A period of partial disability usually follows active treatment and rehabilitation phases and, during this phase, progress is continued toward maximum efficiency. Efficiency in strength or coordination, for example, in a specific action improves over a period of months, usually until a plateau is reached from which there is little change. During this stage new habits or movement patterns may be developed to replace those permanently disturbed by the disease or injury. Often it is the challenge of the specific task that stimulates this replacement pattern. A reasonable time should be allowed for adjustment to handicaps if complete restoration is not likely; it may then be decided that a given loss represents permanent impairment.

PERMANENT DISABILITY

Impairment of function persisting after active treatment, rehabilitation and adaptive phases are completed is assessed as lasting for all time. Fair assessment of this is a constant challenge, but still is a reasonable responsibility of the doctor. Compensation and pension laws follow scales and tables based fundamentally on loss of body structure. The problem is to translate a partial loss of limb function into practical terms. Amputations from time immemorial have been the

basis for computing disability, and tables worked out on a percentage basis have been developed on this premise. However, there is a further factor of significance in the form of functional worth rather than pure structural loss that is most important. Furthermore, if it is feasible, some gradation according to occupation or situational influences may be desirable.

In the final analysis, however, the surgeon will have fulfilled his responsibility if he identifies the residual structural defect and interprets it in terms of limb function, leaving any additional gradations such as situational influence to the locally concerned authorities. The United States Veterans Bureau and other authorities, such as McBride, have made a fundamental contribution to analysis of functional incapacity as related to occupation; the reader is referred to these contributions for amplification of the interpretation of impairment.

LEGAL RESPONSIBILITIES

The surgeon will be expected to prepare a proper report, one which defines the injury and the patient's incapacity in terms that may be understood by the lawyer and which sets forth a clear conclusion regarding the injury. He may be asked to testify, in which case he will be expected to be able to present the nature of the damage resulting from the accident, the possibilities of reconstruction and rehabilitation, the result of the healing process, the extent of interference with the patient's working and leisure activities, and the permanence of these changes.

INVESTIGATION OF PHYSICAL IMPAIRMENT

In expressing an opinion and substantiating it, the surgeon relies on a good working knowledge of the mechanism of common injuries and their manifestations as well as the likely degree of success following surgical reconstruction. Therefore, he requires an accurate history, particularly of the injury mechanism, a thorough physical assessment, all the pertinent x-rays, and reports of any special investigations. Specific considerations arise in automobile and industrial accidents which lead to somewhat differing presentations, so that it is best to consider these under separate headings. In each instance, however, there is a fundamental plan to be followed, dealing with special points in the history, investigation of the episode of the injury and the patient's responses to therapy and the process of rehabilitation.

NECK INJURIES

Assessment of the "stop-light" sprain has become a frequent task. The classification and manifestations of these injuries has been considered in the chapter on automobile injuries and should be reviewed for full understanding of this problem (see Chapter XII).

Important Points in the History. Much more information regarding the incident is required than the patient's usual description of being "hit from behind." The points to be emphasized are the severity of the impact, the direction from which it came, the position of the head at the time of impact, and the patient's relationship to other structures in the car. In many cases simple observations are extremely helpful in determining the amount of violence that was involved. A query may be made as to whether the patient was wearing glasses that were knocked off, or whether the seat was broken or adjacent passengers were similarly involved. Many patients indicate they were "knocked out" by the accident, but concussion is not common in the usual extension-flexion mechanism and, as a rule, these patients mean that they were confused or somewhat dazed. It is important to define such an experience as accurately as possible.

Onset of Symptoms. In most instances these patients are not seriously disabled. They are able to get out of the car, go to the hospital for emergency treatment and x-ray and be discharged to the care of their personal physician. Some soreness locally at the back of the neck is appreciated initially, but later, usually some hours afterward, more severe stiffness may set in. Older patients who already have some spine degeneration may have some symptoms that extend to the upper limbs. These symptoms persist in varying degrees, depending upon the severity of the impact. Some 72 hours following the injury, as the patient takes stock of his state, he may be conscious of pain extending to the shoulder, persistent discomfort in the shoulder-neck region, pain through the front of the chest, pain implicating the anterior neck,

difficulty in swallowing, a sensation of fullness in the face or generalized headache.

Physical Findings. In the initial stages true limitation of neck bending is almost always present. When there are no signs of nerve root involvement, it should not persist for longer than three to four months. When the patient is seen for impairment assessment, it usually is some months after the injury.

Study should be made of both the neck segments, that is, the occipital axial dimension, indicated by rotatory restriction, and the lower segment, C.3–C.7, where loss of flexion extension usually ensues. The latter is the more common persisting sign.

Points of local tenderness related to the ligamentum nuchae and suspensory muscles should be identified. The range of rotation is 60 degrees to either side and 45 degrees forward and backward flexion, with lateral flexion normally 60 to 70 degrees from the midline. Deformity is rarely present, but the neck may be held rigidly as a result of muscle spasm. The one abnormality which should not be ignored and yet may be overlooked is loss of rotation due to implication of the occipito-axial segment. Rarely subluxation of a posterior facet in the lower segment is present. This will be identified by restriction of flexion and pain on extension. Often there is difficulty in getting the head and neck back to the normal point of extension.

These injuries are a result of the sudden cessation of motion, not of the sudden acceleration of motion; it is the abnormal braking mechanism, not an abnormal moving mechanism, that develops as a result of the impact.

ASSESSMENT OF MOTOR SYSTEM. The erector spinae group and the suspensory muscles should be assessed carefully. Muscle atrophy is rare in a usual extension-flexion injury, but pre-existing conditions can produce it and the findings may be misinterpreted. Many individuals also have a natural atony of the erector spinae group, leaving the underlying area unduly sensitive to further insult.

Involvement of the nerve supply to the shoulder group of sufficient severity to produce paralysis or atrophy is rare in a pure neck injury. Implication of intrinsic muscles of the hand is much more frequent, but this is never an early change. If it should be noted immediately after the injury, it is an antecedent development. The thenar group is the one most often involved.

Electrodiagnosis plays an important role in identifying motor lesions from cervical trauma. Significant root insult may be identified by electrical changes in the cervical erector spinae muscles. The posterior branch of the spinal nerve comes off beyond the point of disc and foraminal pressure, so that if it is disturbed, definite involvement of the nerve root has occurred in the neck injury mechanism. The presence of consistent fibrillation potentials coming from semispinalis and spinous zones can be detected accurately and is most significant.

SENSORY CHANGES. A search for sensory changes should always be made. Such changes are usually apparent in the hand if sufficient force has been involved to implicate the nerve root. Subjective numbness with some alteration in appreciation of touch and pinprick is the usual finding in the zone of autogenous supply. Sixth root change implicates the thumb and index finger; the seventh root, usually some combination of the second, third and fourth fingers; and the eighth root, the fourth and fifth fingers. These are always superficial losses, true anesthesia of the part being exceedingly rare. When anesthesia is present, involvement of the supply much more peripherally, at a point beyond the foramen, should be suspected rather than the vertebral column zone. In all these injuries the anterior portion of the neck should be assessed for brachial plexus changes and cervical ribs. The elbows and wrists should also be examined to be certain there are no old abnormalities apart from the neck that might produce changes in the hand which could be misinterpreted as being the result of an extension-flexion injury. The common example of this is old fractures in the region of the elbow, implicating the ulnar nerve. Cervical ribs are also often overlooked, but when they are present, they must be counted as an additional element in the injury mechanism. When an extra rib is present, signs and symptoms emanating from the front of the neck are much more commonly interpreted than when this abnormality is not present.

ASSESSMENT OF TENDON REFLEXES. The biceps and triceps jerks should always be assessed. This must be done properly for the results to be of significance. Loss of either is important. The biceps is the one more often implicated. If no response is obtained the first time, it should be tested repeatedly to make sure it is truly absent. In the author's experience, the reflexes are not often implicated in the usual extension-flexion injury, but the tests should be made routinely. Loss of the biceps reflex implicates the C.5–C.6 roots, and loss of the triceps implicates the C.7 root.

SHOULDER INVESTIGATION

Most shoulder injuries requiring assessment are a result of industrial accidents rather than being stop-light sprains. Fractures and dislocations present a straightforward pattern of impairment not requiring extensive investigation. Trauma to the shoulder is much more likely to involve the soft tissues, and the result can be significant so that a careful study of shoulder function is required.

Pertinent History in Shoulder Accidents. Complaints presented by an industrial claimant preparatory to legal action must be sifted carefully. They differ considerably at times from those of the private patient presenting with a similar lesion. The friendly approach and generous cooperation, no matter what responsibilities are held by the examiner, should be maintained. An attitude of outright resentment on the part of the patient may be encountered, and it is the responsibility of the examiner to cope with this effectively. If this is not accomplished, false conclusions may be drawn and can be a source of embarrassment later in court or at commission investigations.

INJURY EPISODE. Particular attention in the case of an injured workman is needed to pass a just opinion regarding settlement of compensation or insurance. In many instances a lay board rightfully decides this point, but questions are frequently put to the doctor as to whether the history of an accident that is given could have resulted in the injury or disability under investigation. Attention to the following points will be of assistance in settling this.

Date and Time of Initial Disturbance. From the standpoint of accurate reporting, all observations should be carefully documented. Most patients with significant disability can recall very clearly when they were hurt and can recount the circumstances surrounding the incident. When no definite time of episode can be recalled, more investigation is needed to relate the complaint to a given occupation. For example, a fall or blow on the shoulder is a common incident. Should a history be given of pain coming on gradually in the shoulder, it is less likely that there is an occupational association. Investigation may show a well established cervical rib.

There are activities which gradually produce shoulder symptoms, and frequently a relatively minor episode is the true precipitating factor. In occupations carried out by painters, decorators, plasterers, hoistmen and bricklayers, there is constant use of the arms at shoulder level or in the overhead position, so that some wear and tear on the intrinsic shoulder mechanism, like the rotator cuff, can reasonably be anticipated. Gradual onset of pain in the shoulder in such an occupation might reasonably be related to the work without an obvious more severe traumatic episode.

Observations as to the patient's precise routine at a given job may be important. If a man who has been employed at a routine sorting operation is shifted to a post requiring the use of a heavy pneumatic drill, it might reasonably be expected that there would be some physical effects.

Severity of Initial Disturbance. In most instances a patient seeks treatment early for significant discomfort and notifies his employer immediately of incapacity. Failure to document an injury or incapacity or to seek treatment suggests a not particularly disabling episode. If the patient reports the accident and seeks medical help, eligibility for compensation is on firm ground.

Extent of Incapacity. In legal controversies, particularly, the examiner should document the type and length of treatment. A history of immobilization in a plaster spica for six months, as against a sling for six days, is accepted as indicating a more severe injury. Attention is paid to the length of time away from work in the light of the treatment prescribed. A simple contusion of the shoulder should not require six weeks away from work, nor should a fracture of a clavicle prevent a housewife from resuming her duties for six months. There is a well established time for normal healing with which the examiner should be familiar.

Significance of Pain and Tenderness. The significance of the complaint of pain is altered in this examination, and it is the examiner's responsibility to gauge the sincerity and the severity. Complaints should be substantiated by clinical signs. In the case of pain, the finding of tenderness is most significant. Most medical men develop a knack of telling whether a patient's story is exaggerated, and whether the description of the discomfort fits into properly recognized patterns. There are some common complaints that may be elicited from almost all patients of a certain age. Backache and aching shoulders are such examples. Women, particularly, are prone to complain of vague shoulder-neck ache when questioned. This rarely has an acute component, as would be expected from a significant traumatic incident, and is more often related to neck than to arm action. True tenderness is usually accompanied by accessory changes that reinforce the impression of discomfort, such as facial contortions, muscle spasms, withdrawal and protective acts. Once precisely painful points are located, they should be marked and tested again later in the examination, possibly with the patient's attention diverted so that the constancy of the point of suspected sensitivity is established.

Pain and tenderness are significant from the disability standpoint because they interfere with normal function. A workman loses confidence in his ability to carry out certain acts and, when this happens, strain falls on accessory structures in an effort to compensate for this loss. The result is awkwardness and inevitable inefficiency. A patient with posttraumatic acromioclavicular arthritis, for example, will stop lifting the arm above the shoulder to avoid the pain. When some act is suddenly necessary and involves this movement and he is unprepared for it, pain results and he may let go whatever he is holding. This makes safety a factor, since a workman with a potential painful arc may be a hazard to others as well as himself. Similarly, sudden onset of shocking or severe shoulder pain may cause a housewife to stumble from a chair or stool on which she is standing to put up curtains or to dust the ceiling. The patient with a fused shoulder uses girdle muscles like the trapezius much more than normal and, consequently, may develop an aching neck-shoulder pain, which then becomes a fatigue factor and diminishes his efficiency.

Significance of Limitation of Movement. Loss of shoulder movement is a significant disability. The purpose of this joint is to enhance the effectiveness of the hand, so that far greater incapacity ensues when it is stiff than just loss of the shoulder joint action alone. Movement of the arm as a whole, and then with the scapula fixed, should be as-

girdle and body rotation replace loss of joint rotation

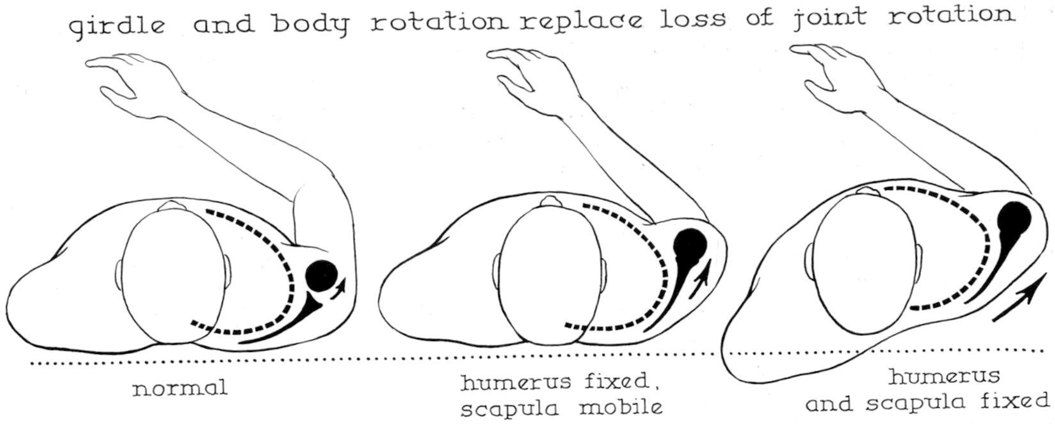

normal

humerus fixed,
scapula mobile

humerus
and scapula fixed

Figure 18-1 Substitution when the shoulder is fused.

sessed. Mobility of the scapula masks gleno-humeral movement.

The movements of particular importance about the shoulder are flexion and external rotation. Abduction is significant but can be compensated for by bending or rotating the whole body (Fig. 18-1). External rotation is hampered by capsular adhesions mostly and is difficult to replace. Internal rotation may be replaced, however, by abduction and girdle rotation because the scapula may be levered posteriorly in a winging action, but it cannot go in the opposite direction to replace external rotation. A range of 180 degrees for circumduction is accepted as normal, and loss of 10 to 15 degrees at the end of this range may not be of great significance. Practice and use will likely compensate so that little real permanent impairment materializes. When the range is decreased to 90 degrees, about 20 per cent of the function of the extremity is lost. Most work is done at a level below the eyes, so that if the arm can be raised to the shoulder level most manual work can be performed.

When the shoulder is fused, resultant use of the upper extremity then depends upon the amount of motion that can be obtained by movement of the scapula on the chest (Fig. 18-2). The optimum position for ankylosis of the shoulder is 60 degrees abduction, 10 to 15 degrees flexion and neutral rotation, and in this position, the disability is about 30 per cent. However, if there is no movement of the scapula and it is fixed, disability increases to 45 per cent. When the shoulder is fixed above or below the optimum position, disability is increased to 50 to 60 per cent. When scapular motion is lost in addition,

incapacity of the extremity rises to 65 to 70 per cent.

Deformity. Altered contour arises chiefly from malunion of fractures and is a source of disability cosmetically and functionally. Appearance of the shoulder is rarely appreciably permanently altered and is of somewhat less consequence in a workman. The problem arises chiefly in fractures of the clavicle in young women, and here it should be remembered that in most instances a seemingly unsightly mass of callus usually recedes appreciably. Malunion of the humerus is a deformity interfering with function. The chief source is a fracture of the surgical neck which unites in too much internal rotation, so that the patient has difficulty in getting the hand to the mouth without flexing the neck.

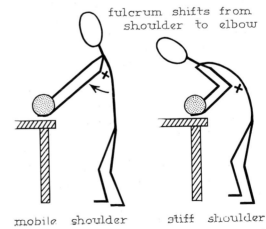

fulcrum shifts from
shoulder to elbow

mobile shoulder   stiff shoulder

Figure 18-2 When the shoulder is fused or ankylosed, the body substitutes through flexion of the spine to assist in such activities as lifting.

Weakness and Muscle Atrophy. Like the association of tenderness with the complaint of pain, so does weakness become significant when muscle atrophy is apparent. Weakness is a universal association of injury but needs to be carefully assessed. In establishing a diagnosis it may not be quite so prominent, but in estimating permanent impairment it assumes greater importance. However, some recovery and improvement may reasonably be expected with time after most injuries. Generalized atrophy is common and of less importance, but localized wasting is of much more consequence. It indicates individual muscle loss, and the state of innervation in particular should be assessed before the extent of permanent disability is estimated.

Loss of Sensation. Nerve damage is not uncommon, and sensory loss should be looked for carefully. Plexus injuries have been dealt with in detail in the chapter on nerve injuries. Isolated nerve injuries producing sensory changes include axillary, musculocutaneous and posterior cord lesions. It is the posterior cord lesions that most often result in permanent impairment. For precise assessment of such injuries, the chapter on nerve lesions should be consulted.

REFERENCES

A guide to the evaluation of permanent impairment of the extremities and back. J.A.M.A. Feb 15, 1958.

American Academy of Orthopedic Surgeons: Manual for Orthopedic Surgeons in Evaluating Permanent Physical Impairment.

Bateman, J. E.: Disability evaluation about the shoulder. Surg. Clin. N. Amer. *43*:1721–1726, 1963.

Marchiano, G., et al.: Contribution to the radiologic study of habitual dislocation of the shoulder and medico-legal considerations. G. Med. Milit. *115*:372–379, 1965.

McBride, E. D.: Disability Evaluation. 5th ed. Philadelphia, J. B. Lippincott Co., 1953.

Medical Society of North Carolina: Guide for Permanent Disability Evaluation of Industrial Accidents. 1960.

Rice, C. O.: Industrial Disabilities. Springfield, Ill., Charles C Thomas, 1952.

Rudd, J. L.: Need for better cervical neck traction. Med. Trial. Techn. Quart. *11*:27–36, 1965.

Chapter XIX

PERCENTAGE CALCULATION OF DISABILITY FROM COMMON INJURIES

Perhaps the commonest mistake that is made in assessing disability is to attempt to do it before treatment has been completed. Proper timing requires a review of the whole injury process, including the periods of active treatment, rehabilitation and redevelopment or accommodation.

In most instances the plan of management is quite straightforward and no confusion arises in delineating the various phases. In complicated cases, however, the contribution and efficiency of certain reconstructive procedures may not have been taken into consideration. Finally, most authorities today have agreed that treatment now includes the rehabilitation phase and, in some instances, this is extended to redevelopment and re-education of a disabled workman.

Most injured persons, both civilian and industrial, return to their former jobs, even when they have some permanent impairment. How they fit into the former position or how much the new impairment will interfere can be assessed only by a trial run. If this process of adaptation is financially detrimental, some compensation on a partial basis is only fair. This means that the report on the injury may not be finalized until some months after active treatment has been completed. An important corollary of this is apparent and of extreme importance to the patient; scars may break down, joints may become painful or fatigued or complications attendant on an initial insult may appear, thereby altering the significance of the incapacity. Scientific re-education of the injured worker may decrease this incapacity. There are industries making a determined effort to use the injured worker efficiently so as to avoid manpower loss.

MECHANISM OF ESTIMATING IMPAIRMENT IN THE SHOULDER

When a patient has reached a plateau of function and it is about time to measure his disability, certain fundamental principles should be followed. The defect has to be measured and then interpreted in terms of its percentage interference with the function of the body as a whole.

MEASURING THE DEFECT

The process of measuring the physical deviation from the norm requires some explanation. In all extremity assessment, interference with normal activity is principally reflected in loss of joint action. This may be the result of direct joint damage, muscle weakness or paralysis, or interference with control of the part. However, the result of any of this damage is most often apparent in abnormal joint action, so that measuring this module serves as a common denominator in identifying the defect. In the upper portion of the arm, alteration in shoulder action is quite a demonstrable entity.

A further principle requires acceptance. To simplify and standardize interpretation, the measurement is done in terms of the major joint action. In the shoulder, particularly, there is a whole system of joints, and it is obviously impractical to precisely implicate each one in the assessment. More than one direction of action or range of motion may be hampered following a given injury, but measuring each small loss in attempting to demarcate all of them is not feasible. By common consent, and as a result of practical observation, if the major loss is assessed properly, it is a reasonable indication of the defect. To make such measurement more representative it is customary to use the combined range of the complete joint action as the basic norm for comparison. In the shoulder, then, the arc of circumduction, which totals 200 degrees, is used as basic, and the degree of this arc lost constitutes the defect or the actual physical loss of the shoulder action.

RELATING THE PHYSICAL LOSS TO THE SEGMENT OF THE BODY

The usefulness of a limb to the rest of the body has always been calculated from experience with amputations. This formed the basis for the original wartime pension awards, and the principles of this mechanism have filtered through to our present-day system. This accumulated experience has resulted in the acceptance of certain basic values for the arm and the leg. In more recent times industrial commissions and compensation boards have established working values for parts or segments of the limbs. These segmental values are now used as the norm, and against these the abnormal is compared.

MATHEMATICAL CALCULATION

As previously mentioned, the functional arc of the shoulder is 200 degrees, which comprises 150 degrees of elevation from the side to vertically above the head and a further 45 degrees of backward extension. The value of the shoulder as a segment of the upper limb is set at 60 per cent. This figure is arrived at by averaging figures of many authorities and is related to the value of total loss of limb at this level. It may well be argued that the remainder of the extremity would be "worth" much more than 40 per cent, so how can the shoulder alone be "worth" 60 per cent? The answer to this is that we are concerned with the effect of what is lost, not what remains. Experience has shown that the awkwardness, incapacity, disturbance of function and necessary over-activity of the remainder that result from the total loss of the shoulder segment is 60 per cent of the extremity's usefulness. It is the negative factor that must be measured, not the remaining positive one. The mathematical principles of estimating incapacity of the shoulder from an injury that has resulted in a loss of 100 degrees of circumduction only would be $100/200$ degrees $\times 60 = 30$ per cent of the limb. For practical purposes, upper and lower limbs are considered equal, so the body percentage of such an injury would be $50/100$ degrees $\times 30 = 15$ per cent of the body.

ASSESSMENT OF INDIVIDUAL SHOULDER COMPONENTS

The shoulder is really a system of joints, the glenohumeral, acromioclavicular and sternoclavicular, and, in addition, there are two associated mechanisms which in a way serve as joints, the scapulothoracic and bicipital. Identification of these components assists in the breakdown of total shoulder activity. It is of further assistance in assessing certain injuries that involve one but not all of these mechanisms that must be expressed in terms of the total joint function.

The glenohumeral joint is considered as

50 per cent of the total system of shoulder function. It is well recognized that total loss of glenohumeral action such as occurs following an arthrodesis of the shoulder does not completely wipe out overall shoulder action. A workman can still make use of his fused shoulder by swinging the girdle as a whole, moving the scapula on the chest wall. If the scapula rotators are still acting, he retains considerable usefulness of the shoulder. Similarly, the defect from poliomyelitis in which all shoulder muscles are paralyzed, including those moving the scapula, is of much greater magnitude than would be the loss of the glenohumeral action only.

The precise act of glenohumeral range is 180 degrees, consisting of 150 degrees of elevation before the scapula starts to move and 30 degrees of extension, producing a total arc of 180 degrees. The acromioclavicular joint is part of this system and has a functional arc of 45 degrees. Its contribution to the whole is taken from the 50 per cent remaining from glenohumeral action and comprises approximately one third of that remainder, or about 16 per cent.

The scapulothoracic joint contributes an arc of 60 degrees, and is rated as one third of 50 per cent of the shoulder also. The remaining anatomical divisions are of less importance in the overall picture. The sternoclavicular joint and biceps mechanism may be considered to be one half as important as the other two segments and, therefore, comprise one sixth of the allotted 50 per cent, apart from glenohumeral action.

COMMON INJURIES TABLE

Having assimilated the principles and identified the segmental and relative values, the examiner still has the problem of translating common injury defects into these terms. This requires a study of the individual injury's effect on the cardinal parts of the whole shoulder complex. In other words, the injury must be thought of in terms of its major anatomical interference, so that it may be related to the whole. A fracture of the outer end of the clavicle obviously effects the acromioclavicular joint more than it does the glenohumeral joint. A fracture of the upper end of the humerus mainly implicates the glenohumeral joint, and so on. It is possible to relate nearly all common injuries to a zone of particular implication and, therefore, use this as the yardstick. In the ensuing discussion, common entities have been selected.

FRACTURES OF THE UPPER END OF THE HUMERUS

The incapacity resulting from these injuries, including fractures of tuberosities, fractures of the head of the humerus, fractures of the surgical neck and fracture dislocations of the humerus, is nearly always reflected in loss of glenohumeral motion. The glenohumeral functional arc is 180 degrees. The amount of loss motion in the arc of circumduction is measured as follows:

> Loss of motion over functional arc
> multiplied by glenohumeral contribution to the whole shoulder,
> multiplied by the shoulder segment of whole limb,
> multiplied by relation of limb to whole body.

For example: $90/180$ degrees $\times 50/100 \times 60/100 \times 50 = 7.5$ per cent. If a patient has lost half his normal range of motion at the glenohumeral joint following a fracture, it would still represent only a part of the contribution to the shoulder girdle, and this, in turn, is only a part of the whole limb, which in turn is only part of the whole body.

FRACTURES OF THE TUBEROSITIES

These are important because of their effect on abduction and possible interference with action of the rotator cuff. These considerations apply usually to young active wage-earners. A fracture without displacement will unite in four weeks, and a further period of two to four weeks will allow resumption of work. Fractures with displacement, which need surgical excision and cuff repair, cause more prolonged disability, usually a period of three to four months. Full range of motion is commonly regained. Any loss can be calculated precisely according to the fraction mechanism indicated previously.

FRACTURES OF THE SURGICAL NECK

Workmen do not frequently suffer this injury, but it is common in older people who are not working and so is not a serious problem from an occupational standpoint. When it occurs in an elderly workman, movement is started early and in six weeks a comminuted and little displaced fracture is united. In younger men with more complicated displacement, immobilization is necessary for eight to ten weeks, and a further period of four to six weeks is required to restore movement well enough for resumption of work. Similar considerations apply to fractures of the anatomical neck. Fracture dislocation is a most serious injury, usually requiring open operation. The period of total incapacity then runs 10 to 12 weeks before union may be expected and, following this, it is frequently eight to ten weeks before suitable function is restored.

MECHANISM OF DISABILITY

The specific alterations which lead to the loss of joint motion in fractures of the upper end of the humerus are angulation and alteration in joint surfaces, articular and periarticular contractures, delayed union and nonunion. Any one of these factors may be followed by considerable joint stiffness, resulting in diminished excursion. Frequently a fracture leaves such a short proximal segment close to the joint that it is easily involved in contracture of periarticular structures. Older people, particularly, develop limitation of movement from periarticular adhesions. Mobility of the scapula is the most important compensating mechanism and it decreases impairment considerably. Pain and weakness enhance the disability. The most serious complication is osteoarthritis from gross distortion of the joint surfaces. Almost all movement may be lost in such instances and, when this occurs, these joints should be assessed for all practical purposes as if they were completely ankylosed. Arthrodesis of the shoulder is usually assessed at from 30 to 40 per cent, depending upon the arm involved and the position of fixation. The optimum position is 60 degrees abduction and 10 to 15 degrees flexion. Below this level, function of the hand is limited. Often these patients complain of pain resulting from the strain of constant rotation of the scapula and the necessity for using the accessory muscles excessively.

IMPAIRMENT FROM DISLOCATIONS ABOUT THE SHOULDER

Simple dislocation without complication responds well to conservative treatment and rarely leaves permanent impairment. After reduction most patients are able to resume moderate use of the shoulder at the end of four weeks and full use at the end of two months. The important complications are fractures of the tuberosity, rupture of the rotator cuff, axillary nerve paralysis and the development of recurrent dislocation.

All these complications may introduce an element of impairment. Fractures of the tuberosity require six to eight weeks to unite and a further period of roughly four weeks to recover good movement and power. In a fracture of the tuberosity with a small displaced fragment, it may be excised; the period of incapacity is not usually longer than six to eight weeks. Movement to a right angle returns quickly, but full circumduction may require a further six to eight weeks. Permanent limitation of motion is not common, and a few degrees loss at the end of the range is not significant.

Dislocation may be complicated by damage to the rotator cuff involving the supraspinatus or the subscapularis. Following treatment of the dislocation, this results in an additional period of disability amounting to the length of time required for treatment of a cuff lesion. Disability then is rated as discussed under cuff tears.

Disability from axillary nerve paralysis is rarely permanent. The patient usually recovers in six to eight weeks, but sometimes four to six months is required. In some instances surgical exploration is required; the effects of permanent paralysis are discussed in the section on nerve injuries.

Recurrent dislocation is a potent source of permanent impairment. When treated by operations such as are described in Chapter XI, the operations are usually successful, so that the impairment is significantly decreased. The period of complete incapacity is about six weeks, and following a further six weeks of therapy most of the shoulder movement is recovered. Permanent impairment is due to limitation of movement. Loss of a small amount of external rotation is a frequent occurrence and possibly desirable, but is not usually regarded as functionally significant. When weakness and limitation of abduction to 90 degrees is present, the resulting impairment, as calculated previously, would be in the neighborhood of 15 per cent of the part.

Untreated recurrent dislocation is a serious permanent disability. In industry it is a hazard to the worker and also to his fellow employees because of the safety element. In a casual motion of lifting or reaching, the shoulder may slip out of joint, with serious consequences. For this reason, operative repair always should be recommended. The disability has been assessed at 35 per cent of the part when the condition of recurrent dislocation exists.

Acromioclavicular Dislocation. Simple dislocations, well treated, do not normally lead to permanent impairment. The period of incapacity varies from four to eight weeks, depending upon the type of treatment employed. When rupture of the suspensory ligaments has occurred, a longer period of treatment is required, usually six to ten weeks.

Chronic or recurrent dislocation in which reconstruction of the conoid and trapezoid ligaments is necessary involves limitation of heavy activity for three to four months. Some permanent impairment may result from this injury because of weakness of the shoulder, particularly in overhead activities. In untreated cases this amounts to something less than the total contribution of the acromioclavicular motion, which is 15 per cent of the part.

Sternoclavicular Dislocations. Dislocation is relatively easily reduced in the sternoclavicular joint and usually remains quite stable. After reduction, disability is uncommon. Most activities are feasible three weeks after reduction, but for a further three weeks some discomfort on abduction and flexion of the shoulder may be encountered.

Permanent impairment follows unreduced dislocations. Pain is appreciated through the midrange of abduction and flexion particularly, and power in the shoulder is decreased. The unsightly appearance adds to the impairment, leading to incapacity of 15 to 20 per cent of the part. After reduction and fixation some sternoclavicular arthritis may ensue or a moderate amount of instability persist, resulting in disability of 10 to 12 per cent of the part.

Contusions, Sprains and Fibrositis Assessment. In most instances proper early treatment prevents permanent impairment from injuries like these. Time lost from work reaches formidable figures if the lesions are neglected or not treated properly. In bruises and sprains a few muscle fibers are torn, usually those close to bony attachments; they heal with rest, relief of pain and avoidance of irritating movements. The sooner active motion is started after acute pain subsides, the better will be the resulting activity of the shoulder girdle. Local anesthetic infiltrations into the trigger zones and physiotherapy improve these conditions quickly; disability results from too long a rest or rest without proper exercise.

Seven to ten days should be the maximum period of incapacity. In some instances a traumatic origin is suggested in fibrositis, there being small fascial herniations leading to some permanent scarring and impairment. Assiduous treatment helps these lesions also, and disability should not last longer than a matter of days.

Traumatic Tendinitis. Recurrent sprains or similar straining activities on the shoulder may produce the entity referred to as a traumatic tendinitis. As a rule, these patients have little total impairment and are able to carry on at their occupations, but occasionally this is not so. During the acute phase, particularly if there is the additional irritation of a calcified deposit, a short period of total incapacity may develop.

The speed and efficiency of active treatment control the impairment to a large extent. Most patients respond to systemic medications, physiotherapy and local injections. Recovery in a period of two to four weeks without significant permanent disability is frequent. Some patients are unable to tolerate the pain and limitation of motion and require surgical measures, particularly if adhesive capsulitis develops. The period of incapacitation is then extended materially.

Patients who require surgical exploration are typically totally incapacitated for a period of six to eight weeks and gradually regain use of the limb over a period of a further four to six weeks. Significant residual impairment is unusual but, if it occurs, is measured according to the amount of glenohumeral motion which is lost.

Ruptures of the Rotator Cuff. The effect of cuff damage is to weaken shoulder action and to lead to limitation of glenohumeral function. These injuries are assessed on the basis of glenohumeral function, which represents 50 per cent of total shoulder action. The patient who exhibits 10 to 15 degrees limitation does not have significant impairment. Even in the most extensive injuries, recovery of motion to at least 90 degrees following surgical repair may be anticipated. Many shoulders recover motion to a right angle when a cuff tear has been repaired. The interference resulting from a massive full thickness tear, therefore, would be calculated as follows:

$$2/3 \times 30 \times 50/100 = 20 \text{ per cent of the limb}$$

or 10 per cent of the body. Additional consideration is often necessary after a cuff has been repaired. The basic function is still plotted on loss of glenohumeral function. Possibly the patient has motion in circumduction only to 90 degrees; this would then mean $90/180 \times 50/100$ of 60 per cent = 15 per cent of the limb or 7.5 per cent of the body.

Untreated Lesions and Complete Tears. Disability is extensive in this group and the theory of leaving such injuries alone, expecting that they will recover in a period of two years, is fallacious. It is true that one may hear no more from these patients, but if they are followed and examined it will be found that the use of the shoulder is significantly impaired. The attitude of doing nothing for them is to be condemned. Frequently these patients have only 25 to 35 degrees glenohumeral abduction. If the scapula is movable, they may reach 60 degrees by using a girdle type of arm swing. This means that use of the hand and forearm is significantly limited. The elbow must bend at the waist level, so there is serious interference with reaching, throwing and hoisting. Gripping and holding at the waist level is not hampered because it is in the line of fixation. Workmen in occupations such as construction, carpentry, painting and bricklaying will be incapacitated. In addition to the difficulty in performing work, the inability to put the hand and arm out at the side for protection, as in falling, is an added hazard at home as well as in industry. Bench work is feasible but is also hampered if the workman cannot rest the arm sufficiently to make considerable use of the opposite one. The disability is a little less when it is not the master hand that is involved since the injured arm can still be used as the holding member. Untreated tears have a permanent disability of 30 to 40 per cent of the extremity. If repair is performed and motion is recovered even to a right angle, the permanent impairment is decreased by 50 per cent. In all instances, it has been the author's experience that pain is materially decreased following surgery.

Bicipital Injuries. Rupture of the long head of the biceps or traumatic tendinitis is a not uncommon lesion. In the elderly individual who is not earning his living, the resulting weakness in the shoulder function and elbow flexion may not be significant. Disability lasts two to three weeks and no significant permanent impairment develops. In the young workman, however, the loss of function of the long head of the biceps weakens elbow flexion and also diminishes the power of forward flexion of the shoulder. The more chronic lesions, such as recurrent slipping of the long head of the tendon or ruptures of the intratubercular ligament, require surgery. This entails a period of total incapacity of roughly six weeks, followed by a further period of roughly four weeks during which extensive recovery may be anticipated. In rupture of the long head of the biceps, transplantation to the coracoid process is recommended; this entails a period of disability of four to six weeks followed by a period of two to four weeks of gradual recovery of function. The surgery does not leave a normal shoulder and some weakness in forward flexion occurs, particularly in the young workman. As a rule, this is not more than 5 per cent. When the condition is untreated, there is more interference with shoulder function, and disability may increase to 15 to 20 per cent of the part.

Frozen Shoulder or Adhesive Capsulitis. Significant limitation of glenohumeral function may be a complication of many injuries to the shoulder, and this has been interpreted under the specific lesions. In addition, the shoulder may be implicated when the main injury is at some distance, for example, at the elbow, in the forearm or in the wrist. A simple Colles fracture may recover well, but if the shoulder is neglected during the period of rehabilitation, significant impairment results because of development of adhesive capsulitis. This type of contracture is preventable, but once established, it may be the source of permanent impairment. The majority of these problems occur in the older age group, which makes the possibility of adaptation still more difficult.

Mechanism of Disability—Frozen Shoulder. The gluing of the capsule to the head of the humerus limits motion in all directions, and this is followed by wasting and weakness of the important muscles about the shoulder. Disuse atrophy prolongs the disability and a vicious cycle begins. In a frozen shoulder the effectiveness of the hand is seriously compromised, the forearm becomes the lever, and the extent of usefulness is then limited to the range through which the forearm may be operated. The elbow is held at the side and the loss of rotation at the shoulder further limits the rotatory range of the hand.

Some adaptation and compensation are obtained by improving the power and the use of accessory muscles like the trapezius. The pectoralis major also assists in pulling the shoulder girdle forward. When these accessory muscles are trained to increase movement, there is increased stress and strain on these muscles, which may then be the seat of further pain, adding to the disability. Neck muscles participate in this substitution process also, and tension is increased by the unconscious bending of the neck to help in flexion and abduction when a girdle action is used. Neck pain and headache may then develop also.

The underlying cause of the contracture controls the extent of the permanent impairment. In addition, the length of time the contracture has been present and the assiduousness of treatment are controlling factors. In an adhesive capsulitis or frozen shoulder established for six to eight months, it is extremely difficult to restore glenohumeral motion, apart from resorting to surgical measures should other conditions make this feasible. In the established condition, disability is about 30 per cent, similar to that in an ankylosis of the shoulder. When there is a painful element in addition to the freezing, impairment is increased to 50 to 60 per cent of the extremity.

ASSESSMENT OF IMPAIRMENT IN FRACTURES OF THE CLAVICLE

In a forward fall, which is the commonest mechanism of injury, force is rapidly transmitted from hand to shoulder, with the impact being taken, usually, at the junction of the middle and outer third of the clavicle. It is at this point that the shape of the clavicle alters in two ways: it is the junction zone of the double curve, and the cross section of the bone alters at this point from flat laterally to tubular medially. These changes favor localization of fractures in this region. The resulting deformity comprises shortening, overriding of fragments and a forward slumping of the shoulder.

Treatment Period. The treatment period in an adult requires about eight weeks for solid union and restoration of limb movement. During this time, depending upon the method of treatment, the patient is partially disabled. If the fracture has been treated by the application of a plaster yolk, few purposeful activities are possible, but if operative fixation is carried out, there is usually an earlier resumption of at least light duties. Office work is possible at an early stage, but an automobile mechanic will be off work for eight to ten weeks. The often stated academic period of four weeks is really not long enough for solidification and restoration of function in an adult.

Permanent Impairment. No permanent impairment results from good union and reasonable alignment. Large masses of callus rarely persist as significant deterrents to function. Shortening, overriding and poor alignment are the commonest sources of impairment. Occupation governs somewhat how much such derangement interferes with working ability. Workmen like carpenters or painters, with much overhead work, have a somewhat longer period of partial disability. Those using the shoulder for carrying heavy objects will have persistent tenderness for six to 12 months after the fracture has healed.

Serious complications like malunion and nonunion that require surgery lengthen the temporary total disability to at least six months, and the chances of permanent disability are also increased. Complications such as infection, disfiguring scars and persistent weakness are a risk of major reconstruction in this area. Contrary to an old longstanding impression, nonunion of the clavicle is not rare. In cases with slight residual limitation of shoulder motion or muscle weakness, an assessment of 5 per cent of the arm is made, and this is increased to 10 to 15 per cent in mal- and nonunion. It may be argued that complete congenital absence of the clavicle is sometimes observed and causes little disability. Such a premise is fallacious, however, because it applies only to patients who have had a deformity from birth and have been able to learn to accommodate to it during the formative years. Those who have had a clavicle and lost it are seriously disabled. Partial loss of the clavicle from too extensive resection is also disabling, leaving a defect of 25 per cent of the limb, because of the instability from the loss of suspensory ligaments.

ASSESSMENT OF IMPAIRMENT IN FRACTURES OF THE SCAPULA

The scapula participates in shoulder-arm motion, so that disturbance in contour and motion will hamper shoulder motion activities.

Mechanism of Impairment. Direct violence from a blow on the top or posterior aspect of the shoulder is the common cause of fractures of the neck, acromion or body of the scapula. These unite quickly, usually in six to eight weeks, and a period of two to four weeks more restores function. Permanent impairment is not frequent but can arise in two types of fractures.

FRACTURE OF THE NECK WITH PERSISTENT DISPLACEMENT OF THE GLENOID. In this instance limitation of motion of the humerus in the glenoid arises as a result of altered alignment or position of the fulcrum of action and also as a result of irregularities of the glenoid articulating surface. Workmen needing above-shoulder motion, such as in painting or plastering, are hampered somewhat, but it is rarely necessary for the patient to change his occupation. Permanent impairment for 8 to 20 per cent of the arm results, depending upon the degree of the shoulder limitations.

FRACTURES OF THE BODY, INVOLVING THE VERTEBRAL MARGIN OF THE SCAPULA. In this instance irregularities in the medial border of the scapula, which may develop in comminuted fractures, leads to impingement of the vertebral body on the soft parts. A chronic irritation results, with a varying amount of pain, crepitus and limitation of motion. Sometimes this can be rectified by excision of the irregular zones. When the changes are permanent, incapacity implicates the scapulothoracic girdle contribution and usually is in the range of 5 to 10 per cent of the limb.

IMPAIRMENT RESULTING FROM EXCISION OF BONES OF THE SHOULDER GIRDLE

In some instances trauma or disease so implicates a part or all of a bone contributing to the shoulder that it must be excised. The need to estimate incapacity arises chiefly after injury.

Clavicle

Complete Absence. In Chapter I the various congenital abnormalities are discussed. As a rule, when such a deformity is present from birth, adaptation accomplishes so much that little impairment results. When the loss occurs later in life, adaptation contributes significantly but less completely. The source of the impairment is loss of stability and loss of the regulatory action of suspensory ligaments. Impairment then is somewhat akin to a flail shoulder and may amount to 60 per cent of the part. Fascial suspension as is carried out for a sagging shoulder materially diminishes the impairment, decreasing it approximately 50 per cent.

Partial Excision, Inner Portion. Little disability results from excision of the inner end of the clavicle. In conditions such as sternoclavicular arthritis or unreduced dislocation, the operation may be carried out to improve the residual deformity and impairment. The treatment period covers three to six weeks, and the residual incapacity is about 5 per cent.

Partial Excision, Outer Portion. Removal of the outer half of the clavicle is disabling. Severe sagging shoulder results owing to irreparable loss of the suspensory ligaments. There are two elements comprising the permanent disability: The initial and less serious one is the altered appearance, since the unanchored lateral end of the clavicle usually protrudes upward, producing an unsightly alteration of the normal contour. The more disabling complication develops gradually. As the shoulder sags, increasing tension and pressure follow the neurovascular bundle, and eventually impairment of nerve function may compromise the whole upper limb. Shoulder action is also impaired by the loss of stability. Weakness in forearm and hand results from the brachial plexus irritation. If the condition is untreated, the disability amounts to 55 to 65 per cent of the extremity. Considerable improvement follows reconstruction. Movement to a right angle is possible, and the radiating symptoms are materially diminished. Disability is then estimated at 20 to 30 per cent of the part.

Acromioclavicular arthroplasty, on the other hand, is a frequent surgical procedure and does not impair shoulder action in the same way or to the same degree. In this instance, a small segment of only one half inch of the outer end of clavicle is excised and the joint ligaments are largely preserved, so that instability does not develop. When this is done, however, it does not leave a completely normal joint, and some small degree of impairment, 5 to 7.5 per cent of the part, may be calculated.

IMPAIRMENT RESULTING FROM LOSS OF THE SCAPULA

Infrequently it is necessary to remove the scapula completely, as for example in certain tumors, but almost never as a result of trauma. Loss of the scapula is disabling and results in incapacity similar to a flail shoulder, or about 60 to 70 per cent of the part.

IMPAIRMENT FROM LOSS OF THE UPPER END OF THE HUMERUS

Loss of the upper end of the humerus results from certain fractures, resection of tumors and, in some cases, arthritis. When a poorly controlled lax shoulder results, the impairment is greater than that following arthrodesis. Weakness, pain and loss of stability result in an impairment of 50 to 60 per cent.

In recent years this defect has been materially diminished by prosthetic replacement. The upper end of the humerus may be successfully replaced by a vitallium prosthesis. The effect of this replacement is to improve the appearance, diminish the instability, and contribute a degree of function. In most instances it is the loss of the soft tissues such as the rotator cuff and subscapularis which materially interferes with function. As in the case of assessing the effects of prosthetic replacement in the lower limb, it is felt that a shoulder which requires a prosthesis is vulnerable on many sides and that, for practical purposes, the assessment should be as if no normal shoulder function remained, or roughly 60 per cent of the extremity. In actual practice, however, the use of the prosthesis may materially improve the condition, diminishing pain and improving function. When good movement may be developed to a right angle, for example, the incapacity is reduced 20 to 25 per cent.

IMPAIRMENT RESULTING FROM NERVE INJURY ABOUT THE SHOULDER

Nerve injuries about the shoulder are common and a frequent source of permanent impairment. Many large and important nerves course through this area and may be involved in many injury mechanisms. In some instances the use of the electromyograph is extremely helpful in identifying the lesion and predicting the likelihood of recovery following surgical reconstruction.

Brachial Plexus Injuries. Serious impairment from either closed traction injuries or the less frequent open laceration is not infrequently encountered. In some instances nerve damage is a part of multiple injuries, such as a fracture of the upper end of the humerus or fracture of the clavicle. It is extremely important to initiate management of the nerve injury as early as possible; this has been emphasized in the chapter on nerve injuries. The period of total incapacity in these injuries is extensive, and nearly all are followed by some permanent impairment.

Total Plexus Avulsion. Traction lesions are the commonest source of this extremely serious injury and leave an arm 100 per cent disabled. Not only is there total loss of function of the limb, but the element of pain may be considerable. Traction injuries such as root avulsion are notorious sources of persistent arthralgia. When this complication is present, the interference with normal working ability spreads far beyond the loss of power and sensation of the individual limb. An element of at least a further 50 per cent incapacity of the limb should be added and, in some instances, the persistence of the arthralgia completely interferes with the resumption of gainful employment.

A further complication is that, as a rule, amputation in the region of the midshaft of the humerus or at the supracondylar level is needed to remove an insensitive, flail extremity, which, if retained, becomes a further liability.

C.5–C.6 Paralysis. Permanent loss of the function of these roots means a total loss of shoulder function. An arthrodesis or a trapezius transfer, as outlined in the chapter on nerve injuries, is required. The usual assessment of complete loss of C.5–C.6 is in the range of 65 to 75 per cent of the extremity. Arthrodesis diminishes this figure, as does also the trapezius transfer to approximately the same degree.

C.7–C.8 and T.1 Permanent Paralysis. Paralysis of the lower roots implicates the hand. There are various reconstructive procedures available which should always be evaluated. When replacement is minimal, and if anesthesia of the hand is present, it should be assessed as a forearm amputation, or roughly 50 to 60 per cent of the limb.

Trapezius Paralysis. Permanent paralysis of the trapezius leaves a serious defect. Not only is the loss of the muscle substance unsightly, but these patients complain of a dragging ache in the shoulder, so much so that sometimes wearing a heavy coat is most uncomfortable. The loss of the trapezius function seriously interferes with abduction and flexion of the arm, because of the absence of the powerful stabilizing action of the trapezius in clamping the scapula to the chest wall. In untreated patients disability is in the region of 30 to 35 per cent. When a successful trapezius suspension is performed, disability decreases to approximately 20 per cent.

Serratus Anterior Paralysis. Similar considerations to those observed with reference to the trapezius pertain in permanent damage to the long thoracic nerve. The aching pain is less with a serratus paralysis, and the weakness is not quite so pronounced. Surgical reconstruction in the form of a fascial sling procedure, which clamps the scapula to the chest, may be carried out. Impairment in irreparable lesions is usually in the range of 20 per cent of the limb.

Deltoid Paralysis. The deltoid is the most powerful muscle about the shoulder and its loss is disabling. Weakness and diminished control in abduction, flexion and circumduction result. The extent of permanent impairment is controlled by the effectiveness of the accessory muscles. When the biceps, triceps, pectorals, trapezius and rotator groups are functioning, the deltoid may be effectively replaced, and apparently minimal impairment results. However, as a rule, in these instances the loss of power is significant, and although the patient may be able to lift the arm against gravity, he is unable to carry out strenuous activities.

There are reconstructive procedures such as the trapezius transfer which diminish the permanent impairment. Permanent complete paralysis leaves disability in the range of 30 to 40 per cent of the limb.

Suprascapular Nerve. Abduction and rotation of the humerus are impaired, leaving an impairment of 10 to 15 per cent.

Musculocutaneous Nerve. Crushing injuries to the forearm may implicate this nerve unexpectedly. Permanent paralysis leaves weakness in flexion of the elbow. This is diminished by the contribution of the flexors of the forearm, but considerable weakness still results. The lesion above the muscular branches leaves an impairment in the nature of 30 to 40 per cent. Injury below the branches, however, leaves only loss of a little sensation along the outer aspect of the forearm, which usually is gradually obliterated by ingrowth from the sides, so that little impairment accrues.

Radial Paralysis. Loss of extensor power of the elbow and/or wrist is disabling. Inability to extend the wrist and fingers prevents the hand from assuming the position of slight dorsiflexion at the wrist which is so important in maintaining the strength of the grasp position. The salient feature is that tendon transfer and arthrodesis of the wrist compensate for this defect considerably. In permanent wrist drop, disability is in the range of 45 to 55 per cent; after a good tendon transfer, this may be reduced to 15 to 20 per cent.

Triceps Paralysis. Loss of active extension limits such activities as pitching, stretching and holding. To a degree, gravity compensates in many acts, but the loss of strength will be noticed. Permanent impairment is in the range of 5 to 15 per cent.

Median Paralysis. Both the motor and sensory components are vital in this nerve, and irreparable lesions are seriously incapacitating. Tendon and nerve transfers, as outlined in earlier chapters, effect considerable replacement. The sensory loss is particularly disabling because we use the index finger and the thumb so much in the acts of feeling. In complete lesions above the elbow, disability is roughly 60 per cent, and below the elbow, roughly 40 per cent.

Ulnar Nerve Paralysis. Ulnar nerve lesions are more common than any other nerve injury in the upper limb. The motor loss is the most incapacitating feature. A weak, thin, deformed hand results. Tendon transfer may be performed, which diminishes the impairment about 50 per cent. Impairment is usually assessed at roughly 40 to 50 per cent of the part because of the resulting weakness in the hand and fingers.

ASSESSMENT OF IMPAIRMENT IN NECK INJURIES

In neck injuries impairment is a composite modality involving some measurable components and others not so easily assessed (see Chapter XII). Loss of neck motion is readily measured, and residual motor and sensory loss can also be computed (Table 19–1). Estimation of the pain element is much more difficult. In addition, the neck is

Table 19–1 ASSESSMENT OF IMPAIRMENT IN NECK INJURIES

Soft Tissue Injuries (Stop-light Sprain)

1. Recovery without symptoms: No percentage.
2. Complaint of persistent neck pain, no decrease in motion, no other physical findings: 5 to 10 per cent of body.
3. Persistent neck pain plus restriction of motion, rotation, flexion, extension or both: 25 per cent loss, 10 to 15 per cent of body.
4. Persistent pain plus marked restriction of motion amounting to 25 to 50 per cent: 15 to 30 per cent of body.

Upper Segment Injuries (Fractures of Atlas, Axis, Odontoid and Posterior Elements)

1. Loss of motion up to 25 per cent: 10 to 12 per cent of body.
2. Loss of motion up to 50 per cent: 20 to 25 per cent of body.
3. Complete ankylosis, upper segment: 40 to 50 per cent of body.

Fractures of the Lower Segment (Cervical Spine, C.3–C.7)

1. Compression of body, no neurological sequelae: 10 per cent.
2. Fractures of two vertebral bodies with no neurological sequelae: 15 per cent.
3. Fractures plus restricted motion in addition to the above:
   Moderate, 25 to 50 per cent; marked, to 50 per cent or more.
   One vertebral body, 15 to 20 per cent; two vertebral bodies, 20 to 25 per cent.
4. Fractures, posterior elements only: 10 per cent.
5. Fractures of posterior elements in addition to the above body involvement: 5 to 10 per cent.
6. Operative stabilization as in anterior interbody fusion:
   No residual pain or neurological change, 15 per cent.
   Fusion plus residual pain and some neurological sign, up to 30 per cent.

a compound structure with elements serving multiple functions as well as the total unit, contributing significantly to the function of the shoulder at one end and to the head at the other (Fig. 19–1).

PRINCIPLES OF NECK FUNCTION

In a normal spine weight bearing is accomplished by bony structures in balance. These, in turn, are retained in this position by the ligaments. The motion of these parts is then produced by the muscles, which also assist in the balance process. Since the neck is but a part of the spine, alterations in this region may be followed by compensatory changes elsewhere; for example, the normal cervical lordosis, if lost, initiates compensatory alterations above and below. These changes may be at some distance, but the mobility of the cervical segments establishes it along with the lumbar region as a zone of compensation. Some initial extension at the atlanto-occipital joint may be necessary, or an increased lordosis in the lumbar region may develop in response to changes in the area between these levels in order to keep the head and eyes at effortless levels.

In sorting out neck action the principle of recognizing two separate segments of function has important practical applications and assists particularly in the estimation of impairment (Fig. 19–2). We can recognize an upper segment consisting of the occiput, C.1 and C.2, which is primarily concerned with the control of the head action and in particular with rotatory motion in the cervical spine. The lower segment consisting of bodies C.3 to C.7 is concerned much more with flexion and extension and the maintenance of spinal balance and does not contribute nearly so much to activities that are principally the responsibility of the upper segment. Permanent physical change involving the upper segment may then be recognized as implicating specific function in this region, but changes in the lower segment, in addition to the local alteration, implicate structures and function extending in the opposite direction to the shoulder, arm and hand. To be sure, at the level of functional

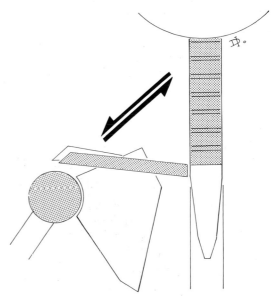

Figure 19–1 Shoulder-neck aggregate.

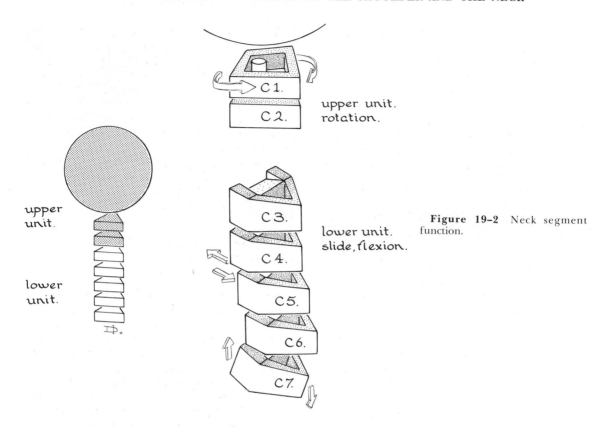

Figure 19-2 Neck segment function.

transition in segments C.2, C.3 and C.4, there may be some overriding of minor function, but by and large the upper segment contributes to symptoms and signs related to occiput, head and face, whereas the segments below implicate the neck, shoulder and upper arm.

ASSESSMENT OF INJURIES IN THE UPPER SEGMENT, OCCIPUT, C.1 AND C.2

The occipito-atlanto-axial unit is implicated in fractures and dislocations, and such injuries may leave significant persistent change. Permanent impairment is principally estimated in terms of loss of motion; the element of pain is relatively less prominent, but extension of discomfort to the jaws, face and temporal region, as well as headache, may accompany these injuries.

FRACTURES OF ATLAS AND AXIS

The disabling residual change from these injuries is interference with rotatory motion. Normally the head rotates throughout an arch of 120 degrees, with 60 degrees to each side. This is extremely important in the safe operation of an automobile. In many areas the driving laws require head turning rather than mirror viewing in moving from one traffic lane to another because of the numerous small cars now on the road.

These fractures usually heal without deformity, but some loss of motion is common because the whole segment must be immobilized to allow proper healing. Some substitution is available through lateral bending and trunk rotation, so that head turning is not totally lost even in occipitocervical fusions.

Estimation of Impairment. Loss of 25 per cent motion amounts to 10 to 12 per cent of body; loss of 50 per cent rotation, 20 to 25 per cent of body; complete ankylosis, 40 to 50 per cent of body. Included in these figures would be the results of fractures of the atlas, the odontoid and the body and posterior elements of the axis.

Neural involvement may be a complication that leads to quadriplegia, which is 100 per cent disability. The nerve root factor is added to the loss of movement factor. When a total arm is involved, 50 per cent is added; both arms or one arm and one leg, hemiplegia, also constitutes 100 per cent impairment. Rarely is there individual root loss of significance in this upper segment, the signs being more of cord implication. In some instances there is the addition of pain extending to the root of the ear and the side of the face. As a rule, this element subsides with the healing process, but when it persists at a significant level it may be considered to add a further figure of 50 per cent of the residual defect. The serious neural changes are the result of cord implication but may be of transient duration.

ASSESSMENT OF LOWER CERVICAL SPINE SEGMENT IMPAIRMENT

Fractures and dislocations in cervical vertebrae C.3–C.7 are common and frequently result in permanent impairment. The elements of disability include loss of motion, pain and neural involvement.

Motion Loss. The normal range is 90 degrees flexion extension and 90 degrees lateral bending. Fractures and dislocations of vertebral bodies, laminae and spinous processes may heal with interference in these actions. Owing to the wide range of reserve action, if one segment is lost, extensive loss may not be apparent because of substitution from the segments above or below.

When two vertebral bodies have been fused as in anterior interbody fusion, remarkably little loss of motion accrues, as a rule. Fusion of the posterior elements appears more disabling, although radiologically the same degree of motion loss has occurred. Up to 50 per cent loss of flexion extension or lateral bending is assessed as 25 to 30 per cent of the body. Little significance is attached to the particular element that was involved either in body or in posterior arch element. Some difference is accepted in the likely period of temporary total disability, it being greater in fractures of the body than when the posterior arch is involved, as a rule.

ASSESSMENT OF IMPAIRMENT IN SOFT TISSUE INJURIES (STOP-LIGHT SPRAINS)

Musculotendinous and ligamentous injuries comprise the bulk of lesions for which assessment is required. In most instances when a rear-end impact has been sufficient to produce frank stiffness and limitation of motion, some ligamentous damage has occurred. In many presentations of this subject, the extensor element has been depicted as the injuring one. However, a careful analysis of the injury mechanism focuses attention on the terminal phase of the act, which is the forward flexion jolt, resulting from the precipitant stopping of the vehicle which has

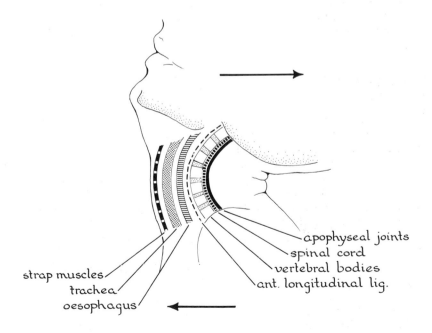

apophyseal joints
spinal cord
vertebral bodies
ant. longitudinal lig.

strap muscles
trachea
oesophagus

WHIPLASH - POSTERIOR SWING ACCELERATION

Figure 19-3 Soft tissue layers involved in extension-flexion lesions.

been hit. It is the posterior elements that are put on the stretch in the forward flexion, and it is in this region that symptoms persist. Often the impairment is subjective pain that is suboccipital, midcervical or in the shoulder-neck angle. The acute discomfort subsides in a matter of weeks, but a more persisting aching element, usually implicating the shoulder-neck zone but not accompanied by any limitation of neck motion, may last for a period of four to six months (Figs. 19–3 to 19–5).

Assessment

1. Persistent neck pain, no motion, restriction or other physical findings, 5 to 10 per cent of body.

2. Persistent neck pain, plus restriction of rotation or flexion extension, amounting to 25 to 50 per cent of neck motion, 10 to 15 per cent of body.

3. Pain plus marked restriction of motion, 50 per cent of neck motion, 15 to 30 per cent of body, usually plus some radiating symptoms.

PREPARATIONS FOR LEGAL DISCUSSION – PRETRIAL CONSULTATION AND TESTIFYING

Neck injuries become a source of legal controversy in so many instances that it behooves all who undertake the responsibility of treating them to prepare themselves adequately for discussions with legal advisors. In the beginning it should be realized that these matters are of great importance to the patient and to the lawyers concerned. If the practitioner has assumed the responsibility of treating a patient and that patient requires legal presentation of the findings resulting from the injury, his treatment, his progress and the result that was obtained, the doctor should assume these responsibilities as part of the service he owes his patient. The doctor who refuses to accept this responsibility is not performing his duties properly.

The legal interests should be held in proper regard, because members of a fellow profession have a right to expect cooperation. These principles apply to the interests of both plaintiff and defendant.

Preparations for a pretrial discussion or for testifying should be thorough from the standpoint of providing adequate notes, x-ray and laboratory findings and the final outcome for the patient. Many errors are made by doctors in underestimating the capacity of competent lawyers to understand and assimilate the medical facts of these problems. It may be necessary to guide a lawyer somewhat in his interpretation by reading what he has prepared, but this can always be performed in proper fashion. Should the positions be reversed, most doctors today would find themselves at a

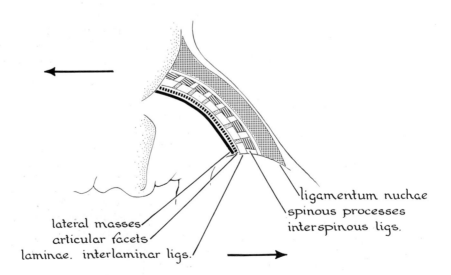

lateral masses
articular facets
laminae. interlaminar ligs.

ligamentum nuchae
spinous processes
interspinous ligs.

WHIPLASH - FORWARD SWING - DECELERATION

Figure 19–4   Soft tissue layers involved in flexion-extension lesions.

LIGAMENTS LIMITING FLEXION

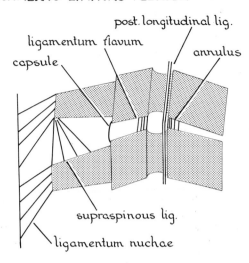

LIGAMENTS LIMITING EXTENSION

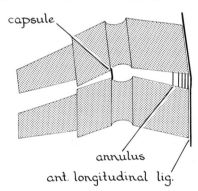

Figure 19–5 Principal ligaments involved in flexion and extension injuries.

serious disadvantage, so that it behooves us to explain with patience and intelligence.

Some lawyers have become quite familiar with these problems and may dwell on them at length. In these circumstances the medical man should treat this performance respectfully, showing a spirit of cooperation rather than resentment.

Pretrial consultation with the lawyer is an extremely worthwhile procedure. In some instances it may facilitate settlement of the controversy without a trial simply because better understanding of the injuries has been presented and also because there has been a clear interpretation of the evidence and the body changes on which it is based. In all instances consultation improves the comprehension of the lawyer and helps him to assist the doctor in court, which is important.

In no way should such preparation be con-

sidered unorthodox or inappropriate. Should the doctor be queried and cross-examined in court as to whether a pretrial consultation has taken place, there is no reason whatsoever to conceal it; rather, it is an evidence of a sincere effort to present the facts clearly and justly to jury and judge. In all fairness to the doctor involved, he may make an appropriate charge for such a consultation; in no way should it be regarded as a curbstone consultation for which the expenditure of his time and thought is not to be recognized.

In most instances physicians who are called to give testimony have adequate background and an up-to-date knowledge of the injuries in question. Should this not be the case, it is of paramount importance that the doctor consult the recent literature and be sure that his own background of knowledge is complete regarding all facets of the subject to be discussed; he may be certain that those asking the questions will have made such an effort. Should it be necessary to testify, the surgeon is fortified by this preparation, and he can deal effectively with any problems that should arise. Not only does this improve the interpretation of the facts for the jury and judge, but it lessens considerably the time required in the witness box.

GUIDELINES TO TESTIFYING

Presenting evidence in court has become a significant responsibility of the medical profession. It is felt that there are certain fundamental rules for preparation and presentation that may be followed with advantage. The following are guidelines applied particularly to orthopedic problems, and neck and shoulder lesions in particular. For other applications and a more extensive knowledge of the subject, the reader is referred to an excellent book, *The Law of Medical Practice* by B. Shartel and M. L. Plant, professors of law at the University of Michigan, and published by Charles C Thomas.

1. The pretrial consultation is of inestimable value. It provides a solid groundwork for understanding with the lawyer involved, brings to light any discrepancy that might appear, and often makes court appearance unnecessary.

2. The presenting of evidence should be regarded as a reasonable responsibility of the doctor if he has treated the patient. If he is appearing as an expert witness, having

assessed the results of the injury and care by others, he should realize he is helping to facilitate the administration of justice.

3. The court requires some evidence of the witness's qualifications and it is helpful to have these readily available in a typewritten curriculum vitae which may be read in detail or simply summarized, according to the wishes of the court.

4. In many instances, particularly because he is an expert witness, the lawyer will simply let the doctor tell the story of the injury, the treatment and the progress. The doctor should be prepared to do this, preferably from memory or with reference to a few notes.

5. Presentation in court by reading prepared notes may be adequate but is not nearly so effective. Such documents when taken into the witness stand may be examined by the opposition or retained as part of the court record, so they must be very carefully scrutinized before presentation. Notes have the disadvantage of possibly not providing answers to questions which might be asked by the opposition so that, in the end, presentation of important evidence may be necessary without any help from these documents. It is better to rely upon more effective preparation.

6. Evidence should be presented in an honest and straightforward fashion. If the injuries are not extensive, they should be referred to in this fashion; if a good result has accrued from the treatment provided, this should be stated.

7. In presenting the evidence, all statements should be enunciated clearly and slowly, with the material directed toward the jury, but in such a fashion that the judge may hear and assimilate it. Since many facts in the preparation need to be written down, it may be presented at a leisurely pace, both for emphasis and to facilitate recording.

8. It is of extreme importance to refer to parts of the body, operations and treatment procedures in language that the jury can understand. By and large, laymen have little knowledge of anatomical terms and physiological or pathological reactions, so that it behooves the witness to clarify these in understandable language.

9. Occasions may arise when it is helpful to show the jury anatomical specimens, such as a short segment of the spine, so that they may more clearly understand the relations of bones, joints and intervertebral discs. If this is done, the explanation should be in as simple terms as possible so as not to burden the listeners with technical terms not easily comprehended.

10. Privileges vary considerably as to whether x-rays may be presented as evidence, but in explaining injuries to the neck and shoulder they are of particular significance. By and large it is reasonable to refer to significant changes which appear in the x-rays, but again the relative importance of these should be pointed out to the judge and the jury. Even a normal x-ray may confuse some members of the jury, so if they are to be used, they must be referred to in the proper context. X-rays are routine and, as a rule, reveal a great many more normal than abnormal elements. The taking of an x-ray does not necessarily connote the seriousness of a problem; it is simply an accurate means of investigating bone and joint changes.

It is extremely important if x-rays are to be used not to discuss what are essentially normal abnormalities. All cervical spines exhibit some signs of deterioration beyond the age of 35, and such changes should not be presented in an unfair light to the jury. On the other hand, if early x-rays of a young patient following a severe rear-end collision clearly show obliteration of the normal lordotic curve, this is significant and it is in order to present it, even though it is a relatively small change. However, the explanation will be of more importance than the x-ray.

11. Cross examination is often feared as an ordeal by the witness, but this does not need to be the case. If there has been adequate preparation, only pertinent aspects need be covered. Neither the judge nor the lawyer involved will allow irrelevant subjects to be introduced. Elaborate answers are not necessary and, by and large, the shorter and more direct answer, the more effective it is.

12. Ambiguous questions may be asked, and the witness should be prepared to deal with these in proper fashion. He has every right to sort a question out and to indicate that it must be answered in segments since it might not be answered completely truthfully unless this is done.

13. Opposing lawyers frequently attempt to stampede a witness into giving a yes or no answer to a particular question. In some instances this is quite feasible, but when it is not or when it is undesirable or ambiguous,

Table 19–2 SUMMARY OF ASSESSMENT OF DISABILITY ABOUT THE SHOULDER

	Per Cent
Arthrodesis in optimum position	30–35
Arthrodesis but scapula fixed	45
Arthrodesis at the side	65–75
Ruptures of the rotator cuff	
With treatment and power to 90°	15–20
Untreated	30–40
Frozen shoulder	
No pain, position is usually less than optimum	30–40
With pain	50–60
Fractures of the clavicle	
Slight limitation of shoulder movement	5
Slight limitation of movement plus malunion	10–15
Fractures of the scapula	
Neck with articular involvement	10–20
Vertebral border	5–10
Fractures of upper end of humerus	
Tuberosity, with movement limited to 90°	12–18
Surgical neck, flexion and abduction to 90°	15–20
Flexion and abduction to 60°	20–25
Ankylosis at the side	30–40
Glenohumeral dislocations	
Simple, abduction limited to 90°	15–20
Recurrent dislocation, treated but with limitation to 90°	15–20
Recurrent dislocation, untreated	35–40
Acromioclavicular dislocations	
Recurrent dislocation	10–15
Sternoclavicular dislocation	
Chronic	15–20
Treated	10
Loss of bones about the shoulder	
Clavicle	
Complete	60
Medial half	5
Lateral half	50–55
Scapula (complete)	60–70
Humerus	
Upper end, complete	60–70
With arthroplasty	20–25
With arthrodesis	30–40
Nerve Lesions	
Trapezius paralysis, complete, untreated	30–35
Treated by suspension	20
Serratus paralysis, complete	20
Deltoid paralysis	30–40
Treated by tendon transfer	Approx. 20
Plexus lesions	
Paralysis of abductors, complete	55–60
Paralysis treated by arthrodesis	35–40
Paralysis treated by tendon transfer	25–30
Suprascapular nerve	10–15
Musculocutaneous nerve, complete	30–40
Triceps paralysis	5–15
Complete plexus paralysis	100
Radial paralysis, complete	45–55
Treated by tendon transfer	10–15
Median paralysis, complete at shoulder level	60
Ulnar paralysis, complete at shoulder level	40–50

The preceding figures apply to extremity only. Disability in terms of the body as a whole is usually estimated at approximately 50 per cent of these figures.

it is quite proper to state firmly that yes or no is not the complete answer to this question and that a fuller explanation is required. If this is remembered, it will not be possible for the issue to become improperly confused.

14. A frequent approach in cross-examination by a lawyer is reference to testimony or opinion contrary to that of the witness, expressed by another doctor or some senior authority. This should not present any problem since you will have given your opinion based on your examination of the patient at a given time and on the responses which that patient has made. Allowance may be given for the examinations carried out at a different interval during the treatment period or the period of rehabilitation. Similarly, patients' responses may vary from time to time and under different circumstances. By and large, when there are physical findings that support a given opinion, this is reasonable substantiation.

Similar considerations apply if it is suggested that a different opinion was expressed by yourself on another occasion. No two patients are the same and no two injury forces are precisely alike. Similarly, the variation in treatment program and individual patient response is beyond your control.

15. One of the prime tricks of lawyers in cross-examination is to make the witness angry, so that he blurts out inadequate or insecure responses. It should be borne in mind that the properly prepared medical witness has a vastly superior knowledge and background on the subject under discussion; if resort is made to such tactics, that background may be drawn upon. Most able attorneys refrain from these tactics because the well prepared and expert witness may take advantage of the questions on cross-examination to expand the evidence and elaborate in a fashion not previously carried out.

16. Frequently it is desirable to be as precise as possible in the estimation of impairment. Both judge and jury have the feeling that if a witness can talk in terms of percentage impairment, he has a background of knowledge on the subject which is significant. The witness under these circumstances may well be asked the source of his information, and he should be prepared to expound or at least to state a usual process for the estimation of impairment. The court recognizes that there are authorities and established contributions to literature which may be drawn upon as a background for this mechanism, and it is quite in order to state this. When a witness has a thorough understanding of the process of estimation, no problems arise and it contributes significantly to his stature in the presentation.

REFERENCES

Bateman, J. E.: Disability evaluation in the upper limb. Lawyer's Med. J. *1*:91, 1966.

Day, A. J., et al.: Recurrent dislocation of the shoulder. A comparison of the Bankart and Magnuson procedures after 16 years. Clin. Orthop. *45*:123–126, 1966.

Gjores, J. E., et al.: Prognosis in primary dislocation of the shoulder. Acta Chir. Scand. *129*:468–470, 1965.

Rice, C. O.: Industrial Disabilities of the Extremities. Springfield, Ill., Charles C Thomas, 1952.

Shartel, B., and Plant, M. L. (ed.): The Law of Medical Practice. Springfield, Ill., Charles C Thomas, 1959.

Index